Age-Related Macular Degeneration: Diagnosis and Treatment

Age-Related Macular Degeneration: Diagnosis and Treatment

Editor: Veronica Martin

FOSTER ACADEMICS
www.fosteracademics.com

www.fosteracademics.com

FOSTER ACADEMICS

Cataloging-in-Publication Data

Age-related macular degeneration : diagnosis and treatment / edited by Veronica Martin.
p. cm.
Includes bibliographical references and index.
ISBN 978-1-63242-755-7
1. Retinal degeneration. 2. Retinal degeneration--Diagnosis. 3. Retinal degeneration--Treatment.
4. Retinal degeneration--Age factors. 5. Retina--Diseases. I. Martin, Veronica.
RE661.D3 A34 2019
617.735--dc23

Foster Academics,
118-35 Queens Blvd., Suite 400,
Forest Hills, NY 11375, USA

ISBN 978-1-63242-755-7 (Hardback)

Contents

Preface

Age-related macular degeneration (AMD) is the clinical condition, which results in blurred vision or vision loss at the center of the visual field, due to a damage to the macula. Such a loss of central vision can make it difficult to recognize faces, read, drive or perform activities of daily life. Visual hallucinations are also common in people with this condition. It typically occurs in older people, but may be prevented by exercising and adhering to a good diet. Depending on the severity of AMD, it can be early, intermediate and late AMD. The diagnosis of AMD is through an eye examination. There is no treatment for vision loss but the management strategy strives to slow down the progression of AMD, by removing risk factors. This happens through mineral and antioxidant supplementation, and vascular endothelial growth factor inhibitors, among others. This book contains some path-breaking studies in age-related macular degeneration. It unfolds the innovative aspects in the diagnosis and treatment of this disease. This book will help the readers in keeping pace with the rapid changes in this field. The readers would gain knowledge that would broaden their perspective about this medical condition.

After months of intensive research and writing, this book is the end result of all who devoted their time and efforts in the initiation and progress of this book. It will surely be a source of reference in enhancing the required knowledge of the new developments in the area. During the course of developing this book, certain measures such as accuracy, authenticity and research focused analytical studies were given preference in order to produce a comprehensive book in the area of study.

This book would not have been possible without the efforts of the authors and the publisher. I extend my sincere thanks to them. Secondly, I express my gratitude to my family and well-wishers. And most importantly, I thank my students for constantly expressing their willingness and curiosity in enhancing their knowledge in the field, which encourages me to take up further research projects for the advancement of the area.

Editor

1

Protection of Retina by αB Crystallin in Sodium Iodate Induced Retinal Degeneration

Peng Zhou[1], Ram Kannan[1], Christine Spee[3], Parameswaran G. Sreekumar[1], Guorui Dou[1], David R. Hinton[2,3]*

1 Doheny Eye Institute, Los Angeles, California, United States of America, **2** Departments of Pathology, Keck School of Medicine of the University of Southern California, Los Angeles, California, United States of America, **3** Ophthalmology, Keck School of Medicine of the University of Southern California, Los Angeles, California, United States of America

Abstract

Age-related macular degeneration (AMD) is a leading cause of blindness in the developed world. The retinal pigment epithelium (RPE) is a critical site of pathology in AMD and αB crystallin expression is increased in RPE and associated drusen in AMD. The purpose of this study was to investigate the role of αB crystallin in sodium iodate ($NaIO_3$)-induced retinal degeneration, a model of AMD in which the primary site of pathology is the RPE. Dose dependent effects of intravenous $NaIO_3$ (20-70 mg/kg) on development of retinal degeneration (fundus photography) and RPE and retinal neuronal loss (histology) were determined in wild type and αB crystallin knockout mice. Absence of αB crystallin augmented retinal degeneration in low dose (20 mg/kg) $NaIO_3$-treated mice and increased retinal cell apoptosis which was mainly localized to the RPE layer. Generation of reactive oxygen species (ROS) was observed with $NaIO_3$ in mouse and human RPE which increased further after αB crystallin knockout or siRNA knockdown, respectively. $NaIO_3$ upregulated AKT phosphorylation and peroxisome proliferator-activator receptor-γ ($PPAR_\gamma$) which was suppressed after αB crystallin siRNA knockdown. Further, $PPAR_\gamma$ ligand inhibited $NaIO_3$-induced ROS generation. Our data suggest that αB crystallin plays a critical role in protection of $NaIO_3$-induced oxidative stress and retinal degeneration in part through upregulation of AKT phosphorylation and $PPAR_\gamma$ expression.

Editor: Raghavan Raju, Georgia Regents University, United States of America

Funding: Supported in part by grants EY01545 (DRH) and by core grant EY03040, the Arnold and Mabel Beckman Foundation, and an unrestricted grant to the Department of Ophthalmology from Research to Prevent Blindness Inc., New York, NY. The funders had no role in study design, data collection and analysis, decision to publish, or preparation of the manuscript.

Competing Interests: The authors have declared that no competing interests exist.

* E-mail: dhinton@usc.edu

Introduction

Age-related macular degeneration (AMD) is characterized by progressive degeneration of the macular region of the retina resulting in loss of central vision. AMD is the leading cause of irreversible blindness in the developed world [1]. Clinically, AMD manifests in two forms; a non-exudative dry form and an exudative, neovascular wet form [1,2]. Geographic atrophy (GA) is an advanced form of dry AMD with extensive atrophy and loss of the retinal pigment epithelium (RPE) and overlying photoreceptors and is responsible for 10–20% of cases of legal blindness from AMD [3,4]. At present, there is no available effective treatment for GA.

A number of murine models have been generated that simulate features of dry AMD including RPE degeneration, lipofuscin accumulation, subretinal deposits, and loss of photoreceptors [5–12]. Our laboratory recently showed that bone morphogenetic protein-4 (BMP-4) is highly expressed in dry AMD and mediates oxidative stress-induced senescence in RPE in in vitro dry AMD thus serving as a molecular switch between atrophic and neovascular AMD [13,14]. Localized RPE debridement or genetic ablation of RPE can lead to a profound reduction in RPE cells and consequent loss of photoreceptors [15]. Retinotoxicity can also be induced by endogenous and exogenous agents in laboratory animals. Mice receiving polyinosine-polycytidylic acid (Poly I: C) had morphological changes similar to that of humans with dry ARMD exhibiting soft and/or hard Drusen, GA [16]. Recently, the conditional ablation of the microRNA processing enzyme DICER1 was shown to induce RPE degeneration in mice [17]. Genetic or pharmacological inhibition of inflammasome components (NLRP3, MYD88) was reported to prevent RPE degeneration induced by DICER1 loss or AluRNA exposure [18]. While most of the animal models for GA mentioned above are long-term involving prolonged treatment regimens, the $NaIO_3$-induced retinal degeneration model has proven to be a convenient and widely used model, because it is rapid, reproducible and has a primary site of pathology in the RPE [6,19–22]. Thus, in the present study, we have utilized the $NaIO_3$ model in 129S6/SvEvTac mice to study mechanisms of retinal degeneration.

Crystallins are members of the small heat shock protein (sHSP) family, and αB crystallin has been found to have high chaperone efficiency, and bind misfolded proteins with high affinity and stoichiometry [23]. An increased expression of αB crystallin was found in RPE and associated drusen in dry AMD [24,25]. Both αA and αB crystallin are expressed in the mouse retina [26–28]. Mice lacking αB crystallin have provided considerable insights into the functional roles of this protein [29]. Our laboratory has shown that RPE cells from mice lacking αB crystallin are more susceptible to oxidative and endoplasmic reticulum stress as compared to wild type RPE [28,30,31]. Further we found that RPE cells overexpressing αB crystallin showed resistance to apoptosis, suggesting that αB crystallin may prevent stress-induced cell death [32]. Recently, evidence for the secretion of αB crystallin by RPE exosomes and protection of neighboring photoreceptors and RPE by exogenous αB crystallin was presented by our laboratory [33] suggesting that αB crystallin has significant potential in retinal therapy.

This study was undertaken to investigate the role of αB crystallin in a model of $NaIO_3$ induced retinal degeneration in 129S6/SvEvTac mice. Further, using cultured mouse and human RPE cells, we also investigated the mechanism of regulation of cell death from $NaIO_3$-induced oxidative stress by αB crystallin. Our major finding is that absence of αB crystallin in αB crystallin knockout mice causes more severe degeneration of the retina in $NaIO_3$-treated mice as compared to wild type mice treated with $NaIO_3$. Further, our studies also suggest that αB crystallin plays a critical role in protection of $NaIO_3$-induced oxidative stress and retinal degeneration in part through upregulation of AKT phosphorylation and $PPAR_\gamma$ expression.

Results

Selection of optimal *in vivo* dose and duration of $NaIO_3$ treatment

Preliminary experiments were performed to select an optimal dosage of $NaIO_3$ that was used in all subsequent *in vivo* experiments in mice. We tested the effect of a single intravenous injection of 20, 35, 50 and 70 mg/kg $NaIO_3$ for 1, 2 and 3 weeks on retinal morphology. The histologic data from varying doses of $NaIO_3$ treatment are presented in Figure 1. $NaIO_3$-induced retinal degeneration increased with the dose. The extent of degeneration was absent to mild with 20 mg/kg, moderate with 35 and 50 mg/kg and was severe with 70 mg/kg dose 3 week after $NaIO_3$ treatment (Figure 1). We chose the 20 mg/kg $NaIO_3$ dose that produced no more than mild degeneration in all our subsequent experiments to enable studying the exacerbating effects of αB crystallin knockout on retinal damage (see below). While high doses of $NaIO_3$ resulted in retinal degeneration as early as 1 week post-injection, the low dose (20 mg/kg) $NaIO_3$ showed damage localized to the RPE at the 3 week time-point (Fig S1).

Fundus photography shows accelerated $NaIO_3$-induced retinal degeneration in αB crystallin knockout mice

To determine the extent of $NaIO_3$-induced retinal degeneration, we compared the fundus photographs of mice from PBS-treated WT, $NaIO_3$-treated WT, PBS-treated αB crystallin knockout, and $NaIO_3$-treated αB crystallin knockout groups at the end of 3 weeks. The dose of $NaIO_3$ in these studies was 20 mg/kg. The retinal degeneration induced by $NaIO_3$ in mice appeared as patchy white retinal lesions when observed by fundus photography (Fig. 2).

The fundus photographs of thirteen out of fourteen $NaIO_3$-treated αB crystallin knockout mice showed patchy retinal degeneration three weeks after injection (Fig.2D, E). Only three out of fourteen eyes of $NaIO_3$-treated wild type mice showed retinal degeneration (Fig 2B, E). Thus, the difference in the number of mice with retinal degeneration between $NaIO_3$-treated αB crystallin knockout mice and $NaIO_3$-treated wild type mice was highly significant ($P<0.001$). No apparent degeneration could be seen in control, untreated wild type or αB crystallin knockout retina.

Histopathology shows accelerated $NaIO_3$-induced degeneration in αB crystallin knockout mice

The primary site of pathology after $NaIO_3$ injection (20 mg/kg) was the RPE layer; we observed that the RPE layer was discontiguous and damaged in all αB crystallin knockout mice, while only two out of seven wild type mice showed these changes in the RPE (Fig. 3). Using TUNEL staining we confirmed that with $NaIO_3$ (20 mg/kg; 3 week time point) cell death was localized to the RPE layer in the αB crystallin knockout mice (Figure S2). Significant differences were found between $NaIO_3$-treated wild type mice and $NaIO_3$-treated αB crystallin knockout mice in the extent of RPE degeneration ($P<0.01$). Retinas from αB crystallin knockout mice (Fig. 3D) revealed more severe degeneration from $NaIO_3$ injection as compared to wild-type retinas (Fig. 3B). Total retinal thickness was significantly decreased ($P<0.01$) in αB crystallin knockout mice with $NaIO_3$ treatment as compared to untreated αB crystallin knockout group ($P<0.01$). In contrast, in wild type mice, no significant difference in retinal thickness after treatment with $NaIO_3$ was found vs. untreated controls. (Fig. 3F). An assessment of the localization of retinal damage by $NaIO_3$ was made by counting the number of nuclei in the inner nuclear layer (INL), outer nuclear layer (ONL) and ganglion cell layer (GCL) of wild type and αB crystallin knockout retina (Fig. 3G–I). This analysis revealed that the loss of nuclei was more prominent at 3 weeks post-$NaIO_3$ injection in αB crystallin knockout retina vs. that of wild type. The number of nuclei per unit area showed a significant decrease with $NaIO_3$ injection in the ONL of αB crystallin knockout mice which was statistically significant ($P<0.01$; Fig. 3I). No significant differences in the number of nuclei in any of the other nuclear layers (GCL, INL) were found between the $NaIO_3$-injected and PBS-injected groups of wild type mice (Fig. 3-G,H).

Reduced ERG amplitudes in $NaIO_3$-treated αB crystallin knockout mice

To determine whether the absence of αB crystallin had an effect on the retinal function of $NaIO_3$-treated mice, we compared mesopic (mixed rod and cone) ERG responses. These studies to assess the functional response of neural retina were performed in four groups of mice (PBS-treated WT, $NaIO_3$-treated WT, PBS-treated αB crystallin knockout, and $NaIO_3$-treated αB crystallin knockout) that received a dose of 20 mg/kg $NaIO_3$ at the end of 3 weeks. Significant differences were observed in the ERGs of $NaIO_3$-treated αB crystallin knockout mice compared with the PBS-treated αB crystallin knockout mice (Fig 4A). The amplitude of the *a* wave of the ERG, that originates from the photoreceptors, of $NaIO_3$-treated αB crystallin knockout mice decreased by 68.3% compared with that of PBS-treated αB crystallin knockout mice (Fig 4B). The amplitude of the *b* wave of the ERG, (that originates from the bipolar cells), of $NaIO_3$-treated αB crystallin knockout mice decreased by 55.3% compared with that of PBS-treated αB crystallin knockout mice (Fig 4C). No significant differences were found between the ERGs of the $NaIO_3$-treated and control wild type mice at this low dose (Fig 4B,C).

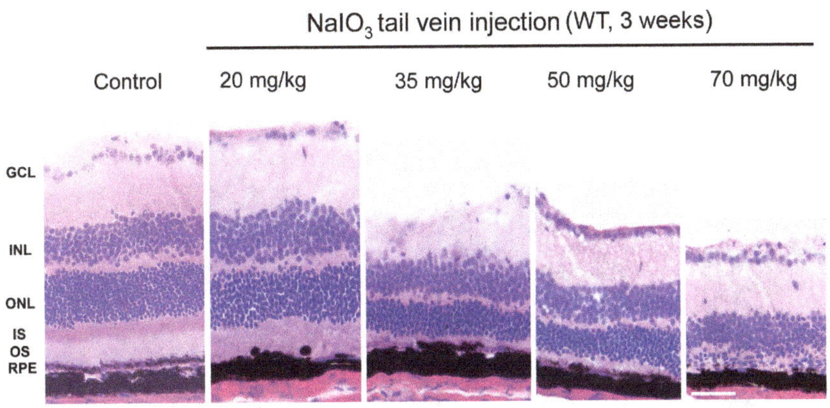

Figure 1. H & E staining of retina showing dose dependent effect of $NaIO_3$ in 129S6/SvEvTac wild type (WT) mice. The intravenous $NaIO_3$ doses used were 20, 35, 50 and 70 mg/kg body weight. Mice were euthanized after 3 weeks of treatment, eyes were enucleated, frozen sections of retinal were obtained, and H & E staining was performed. Most mice treated with 20 mg/kg showed an intact layer of contiguous RPE although occasional mice showed focal RPE degeneration and loss at the end of 3 weeks (as shown in this figure). The higher doses showed moderate and severe damage to the RPE cell layer, and outer nuclear layer. GCL: ganglion cell layer; ONL: outer nuclear layer; INL: inner nuclear layer; IS: inner segment; OS: outer segment. Bar equals 75 μm.

Increased production of reactive oxygen species (ROS) in αB crystallin knockout RPE and cultured human RPE cells transfected with αB crystallin siRNA after $NaIO_3$ treatment

These experiments were performed in both mouse and human RPE cultured in 0.5% FBS-containing DMEM; cells were treated with 200 μg/ml $NaIO_3$ for 24 h. Treatment with $NaIO_3$ induced ROS production in RPE from WT mice which was not found in untreated controls (Fig. 5A–B). ROS partially co-localized with mitochondria. The ROS production was even higher in αB crystallin knockout RPE after $NaIO_3$ treatment (arrows, Fig. 5D). Negligible ROS was produced in αB crystallin knockout RPE without $NaIO_3$ (Fig.5C). To further evaluate the effect of $NaIO_3$ on ROS production, we studied primary human RPE cells after αB crystallin knockdown. The percentage of knockdown of αB crystallin in human RPE by siRNA transfection was about 80% as determined by Western blot analysis (Fig 5E). Treatment with $NaIO_3$ resulted in a pronounced intracellular generation of ROS that was predominantly localized to the mitochondria in αB crystallin siRNA-transfected RPE cells (Fig. 5I–K). However, the staining for ROS was much less prominent in $NaIO_3$-treated RPE cells with scrambled siRNA (Fig. 5F–H). Thus, these results show that knockout or siRNA knockdown of αB crystallin results in increased generation of ROS in RPE cells treated with $NaIO_3$.

Mode of cell death in RPE exposed to low dose of $NaIO_3$ is not by necrosis

Propidium iodide (PI) staining was performed to assess necrotic features in RPE cells incubated with different doses of $NaIO_3$. The $NaIO_3$ treatment of RPE was performed for 24 h in 0.5% FBS-containing DMEM at doses of 200, 500, or 1000 μg/ml, respectively. Confocal microscopy images are presented in Fig. 6 (A–H) that show PI staining in control (scrambled siRNA) RPE nuclei (Fig. 6A–D) and αB crystallin siRNA-transfected RPE nuclei (Fig. 6E–H) with or without $NaIO_3$ treatment. No significant differences were found in the number of PI positive cells between control group and the group treated with 200 μg/ml of $NaIO_3$ in both scrambled siRNA and αB crystallin siRNA-transfected human RPE cells. Treatment with 500 and 1000 μg/ml of $NaIO_3$ resulted in increased PI positive cells both in scrambled siRNA RPE and αB crystallin siRNA pretreated RPE ($P<0.01$). However, no significant differences were found between the number of PI positive cells in control RPE and αB crystallin siRNA-transfected groups (Fig. 6I). Therefore, it can be concluded that high dose $NaIO_3$ (500 μg/ml and 1000 μg/ml) induced predominantly RPE cell necrosis, while induction of necrosis was negligible or insignificant with low dose $NaIO_3$ (200 μg/ml).

Increased apoptosis in αB crystallin siRNA-transfected RPE with low dose $NaIO_3$

TUNEL staining was performed to assess the extent of apoptosis with $NaIO_3$ in RPE cells. Fig. 7 shows TUNEL staining in control RPE cells (Fig. 7A–B) and αB crystallin siRNA-transfected RPE cells (Fig. 7C–D) treated with a low dose (200 μg/ml) of $NaIO_3$. The duration of $NaIO_3$ exposure of RPE in 0.5% FBS-containing DMEM was 24 h. Treatment with 200 μg/ml $NaIO_3$ resulted in increased TUNEL-positive cells with αB crystallin siRNA-transfection as compared with scrambled siRNA controls (Fig. 7E) ($P<0.01$). However, no significant difference was found between control and $NaIO_3$-treated RPE cells without αB crystallin siRNA-transfection. Thus $NaIO_3$ induces apoptosis in αB crystallin siRNA-transfected RPE cells that were exposed to low doses.

Increased caspase 3 activation with $NaIO_3$ and αB crystallin siRNA

Cleaved caspase 3 staining was performed to confirm that the mechanism of cell death was by apoptosis. Fig. 8 shows immunostaining of cleaved caspase 3 in control human RPE cells (Fig. 8A B) and αB crystallin siRNA-transfected RPE cells (Fig. 8C–D) treated with low dose $NaIO_3$. The duration and dose of $NaIO_3$ exposure of RPE in 0.5% FBS-containing DMEM was 24 h and 200 μg/ml. Treatment of RPE cells with 200 μg/ml $NaIO_3$ resulted in an increase in the number of cleaved caspase 3-positive cells with αB crystallin siRNA-transfection as compared to scrambled siRNA controls (Fig. 8E) ($P<0.01$). However, no significant difference was found between control and $NaIO_3$ treated RPE cells without αB crystallin siRNA-transfection. This indicates that apoptosis with low dose $NaIO_3$ (200 μg/ml) in αB crystallin siRNA-transfected RPE cells occurs via caspase 3 activation.

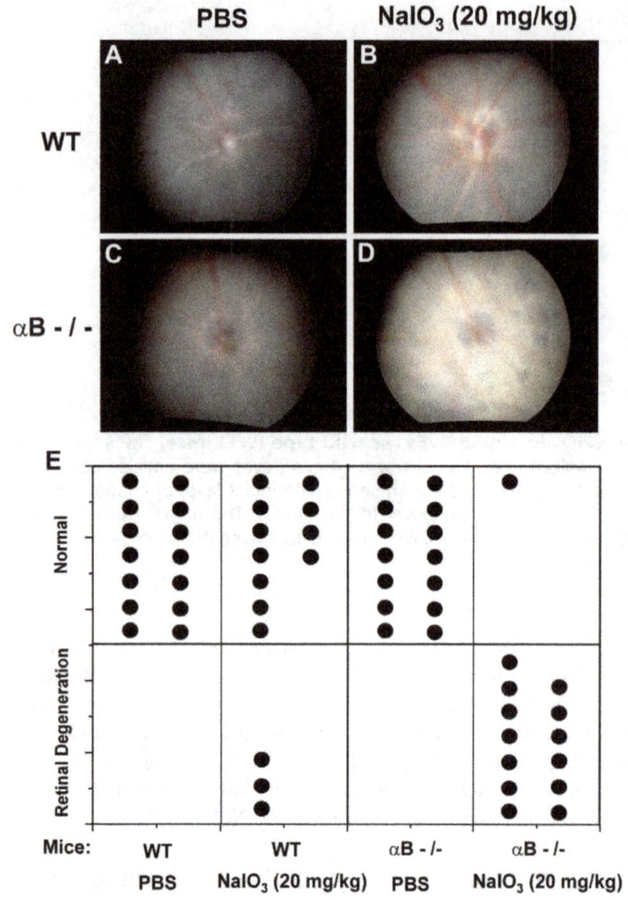

Figure 2. Fundus photograph of control and $NaIO_3$-treated αB crystallin knockout mice (αB-/-). Three weeks after tail vein injection of 20 mg/kg $NaIO_3$, fundus photograph was taken in PBS-treated wild type (WT) (A), $NaIO_3$-treated WT (B), PBS-treated αB-/- (C), and $NaIO_3$-treated αB-/- (D) mice. Arrows indicate sites of retinal degeneration. Thirteen $NaIO_3$-treated αB-/- mice showed patchy retinal degeneration three weeks after $NaIO_3$ injection (E). Only three out of fourteen eyes of $NaIO_3$-treated WT mice showed retinal degeneration (E). A statistically significant difference was found between $NaIO_3$-treated αB-/- and $NaIO_3$-treated WT mice ($P<0.001$).

Signaling molecules associated with $NaIO_3$-induced RPE cell death

We investigated the mechanism of the exacerbation of $NaIO_3$-induced RPE cell apoptosis in the absence of αB crystallin by analyzing several apoptotic signaling proteins (Fig. 9). Expression of phosphorylated AKT at serine 473 increased after treatment with low dose (200 μg/ml) $NaIO_3$ (Fig. 9B). However, the increase of phospho-AKT was much lower in αB crystallin siRNA-transfected RPE cells treated with $NaIO_3$ compared to controls. A similar trend was observed for phospho-GSK 3β and phosphorylated -c-Raf, signaling proteins downstream of AKT. Low dose $NaIO_3$ markedly increased $PPAR_\gamma$ expression in scrambled transfected RPE cells, while this increase could not be seen in αB crystallin siRNA-transfected RPE cells (Fig. 9C). However, no significant changes were evident with $NaIO_3$ treatment in phospho-PDK1, a kinase upstream of AKT (Fig. 9A). This suggests that AKT may be the point of interaction with $NaIO_3$ in the AKT signaling pathway (Fig. 9A).

The treatment with low dose (200 μg/ml) $NaIO_3$ increased $PPAR_\gamma$ expression in RPE. The increased expression of $PPAR_\gamma$ possibly exerts a reactive protective role, as we observed A-PAF, a $PPAR_\gamma$ ligand, significantly decreased the generation of ROS (Fig. 10A). On the other hand, GW9662, a $PPAR_\gamma$ antagonist, caused a significant increase in $NaIO_3$-induced production of ROS ($P<0.01$; Fig. 10B). The increase in $PPAR_\gamma$ by $NaIO_3$ was attenuated in $NaIO_3$-treated αB crystallin siRNA-transfected RPE cells thereby compromising the protective defense by $PPAR_\gamma$ under these conditions (Fig. 10A, B).

Discussion

In an attempt to understand the protective role of αB crystallin in stress-induced RPE degeneration, we have investigated the effect of suppression of αB crystallin on apoptosis and have studied the signaling mechanisms associated with this phenomenon. For this purpose, we used a murine model of $NaIO_3$-induced retinal degeneration *in vivo* and cell death in human RPE *in vitro*.

$NaIO_3$ has been previously shown to induce selective degeneration of the RPE and consequent retinal degeneration [6,19,20]. A low dose of $NaIO_3$ was used to induce retinal degeneration in this study. No significant retinal degeneration was found on fundus photography in wild type mice three weeks after tail vein injection of low dose $NaIO_3$, while 93.7% (15/16) eyes of αB crystallin knockout mice exhibited retinal degeneration after the same treatment. A much higher dose and duration of treatment (100 mg/kg $NaIO_3$; 6 weeks) was required in ICR strain of mice to induce changes in morphology in the retina [21] indicating that differences among mouse strains can also play a role [19–21]. Furthermore, previous ultrastructural and TUNEL labeling studies showed that RPE cell death induced by 100 mg/kg $NaIO_3$ was from necrosis and that of the photoreceptors was from apoptosis [21]. In the present study, increased RPE apoptosis was found in low dose $NaIO_3$-treated RPE cells from αB crystallin knockout mice and in human RPE after αB crystallin knockdown; however, necrosis was minimal. Necrotic cells increased in a dose dependent manner with high dose of $NaIO_3$. Therefore, we may conclude that low dose of $NaIO_3$ induces RPE cell apoptosis, while high dose of $NaIO_3$ results in RPE cell necrosis.

The role of αB crystallin in cellular protection is becoming increasingly important because αB crystallin acts on a variety of cellular processes [23,27]. Newer studies have taken advantage of αB crystallin's antiapoptotic and anti-inflammatory properties in devising therapy [34,35]. For example, intravenous administration of αB crystallin in mice was found to reduce inflammation and thus play a protective role in experimental autoimmune demyelination [34,36]. αB crystallin may play an important role in protection of retinal neurons from damage by metabolic and environmental stress as seen by evidence of elevated crystallin expression in light damaged photoreceptors and in models of retinal degeneration [37,38]. αB crystallin could be important in the development of, or in response to, AMD since αB crystallin was found to be accumulated in RPE, drusen and Bruch membrane tissues from AMD patients [23,24]. In a recent study, we found that αB crystallin is secreted via exosomes by RPE cells and presented evidence for its extracellular function in protecting neighboring RPE cells and photoreceptors from oxidative injury [33].

In our present studies, we found that lack of αB crystallin accelerated and augmented the retinal degeneration in $NaIO_3$-treated mice *in vivo* and was associated with increased RPE cell apoptosis *in vitro*. In previous studies from our laboratories, we had reported that lack of αB crystallin renders RPE cells more susceptible to apoptosis from oxidative stress induced by H_2O_2 [28]. Similarly, when RPE cells were exposed to ER stress,

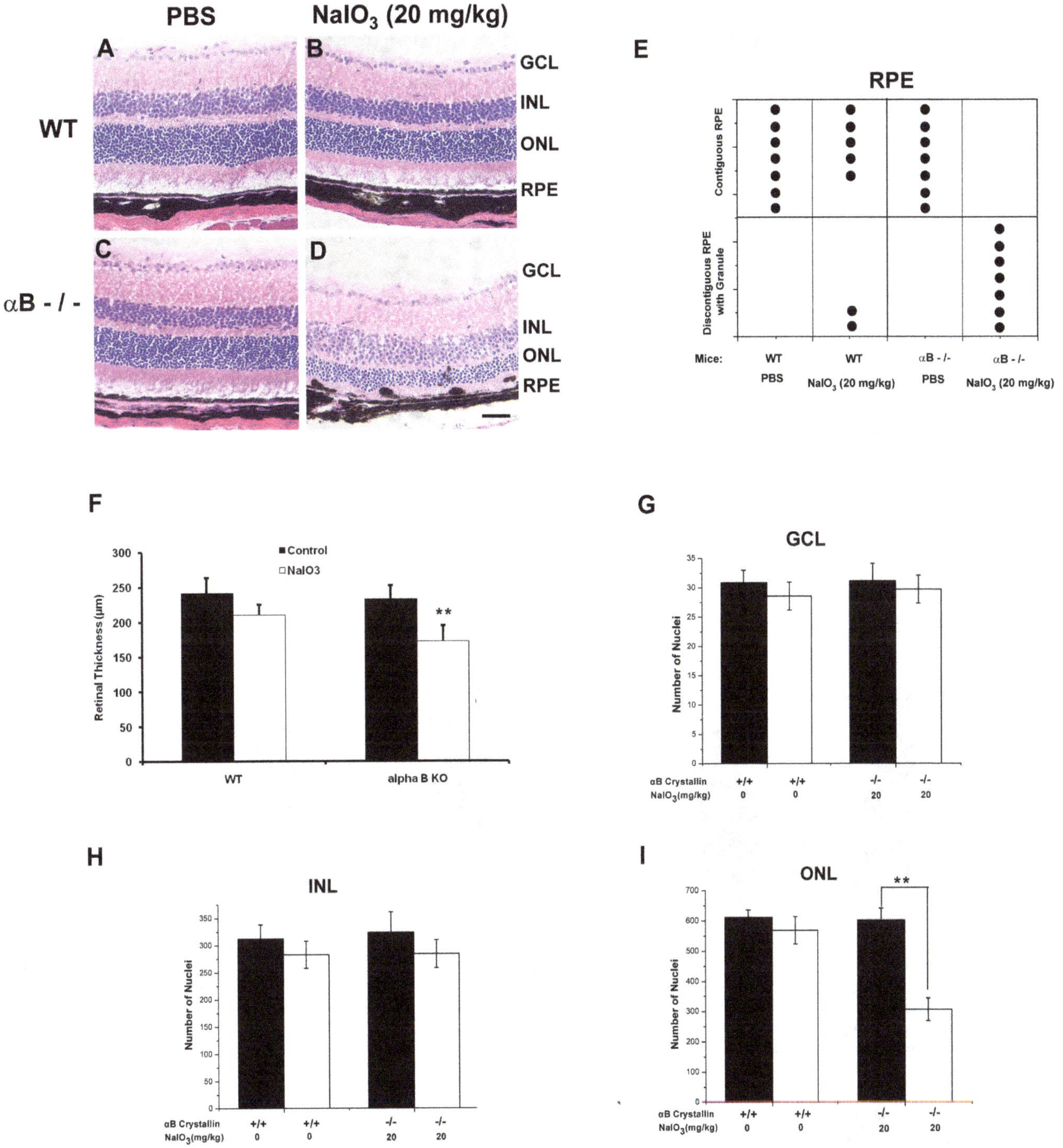

Figure 3. Histopathology of retina from control and $NaIO_3$-treated αB crystallin knockout (αB-/-) mice. Three weeks after tail vein injection of 20 mg/kg $NaIO_3$, eyes were enucleated and frozen sections were stained with H&E. The four experimental groups of mice were PBS-treated WT (A), $NaIO_3$-treated WT (B), PBS-treated αB-/- (C), and $NaIO_3$-treated αB-/- (D). The RPE layer in αB-/- mice with $NaIO_3$ injection were discontiguous and damaged. Only two out of seven WT mice showed discontiguous and damaged RPE (E). Bar graph showing retinal thickness (μm) with and without $NaIO_3$ in WT and αB-/- mice. (F). Retinal thickness was significantly lower ($P<0.01$) in $NaIO_3$ treated αB-/- mice when compared to the corresponding WT group. No significant differences in the number of nuclei in the ganglion cell layer, outer nuclear layer or inner nuclear layer were found between the $NaIO_3$-injected and PBS-injected WT mice (G–H). The number of nuclei per unit area in the outer nuclear layer of $NaIO_3$ injected αB-/- mice showed a significant decrease ($P<0.01$) as compared to control without $NaIO_3$ injection (I). RPE: RPE cell layer; ONL: outer nuclear layer; INL: inner nuclear layer; GCL: ganglion cell layer. Data are mean ± SEM, n = 7/group, **$P<0.01$. Bar equals 75 μm.

apoptosis ensues and αB crystallin regulated ER-stress induced cell death [31]. Silencing of αB crystallin by siRNA knockdown exacerbated apoptosis while overexpression attenuated apoptotic cell death in RPE cells [30,31]. Our present data show that induction of apoptosis by $NaIO_3$ occurs through generation of

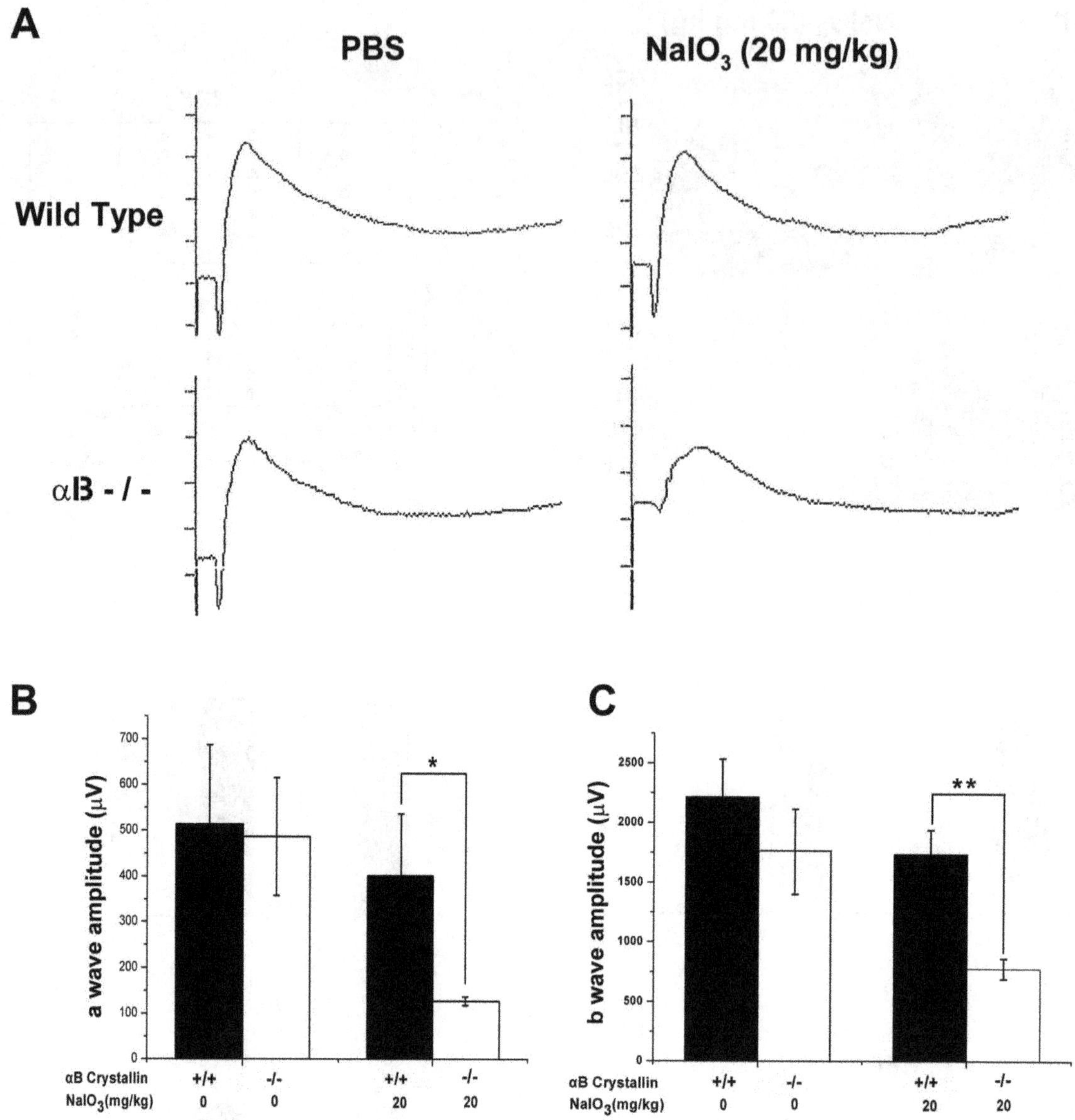

Figure 4. Reduced ERG amplitudes in $NaIO_3$-treated αB crystallin knockout (αB-/-) mice. Three weeks after tail vein injection of 20 mg/kg body weight $NaIO_3$, mesopic ERG responses were recorded in PBS-treated WT, $NaIO_3$-treated WT, PBS-treated αB-/-, and $NaIO_3$-treated αB-/- mice (representative ERGs shown in A). The amplitudes of *a* wave of the ERG of $NaIO_3$-treated αB-/- mice decreased by 68.3% compared with that of PBS-treated αB-/- mice (B). The amplitudes of *b* wave of the ERG of $NaIO_3$-treated αB-/- mice decreased by 55.3%, compared with that of PBS-treated αB-/- mice (C). Data are mean ± SEM, n = 5/group, $^*P<0.05$, $^{**}P<0.01$.

ROS consistent with the known oxidative properties of iodate ions involving mitochondria [6,19,20].

In the αB crystallin knockout mouse, knockout of the αB crystallin gene also disrupted the closely related gene HSPB2 [29]. However, while HSPB2 is expressed in muscle tissues, our previous work established that HSPB2 is not expressed in normal or pathologic murine posterior eye cups, including the retina and RPE [29,39]. Therefore, loss of HSPB2 has no effect on the evaluation of αB crystallin knockout in studies of retinal degeneration.

It was reported that there was no apparent phenotype in the retina of αB crystallin knockout mice [29]; however, our recent studies found that while the histology of the neural retina was unaffected, there was a mild decrease in retinal vessel density in the inner plexiform layer in αB crystallin knockout mice compared to wild type [39]. We found that absence of αB crystallin accelerated and augmented the degeneration of the retina in $NaIO_3$ treated mice in this study. Further, apoptosis was exacerbated in RPE after αB crystallin siRNA knockdown. For example, we observed increased production of ROS in RPE cells from αB crystallin knockout mice and human RPE cells transfected with αB crystallin siRNA upon $NaIO_3$ treatment. These results suggest that while an apparent retinal phenotype could not be found *in vivo* in normal conditions, suppression of αB crystallin does indeed cause injury and death at a cellular level in RPE after oxidative stress. Furthermore, the mode of cell death was via apoptosis and necrosis was not seen in RPE cells treated with low $NaIO_3$ doses.

It is of interest that very recently it was shown that knockout of αA crystallin also exacerbates retinal degeneration in the $NaIO_3$ model [40]. We have previously shown that αB crystallin is expressed at much higher levels in RPE than αA crystallin but that

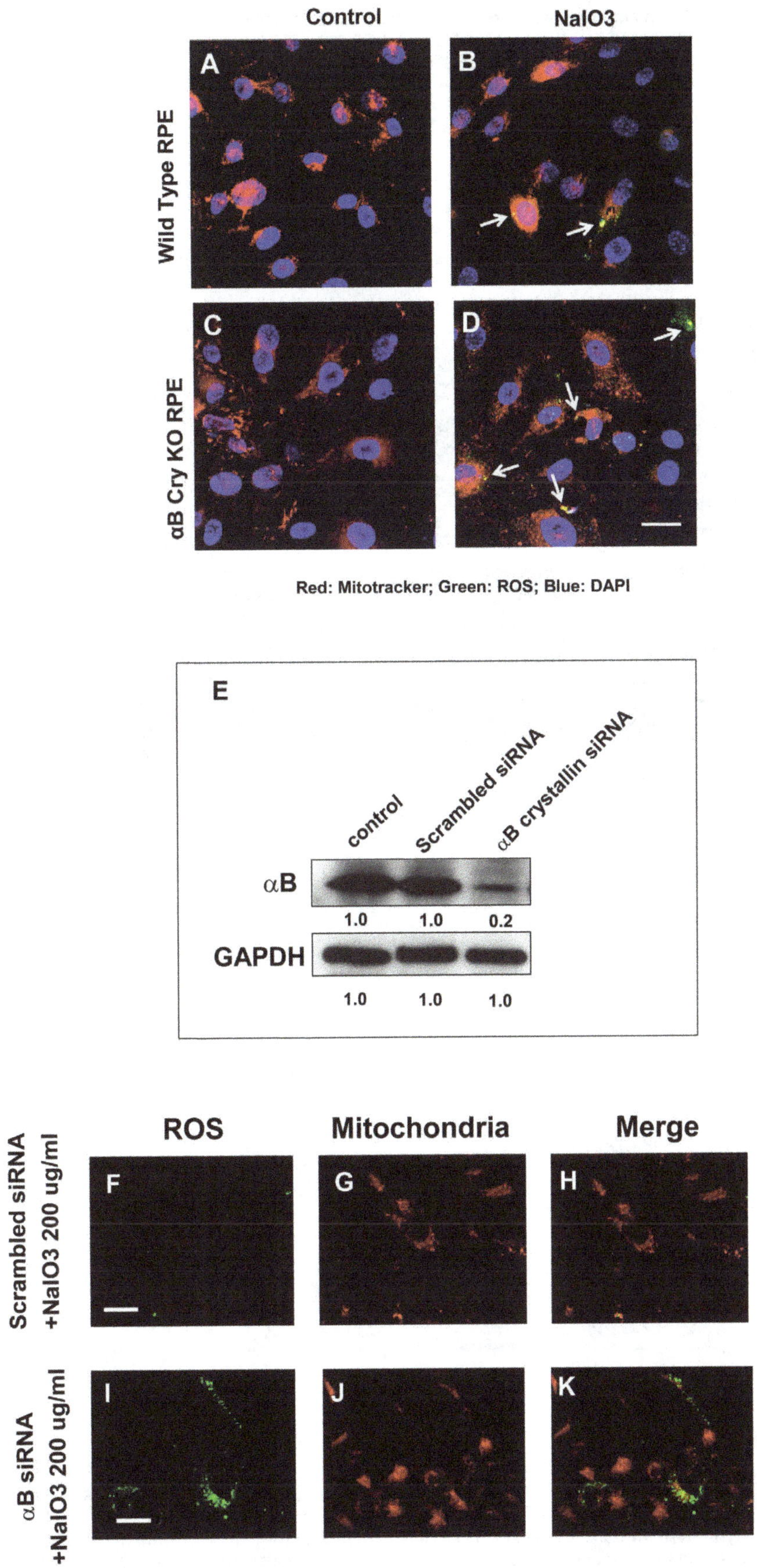

Figure 5. Increased production of reactive oxygen species (ROS) in mouse primary RPE cells and human RPE cells transfected with αB crystallin (αB-/-) siRNA after $NaIO_3$ treatment. Confluent mouse RPE cells from αB-/- and WT mice were treated with 200 µg/ml $NaIO_3$ for

24 h. In panels A–D, DAPI is shown in blue, ROS staining in green and mitotracker in red. ROS staining was observed in WT RPE cells treated with $NaIO_3$ (A–B). RPE cells from αB-/- mice (C–D, see white arrows) showed increased accumulation of ROS that partially colocalized with mitochondria. For studies with human RPE cells, αB crystallin was knocked down (~80%) by siRNA transfection (Fig. 5E). Increased ROS production was observed in αB crystallin si-RNA transfected human RPE cells with $NaIO_3$ as compared to scrambled siRNA transfected cells which showed negligible ROS staining (I–K). (F–H). Scale bars represent 20 μm for A–D and 10 μm for F–K, respectively.

knockout of either αA or αB crystallin in RPE renders them more susceptible to oxidative stress [28]. Thus, it might be interesting to study the effects of double knockout of αA and αB crystallin on the extent of retinal degeneration in this model.

We used human RPE cultures *in vitro* to elucidate the mechanism of $NaIO_3$ induced apoptosis under conditions of αB crystallin deficiency. PPAR-$_\gamma$, a member of a nuclear receptor superfamily, plays a key role in numerous cellular functions and is

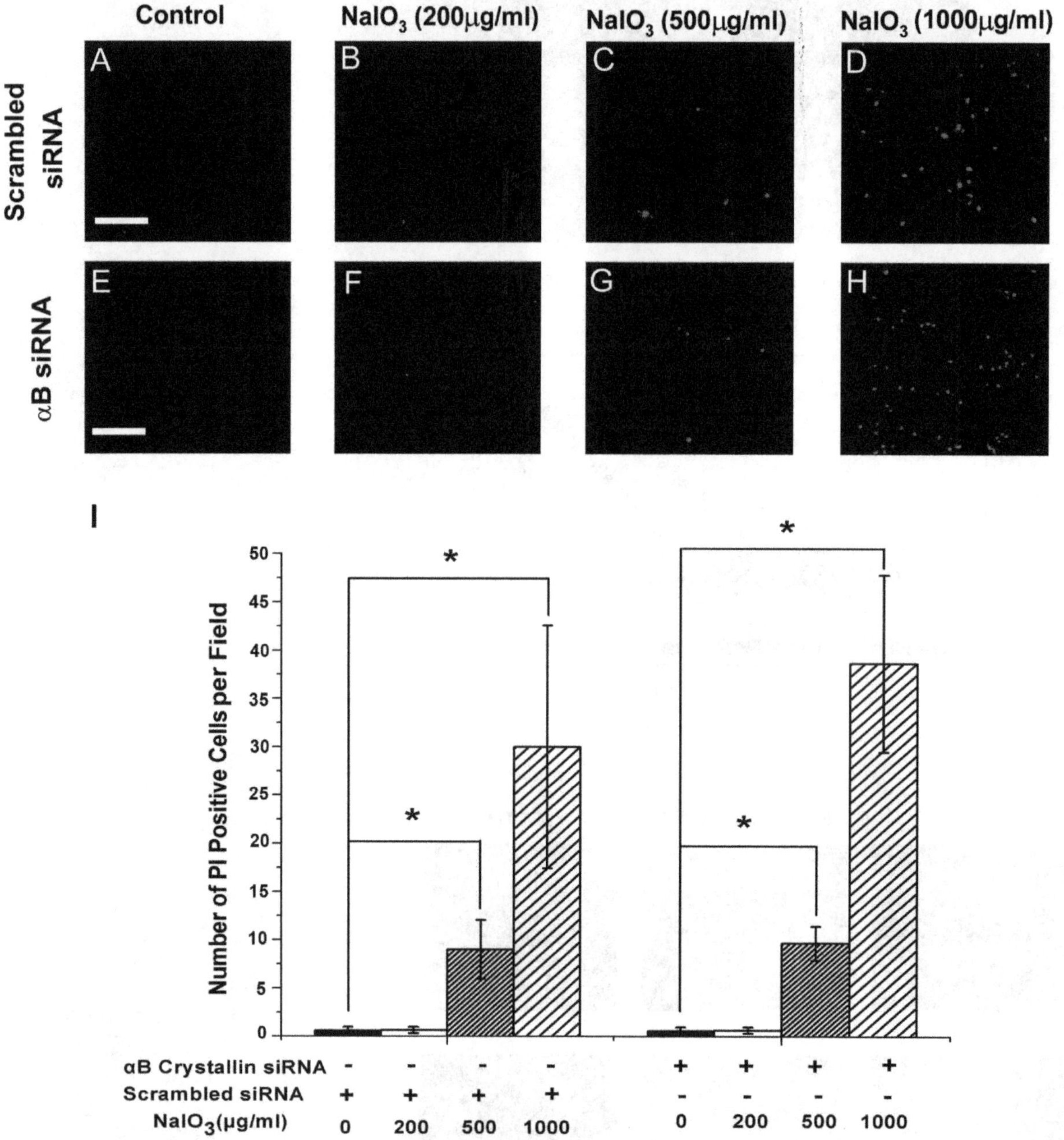

Figure 6. Occurrence of necrosis with high doses of $NaIO_3$ in human RPE cells. Forty-eight hours after scrambled siRNA or αB crystallin siRNA transfection, RPE cells were treated with 200, 500, 1000 μg/ml $NaIO_3$ for 24hours. Propidium iodide (PI) staining positive cells were determined in scrambled siRNA-transfected RPE cells (A–D) and αB crystallin siRNA-transfected human RPE cells (E–H) treated with $NaIO_3$. Treatment with 500 and 1000 μg/ml of $NaIO_3$ resulted in increased PI positive cells both in control RPE cells and αB crystallin siRNA pretreated human RPE cells (I). However, no significant differences were found between the number of PI positive cells in control RPE groups and αB crystallin siRNA-transfected group (I). Data are mean ± SEM from three individual experiments, αB siRNA refers to αB crystallin siRNA. *$P<0.05$. Scale bar = 40 μm.

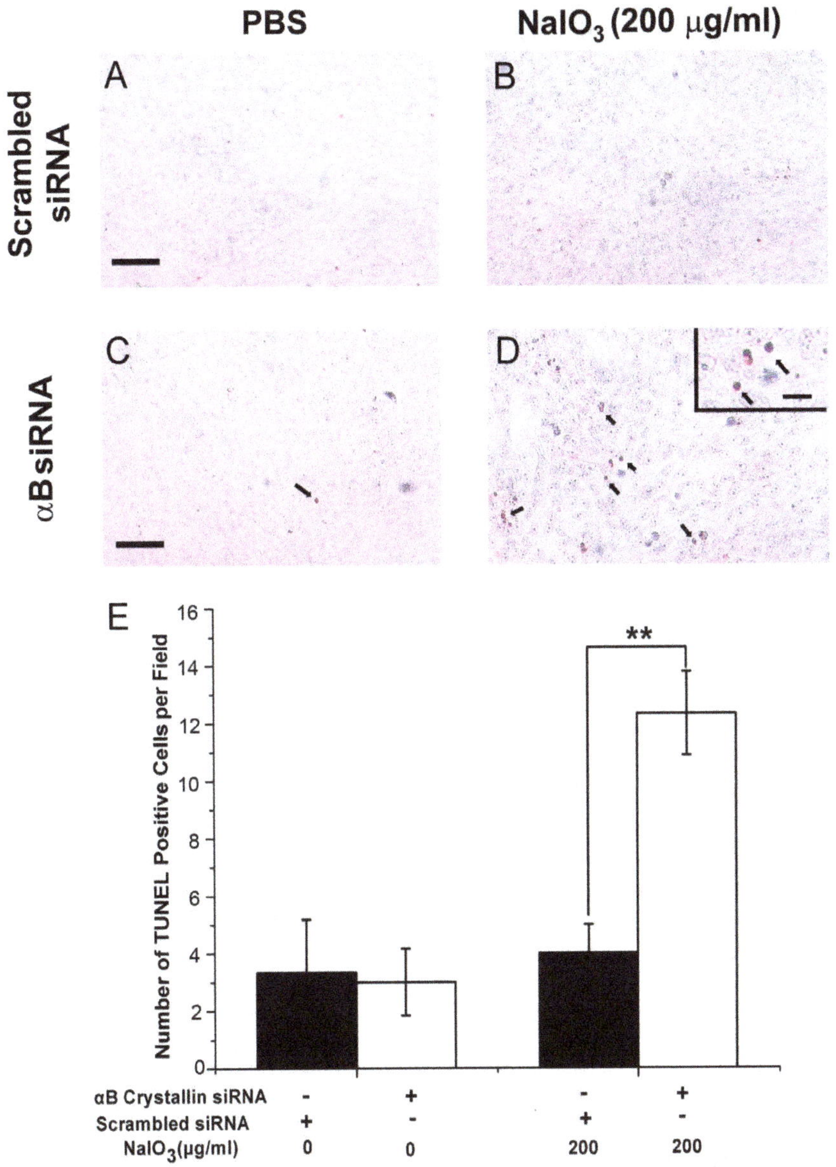

Figure 7. Induction of apoptosis in RPE cells with low dose of $NaIO_3$. Forty-eight hours after scrambled siRNA or αB crystallin siRNA transfection, human RPE cells were treated with 200 µg/ml $NaIO_3$ for 24 hours. TUNEL staining was performed in scrambled siRNA-transfected human RPE cells (A, B) and αB crystallin siRNA-transfected human RPE cells (C, D). Treatment with $NaIO_3$ resulted in increased TUNEL-positive cells with αB crystallin siRNA-transfection as compared with scrambled siRNA controls. (arrows in inset in D and E). Data are mean ± SEM from three individual experiments, αB siRNA refers to αB crystallin siRNA. **$P<0.01$. Scale = 40 µm for A–D and 10 µm for inset in D.

a key regulator of mitochondrial biogenesis and of ROS metabolism [41]. We found that the expression of $PPAR_\gamma$ protein in RPE cells increased after treatment with low dose $NaIO_3$. The increase in $PPAR_\gamma$ expression was significantly lower in αB crystallin siRNA-transfected RPE cells treated with $NaIO_3$. Furthermore, the $PPAR_\gamma$ ligand A-PAF inhibited ROS production in αB crystallin knockdown RPE cells treated with $NaIO_3$. This finding of ROS inhibition by $PPAR_\gamma$ ligand in RPE cells is consistent with some recent reports in other cell types. In mesangial cells, $PPAR_\gamma$ ligand rosiglitazone abolished ROS generation during exposure to high glucose, while inhibition of $PPAR_\gamma$ by GW9662 caused ROS generation in normal glucose [41]. Further, αB crystallin was shown to effectively inhibit both ROS formation and apoptosis in cultured vascular endothelial cells [42]. The ROS-inhibitory function of $PPAR_\gamma$ could arise from the antioxidative properties reported for $PPAR_\gamma$. For example, it was shown recently that thiazolidinediones, synthetic ligands of $PPAR_\gamma$, effectively protected pancreatic beta-cells from oxidative stress by an increase in the expression of the antioxidative enzyme catalase [43]. Similarly, antioxidative, neuroprotective function for $PPAR_\gamma$ was reported in a model of Parkinson's disease [44]. It will be of interest to investigate whether the observed antiapoptotic function of $PPAR_\gamma$ in RPE is linked to any changes in endogenous antioxidant enzymes. In this context, our laboratory has shown that overexpression of αB crystallin protects human RPE from oxidative and ER stress and upregulation of GSH and its biosynthetic enzymes are involved in this process [31,32,45].

The phosphoinositide 3-kinase (PI3K)-Akt pathway serves to coordinate the cellular response and ultimately determine cell fate

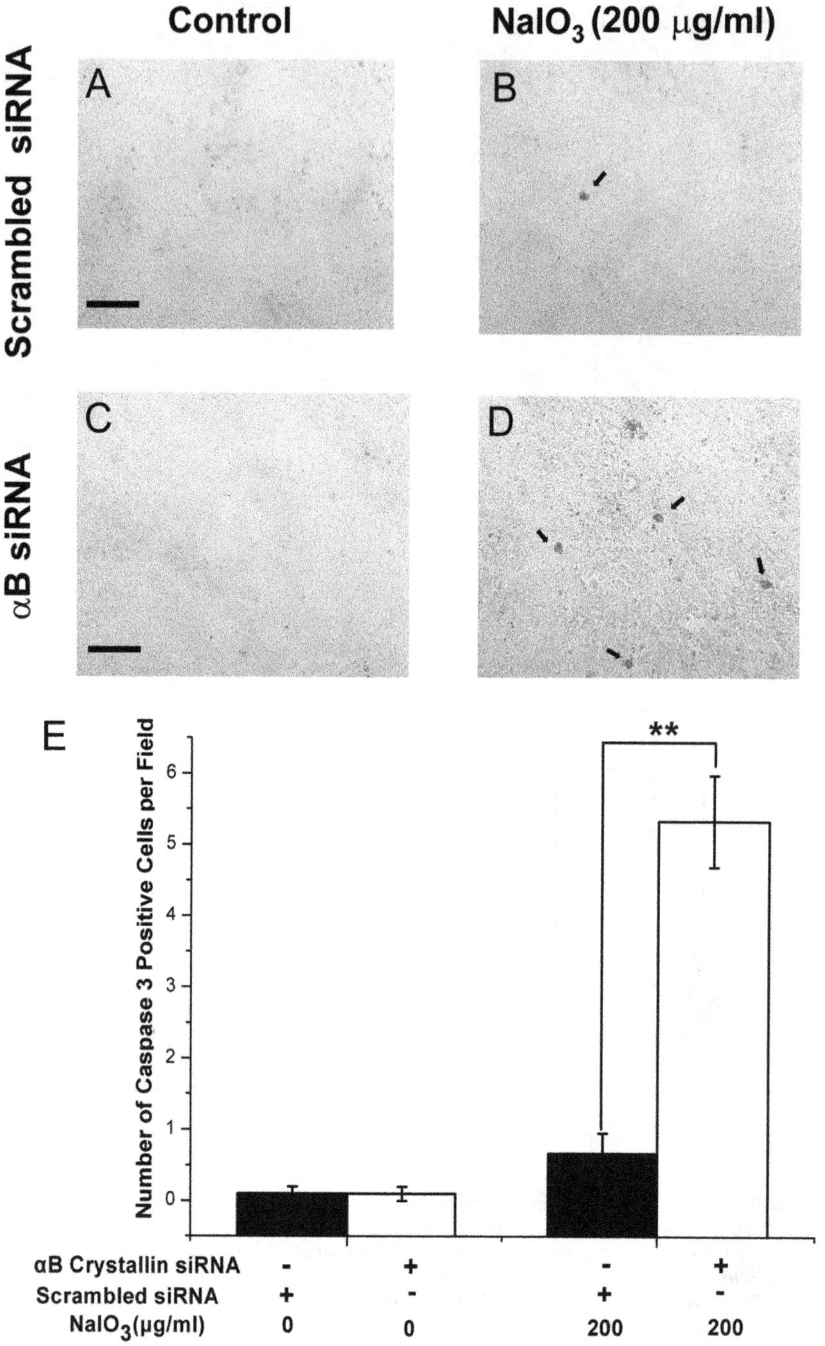

Figure 8. Caspase 3 activation with $NaIO_3$ treatment and increased activation with knockdown of αB crystallin siRNA in human RPE cells. Forty-eight hours after scrambled siRNA or αB crystallin siRNA transfection, human RPE cells were treated with 200 μg/ml $NaIO_3$ for 24 hours. Cleaved caspase 3 staining was performed in scrambled siRNA-transfected human RPE cells (A, B) and αB crystallin siRNA-transfected human RPE cells (C, D). Treatment with 200 μg/ml of $NaIO_3$ resulted in increased amount of cleaved caspase 3-positive cells with αB crystallin siRNA-transfection vs. scrambled siRNA controls (E). Data are mean ± SEM from three individual experiments, αB siRNA refers to αB crystallin siRNA in panels C and D. **$P < 0.01$. Scale bar = 40 μm.

[46]. Akt activation enhances RPE cell survival. It was reported that H_2O_2 induced PI3K and thereby activated Akt in human RPE cells [47]. AKT activation occurs through direct oxidation of phosphatase tensin homologue (PTEN) in acute oxidative stress [48]. We found in the present study that phosphorylated Akt and the signaling proteins downstream of AKT increased in RPE cells after treatment with $NaIO_3$, Further, knockdown of αB crystallin by siRNA suppressed the activation of Akt. Together, these data suggest αB crystallin mediated protection of RPE cells from $NaIO_3$ induced oxidative stress involves AKT. Working with HeLa cells, Pasupuleti et al. found evidence for activation of the PI3K/Akt cell survival pathway by alphaA crystallin by promoting phosphorylation of PDK1, AKT and PTEN [49]. It is of interest that Zhao et al reported that RPE dedifferentiation and hypertrophy in a model

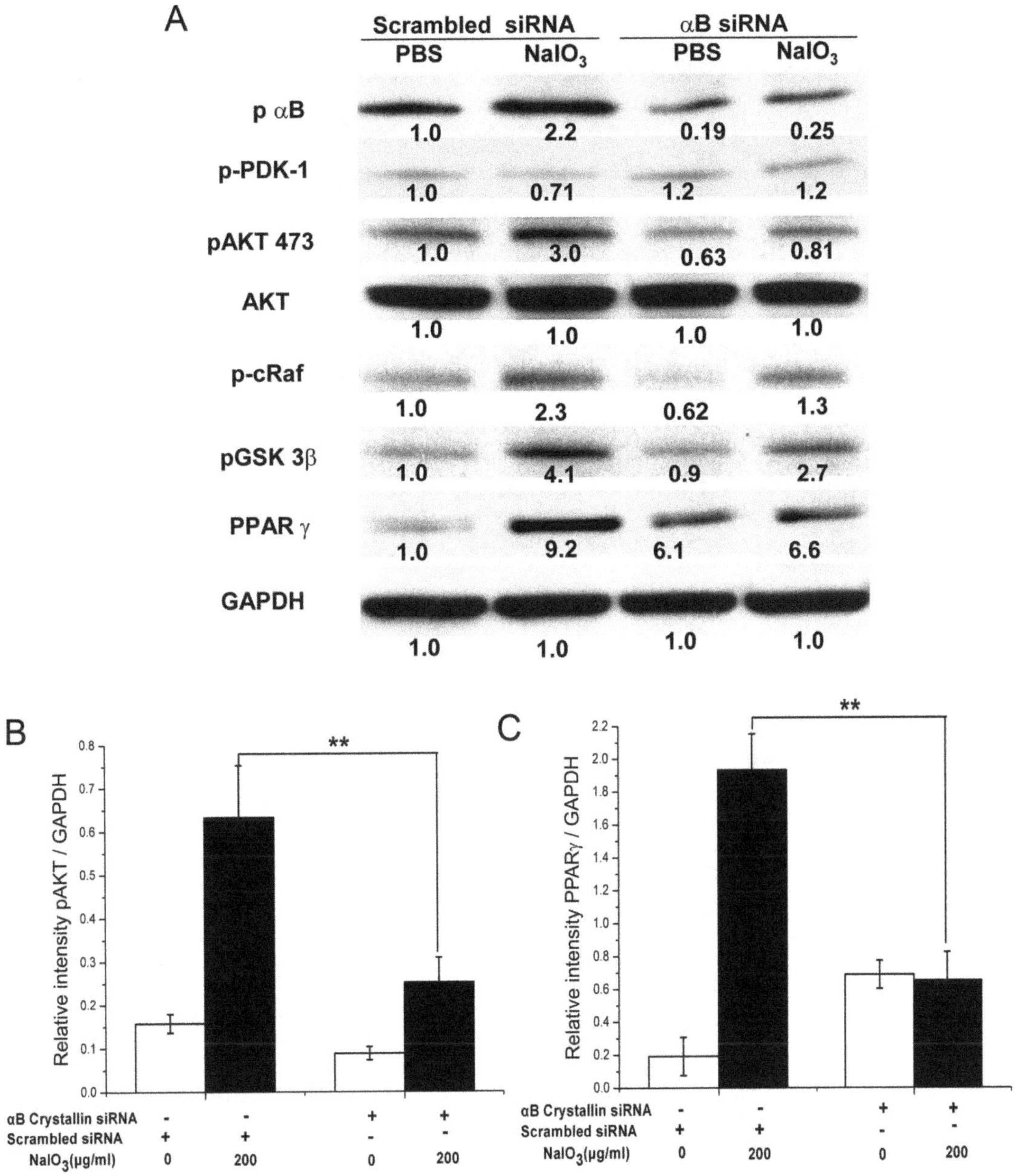

Figure 9. Western blot analysis showing changes in expression of signaling molecules with $NaIO_3$. Forty-eight hours after scrambled siRNA or αB crystallin siRNA transfection, human RPE cells were treated with 200 μg/ml $NaIO_3$ for 24 hours. Cells were lysed and western blot was performed. (A) Phosphorylated level of AKT at serine 473 increased after the treatment of low dose (200 μg/ml) $NaIO_3$ (B). The increase of phospho-AKT was lower in αB crystallin siRNA-transfected RPE cells treated with $NaIO_3$. Similar trends were found for phospho-GSK 3β and phospho-c-Raf, and $PPAR_\gamma$ and quantification is shown for $PPAR_\gamma$ in (C). However, no significant changes were found in phospho-PDK1, a kinase upstream of AKT. All experiments were performed three times and representative gels are presented. Protein expression levels were measured by Bandscan software, normalized to GAPDH, and labeled under each corresponding band. The bars for group B and C for pAKT and $PPAR_\gamma$ are derived from 3 individual experiments. αB siRNA refers to αB crystallin siRNA. pαB in panel A refers to phosphorylated αB crystallin. $^{**}P<0.01$.

of oxidative phosphorylation (OXPHOS) deficiency or $NaIO_3$ administration to B6 mice resulted in the stimulation of AKT/mammalian target of rapamycin (AKT/mTOR pathway [7]. Further, evidence for RPE oxidative damage and a rapid reduction of RPE65 and several other RPE-characteristic proteins was found [7]. This led the authors to suggest that mTOR pathway inhibition could be an effective therapeutic strategy for retinal degenerative diseases involving RPE stress [50].

In conclusion, our data show that αB crystallin plays a critical role in protection of $NaIO_3$ induced oxidative and retinal degeneration in part through upregulation of AKT phosphorylation and $PPAR_\gamma$ expression.

Materials and Methods

Ethics statement

This study conforms to applicable regulatory guidelines at the University of Southern California, principles of human subject

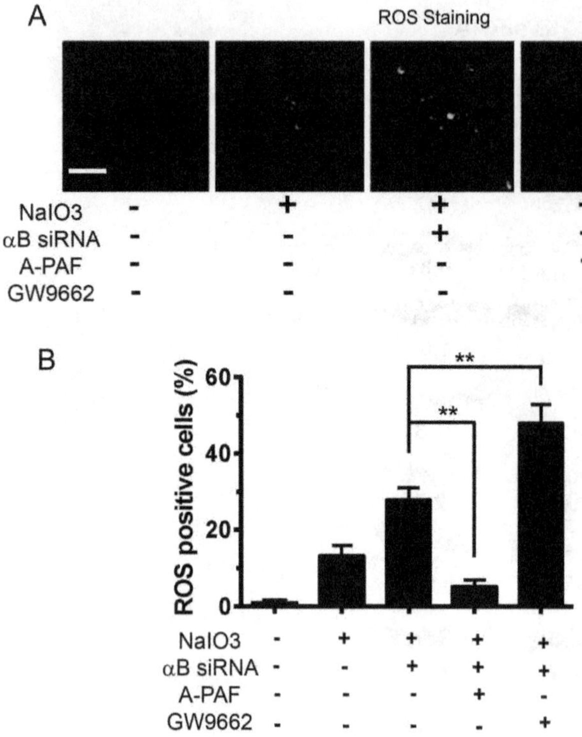

Figure 10. Detection of reactive oxygen species (ROS) in the presence and absence of PPAR$_\gamma$ ligand/antagonist. Increased production of ROS was observed in RPE cells transfected with αB crystallin siRNA upon $NaIO_3$ treatment as compared to control group. A-PAF, a PPAR$_\gamma$ ligand, suppressed ROS production significantly ($P<0.01$) in αB crystallin siRNA transfected cells treated with $NaIO_3$ (A). On the other hand, GW9662, a PPAR$_\gamma$ antagonist significantly increased ROS positive cells in αB crystallin siRNA transfected cells treated with $NaIO_3$. ROS positive cells were quantified from four random images derived from 4 individual experiments. αB siRNA refers to αB Crystallin siRNA. (B). Scale bar = 40 μm. **$P<0.01$.

protection in the Declaration of Helsinki and principles of animal research in the Association for Research in Vision and Ophthalmology and Statement for the Use of Animals in Ophthalmic and Vision Research. All procedures with mice were performed in compliance with the Keck School of Medicine Institutional Animal Care and Use Committee approved protocols and the ARVO Statement for the Use of Animals in Ophthalmic and Vision Research. The Institutional Review Board (IRB) approved our use of human RPE cells under protocol #HS-947005 (valid until April 4, 2014). Human fetal eyes (16–18 weeks of gestation) were obtained from advanced Bioscience Resources Inc. (ABR, Alameda, CA) and written informed consent was obtained from all donors. The University of Southern California Institutional Animal Care committee approved our animal studies under protocol #11710 (valid until October 18, 2014).

The 129S6/SvEvTac wild type mice were purchased from Taconic Farms (Germantown, NY), and the αB crystallin knockout mice in 129S6/SvEvTac background were obtained from the National Eye Institute [28,29]. Mice aged between 6 and 8 weeks maintained on a standard laboratory chow in an air-conditioned room equipped with a 12-hour light/12-hour dark cycle were used in all studies.

Experimental groups and $NaIO_3$ treatment

The mice were divided into four groups of seven mice per group: control wild type (PBS-treated WT), $NaIO_3$-treated wild type ($NaIO_3$-treated WT), control (PBS) αB crystallin knockout mice, and $NaIO_3$-treated αB crystallin knockout mice.

Experiments to determine the dose and time-dependent effect of $NaIO_3$ were performed using doses of 20 mg/kg, 35 mg/kg, 50 mg/kg and 70 mg/kg body weight and duration of the study was one week to three weeks post $NaIO_3$ administration. Briefly, varying doses of sodium iodate ($NaIO_3$; Sigma, St. Louis, MO) diluted with Phosphate buffered saline (PBS) were injected through the tail vein to restrained mice. Animals injected with equivalent volumes of PBS served as controls. Electroretinography and fundus photograph (see below) were assessed 21 days post-injection. After the tests were performed, mice were euthanized with CO_2 and their eyes processed for histology.

Electroretinography (ERG)

Mice were dark-adapted overnight and anesthetized by intraperitoneal injection of ketamine (100 mg/kg body weight) and xylazine (10 mg/kg body weight). Pupils were dilated with topical administration of 2.5% phenylephrine containing 0.5% tropicamide, and the cornea was anesthetized with 0.5% proparacaine. Mesopic ERGs were measured using a non-attenuated light stimulus. To measure cone responses, a 6 lux white background light was delivered through the other arm of the coaxial cable to suppress rod responses, and a non-attenuated light stimulus was applied. *a*-Wave amplitude was measured from the baseline to the trough of the *a*-wave, while *b*-wave amplitude was measured from the trough of the *a*-wave to the peak of the *b*-wave [51].

Fundus photography

Mice were anesthetized by administration of ketamine and xylazine as described above. Pupils were dilated and the cornea was anesthetized with 0.5% proparacaine. Images were captured using a 35 mm Kowa hand-held fundus camera (Genesis, Tokyo, Japan).

Histopathologic analysis

Eyes were enucleated and the anterior segments were removed. The remaining posterior eye cups were snap-frozen in tissue freezing medium (Triangle Biomedical Sciences, Durham, NC), Optimal cutting temperature (OCT). Cryostat Sections (8 μm) were stained with hematoxylin and eosin (H&E), to assess the histopathologic changes.

Mouse retinal sections were scanned and retinal thickness was measured (Aperio ScanScope; Leica Biosystems) using Aperio software. Cell numbers in RPE layer, GCL layer, INL layer and ONL layer were determined by counting the nuclei in a 50 μm wide region of retinal section located at equal distance from the ora serrata and the optic disc. For each group, three eyes were dissected. For each, three different regions were counted by Image J 4.3.2 (NIH Image). Average cell numbers and standard deviation were calculated using Statlab (SPSS Inc, Chicago, Illinois, USA).

Human and mouse RPE cell cultures

All procedures conformed to the Declaration of Helsinki for research involving human subjects and were performed with the approval of the institutional review board (IRB) of the University of Southern California. Human RPE cells were isolated from fetal human eyes of 16–18 wks gestation (Advanced Bioscience Resources, Inc., Alameda, CA) as previously described [52,53]. Cells were cultured in DMEM (Fisher Scientific, Pittsburgh, PA) with 2 mM L-glutamine, 100 U/ml penicillin, 100 μg/ml streptomycin (Sigma, St. Louis, MO), and 10% heat-inactivated fetal bovine serum (FBS, Irvine Scientific, Santa Ana, CA). The preparations contained >95% RPE cells (cytokeratin-positive). Cells used were from passages 2 to 4. Primary mouse RPE cells were isolated as previously described [54]. Primary mouse RPE cells were isolated from 4 to 6 week old WT (129S6/SvEvTac) and αB crystallin knockout mice. RPE cells were cultured in DMEM containing 20% FBS and antibiotics until confluent and P3 cells were used for experiments.

αB crystallin small interfering RNA (siRNA) transfection

Human RPE cells were switched to DMEM containing 0.5% FBS shortly before transfection. siRNA targeting αB crystallin was diluted in DMEM without serum. HiPerFect Transfection Reagent (Qiagen, Valencia, CA) was added to the diluted siRNA and mixed by vortexing. After incubation for 10 min at room temperature, the complexes were added dropwise to RPE cells. The final siRNA concentration was 5 nM. The cells were harvested or fixed for further assay 24 hours later. The sequence for siRNA targeting αB crystallin was: sense: r(CCA GGG AGU UCC ACA GGA A)dTdT; antisense:r(UUC CUG UGG AAC UCC CUG G) dTdT; nonsilencing control siRNA (scrambled siRNA): sense r(UUC UCC GAA CGU GUC ACG U) dTdT; antisense:r(ACG UGA CAC GUU CGG AGA A) dTdT. Forty-eight hours after transfection, *in vitro* effects of $NaIO_3$ were studied either with a fixed final concentration 200 μg/ml added to the culture medium or at different doses as specified.

Determination of ROS

To determine the compartmentalized generation of reactive oxygen species (ROS), mitochondria were labeled by a cell-permeable mitochondria-specific red fluorescent dye (Mito-Tracker, Molecular Probes); stained with carboxy-H2-DCFDA (Molecular Probes; 5 μM for 1 h at 37 °C), and rapidly evaluated by confocal microscopy (LSM510, Zeiss, Thornwood, NY, USA) as previously described [28,31]. A yellow color is observed when ROS (green) are colocalized in the mitochondria (red). In some experiments, the effect of treatment with Azelaoyl PAF (A-PAF) (Sigma, St, MO, USA), a $PPAR_\gamma$ ligand at a concentration of 20 μM and GW9662 (Cayman Chemicals, Ann Arbor, Mich, USA), a $PPAR_\gamma$ antagonist, at a concentration of 10 μM was determined [55,56].

Determination of necrosis and apoptosis with $NaIO_3$

Propidium Iodide (PI) stains DNA of necrotic cells [28,31]. Human RPE cells on an eight-well Lab-TekTM chamber were treated with 10 mg/ml PI (Roche Applied Science) for 15 min at 25 °C in the dark. Cells were washed once with ice-cold PBS and observed under a laser scanning confocal microscope (LSM510, Zeiss, Thornwood, NY, USA).

Apoptosis (DNA fragmentation) was detected by the terminal deoxynucleotidyl transferase (TdT)-mediated dUTP-biotin nick end-labeling (TUNEL) method according to the manufacturer's protocol (In situ cell death detection kit-POD; Roche Applied Science). In short, after treatment with several doses of $NaIO_3$ at room temperature, RPE cells on eight-well Lab-TekTM chambers were fixed in 1% paraformaldehyde solution and rinsed with PBS. Cells were then incubated with the TUNEL reaction mixture containing TdT and fluorescence UTP for 1 hour at 37°C in a humidified chamber. The nucleotides incorporated into DNA breaks were detected by applying anti-fluorescein peroxidase (POD) conjugate and peroxidase substrate.

Immunocytochemistry of Cleaved Caspase-3

Human RPE cells on an eight-well Lab-TekTM chamber were fixed in 4% paraformaldehyde for 30 min, and then permeabilized using 0.2% Triton-X 100 at 37°C for 15 min. Blocking was achieved by addition of 1% goat serum for 20 min. The samples were incubated with primary anti-cleaved caspase-3 antibody (Cell Signaling; 1:200) for 1 hr at room temperature. After washing with PBS, secondary biotinylated conjugated goat anti-rabbit antibody (1:400; Vector, Burlingame, CA, USA) was applied to the slides for 30 min at room temperature. After washing with PBS, streptavidin peroxidase (Invitrogen, Camarillo, CA, USA) was applied to the slides for 30 min. 3-Amino-9-Ethylcarbazole (AEC) was added to the slide (AEC Substrate Kit, Invitrogen, Camarillo) which produced a red colored deposit. Sections were examined and photographed with microscope (Leica, Germany).

Western blot analysis

Cells were lysed, supernatants were collected, and proteins were resolved on Tris-HCl 10% polyacrylamide gels (Ready Gel; Bio-Rad, Hercules, CA) at 120 V. The proteins were transferred to PVDF blotting membrane (Millipore, Bedford, MA). The membranes were probed with antibody for phospho-αB crystallin (Ser 59, Stressgen), pan-AKT (C67E4, Cell Signaling), phospho-AKT (Ser 473, Cell Signaling), phospho-PDK1 (Ser 241, Cell Signaling), phospho-c-Raf (Ser 259, Cell signaling), phospho-GSK-3β (Ser 9, Cell Signaling), $PPAR_\gamma$ (Santa Cruz Biotechnology) all at 1:1,000 dilution. Membranes were washed and incubated with a horseradish peroxidase (HRP)-conjugated secondary antibody (1:3,000, Vector Laboratories, Burlingame, CA) for 30 min at room temperature. Images were developed by adding ECL chemiluminescence detection solution (Amersham Pharmacia Biotech, Cleveland, OH). Monoclonal anti mouse GAPDH was used as the loading control.

Statistics

All experiments were performed at least three times. The data were analyzed using the Student's t-test (amplitudes of ERG; number of nuclei of outer nuclear layer, inner nuclear layer and ganglion layer histopathology; ROS; TUNEL; Cleaved caspase 3; and western blot) or Chi-square (fundus photography, RPE layer histopathology) and $P<0.05$ was considered as significant.

Supporting Information

Figure S1 Fundus images showing time-dependent effect of a single dose of $NaIO_3$ on wild type (WT) and αB crystallin -/- (αB-/-) mice. Representative images from a single mouse from WT and αB-/- groups are shown on the left accompanied by data for all experimental animals on the right. Fundus photography was taken one, two and three weeks after tail vein injection of PBS or 20 mg/kg $NaIO_3$. PBS-treated WT and PBS-treated αB -/- did not exhibit any degenerative changes (data not shown). $NaIO_3$-treated WT mice did not show retinal degeneration at any time point (A). However, $NaIO_3$- treated αB-/- mice showed patchy retinal degeneration two and three weeks after $NaIO_3$ injection (B). Arrow indicates the site of patchy retinal degeneration. αB-/- refers to αB crystallin knockout mice.

Figure S2 $NaIO_3$-induced cell death in RPE layer of αB crystallin knockout mouse retina as determined by TUNEL staining. TUNEL staining was performed after WT and αB crystallin knockout mice were injected with 20 mg/kg $NaIO_3$. No TUNEL+ cells were observed in the RPE layer of WT retina while TUNEL+ cells could be easily identified in the RPE layer of αB crystallin knockout retina (white arrow). Scale bar $=50$ μm.

Acknowledgments

We wish to thank Ernesto Barron for assistance with figures.

Author Contributions

Conceived and designed the experiments: PZ RK DRH. Performed the experiments: PZ PGS CS GD. Analyzed the data: PZ PGS RK DRH. Wrote the paper: PZ RK DRH.

References

1. Gehrs KM, Anderson DH, Johnson LV, Hageman GS (2006) Age-related macular degeneration-emerging pathogenic and therapeutic concepts. Ann Med. 38: 450–471.
2. Ambati J, Fowler B (2012) Mechanisms of Age-related macular degeneration. Neuron. 75: 26–39.
3. Bird AC (2010) Therapeutic targets in age-related macular degeneration. J Clin Invest. 120: 3033–3041.
4. Klein ML, Ferris FL 3rd, Armstrong J, Hwang TS, Chew EY, et al. (2008) Retinal precursors and the development of geographic atrophy in age-related macular degeneration. Ophthalmology. 115: 1026–1031.
5. Ramkumar HL, Zhang J, Chan CC (2010) Retinal ultrastructure of murine models of dry age-related macular degeneration. Prog Retin Eye Res 29:169–90.
6. Enzmann V, Row BW, Yamauchi Y, Kheirandish L, Gozal D, et al. (2006) Behavioral and anatomical abnormalities in a sodium iodate-induced model of retinal pigment epithelium degeneration, Exp Eye Res 82:441–448.
7. Zhao C, Yasumura D, Li X, Mathes M, Lloyd M, et al. (2011) mTOR-mediated dedifferentiation of the retinal pigment epithelium initiates photoreceptor degeneration in mice. J Clin Invest 121: 369–383.
8. Markovets AM, Saprunova VB, Zhdankina AA, Fursova AZh, Kolosova NG (2011) Alterations of retinal pigment epithelium cause AMD like retinopathy in senescence-accelerated OXYS rats. Aging (Albany, NY) 3: 44–54.
9. Kolosova NG, Muraleva NA, Zhdankina AA, Stefanova NA, Fursova AZ, et al. (2012) Prevention of age-related macular degeneration-like retinopathy by rapamycin in rats. Amer J Pathol 181:472–477.
10. Malek G, Johnson LV, Mace ME, Saloupis P, Schmechel DE, et al. (2005) Apolipoprotein E allele-dependent pathogenesis: a model for age related macular degeneration. Proc Natl Acad Sci USA 102: 11900–11905.
11. Ding JD, Johnson LV, Herrmann R, Farsiu S, Smith SG, et al. (2011) Antiamyloid therapy protects against retinal pigmented epithelium damage and vision loss in a model of age-related macular degeneration. Proc Natl Acad Sci USA 108: E279–87.
12. Karan G, Lillo C, Yang Z, Cameron DJ, Locke KG, et al. (2005) Lipofuscin accumulation, abnormal electrophysiology, and photoreceptor degeneration in mutant ELOVL4 transgenic mice: a model for macular degeneration. Proc Natl Acad Sci USA 102:4164–4169.
13. Zhu D, Wu J, Spee C, Ryan SJ, Hinton DR (2009) BMP4 mediates oxidative stress-induced cell senescence and is overexpressed in age-related macular degeneration. J Biol Chem 284: 9529–9539.
14. Zhu D, Deng X, Xu J, Hinton DR (2009) What determines the switch between atrophic and neovascular forms of age related macular degeneration? -the role of BMP4 induced senescence. Aging (Albany, NY). 12: 740–745.
15. Longbottom R, Fruttiger M, Douglas RH, Martinez-Barbera JP, Greenwood J (2009) Genetic ablation of retinal pigment epithelial cells reveals the adaptive response of the epithelium and impact on photoreceptors, Proc Natl Acad Sci USA 106:18728–18733.
16. Kleinman ME, Kaneko H, Cho WG, Dridi S, Fowler BJ, et al. (2012) Short-interfering RNAs induce retinal degeneration via TLR3 and IRF3. Mol Ther. 20: 101–108.
17. Kaneko H, Dridi S, Tarallo V, Gelfand BD, Fowler BJ, et al. (2011) DICER1 deficit induces AluRNA toxicity in age-related macular degeneration. Nature 471: 325–330.
18. Tarallo V, Hirano Y, Gelfand BD, Dridi S, Kerur N, et al. (2012) DICER1 loss and Alu RNA induce age-related macular degeneration via the NLRP3 inflammasome and MyD88. Cell 149: 847–859.
19. Franco LM, Zulliger R, Wolf-Schnurrbusch UE, Katagiri Y (2009) Decreased visual function after patchy loss of retinal pigment epithelium induced by low-dose sodium iodate, Invest Ophthalmol Vis Sci. 50:4004–4010.
20. Ringvold A, Olsen EG, Flage T (1981) Transient breakdown of the retinal pigment epithelium diffusion barrier after sodium iodate: a fluorescein angiographic and morphological study in the rabbit, Exp Eye Res 33:361–369.
21. Kiuchi K, Yoshizawa K, Shikata N, Moriguchi K, Tsubura A (2002) Morphologic characteristics of retinal degeneration induced by sodium iodate in mice. Curr Eye Res 25:373–379.
22. Redfern WS, Storey S, Tse K, Hussain Q, Maung KP, et al. (2011) Evaluation of a convenient method of assessing rodent visual function in safety pharmacology studies: effects of sodium iodate on visual acuity and retinal morphology in albino and pigmented rats and mice. J Pharmacol Toxicol Methods 63: 102–114.
23. Kannan R, Sreekumar PG, Hinton DR (2012) Novel roles for alpha crystallins in retinal function and disease. Prog Retin Eye Res 31: 576–604.
24. Nakata K, Crabb JW, Hollyfield JG (2005) Crystallin distribution in Bruch's membrane-choroid complex from AMD and age-matched donor eyes. Exp Eye Res 80:821–826.
25. De S, Rabin DM, Salero E, Lederman PL, Temple S, et al. (2007) Human retinal pigment epithelium cell changes and expression of alphaB-crystallin: a biomarker for retinal pigment epithelium cell change in age-related macular degeneration. Arch Ophthalmol. 125: 641–645.
26. Xi J, Farjo R, Yoshida S, Kern TS, Swaroop A, et al. (2003) A comprehensive analysis of the expression of crystallins in mouse retina, Mol Vis 9:410–419.
27. Fort PE, Lampi KJ (2011) New focus on alpha-crystallins in retinal neurodegenerative diseases. Exp Eye Res. 92: 98–103.
28. Yaung J, Jin M, Barron E, Spee C, Wawrousek EF, et al. (2007) alpha-Crystallin distribution in retinal pigment epithelium and effect of gene knockouts on sensitivity to oxidative stress. Mol Vis.13:566–577
29. Brady JP, Garland DL, Green DE, Tamm ER, Giblin FJ (2001) AlphaB-crystallin in lens development and muscle integrity: a gene knockout approach, Invest Ophthalmol Vis Sci. 42:2924–2934.
30. Yaung J, Kannan R, Wawrousek EF, Spee C, Sreekumar PG, et al. (2008) Exacerbation of retinal degeneration in the absence of alpha crystallins in an in vivo model of chemically induced hypoxia. Exp Eye Res. 86: 355–365.
31. Dou G, Sreekumar PG, Spee C, He S, Ryan SJ (2012) Deficiency of alphaB crystallin augments ER Stress-induced apoptosis by enhancing mitochondrial dysfunction. Free Radic Bio Med. 53: 1111–1122.
32. Sreekumar PG, Spee C, Ryan SJ, Cole SPC, Kannan R, et al. (2012) Mechanism of RPE cell death in alpha-crystallin deficient mice: A novel and critical role for MRP1-mediated GSH efflux. PLoS ONE. 7(3):e33420. doi:10.137/journal.pone.0033420
33. Sreekumar PG, Kannan R, Kitamura M, Spee C, Barron E, et al. (2010) AlphaB crystallin is apically secreted within exosomes by polarized human retinal pigment epithelium and provides neuroprotection to adjacent cells. PLoS ONE 5(10): e12578. doi:10.1371.journal.pone.0012578
34. Ousman SS, Tomooka BH, van Noort JM, Wawrousek EF, O'Connor KC (2007) Protective and therapeutic role for alphaB-crystallin in autoimmune demyelination. Nature 448: 474–479.

35. Brownell SE, Becker RA, Steinman L (2012) The protective and therapeutic function of small heat shock proteins in neurological diseases. Front Immunol. 3: 74.
36. Rothbard JB, Kumellas MP, Brownell S, Adams CM, Su L et al (2012) Therapeutic effects of systemic administration of chaperone alphaB crystallin associated with binding proinflammatory plasma proteins. J Biol Chem 287: 9708–9721.
37. Organisciak D, Darrow R, Gu X, Barsalou L, Crabb JW (2006) Genetic, age and light mediated effects on crystallin protein expression in the retina, Photochem Photobiol 82:1088–1096.
38. Sakaguchi H, Miyagi M, Darrow RM, Crabb JS, Hollyfield JG (2003) Intense light exposure changes the crystallin content in retina, Exp Eye Res 76:131–133.
39. Kase S, He S, Sonoda S, Kitamura M, Spee C, et al. (2010) alphaB-crystallin regulation of angiogenesis by modulation of VEGF, Blood. 115:3398–3406.
40. Zhou P, Ye H-F, Jiang Y-X, Yang J, Zhu X-J, et al. (2012) AlphaA crystallin may protect against geographic atrophy-meta analysis of cataract vs cataract surgery for geographic atrophy and experimental studies. PLoS ONE 7(8): e43173, doi:10.1371/journal.pone.0043173
41. Whiteside C, Wang H, Xia L, Munk S, Goldberg HJ, et al. (2009) Rosiglitazone prevents high glucose-induced vascular endothelial growth factor and collagen IV expression in cultured mesangial cells, Exp Diabetes Res 2009:910783
42. Liu B, Bhat M, Nagaraj RH (2011) AlphaB-crystallin inhibits glucose-induced apoptosis in vascular endothelial cells, Biochem Biophys Res Commun 321:254–258.
43. Chung SS, Kim M, Lee JS, Ahn BY, Jung HS (2011) Mechanism for antioxidative effects of thiazolidinediones in pancreatic beta-cells. Am J Physiol Endocrinol Metab 311: E912–11.
44. Martin HL, Mounsey RB, Mustafa S, Sathe K, Teismann P (2012) Pharmacological manipulation of peroxisome proliferator activator receptor gamma (PPAR gamma) reveals a role for anti-oxidant protection in a model of Parkinson's disease. Exp Neurol 235: 528–538.
45. Sreekumar PG, Hinton DR, Kannan R (2012) Glutathione metabolism and its contribution to antiapoptotic properties of alpha-crystallins in the retina. In Studies on Retinal and Choroidal Disorders (Stratton RD, Hauswirth WW, Gardner TW, eds.Humana Press) Chapter 9, p. 181–202.
46. Datta SR, Dudek H, Tao Y, Masters S, Fu H (1997) Akt phosphorylation of BAD couples survival signals to the cell-intrinsic death machinery. Cell 91:231–241.
47. Yang P, Peairs JJ, Tano R, Jaffe GJ (2006) Oxidant-mediated Akt activation in human RPE cells, Invest Ophthalmol Vis Sci 47:4598–4606.
48. Kim JW, Kang KH, Burrola P, Mak TW, Lemke G (2008) Retinal degeneration triggered by inactivation of PTEN in the retinal pigment epithelium. Genes Dev 22: 3147–3157.
49. Pasupuleti N, Matsuyama S, Voss O, Doseff AI, Song K, et al. (2010) The anti-apoptotic function of human alphaA-crystallin is directly related to its chaperone activity. Cell Death and Disease. 1, e31; doi: 10;1038/cddis.2010.3
50. Zhu C, Vollrath D (2011) mTOR pathway activation in age-related retinal disease. Aging 3: 346–347.
51. Zhu X, Wu K, Rife L, Cawley NX, Brown B, et al. (2005) Carboxypeptidase E is required for normal synaptic transmission from photoreceptors to the inner retina. J Neurochem. 95: 1351–1362.
52. Sonoda S, Spee C, Barron E, Ryan SJ, Kannan R, et al. (2009) A protocol for the culture and differentiation of highly polarized human retinal pigment epithelial cells. Nat Protoc 4:662–673.
53. Sonoda S, Sreekumar PG, Kase S, Spee C, Ryan SJ, et al. (2010) Attainment of polarity promotes growth factor secretion by retinal pigment epithelial cells: relevance to age-related macular degeneration. Aging 2: 28–42.
54. Kerur N, Hirano Y, Tarallo V, Fowler BJ, Bastos-Carvalho A, et al. (2013) TLR-independent and P2X7-dependent signaling mediate Alu RNA-induced NLRP3 inflammasome activation in geographic atrophy. Invest Ophthalmol Vis Sci 54:7395–7401.
55. Murata T, He S, Hangai M, Ishibashi T, Xi XP, et al. (2000) Peroxisome proliferator-activated receptor-gamma ligands inhibit choroidal neovascularization, Invest Ophthalmol Vis Sci 41:2309–2317.
56. Cheng HC, Ho TC, Chen SL, Lai HY, Hong KF, et al. (2008) Troglitazone suppresses transforming growth factor beta-mediated fibrogenesis in retinal pigment epithelial cells. Mol Vis14:95–104.

2

A Safety Review and Meta-Analyses of Bevacizumab and Ranibizumab: Off-Label versus Goldstandard

Christine Schmucker[1]*, Christoph Ehlken[2], Hansjuergen T. Agostini[2], Gerd Antes[1], Gerta Ruecker[3], Monika Lelgemann[4], Yoon K. Loke[5]

1 German Cochrane Institute, Institute of Medical Biometry and Medical Informatics, Department of Medical Biometry and Statistics, University Medical Centre Freiburg, Freiburg, Germany, **2** University Eye Hospital, University Medical Centre Freiburg, Freiburg, Germany, **3** Institute of Medical Biometry and Medical Informatics, Department of Medical Biometry and Statistics, University Medical Centre Freiburg, Freiburg, Germany, **4** Medical Advisory Service of the German Health Insurance Funds, Essen, Germany, **5** School of Medicine, University of East Anglia, Norwich, United Kingdom

Abstract

Background: We set out a systemic review to evaluate whether off-label bevacizumab is as safe as licensed ranibizumab, and whether bevacizumab can be justifiably offered to patients as a treatment for age-related macular degeneration with robust evidence of no differential risk.

Methods and Findings: Medline, Embase and the Cochrane Library were searched with no limitations of language and year of publication. We included RCTs with a minimum follow-up of one year which investigated bevacizumab or ranibizumab in direct comparison or against any other control group (indirect comparison). Direct comparison (3 trials, 1333 patients): The one year data show a significantly higher rate of ocular adverse effects (AE) with bevacizumab compared to ranibizumab (RR = 2.8; 95% CI 1.2–6.5). The proportion of patients with serious infections and gastrointestinal disorders was also higher with bevacizumab than with ranibizumab (RR = 1.3; 95% CI 1.0–1.7). Arterial thromboembolic events were equally distributed among the groups. Indirect comparison: Ranibizumab versus any control (5 trials, 4054 patients): The two year results of three landmark trials showed that while absolute rates of serious ocular AE were low (≤2.1%), relative harm was significantly raised (RR = 3.1; 95% CI 1.1–8.9). A significant increase in nonocular haemorrhage was also observed with ranibizumab (RR = 1.7; 95% CI 1.1–2.7). Bevacizumab versus any control (3 trials, 244 patients): We were unable to judge the safety profile of bevacizumab due to the poor quality of AE monitoring and reporting in the trials.

Conclusions: Evidence from head-to-head trials raises concern about an increased risk of ocular and multiple systemic AE with bevacizumab. Therefore, clinicians and patients should continue to carefully weight up the benefits and harms when choosing between the two treatment options. We also emphasize the need for studies that are powered not just for efficacy, but for defined safety outcomes based on the signals detected in this systematic review.

Editor: Andreas Wedrich, Medical University Graz, Austria

Funding: This research was supported by a grant from the German Federal Ministry of Education and Research (Grant number: 01KG1020, http://www.gesundheitsforschung-bmbf.de/de/4312.php). The funders had no role in study design, data collection and analysis, decision to publish, or preparation of the manuscript.

Competing Interests: The authors have declared that no competing interests exist.

* E-mail: schmucker@cochrane.de

Introduction

Age-related macular degeneration (AMD) is the leading cause of irreversible blindness in people over the age of 50 in the developed world [1]. Although an estimated 80% of patients with AMD have the non-neovascular form [2], the neovascular (wet or exudative) form is responsible for almost 90% of severe visual loss resulting from AMD [3].

Anti-angiogenic therapy, e.g., anti-vascular endothelial growth factors (anti-VEGF), which aims to prevent further neovascularization rather than only destroy it, is the latest approach to the treatment of neovascular AMD. Currently, the most commonly used VEGF antagonists are ranibizumab (Lucentis, Genentech, Inc., South San Francisco, CA) and bevacizumab (Avastin; Genentech, Inc., South San Francisco, CA).

Ranibizumab, which is an antibody fragment form the bevacizumab molecule with an increased binding affinity for all forms of VEGF, has been approved for the treatment of patients with neovascular AMD by the Food and Drug Administration and by the European Mediciens Agency since 2006 and 2007, respectively. The costs of ranibizumab, however, are immense. Using monthly injections with a dose of 0.5 mg, the annual costs come to more than US$23 000 per patient [4].

In contrast to ranibizumab, bevacizumab was not developed for the treatment of AMD and consequently has no regulatory approval for this indication or mode of administration. Bevacizumab is approved for the treatment of specific cancers, e.g., metastatic colorectal cancer. In chemotherapy regimens, bevacizumab is associated with an increased risk of thromboembolic events [5], haemorrhage [6] and mortality [7]. However, intravitreal bevacizumab is administered at a dose of 1 to 2.5 mg, which is at least 150 times less than the systemic dose used in chemotherapy [8]. The first report of intravitreal bevacizumab administration for neovascular AMD was published in 2005 [9]. After this initial report, numerous case series which (apparently) support the efficacy and safety of bevacizumab were published [10–13]. The costs of intravitreal bevacizumab are much less than for ranibizumab. A single dose of bevacizumab costs 40 times less than a single dose of ranibizumab [4]. This cost differential has important economic implications when extrapolated to the more than 250,000 patients who are treated for neovascular AMD annually in the United States. It is obvious that the low costs and the promising results on visual acuity have led to a widespread off-label use of bevacizumab.

Recently, a long awaited head-to-head comparison from the United States has been published [14]. The results of this trial support the effectiveness of bevacizumab and the authors conclude that both anti-VEGF have equivalent effects on visual acuity when administered according to the same schedule.

However, up to now, safety and tolerability of bevacizumab in comparison to ranibizumab have not been sufficiently assessed. For example, our group conducted a critical assessment of bevacizumab mainly based on the large number of published case series [15]. This previous review highlighted that the perceived low rates of adverse effects for bevacizumab are not supported by reliable data from this study design. Therefore, we performed a systematic review based on randomised controlled clinical trials (RCTs), including latest results of head-to-head comparisons, to address the crucial question whether the available information allow us to judge that unlicensed therapy with bevacizumab is as safe as licensed therapy with ranibizumab, and whether clinicians are justified in offering it to their patients with AMD as a medication with no additional risk. Besides comparing both drugs, we also evaluated whether adverse effects are dose-related.

Methods

Search Strategy

We searched Medline, Premedline, Embase and the Cochrane library from inception until May 2011. The search strategy was based on combinations of medical subject headings and keywords and was not restricted to specific languages or years of publication. The search strategy used in Medline is presented in Text S1. Search strategies for other databases were modified to meet the requirements of each database. The literature search also included terms associated with diabetic macular oedema. However, the results of this search will be presented in a separate review. The searches were supplemented by handsearching the bibliographies of included studies and reviews and by contacting the pharmaceutical manufacturer (Genentech) of ranibizumab and bevacizumab. Currently conducted RCTs comparing Avastin® versus Lucentis® were searched both in the register for clinical trials (http://clinicaltrials.gov/) and in the WHO International Clinical Trials Registry Platform (http://www.who.int/ictrp/en/).

Inclusion Criteria

We included randomised Phase III/IV trials which investigated bevacizumab or ranibizumab in direct comparisons (head-to-head studies) or against any other control group (for potential indirect comparison) in patients with neovascular AMD. RCTs which compared different treatment regimens of ranibizumab or bevacizumab were also included in our systematic review. To address long-term harm, such as myocardial infarction or stroke, one year follow-up data had to be available.

Studies which included patients with other indications than exudative AMD, patients previously treated with VEGF inhibitors or patients receiving systemic anti-VEGF therapy were excluded. We also excluded RCTs which enrolled less than 20 patients.

Data Extraction and Quality Assessment

Titles and abstracts were reviewed using the above mentioned selection criteria which were also predefined in our study protocol. Full papers of appropriate studies were obtained for detailed evaluation. Data extraction and quality assessment was carried out after a modified evaluation tool of the Center for Reviews and Dissemination (Chapter 4, Systematic Reviews of Adverse Effects) [16]. Information on the number of participants, ascertainment of exposure (e.g., dosage and frequency of drug administered), follow-up time, comparability of groups, definition of expected adverse effects, method used to collect adverse effects data, ascertainment of outcomes (ocular and systemic adverse effects) and transparency of patient flow were abstracted. All stages of study selection, data extraction and quality assessment were done independently by two reviewers (CS and CE). Any disagreement was resolved by discussion and consensus.

Statistical Analysis

Data from head-to-head studies, studies which compared ranibizumab versus any other treatment than anti-VEGF, and studies which evaluated different dosages of ranibizumab were analysed using the *R* software [17]. This programme was used to compute statistics and generate forest plots to compare safety outcomes of different treatment arms using risk ratios (RR). A chi-square test ($p\text{-value}<0.05$) and an I^2 test were used to test for statistical heterogeneity between studies. We used the fixed effects model (Mantel-Haeszel method) in the meta-analysis of rare events as it has been shown to be the more appropriate and less biased approach compared to the random effects model [18]. A narrative summary was provided for data that were unsuitable for pooling.

Results

Included Studies

The numbers of studies identified at each stage of the systematic review are shown in Figure 1. After removing duplicate references, the searches identified 1185 citations.

The inclusion criteria were met by 11 RCTs [14,19–28] (19 publications [14,19–36]): three head-to-head studies [14,19,20] (three publications) with a total of 1333 patients, five RCTs [21–25] (12 publications [21–25,29–35]) comparing ranibizumab against any other treatment or dosage with a total of 4054 patients, and three RCTs [26–28] (four publications [26–28,36]) comparing bevacizumab against any other treatment with a total of 244 patients.

Study Characteristics

Head-to-head trials. Table 1 shows study characteristic of head-to-head comparisons. The CATT assigned 1208 (1185 finally fulfilled eligibility criteria) patients to receive ranibizumab or bevacizumab on either a monthly schedule or as needed with monthly evaluation [14]. The studies of Biswas et al. [19] and Subramanian et al. [20] were smaller and included 120 and 28 patients, respectively. In these two trials, patients received bevacizumab or ranibizumab monthly for the first three months, followed by a *pro re nata* schedule.

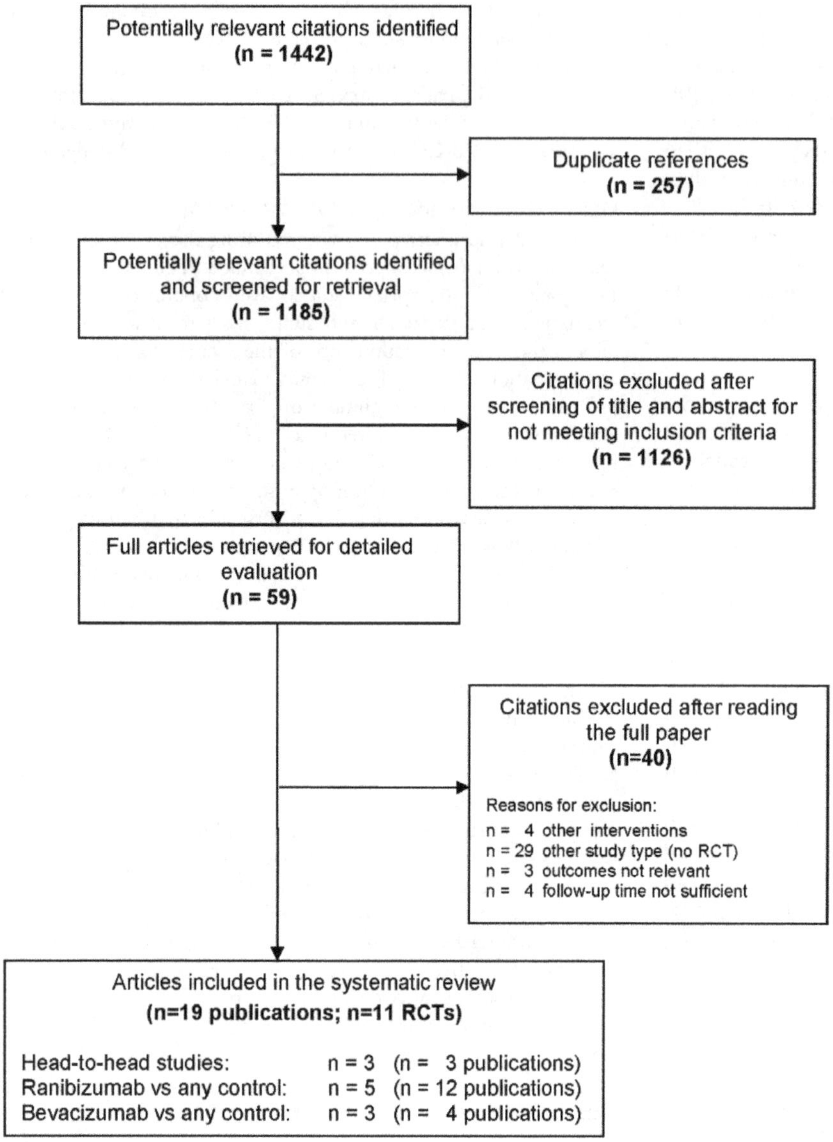

Figure 1. Flow chart of literature search and study selection.

Ranibizumab trials for indirect comparison or dose-relationship evaluation. Characteristics of RCTs of ranibizumab are presented in Table 2. The ANCHOR trial compared monthly ranibizumab injections with photodynamic therapy (PDT) and enrolled 423 patients [21]. The MARINA study enrolled 716 patients and compared monthly intravitreal ranibizumab with sham injections [22]. The PIER study also used sham as a comparator and enrolled 184 patients [23]. In contrast to the MARINA study, treated patients received ranibizumab injections once monthly for three consecutive months, followed by a dose administered once every three months. In the SAILOR study, patients were randomised to receive three consecutive monthly injections of 0.3 mg (n = 1169) or 0.5 mg (n = 1209) ranibizumab [24]. After three months, patients were followed by a *pro re nata* schedule. The EXCITE study randomised 353 patients to 0.3 mg quarterly, 0.5 mg quarterly, or 0.3 mg monthly doses of ranibizumab [25]. Treatment comprised a loading phase (three consecutive monthly injections) followed by a nine month maintenance phase (with monthly or quarterly injections).

Bevacizumab trials for indirect comparison or dose-relationship evaluation. Study characteristics of RCTs comparing bevacizumab with other treatment options are illustrated in Table 3. Sacu et al. assigned 28 patients to bevacizumab or PDT in combination with triamcinolone [26]. Patients received bevacizumab injections once monthly for three consecutive months, followed by a dose administered *pro re nata.* Costagliola et al. enrolled 85 patients and randomised them to bevacizumab as monotherapy or to bevacizumab in combination with PDT [27]. After the first bevacizumab injection retreatment was based on a *pro re nata* schedule. The ABC trial included 131 patients [28]. Bevacizumab was administered once every six weeks. After the first three injections, standardised criteria to decide about retreatment were applied. Patients in the control arm received standard treatment (dependent on the treatment available for different lesion types at the start of the trial).

Table 1. Characteristics of head-to-head studies comparing ranibizumab with bevacizumab (direct comparison).

	Treated patients				Dosage (mg)		Injections per patient (mean)	
Study	Ranibizumab	Bevacizumab	Follow-up (months)	Treatment regime	Ranibizumab	Bevacizumab	Ranibizumab	Bevacizumab
CATT 2011 [14]	599	586	12	monthly or as needed	0.5	1.25	monthly: 11.7±1.5/as needed: 6.9±3.0	monthly: 11.9±1.2/ as needed: 7.7±3.5
Biswas et al. 2011 [19]	60	60	18	monthly for 3 month then as needed	0.5	1.25	5.6	4.3
Subramanian et al. 2010 [20]	8	20	12	monthly for 3 month then as needed	0.5	1.25	4	8

Table 2. Characteristics of RCTs evaluating ranibizumab for indirect comparison.

Study	Included patients	Ranibizumab treated patients	Control treatment	Follow-up (months)	Treatment regime	Dosage (mg)	Injections per patient (mean)
ANCHOR 2009 [21]	423	280	PDT	24	monthly	0.3 and 0.5	24
MARINA 2006 [22]	716	478	sham	24	monthly	0.3 and 0.5	21
PIER 2010 [23]	184	121	sham	24	monthly for 3 month then every 3 month	0.3 and 0.5	nr
SAILOR 2009* [24]	2378	0.3 mg: 1169/0.5 mg: 1209	different dosages of ranibizumab	12	monthly for 3 month then as needed	0.3 and 0.5	4.6 (both groups)
EXCITE 2011 [25]	353	0.3 mg quarterly: 120/0.5 mg quarterly: 118/0.3 mg monthly: 115	different dosages of ranibizumab	12	monthly for 3 month then quarterly vs monthly	0.3 and 0.5	5.7 (0.3 mg quarterly)/5.5 (0.5 mg quarterly)/11.4 (0.3 mg monthly)

Nr: Not reported, PDT: Photodynamic therapy.
**Cohort I* enrolled randomised patients, therefore, we included this group in the systematic review.

Table 3. Characteristics of RCTs evaluating bevacizumab for indirect comparison.

Study	Included patients	Bevacizumab treated patients	Control treatment	Follow-up (months)	Treatment regime	Dosage (mg)	Injections per patient (mean)
Sacu et al. 2009 [26]	28	14	PDT+T	12	monthly for 3 month then as needed	1.0	6.8
Costagliola et al. 2010 [27]	85	45	PDT+B	12	as needed	1.25	4.6
ABC Trial 2010 [28]	131	65	usual care	12	once every 6 weeks then as needed	1.25	7.1

B: Bevacizumab, PDT: Photodynamic therapy, T: Triamcinolone.

Ocular Adverse Effects

Head-to-head trials. In the CATT [14], serious ocular adverse effects rates reported with intravitreal anti-VEGF were: endophthalmitis *(ranibizumab: ≤0.7%, bevacizumab: ≤1.4%)*, uveitis *(ranibizumab: ≤0.3%, bevacizumab: ≤0.7%)*, retinal/choroidal detachment *(ranibizumab: 0.0%, bevacizumab: ≤1.0%)*, retinal tear *(ranibizumab: ≤0.3%, bevacizumab: ≤0.3%)*, ocular vessel embolism or occlusion *(ranibizumab: ≤0.7%, bevacizumab: ≤0.7%)* and vitreous haemorrhage *(ranibizumab: ≤0.3%, bevacizumab: ≤0.3%)* both for the monthly and as needed scheme (Table 4). A pooled analysis of serious ocular adverse effects indicated a significantly increased RR for bevacizumab when compared to ranibizumab (RR = 2.8; 95% CI 1.2–6.5; Figure 2a).

The two head-to-head studies with comparatively low patient numbers did not indicate major safety concerns: Subramanian et al. [20] reported zero rates for serious ocular adverse effects and Biswas et al. [19] reported only minor complications without specifying them (the rate for ranibizumab was 7.3% and for bevacizumab 11.1%).

Ranibizumab trials for indirect comparison. Intravitreal ranibizumab injections have been associated with endophthalmitis (≤2.1%), uveitis (≤1.3%), retinal detachment (≤1.5%), retinal tear (≤1.7%), traumatic lens damage (≤0.9%) and vitreous haemorrhage (≤1.5%) (Table 5) [21,22,23,24,25].

A pooled analysis of the ANCHOR [21], MARINA [22] and PIER [23] study showed that while absolute rates of serious ocular adverse effects were low, relative harm was significantly raised compared to controls (RR = 3.1; 95% CI 1.1–8.9; Figure 3a). In addition, these three landmark trials reported a transient increase in intraocular pressure in the study eye after intravitreal injections.

Bevacizumab trials for indirect comparison. Serious ocular adverse events associated with bevacizumab were uncommon (Table 6). There were no reported cases of endophthalmitis, retinal detachment, retinal tear and traumatic lens damage. One trial reported a single case of vitreous haemorrhage (2%) and two cases of uveitis (3%) [28].

Dose-relationship evaluation. The incidence of serious ocular adverse effects was low and the magnitude of risk did not appear to be increased with higher doses of ranibizumab as compared to the lower dose (RR = 0.9; 95% CI 0.5–1.6; Figure 4a). We were unable to judge the safety profile for different time frames due to the large variety of applications schemata used in the ranibizumab trials. No safety conclusions can be drawn for the optimal dose-relationship of bevacizumab due to a lack of data.

Nonocular Adverse Effects

Head-to-head trials. In the CATT [14] and in the study of Subramanian et al. [20] more patients died in the bevacizumab than in the ranibizumab group (5.1% *versus* 3.0% and 7.1% *versus* 0.0%. respectively) (Table 7). However, these differences were not statistically significant (RR = 1.7; 95% CI 0.8–3.8; Figure 2d). Nonfatal arterial thromboembolic events (myocardial infarction and stroke) were similar distributed among the treatments groups (approximately 1%; RR = 0.8; 95% CI 0.3–2.1; Figure 2b). In contrast, the proportion of patients with serious systemic adverse effects (primarily hospitalisations due to infections such as pneumonia or urinary tract infections and gastrointestinal disorders such as haemorrhage, nausea and vomiting) was significantly higher with bevacizumab than with ranibizumab (RR = 1.3; 95% CI 1.0–1.7; cumulative data from CATT publication). The rate of serious nonocular haemorrhage (duodenal ulcer haemorrhage, gastric ulcer haemorrhage, lower gastrointestinal haemorrhage and rectal haemorrhage) was

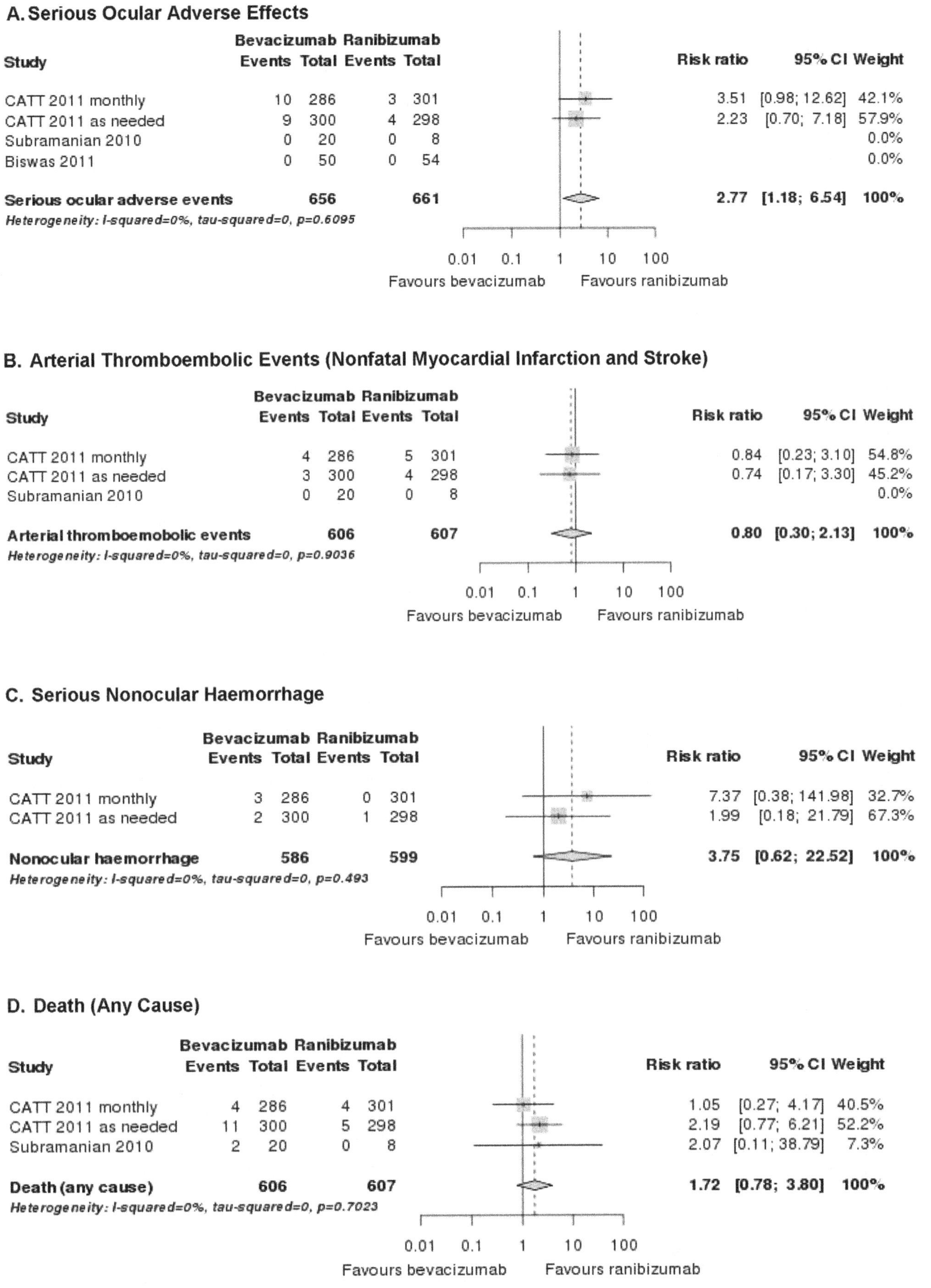

Figure 2. Forest plots: pooled results of head-to-head studies for different safety outcomes.

Table 4. Rates of ocular adverse effects of head-to-head studies (direct comparison).

Study	Endophthalmitis (%)		Uveitis (%)		Retinal/choroidal detachment (%)		Retinal tear (%)		Ocular vessel embolism/ occlusion (%)		Vitreous haemorrhage (%)	
	Ranibizumab	Bevacizumab	Ranibizumab	Bevacizumab	Ranibizumab	Bevacizumab	Ranibizumab	Bevacizumab	Ranibizumab	Bevacizumab	Ranibizumab	Bevacizumab
CATT 2011 monthly [14]	0.7	1.4	0.3*	0.3*	0.0	0.7	0.0	0.3	0.0	0.7	0.0	0.0
CATT 2011 as needed [14]	0.0	0.0	0.0*	0.7*	0.0	1.0	0.3	0.3	0.7	0.7	0.3	0.3
Biswas et al. 2011 [19]	nr	nr	nr	nr	nr	nr	nr	nr	nr	nr	nr	nr
Subramanian et al. 2010 [20]	0.0	0.0	0.0	0.0	0.0	0.0	nr	nr	nr	nr	0.0	0.0

Nr: Not reported.
*Percentage refers to uveitis, scleritis, and anterior chamber inflammation.

Table 5. Rates of ocular adverse effects of RCTs evaluating ranibizumab for indirect comparison and dose-relationship evaluation.

Study	Endophthalmitis (%)			Uveitis (%)			Retinal detachment (%)			Retinal tear (%)			Lens damage (traumatic) (%)			Vitreous haemorrhage (%)		
	0.3 mg	0.5 mg	PDT	0.3 mg	0.5 mg	PDT	0.3 mg	0.5 mg	PDT	0.3 mg	0.5 mg	PDT	0.3 mg	0.5 mg	PDT	0.3 mg	0.5 mg	PDT
ANCHOR 2009 [21]	**0.0**	**2.1**	**0.0**	**0.0**	**0.7**	**0.0**	**1.5**	**0.0**	**0.7**	**0.0**	**0.7**	**0.0**	**0.0**	**0.0**	**0.0**	**1.5**	**0.0**	**0.0**
	0.3 mg	0.5 mg	Sham	0.3 mg	0.5 mg	Sham	0.3 mg	0.5 mg	Sham	0.3 mg	0.5 mg	Sham	0.3 mg	0.5 mg	Sham	0.3 mg	0.5 mg	Sham
MARINA 2006 [22]	**0.8**	**1.3**	**0.0**	**1.3**	**1.3**	**0.0**	**0.0**	**0.0**	**0.4**	**0.4**	**0.4**	**0.0**	**0.0**	**0.4**	**0.0**	**0.4**	**0.4**	**0.8**
PIER 2010 [23]	**0.0**	**0.0**	**0.0**	**0.0**	**0.0**	**0.0**	**0.0**	**0.0**	**0.0**	**0.0**	**0.0**	**0.0**	**0.0**	**0.0**	**0.0**	**nr**	**nr**	**nr**
	0.3 mg	0.5 mg		0.3 mg	0.5 mg		0.3 mg	0.5 mg		0.3 mg	0.5 mg		0.3 mg	0.5 mg		0.3 mg	0.5 mg	
SAILOR 2009 [24]	**0.2**	**0.4**		**0.1**	**0.2**		**0.1**	**0.0**		**0.0**	**0.1**		**0.1**	**0.1**		**0.3**	**0.1**	
	0.3 mg*	0.5 mg*	0.3 mg#	0.3 mg*	0.5 mg*	0.3 mg#	0.3 mg*	0.5 mg*	0.3 mg#	0.3 mg*	0.5 mg*	0.3 mg#	0.3 mg*	0.5 mg*	0.3 mg#	0.3 mg*	0.5 mg*	0.3 mg#
EXCITE 2011 [25]	**nr**	**nr**	**nr**	**nr**	**nr**	**nr**	**0.8**	**0.0**	**0.0**	**0.0**	**1.7**	**0.0**	**0.8**	**0.0**	**0.9**	**nr**	**nr**	**nr**

Nr: Not reported.
*Quarterly.
#Monthly.

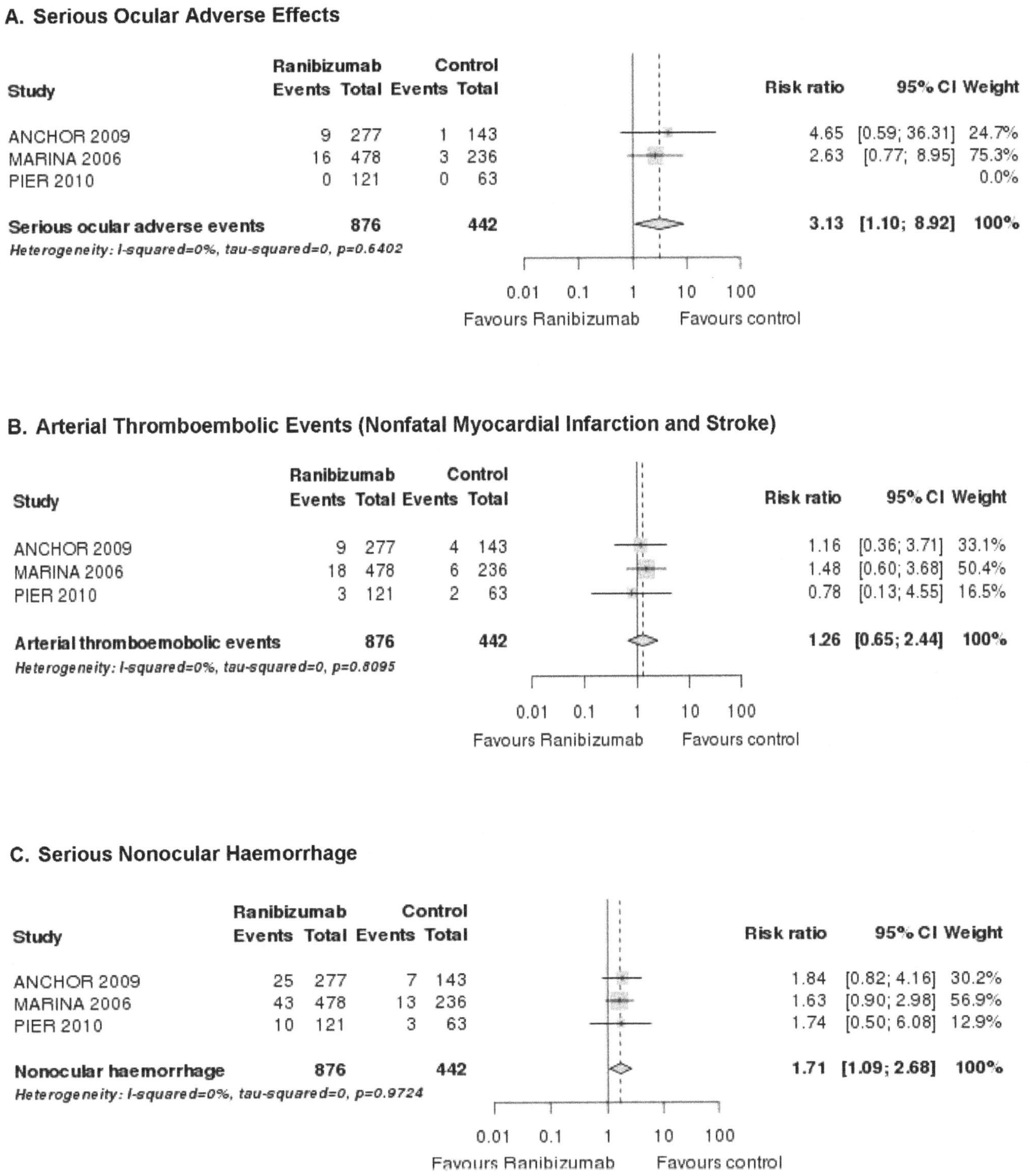

Figure 3. Forest plots: pooled results of RCTs for ranibizumab (any dose vs any control) for different safety outcomes.

numerically, but not statistically significantly higher in the bevacizumab than in the ranibizumab arm (1.0 and 0.7% *versus* 0.0 and 0.3%, respectively [Table 7]). A pooled analysis indicated that there may be a safety signal (RR = 3.8; 95% CI 0.6–22.5; Figure 2c). Biswas et al. did not mention systemic adverse effects in their head-to-head comparison [19].

Ranibizumab trials for indirect comparison. The rates of nonocular serious adverse effects of single RCTs are displayed in Table 8. The rate of key arterial nonfatal thromboembolic effects (myocardial infarction and stroke) during the first and second year of the ANCHOR [21] and MARINA [22] trials was numerically, but not statistically significantly higher in the 0.5 mg arm than in the control arm (3.6% [21] and 2.5% [22], respectively *versus* 1.4%

Table 6. Rates of ocular adverse effects of RCTs evaluating bevacizumab for indirect comparison and dose-relationship evaluation.

Study	Endophthalmitis (%)		Uveitis (%)		Retinal detachment (%)		Retinal tear (%)		Lens damage (traumatic) (%)		Vitreous haemorrhage (%)	
	1.0 mg	PDT+T	1.0 mg	PDT+T	1.0 mg	PDT+T	1.0 mg	PDT+T	1.0 mg	PDT+T	1.0 mg	PDT+T
Sacu et al. 2009 [26]	**0.0**	**0.0**	**0.0**	**0.7**	**1.5**	**0.0**	**0.0**	**0.7**	**0.0**	**0.0**	**1.5**	**0.0**
	1.25 mg	PDT+B	1.25 mg	PDT+B	1.25 mg	PDT+B	1.25 mg	PDT+B	1.25 mg	PDT+B	1.25 mg	PDT+B
Costagliola et al. 2010 [27]	**nr**	**nr**	**nr**	**nr**	**nr**	**nr**	**nr**	**nr**	**nr**	**nr**	**nr**	**nr**
	1.25 mg	UC	1.25 mg	UC	1.25 mg	UC	1.25 mg	UC	1.25 mg	UC	1.25 mg	UC
ABC trial 2010 [28]	**0.0**	**0.0**	**3.0**	**2.0**	**0.0**	**2.0**	**0.0**	**0.0**	**0.0**	**0.0**	**2.0**	**0.0**

B: Bevacizumab. Nr: Not reported. T: Triamcinolone. UC: Usual care.

and 0.8%, respectively). In the ANCHOR [21], MARINA [22] and PIER [23] study, the incidence of serious nonocular haemorrhage (such as gastrointestinal haemorrhage, traumatic subdural haematoma and duodenal ulcer haemorrhage) was also consistently higher in the ranibizumab than in the control groups (2.9% [0.3 mg] [21], 2.1% [0.5 mg] [22] and 9.8% [0.5 mg] [23] *versus* 0.7%, 0.8% and 4.8%). A pooled analysis indicated that this risk reached the standard thresholds for statistical significance (RR = 1.7; 95% CI 1.1–2.7; Figure 3c). Except for the EXCITE study [25], increased infection rates were not reported in the ranibizumab trials.

Bevacizumab trials for indirect comparison. Different to the ranibizumab trials, intravitreal bevacizumab injections were apparently not associated with an increased risk of nonocular haemorrhage (Table 9). However, this assumption is based on limited details concerning the harms reported within the articles: Two trials mentioned generically that no systemic effects were observed [26,27]; and one study reported zero rates for nonocular haemorrhage [28]. Taken together, one bevacizumab trial described a single case (2%) of death and one patient (2%) who experienced a myocardial infarction after intravitreal bevacizumab [28].

Dose-relationship evaluation. The rates of key arterial thromboembolic events were similar across dose groups (RR = 0.9; 95% CI 0.6–1.4; Figure 4b). The rates of nonocular haemorrhage, however, showed a difference between doses, with higher rates in the 0.5 mg dose group compared with the 0.3 mg dose group (Table 8). The total number of events was comparatively small, and the difference was not fully confirmed statistically (RR = 0.6; 95% CI 0.4–1.1; Figure 4c). The incidence of death is not dose related (RR = 0.8; 95% CI 0.5–1.3; Figure 4d). We could not evaluate whether there is a difference in safety outcomes in a less than monthly regimen for ranibizumab due to study heterogeneity. Again, no safety conclusions regarding optimal doses of intravitreal bevacizumab can be drawn due to a lack of data.

Summary of Methodological Quality and Risk of Bias

Head-to-head trials. The methodological quality of the head-to-head studies is presented in Table 10. In one trial patients and investigators were adequately blinded [20]. However, a small sample size, an almost male population and a lack of any description as to how adverse effects were rigorously monitored, as well as the inadequate reporting of actual events does not allow a reliable conclusion on safety outcomes. Similar to Subramanian et al. [20], Biswas et al. [19] also showed large deficiencies in their study methodology. Therefore, no reliable conclusions on safety can be drawn on the basis of these two studies.

The CATT showed no substantial imbalances in the demographic or ocular characteristics of the study groups at baseline [14]. Adverse effects were, in contrast to the two other head-to-head trials, rigorously monitored and adequately reported. Due to the billing status, masking of patients could not be maintained. The adjudication of serious adverse effects could, however, most likely be secured by a medical monitor who reviewed serious adverse effects and was unaware of study group assignment.

It was outstanding that in none of the three head-to-head trials reasons for drop-outs were given. In addition, flow charts documenting the patient flow were missing.

Ranibizumab trials for indirect comparison or dose-relationship evaluation. Three of the ranibizumab trials were of high methodological quality (comparability of groups, adequate blinding, high patient numbers, transparency of patient flow, definition of expected adverse effects and method used to collect adverse effects data; Table 11) [21–23]. The remaining two studies (SAILOR [24] and EXCITE [25]) showed deficiencies in the definition and method used to collect expected adverse effects data.

Bevacizumab trials for indirect comparison or dose-relationship evaluation. Except for the ABC trial [28] the results of RCTs evaluating bevacizumab are of limited values (Table 12). The main limitations stemmed from the lack of blinding and the lack of any description as to how adverse effects were monitored, as well as the inadequate reporting of actual events. In addition to these shortcomings, the overall sample size of bevacizumab treated patients was much lower than for ranibizumab treated patients (244 *versus* 4054 patients).

Discussion

Principal Findings

Head-to-head trials. The study results of head-to-head trials show that the rates of serious ocular adverse effects are low (<1.5%), but they indicate a potential safety risk related to the injection procedure under bevacizumab. Because both ranibizumab and bevacizumab are administered intravitreally and the number of received injections did not differ significantly, the higher risk of ocular adverse effects is either the result of a true difference between the drugs or the method of manufacture. It is

A. Serious Ocular Adverse Effects

Study	0.3mg Events	0.3mg Total	0.5mg Events	0.5mg Total	Risk ratio	95% CI	Weight
ANCHOR 2009	4	137	5	140	0.82	[0.22; 2.98]	18.7%
MARINA 2006	7	238	9	239	0.78	[0.30; 2.06]	34.0%
PIER 2010	0	59	0	61			0.0%
SAILOR 2009	9	1169	10	1209	0.93	[0.38; 2.28]	37.2%
EXCITE 2011	6	235	2	118	1.51	[0.31; 7.35]	10.1%
Serious ocular adverse events		**1838**		**1767**	**0.92**	**[0.53; 1.59]**	**100%**

Heterogeneity: I-squared=0%, tau-squared=0, p=0.916

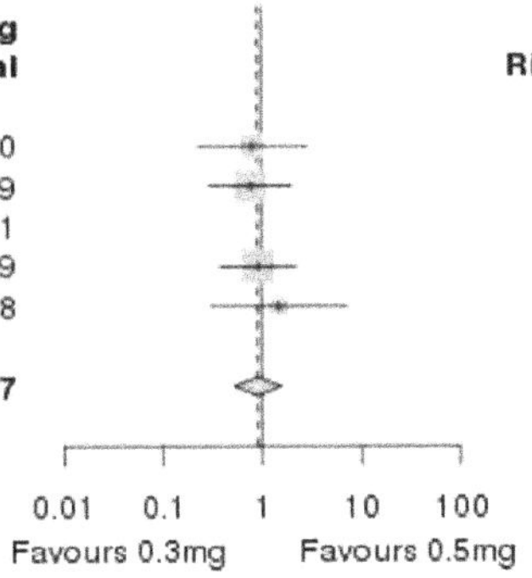

B. Arterial Thromboembolic Events (Nonfatal Myocardial Infarction and Stroke)

Study	0.3mg Events	0.3mg Total	0.5mg Events	0.5mg Total	Risk ratio	95% CI	Weight
ANCHOR 2009	4	137	5	140	0.82	[0.22; 2.98]	11.2%
MARINA 2006	9	238	9	239	1.00	[0.41; 2.49]	20.4%
PIER 2010	0	59	0	61			0.0%
SAILOR 2009	22	1169	30	1209	0.76	[0.44; 1.31]	66.9%
EXCITE 2011	6	235	0	118	6.54	[0.37; 115.14]	1.5%
Arterial thromboembolic events (MI/stroke) nonfatal		**1838**		**1767**	**0.90**	**[0.59; 1.38]**	**100%**

Heterogeneity: I-squared=0%, tau-squared=0, p=0.5124

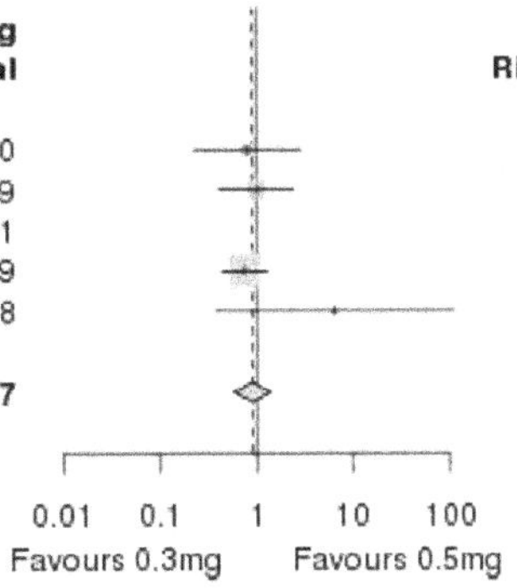

C. Serious Nonocular Haemorrhage

Study	0.3mg Events	0.3mg Total	0.5mg Events	0.5mg Total	Risk ratio	95% CI	Weight
ANCHOR 2009	4	137	3	140	1.36	[0.31; 5.98]	8.0%
MARINA 2006	3	238	5	239	0.60	[0.15; 2.49]	13.5%
PIER 2010	4	59	6	61	0.69	[0.20; 2.32]	16.0%
SAILOR 2009	11	1169	18	1209	0.63	[0.30; 1.33]	48.0%
EXCITE 2011	2	235	4	118	0.25	[0.05; 1.35]	14.4%
Nonocular haemorrhage (serious)		**1838**		**1767**	**0.64**	**[0.39; 1.06]**	**100%**

Heterogeneity: I-squared=0%, tau-squared=0, p=0.6965

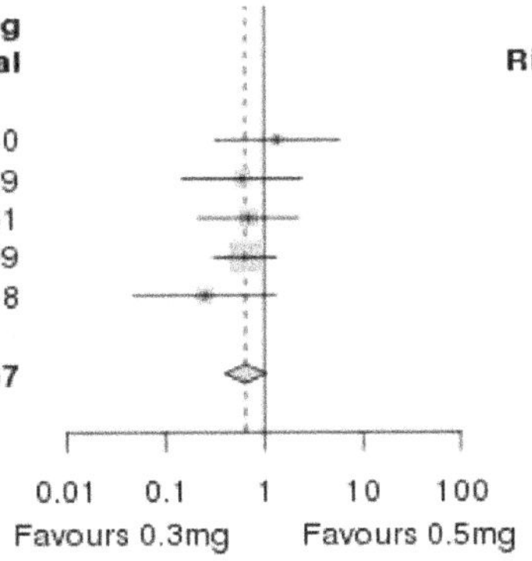

C. Death (Any Cause)

Study	0.3mg Events	0.3mg Total	0.5mg Events	0.5mg Total	Risk ratio	95% CI	Weight
ANCHOR 2009	5	137	3	140	1.70	[0.42; 6.99]	7.1%
MARINA 2006	5	238	6	239	0.84	[0.26; 2.70]	14.4%
PIER 2010	2	59	0	61	5.17	[0.25; 105.41]	1.2%
SAILOR 2009	20	1169	30	1209	0.69	[0.39; 1.21]	70.9%
EXCITE 2011	2	235	2	118	0.50	[0.07; 3.52]	6.4%
Death (any cause)		**1838**		**1767**	**0.82**	**[0.53; 1.29]**	**100%**

Heterogeneity: I-squared=0%, tau-squared=0, p=0.5448

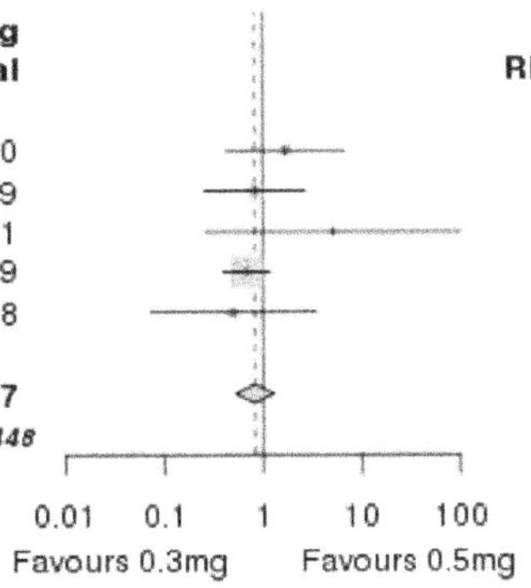

Figure 4. Forest plots: pooled results of ranibizumab 0.3 mg vs 0.5 mg for different safety outcomes.

Table 7. Rates of systemic adverse effects of head-to-head studies (direct comparison).

Study	Death (any cause) (%)		Myocardial infarction (%)		Cerebrovascular accident (%)		Nonocular haemorrhage (%)		Infections (%)	
	Ranibizumab	Bevacizumab	Ranibizumab	Bevacizumab	Ranibizumab	Bevacizumab	Ranibizumab	Bevacizumab	Ranibizumab	Bevacizumab
CATT 2011 monthly [14]	1.3	1.4	0.7	0.7	1.0	0.7	0.0*	1.0*	2.0#	3.8#
CATT 2011 as needed [14]	1.7	3.7	1.0	0.3	0.3	0.7	0.3*	0.7*	4.0#	6.0#
Biswas et al. 2011 [19]	nr	nr	nr	nr	nr	nr	nr	nr	nr	nr
Subramanian et al. 2010 [20]	0.0	7.1**	0.0	0.0	0.0	0.0	nr	nr	nr	nr

Nr: Not reported.
*Data from CATT appendix: they refer to duodenal ulcer haemorrhage, gastric ulcer haemorrhage, (lower) gastrointestinal haemorrhage, rectal haemorrhage.
#Rates refer mainly to pneumonia and urinary tract infections, other infections are not clearly specified.
**Two patients died in the Bevacizumab group (meckel cell carcinoma and unknown cause).

obvious that using an unlicensed drug is less safe than using a licensed one where the regulatory authority monitors quality control of the manufacturer. Therefore, it is likely that the higher rates of ocular adverse effects of bevacizumab could be the result of the compounding procedures used to prepare the syringes containing bevacizumab. Although the rates for ocular safety outcomes were low, it has to be kept in mind that the cumulative risk will increase with repeated injections, i.e., for every new decision, the same risks have to be taken into account.

The pooled relative risk of CATT also indicates a significant signal of a higher hospitalisation rate due to sepsis, pneumonia or gastrointestinal disorders and a possible signal of an increased risk of nonocular haemorrhage following the intravitreal use of bevacizumab [14]. Arterial thromboembolic events and death were, however, not associated with the use of bevacizumab in AMD. Since information on drop outs were missing - a complete follow-up is, however, necessary to determine if those patients who withdrew due to adverse effects are different from those who did not adhere - no final conclusion can be drawn regarding whether these findings were drug-related or due to chance alone. We also cannot exclude the possibility of measured and unmeasured confounders in the CATT that may have influenced the results. There were some minor differences (such as the socioeconomic status and the history of myocardial infarction) in baseline characteristics between the randomised groups but it would be impossible to accurately predict the direction or magnitude of impact that these differences would have on the results. Sepsis, infections, gastrointestinal disorders and haemorrhage are listed as common serious adverse events (≥2% difference between the trial arms in at least one clinical trial) for bevacizumab, therefore, the pattern observed in CATT may not be entirely atypical (http://www.medicines.org.uk/emc/medicine/15748/SPC/). Equally, the potential lack of blinding in CATT may mean that patients and clinicians who were concerned about these recognised events ended up reporting it more frequently with bevacizumab than with ranibizumab.

Ranibizumab and bevacizumab trials for indirect comparison. Our analysis based on three landmark ranibizumab trials indicates a significant increase in nonocular haemorrhage and a significantly higher rate of serious ocular adverse effects under ranibizumab [21–23]. The higher risk of endophthalmitis, retinal detachment/tear and vitreous haemorrhage are not surprising in these trials which used PDT or sham as comparator, because these events are attributable to the injection procedure. Overall, most of the RCTs evaluating ranibizumab fulfil the criteria of reporting adverse effects, but very rare adverse effects, i.e., adverse effects with an incidence rate of less than one in 1000, could not be evaluated because the number of patients was still too small.

In contrast to the RCTs evaluating ranibizumab, the trials evaluating bevacizumab showed methodological limitations (e.g., small sample sizes and inadequate reporting of adverse effects). In addition, generally investigators of RCTs tend to select patients who are fitter, healthier and have lower risks than real-life patients. These factors can lead to an underestimation of adverse effects - especially if we also take into account that higher evidence from phase III/IV ranibizumab trials suggests signals for an increased ocular and systemic vascular and haemorrhagic risk and intravenous bevacizumab for the management of cancer is associated with major systemic adverse effects like thromboembolic events and haemorrhage [5,6]. On the other hand, the risk for developing systemic adverse effects may be much lower in AMD patients who receive a dose of intravitreal bevacizumab

Table 8. Rates of systemic adverse effects of RCTs evaluating ranibizumab for indirect comparison and dose-relationship evaluation.

Study	Death (any cause) (%)			Myocardial infarction (%)			Cerebrovascular accident (%)			Nonocular haemorrhage (%)			Infections (%)		
	0.3 mg	0.5 mg	PDT	0.3 mg	0.5 mg	PDT	0.3 mg	0.5 mg	PDT	0.3 mg	0.5 mg	PDT	0.3 mg	0.5 mg	PDT
ANCHOR 2009 [21]	**3.7**	**2.1**	**3.5**	**0.7**	**3.6**	**1.4**	**2.2**	**0.0**	**1.4**	**2.9**	**2.1**	**0.7**	**nr**	**nr**	**nr**
	0.3 mg	0.5 mg	Sham	0.3 mg	0.5 mg	Sham	0.3 mg	0.5 mg	Sham	0.3 mg	0.5 mg	Sham	0.3 mg	0.5 mg	Sham
MARINA 2006 [22]	**2.1**	**2.5**	**2.5**	**2.5**	**1.3**	**1.7**	**1.3**	**2.5**	**0.8**	**1.3**	**2.1**	**0.8**	**nr**	**nr**	**nr**
PIER 2010 [23]	**3.4**	**0.0**	**1.6**	**0.0**	**0.0**	**1.6**	**0.0**	**0.0**	**0.0**	**6.8**	**9.8**	**4.8**	**nr**	**nr**	**nr**
	0.3 mg	0.5 mg		0.3 mg	0.5 mg		0.3 mg	0.5 mg		0.3 mg	0.5 mg		0.3 mg	0.5 mg	
SAILOR 2009 [24]	**1.7**	**2.4**		**1.2**	**1.2**		**0.7**	**1.2**		**0.9**	**1.5**		**nr**	**nr**	
	0.3 mg*	0.5 mg*	0.3 mg#	0.3 mg*	0.5 mg*	0.3 mg#	0.3 mg*	0.5 mg*	0.3 mg#	0.3 mg*	0.5 mg*	0.3 mg#	0.3 mg*	0.5 mg*	0.3 mg#
EXCITE 2011 [25]	**0.0**	**1.6**	**0.9**	**0.8**	**0.0**	**0.9**	**0.8**	**0.0**	**0.9**	**0.0**	**3.4**	**0.9**	**2.5**	**4.2**	**3.5**

Nr: Not reported.
*Quarterly.
#Monthly.

that is about 0.25% of that used for intravenous treatment [37,38].

Ranibizumab and bevacizumab trials for dose-relationship evaluation. The rates of safety events between 0.5 mg and 0.3 mg ranibizumab were low and did not suggest that the higher dose has a higher risk of ocular adverse effects, arterial thromboembolic events and death. However, there may be a higher rate of nonocular haemorrhage associated with the 0.5 mg dose. The total number of events was small, and the difference was not confirmed fully statistically, but this finding should be monitored via postmarketing surveillance and ongoing trials. Because the 0.5 mg doses of ranibizumab tend to have a slightly greater visual acuity benefit than 0.3 mg doses in patients with neovascular AMD [21,22,24], the decision on how much ranibizumab to use must be decided carefully by the clinician and patient based on the benefit and harm ratio.

Strengths and Limitations

We did not include non-RCTs in this systematic review. The reason behind is that a previous review of our group evaluated safety for ranibizumab and bevacizumab on the basis of observational studies, mainly case reports [15]. However, in the case of bevacizumab follow-up times are too short, sample sizes too small and the monitoring and reporting of adverse outcomes shows large deficiencies, therefore, no reliable conclusions on safety could be drawn using this study design.

We believe that the crucial question whether adverse effects differ between off-label bevacizumab and licensed ranibizumab can only be answered on the basis of head-to-head trials or RCTs

Table 9. Rates of systemic adverse effects of RCTs evaluating bevacizumab for indirect comparison and dose-relationship evaluation.

Study	Death (any cause) (%)		Myocardial infarction (%)		Cerebrovascular accident (%)		Nonocular haemorrhage (%)		Infections (%)	
	1.0 mg	PDT+T	1.0 mg	PDT+T	1.0 mg	PDT+T	1.0 mg	PDT+T	1.0 mg	PDT+T
Sacu et al. 2009 [26]	**nr**	**nr**	**nr**	**nr**	**nr**	**nr**	**nr**	**nr**	**nr**	**nr**
	1.25 mg	PDT+B	1.25 mg	PDT+B	1.25 mg	PDT+B	1.25 mg	PDT+B	1.25 mg	PDT+B
Costagliola et al. 2010 [27]	**nr**	**nr**	**0.0**	**0.0**	**0.0**	**0.0**	**nr**	**nr**	**nr**	**nr**
	1.25 mg	UC	1.25 mg	UC	1.25 mg	UC	1.25 mg	UC	1.25 mg	UC
ABC trial 2010 [28]	**2.0**	**0.0**	**2.0**	**0.0**	**0.0**	**0.0**	**0.0**	**1.0**	**nr**	**nr**

B: Bevacizumab. Nr: Not reported. T: Triamcinolone. UC: Usual care.

Table 10. Methodological quality of head-to-head studies comparing ranibizumab with bevacizumab (direct comparison).

Study	Comparability of groups	Adequate blinding	Definition of expected AE	Definition of method used to collect AE data	Transparency of patient flow	Validity safety
CATT 2011 [14]	yes*	single blind#	yes	yes	unclear	moderate- high
Biswas et al. 2011 [19]	not specified	single blind**	no	no	unclear	low
Subramanian et al. 2010 [20]	no	double blind	in part	no	unclear	low

AE: Adverse effects.
*The CATT showed only minor differences in the socioeconomic status and in the history of myocardial infarction between the randomised groups.
#Outcome assessor and care provider blinded, patient initially masked, billing statement may unmask.
**All assessors were masked. Unclear whether patients were masked.

for indirect comparison with reasonable follow-up times and sample sizes. We are aware that data from RCTs could underestimate adverse effects mainly due to the inclusion of highly selected (non-representative) patients and/or publication bias [39]. In addition, small sample sizes limit the ability to detect rare but serious adverse effects [39]. Therefore, it is likely that the results of this review may have resulted in a lower risk of adverse effects than the true risk.

Other Reviews

A report from the US Food and Drug Administration for intravitreal ranibizumab concluded that there may be a theoretical risk of arterial thromboembolic events [40]. This finding is similar to the result of our meta-analysis of three phase III/IV ranibizumab studies which also shows a possible signal with regard to thromboembolic events (RR = 1.3; 95% CI 0.7–2.4).

Another recent retrospective analysis of 146 942 Medicare case records addressed systemic complications under intravitreal anti-VEGF treatment [41]. Curtis and associates reported higher risks of stroke and all-cause mortality with intravitreal injections of bevacizumab as compared to ranibizumab for the treatment of AMD. Further analysis of the Medicare claims database presented at the 2011 Association for Research in Vision and Ophthalmology (ARVO) annual meeting (Gower EW et al. ARVO 2011 E-Abstract 6644) indicated an 11% higher risk in all-cause mortality and 57% higher risk of haemorrhagic stroke with bevacizumab, with no statistically significant differences in the risk of either myocardial infarction or ischemic stroke. The significance of the results consisted even after adjusting for potential differences in socioeconomic status of the patients.

Van der Reis et al. systematically assessed and compared the incidences of adverse effects of ranibizumab, bevacizumab and pegaptanib [42]. They reported cumulative incidence rates in their review, therefore, we were not able to compare our results with this review directly. However, different to our findings, they summarised that there is no sufficient evidence to conclude that there is a difference between the safety profile of different VEGF inhibitors. The Royal College of Ophthalmologists UK also stated that both drugs have a similar safety profile [43]. This finding is also in contrast to our thorough examinations, which suggests that there remain issues of concern using off-label bevacizumab.

Implications for Clinical Practice

Despite the completion of the one year CATT results, controversies remain regarding the safety profile of bevacizumab. It is unclear whether the observed differences in serious adverse effects between bevacizumab and ranibizumab are due to genuine differences in systemic toxicity, or whether the data has been affected by possible confounding. We conclude that currently it is not possible to rule out a clinically relevant risk for serious adverse effects under the use of unlicensed bevacizumab. The results from the second year of CATT and from other ongoing multicentre comparative clinical trials in Europe (e.g., the IVAN study in Great Britain, the LUCAS study in Norway, the GEFAL study in France, the MANTA study in Austria, or the VIBERA study in Germany) should help to clarify whether these increased risks of adverse effects are related to intravitreal anti-VEGF therapy. If these signals regarding higher rates of adverse effects are

Table 11. Methodological quality of RCTs evaluating ranibizumab for indirect comparison.

Study	Comparability of groups	Adequate blinding	Definition of expected AE	Definition of method used to collect AE data	Transparency of patient flow	Validity safety
ANCHOR 2009 [21]	yes	double blind	yes	yes	yes	high
MARINA 2006 [22]	yes	double blind	yes	yes	yes	high
PIER 2008 [23]	yes	double blind	yes	yes	yes	high
SAILOR 2009 [24]	yes	single (patient)	in part	no	yes	moderate
EXCITE 2011 [25]	in part	double blind	in part	no	yes*	moderate/low

AE: Adverse effects.
*It was outstanding that in the 0.5 mg group 10.2% of patients discontinued because of adverse effects, in the 0.3 mg quarterly group 3.3% and in the 0.3 mg monthly group 4.3%, respectively.

Table 12. Methodological quality of RCTs evaluating bevacizumab for indirect comparison.

Study	Comparability of groups	Adequate blinding	Definition of expected AE	Definition of method used to collect AE data	Transparency of patient flow	Validity safety
Sacu et al. 2009 [26]	in part	open label	no	no	yes	low
Costagliola et al. 2010 [27]	not specified	not specified	no	no	unclear	low
ABC Trial 2010 [28]	in part	double blind	in part	in part	yes	moderate

AE: Adverse effects.

subsequently confirmed to be higher in bevacizumab than in ranibizumab, some of the cost savings with bevacizumab may be negated.

In the meantime, clinicians and patients should continue to carefully weight up the benefits and harms when choosing between the two available treatment options. We also emphasize the need for heightened surveillance for systemic adverse effects with intraocular anti-VEGF injections for AMD and other retinal diseases and studies that are powered not just for efficacy, but for defined safety outcomes based on the signals detected in this systematic review.

Acknowledgments

We thank Edith Motschall of the University Medical Centre Freiburg for conducting the literature search in Medline, Premedline and Embase.

Author Contributions

Conceived and designed the experiments: CS CE HTA GA GR ML YKL. Performed the experiments: CS CE YKL. Analyzed the data: CS CE HTA GA GR ML YKL. Contributed reagents/materials/analysis tools: CS CE HTA GA GR ML YKL. Wrote the paper: CS CE HTA GA GR ML YKL.

References

1. Bressler NM (2004) Age-related macular degeneration is the leading cause of blindness. JAMA 291: 1900–1901.
2. Kahn HA, Leibowitz HM, Ganley JP, Kini MM, Colton T, et al. (1977) The Framingham Eye Study: I. Outline and major prevalence findings. Am J Epidemiol 106: 17–32.
3. Ferris FL, Fine SL, Hyman L (1984) Age-related macular degeneration and blindness due to neovascular maculopathy. Arch Ophthalmol 102: 1640–1642.
4. Steinbrook R (2006) The price of sight - ranibizumab, bevacizumab, and the treatment of macular degeneration. N Engl J Med 355: 1409–1412.
5. US Food and Drug Administration (FDA) MedWatch (2005) Safety: Avastin (bevacizumab). Available: http://www.fda.gov/Safety/MedWatch/SafetyInformation/SafetyAlertsforHumanMedicalProducts/ucm150721.htm via the Internet. Accessed 20 February 2012.
6. Hapani S, Sher A, Chu D, Wu S (2010) Increased risk of serious haemorrhage with bevacizumab in cancer patients: a meta-analysis. Oncology 79: 27–38.
7. Ranpura V, Hapani S, Wu S (2011) Treatment-related mortality with bevacizumab in cancer patients: a meta-analysis. JAMA 305: 487–494.
8. Michels S (2006) Is intravitreal bevacizumab (Avastin) safe? Br J Ophthalmol 90: 1333–1334.
9. Rosenfeld PJ, Moshfeghi AA, Puliafito CA (2005) Optical coherence tomography findings after an intravitreal injection of bevacizumab (Avastin) for neovascular age-related macular degeneration. Ophthalmic Surg Lasers Imaging 36: 331–335.
10. Bashshur ZF, Schakal A, Hamam RN, El Haibi CP, Jaafar RF, et al. (2007) Intravitreal bevacizumab vs verteporfin photodynamic therapy for neovascular age-related macular degeneration. Arch Ophthalmol 125: 1357–1361.
11. Lazic R, Gabric N (2007) Verteporfin therapy and intravitreal bevacizumab combined and alone in choroidal neovascularization due to age-related macular degeneration. Ophthalmology 114: 1179–1185.
12. Wu L, Martinez-Castellanos MA, Quiroz-Mercado H, Arevalo JF, Berrocal MH, et al. (2008) Twelve-month safety of intravitreal injections of bevacizumab (Avastin): results of the Pan-American Collaborative Retina Study Group (PACORES). Graefe's Arch Clin Exp Ophthalmol 246: 81–87.
13. Chen CY, Wong TY, Heriot WJ (2007) Intravitreal Bevacizumab (Avastin) for neovascular age-related macular degeneration: a short-term study. Am J Ophthalmol 143: 510–512.
14. CATT Research Group, Martin DF, Maguire MG, Ying GS, Grunwald JE, et al. (2011) Ranibizumab and bevacizumab for neovascular age-related macular degeneration. N Engl J Med 364: 1897–1908.
15. Schmucker C, Loke YK, Ehlken C, Agostini HT, Hansen LL, et al. (2011) Intravitreal bevacizumab (Avastin) versus ranibizumab (Lucentis) for the treatment of age-related macular degeneration: a safety review. Br J Ophthalmol 95: 308–317.
16. Centre for Reviews and Dissemination (2008) Systematic reviews of adverse effects. In: Systematic Reviews - CRD's guidance for undertaking reviews in health care. York: University of York. pp. 177–198.
17. R Development Core Team (2008) R: A language and environment for statistical computing. Available: http://www.R-project.org via the Internet. Accessed 16 Jan 2012.
18. Bradburn MJ, Deeks JJ, Berlin JA, Russell Localio A (2007) Much ado about nothing: a comparison of the performance of meta-analytical methods with rare events. Stat Med 26: 53–77.
19. Biswas P, Sengupta S, Choudhary R, Home S, Paul A, et al. (2011) Comparative role of intravitreal ranibizumab versus bevacizumab in choroidal neovascular membrane in age-related macular degeneration. Indian J Ophthalmol 59: 191–196.
20. Subramanian ML, Abedi G, Ness S, Ahmed E, Fenberg M, et al. (2010) Bevacizumab vs ranibizumab for age-related macular degeneration: 1-year outcomes of a prospective, double-masked randomised clinical trial. Eye 24: 1708–1715.
21. Brown DM, Michels M, Kaiser PK, Heier JS, Sy JP, et al. (2009) Ranibizumab versus verteporfin photodynamic therapy for neovascular age-related macular degeneration: two-year results of the ANCHOR study. Ophthalmology 116: 57–69.
22. Rosenfeld PJ, Brown DM, Heier JS, Boyer DS, Kaiser PK, et al. (2006) Ranibizumab for neovascular age-related macular degeneration. N Engl J Med 355: 1419–1431.
23. Abraham P, Yue H, Wilson L (2010) Randomized, double-masked, sham-controlled trial of ranibizumab for neovascular age-related macular degeneration: PIER study year 2. Am J Ophthalmol 150: 315–324.
24. Boyer DS, Heier JS, Brown DM, Francom SF, Ianchulev T, et al. (2009) A Phase IIIb study to evaluate the safety of ranibizumab in subjects with neovascular age-related macular degeneration. Ophthalmology 116: 1731–1739.
25. Schmidt-Erfurth U, Eldem B, Guymer R, Korobelnik JF, Schlingemann RO, et al. (2011) Efficacy and safety of monthly versus quarterly ranibizumab treatment in neovascular age-related macular degeneration: the EXCITE study. Ophthalmology 118: 831–839.
26. Sacu S, Michels S, Prager F, Weigert G, Dunavoelgyi R, et al. (2009) Randomised clinical trial of intravitreal Avastin vs photodynamic therapy and intravitreal triamcinolone: long-term results. Eye 23: 2223–2237.

27. Costagliola C, Romano MR, Rinaldi M, dell'Omo R, Chiosi F, et al. (2010) Low fluence rate photodynamic therapy combined with intravitreal bevacizumab for neovascular age-related macular degeneration. Br J Ophthalmol 94: 180–184.
28. Tufail A, Patel PJ, Egan C, Hykin P, da Cruz L, et al. (2010) Bevacizumab for neovascular age related macular degeneration (ABC Trial): multicentre randomised double masked study. BMJ 340: c2459.
29. Brown DM, Kaiser PK, Michels M, Soubrane G, Heier JS, et al. (2006) Ranibizumab versus verteporfin for neovascular age-related macular degeneration. N Engl J Med 355: 1432–1444.
30. Kaiser PK, Brown DM, Zhang K, Hudson HL, Holz FG, et al. (2007) Ranibizumab for predominantly classic neovascular age-related macular degeneration: subgroup analysis of first-year ANCHOR results. Am J Ophthalmol 144: 850–857.
31. Bressler NM, Chang TS, Fine JT, Dolan CM, Ward J, et al. (2009) Improved vision-related function after ranibizumab vs photodynamic therapy: a randomized clinical trial. Arch Ophthalmol 127: 13–21.
32. Boyer DS, Antoszyk AN, Awh CC, Bhisitkul RB, Shapiro H, et al. (2007) Subgroup analysis of the MARINA study of ranibizumab in neovascular age-related macular degeneration. Ophthalmology 114: 246–252.
33. Kaiser PK, Blodi BA, Shapiro H, Acharya NR, MARINA Study Group (2007) Angiographic and optical coherence tomographic results of the MARINA study of ranibizumab in neovascular age-related macular degeneration. Ophthalmology 114: 1868–1875.
34. Chang TS, Bressler NM, Fine JT, Dolan CM, Ward J, et al. (2007) Improved vision-related function after ranibizumab treatment of neovascular age-related macular degeneration: results of a randomized clinical trial. Arch Ophthalmol 125: 1460–1469.
35. Regillo CD, Brown DM, Abraham P, Yue H, Ianchulev T, et al. (2008) Randomized, double-masked, sham-controlled trial of ranibizumab for neovascular age-related macular degnereation: PIER study year 1. Am J Ophthalmol 145: 239–248.
36. Weigert G, Michels S, Sacu S, Varga A, Prager F, et al. (2008) Intravitreal bevacizumab (Avastin) therapy versus photodynamic therapy plus intravitreal triamcinolone for neovascular age-related macular degeneration: 6-month results of a prospective, randomised, controlled clinical study. Br J Ophthalmol 92: 356–360.
37. Bakri SJ, Snyder MR, Reid JM, Pulido JS, Ezzat MK, et al. (2007) Pharmacokinetics of intravitreal ranibizumab (Lucentis). Ophthalmology 114: 2179–2182.
38. Gaudreault J, Fei D, Beyer JC, Ryan A, Rangell L, et al. (2007) Pharmacokinetics and retinal distribution of ranibizumab, a humanized antibody fragment directed against VEGF-A, following intravitreal administration in rabbits. Retina 27: 1260–1266.
39. Chou R, Aronson N, Atkins D, Ismaila AS, Santaguida P, et al. (2010) Assessing harms when comparing medical interventions: AHRQ and the Effective Health-Care Program. J Clin Epidemiol 63: 502–512.
40. Food and Drug Administration (2006) Highlights of prescribing information, Lucentis (Genentech). Available: www.accessdata.fda.gov/drugsatfda_docs/label/2006/125156lbl.pdf via the Internet. Accessed 17 Feb 2012.
41. Curtis LH, Hammill BG, Schulman KA, Cousins SW (2010) Risks of Mortality, Myocardial Infarction, Bleeding, and Stroke Associated With Therapies for Age-Related Macular Degeneration. Arch Ophthalmol 128: 1273–1279.
42. van der Reis MI, La Heij EC, De Jong-Hesse Y, Ringens PJ, Hendrikse F, et al. (2011) A systematic review of the adverse events of intravitreal anti-vascular endothelial growth factor injections. Retina 31: 1449–1469.
43. The Royal College of Ophthalmologists Statement (2011) Bevacizumab (Avastin) use in medical ophthalmology. Available: http://www.rcophth.ac.uk/news.asp?section = 24&sectionTitle = News&itemid = 647 via the Internet. Accessed 02 April 2012.

3

A Prospective Study of Treatment Patterns and 1-Year Outcome of Asian Age-Related Macular Degeneration and Polypoidal Choroidal Vasculopathy

Chui Ming Gemmy Cheung[1,2,3,4]*, Xiang Li[2,5], Ranjana Mathur[1], Shu Yen Lee[1], Choi Mun Chan[1], Ian Yeo[1], Boon Kwang Loh[1], Rachel Williams[6], Edmund Yick-Mun Wong[1], Doric Wong[1], Tien Yin Wong[1,2,3,4]

1 Vitreoretinal Service, Singapore National Eye Centre, Singapore, Singapore, **2** Singapore Eye Research Institute, Singapore, Singapore, **3** Department of Ophthalmology, Yong Loo Lin School of Medicine, National University of Singapore, Singapore, Singapore, **4** Ophthalmology Academic Clinical Program, Duke-NUS Graduate Medical School, Singapore, Singapore, **5** Department of Statistics and Applied Probability, National University of Singapore, Singapore, Singapore, **6** Worldwide Epidemiology, R&D Projects, Clinical Platforms & Sciences, GlaxoSmithKline, Pennsylvania, United States of America

Abstract

Objective: To study the treatment patterns and visual outcome over one year in Asian patients with choroidal neovascular membrane secondary to age-related macular degeneration (AMD-CNV) and polypoidal choroidal vasculopathy (PCV).

Design: Prospective cohort, non-interventional study.

Methods: 132 treatment-naïve patients who received treatment for AMD-CNV and PCV were included. All patients underwent standardized examination procedures including retinal imaging at baseline and follow-up. AMD-CNV and PCV were defined on fundus fluorescein angiography and indocyanine green angiography at baseline. Patients were treated according to standard of care.We report the visual acuity (VA) and optical coherence tomography (OCT) measurements at baseline, month 3 and month 12 The factors influencing month 12 outcomes were analyzed.

Main Outcome Measure: Type of treatment, number of Anti-vascular endothelial growth factor (VEGF) treatments, visual outcome over one year.

Results: Anti-VEGF monotherapy was the initial treatment in 89.1% of AMD-CNV, but only 15.1% of PCV. The mean number of anti-VEGF injections up to month 12 was 3.97 (4.51 AMD-CNV, 3.43 PCV, $p = 0.021$). Baseline OCT, month 3 OCT and month 3 VA were significant in determining continuation of treatment after month 3. At month12, mean VA improved from 0.82 (~20/132) at baseline to 0.68 (~20/96) at month 12 (mean gain 6.5 ETDRS letters, $p = 0.002$). 34.2% of eyes (38/113 eyes) gained ≥15 ETDRS letters and 14.4% (16/113 eyes) lost ≥15 ETDRS letters. There were no significant differences in visual outcome between AMD-CNV and PCV ($p = 0.51$). Factors predictive of month 12 visual outcome were baseline VA, baseline OCT central macular thickness, month 3 VA and age.

Conclusions: There is significant variation in treatment patterns in Asian eyes with exudative maculopathy. There is significant visual improvement in all treatment groups at one year. These data highlight the need for high quality clinical trial data to provide evidence-based management of Asian AMD.

Editor: Pedro Gonzalez, Duke University, United States of America

Funding: This study was supported by National Medical Research Council grant: NMRC/NIG/1003/2009; GlaxoSimthKline Research and Development Protocol WEUSKOP5855. The funders had no role in study design, data collection and analysis, decision to publish, or preparation of the manuscript.

Competing Interests: REW is employed by and holds stock in GlaxoSmithKline. The remaining authors have no competing interest.

* Email: gemmy.cheung.c.m@snec.com.sg

Introduction

Age-related macular degeneration (AMD) is one of the major causes of blindness worldwide [1–4]. The efficacy of ranibizumab, bevacizumab and aflibercept, have been confirmed by landmark clinical trials and these agents are now the mainstay of treatment for exudative AMD [5–11]. However, frequent follow-up and retreatment remain challenging in clinical setting. Data from the US Medicare and several European registries have highlighted these in the form of high treatment discontinuation rate within the first year and low mean number of injections [11–18].

There are few studies which have examined treatment pattern and outcomes of exudative maculopathy specifically in Asians, although it is often assumed that similar results with anti-VEGF therapy can be expected for eyes with choroidal neovascularization secondary to typical AMD (AMD-CNV) while different treatment appears to be required for the polypoidal choroidal vasculopathy (PCV) subtype [19–20]. In addition, lack of government funded reimbursement in many Asian countries, potential differences in patient understanding and expectation, and uncertainties of the role of anti-VEGF mono-therapy in PCV, may all affect the pattern of therapy in an Asian setting [20–24]. Furthermore, because photodynamic therapy (PDT) has been suggested to have superior angiographic, and possibly visual outcome in the PCV subtype [25–28], PDT is recommended as preferred treatment in PCV [29], in contrast to declining usage in Western populations. Therefore, significant heterogeneity remains in the management of Asian eyes with exudative maculopathy, in terms of diagnosis, optimal treatment and outcome.

There are few prospective studies which have examined treatment patterns and outcomes in a "real life" setting in Asians. To address this gap, we performed a prospective observational clinical study to document the current treatment pattern and outcomes of Asian exudative maculopathy, comparing in particular AMD-CNV and PCV.

Methods

Study Design and Population

The Asian AMD Phenotyping Study is a prospectively planned, cohort study approved by the SingHealth Centralized Institutional Review Board (protocol number R697/47/2009). All patients provided written informed consent to participate in this research. Specifically, the Asian AMD Phenotyping Study aimed to investigate prospectively a consecutive series of treatment-naïve Asian patients with exudative maculopathy secondary to AMD-CNV or PCV [30]. Consecutive patients were recruited from the retinal clinic of the Singapore National Eye Centre. Recruitment started on March 01 2010 and is still ongoing.

Clinical Examination and Investigations

Participants received treatment according to standard of care by individual physicians, and treatment was not altered by entering into the study. Patients were followed up prospectively according to clinical need, but minimum reviews at month 1, month 3 and month 12 were mandated by the protocol to ensure minimal data collection. Additional visits were allowed if indicated by clinical needs. All patients underwent a complete standardized ophthalmic examination at baseline and follow-up. This included visual acuity, dilated fundus examination, color fundus photography and optical coherence tomography (OCT), fundus fluorescein angiography (FFA), and indocyanine angiography (ICGA), according to a standardized protocol at baseline.

Fundus photography was performed using a digital mydriatic retinal camera (TRC-50X/IMAGEnet 2000, Topcon, Tokyo, Japan). Spectral domain optical Coherence Tomography (OCT) was performed with the Cirrus OCT (Carl Zeiss Meditec, Dublin, CA) using the 512×128-volume cube setting. Central macular thickness (CMT) was recorded. Fundus angiography with fluorescein and indocyanine green is performed using a fundus camera (TRC-50X/IMAGEnet 2000, Topcon, Tokyo, Japan) or confocal SLO (Heidelberg Retina Angiograph Spectralis; Heidelberg Engineering, Heidelberg, Germany).

Best corrected visual acuity (BCVA) was tested with Snellen chart and converted to LogMAR. Repeat fundus photography and OCT were performed at each follow-up visit and repeat fluorescein and ICGA was performed as deemed appropriate by the treating retinal specialist.

Angiographic Grading

AMD-CNV and PCV were diagnosed clinically and by FFA and ICGA. Both the primary diagnosis and treatment decision were made by the treating clinician, all of whom are fellowship-trained retinal specialist. Presence or absence of CNV was graded using criteria from the Macular Photocoagulation Study [31]. The diagnosis of definitive PCV lesions was based on the angiographic criteria from the Japanese Study Group guidelines, which defined PCV as characteristic polypoidal lesions on ICGA [32] To reflect the 'real-world' scenario, no secondary level grading was used in this analysis.

Treatment Strategies

Treatment was recommended by one of the retinal specialists in the department, all of whom were fellowship-trained. However, patients decided their final treatment after considering their visual need and financial situation. Typically, anti-VEGF therapy was recommended in the presence of subretinal or intraretinal fluid or hemorrhage associated with active AMD-CNV. In cases of PCV, anti-VEGF was recommended where there was significant fluid or hemorrhage subfoveally. In addition, focal laser was recommended if polyps were localized extrafoveally. Where PCV lesions were extensive and not amenable to focal laser, PDT was recommended. Anti-VEGF monotherapy was used in patients who could not afford PDT for subfoveal or juxtafoveal PCV. In selected cases, individual retinal specialist might recommend anti-VEGF monotherapy if polyps were small and vision was good.

Patients were followed-up at intervals determined by their treating physician. A variety of regimens were used, including monthly with prn retreatment, treat-and –extend, and sometimes less frequent follow-up. Retreatment was based on visual acuity, clinical examination and OCT morphology, usually if there is persistent subretinal or intraretinal fluid or hemorrhage. Loading with 3 initial monthly injections was not compulsory.

Anti-VEGF treatment was given intravitreally either as ranibizumab (Lucentis, Novartis) 0.5 mg/0.05 ml or bevacizumab (Avastin, Roche) 1.25 mg/0.05 ml in pre-aliquoted syringes using local compounding pharmacy.

All focal laser treatment was performed by retinal specialists. Generally, treatment was performed with a green laser with a focal contact lens, using the following parameters: 100 to 200 μm spot size, 0.15 to 0.3 millisecond duration to achieve a greyish-white burn to the active polypoidal lesions identified on ICGA. Laser may be repeated at more than one session if closure is felt to be incomplete at follow-up. Laser was not performed on the associated branching network.

PDT was performed with verteporfin (Visudyne, Novartis, Basel, Switzerland) according to the protocol of the TAP study [33]. The greatest linear dimension (GLD) was measured based on FA for CNV lesions, according to TAP protocol. For eyes with PCV, the GLD included the entire area of abnormal choroidal vasculature on the ICGA. The diameter of the laser spot size selected to be 1000 μm more than the GLD. Patients were followed-up 3-monthly after the initial PDT.

Statistical analysis

Statistical analysis was performed using standard statistical software (Statistical Package for Social Science, SPSS version 16, Illinois, Chicago) and R version 2.15.2 (R Development Core Team, Vienna, Austria, 2012). Characteristics of the study population were examined using proportions or means and standard deviation (SD). Wilcoxon rank sum test (Kruskal-Wallis rank sum test if number of groups is more than 2) or Chi-square test (Fisher's exact test if there is any entry with expected number less than 5) was performed to test the difference between diagnosis results (AMD-CNV vs. PCV) or between different treatment patterns. Factors influencing continuation of treatment after month 3 were analyzed by applying recursive partitioning tree model using R package "rpart" (Recursive Partitioning), to the factors of age, gender, initial treatment, OCT CMT (baseline, month 3 and change at month 3) and VA (baseline, month 3 and change at month 3). Decision tree was pruned after built to avoid overfitting.

Linear mixed-effect model was used to analyze longitudinal data of visual acuity over the first year to account for the repeated measurements made on the same eye. Both random and fixed effects of number of injections were added to control the heterogeneous effect among eyes. Stepwise model selection (forward and backward selection) was performed to investigate the effect on visual acuity at month 12, from a set of variables, including age, gender, VA at baseline, VA at month 3, change of VA at month 3, OCT CMT at baseline, OCT CMT at month 3, change of OCT CMT at month 3. Akaike information criterion (AIC) and recursive partitioning and regression tree model were used to select the important predictors for visual acuity at month 12.

Results

From March 1st 2010 to July 31st 2011, a total of 167 study eyes from 167 patients were included (participation rate of 77.7%). The mean age of the subjects was 69.5 years, with a slight male dominance (58.1%). The presenting visual acuity was 0.85 (~20/132). The proportion presenting with 0.3 (~6/12) or better was 13.2%, and the proportion presenting with vision 1.0 (~6/60) or worse was 35.3%. Sixty five eyes (38.9%) had typical AMD-CNV and 102 eyes (61.1%) had PCV. Baseline characteristics are summarized in **Table 1**.

Initial Treatment Pattern for All Eyes

Treatment was initiated between baseline visit and 3-month visit in one hundred and thirty-two eyes (79%). At least 1 anti-VEGF injection was received by 97 of these 132 eyes (73.5%) during the first 3 months (**Table 2**). Of these 97 eyes treated with anti-VEGF, 54 eyes were as monotherapy, and the remainder was in combination with laser (12 eyes) or PDT (29 eyes) or both PDT and laser (2 eyes). After the initial 3 months, only 46.2% (61 eyes) received further treatment, most with continuation of anti-VEGF monotherapy (70.5%, 43 eyes). Data at 1 year was available from 87/97 eyes that were commenced on anti-VEGF therapy. The mean number of injections was 2.46 (3 months), 3.15 (6 months) and 3.97 (12 months) (**Table 3**). The mean cumulative numbers of out-patient visits were 3.08, and 8.03 at month 3 and month 12 (**Table 3**). Among eyes treated with any anti-VEGF, 83.2% received bevacizumab, and the remaining received ranibizumab. Thirty-four out of 41 patients initially treated with PDT remained on follow-up at one year. The mean cumulative number of PDT sessions was 1.29 (range 1–3) during the first year of treatment. Of the 35 eyes that initially did not receive treatment before their month-3 visit, 10 were eventually treated due to increase in activity or patient's change of mind, 8 patients defaulted and the remaining patients continued to be observed.

One-Year Treatment Outcomes for All Eyes

VA at month 12 was available in 113 (of 132) treated patients. The mean VA improved from 0.82 (~20/132) at baseline to 0.68 (~20/96) at month 12 (mean gain 6.5 ETDRS letters, $p = 0.002$, **Table 4, Fig 1**). 34.2% gained ≥15 ETDRS letters and 14.4% lost ≥15 ETDRS letters. VA at month 3 was available in 75 eyes (**Table 4**) and generally are similar to VA at month 12. At month 12, 48% of 98 eyes (including 58.5% of AMd-CNV eyes and 41.3% of PCV eyes) had activity when graded into categories of active and inactive. Central macular thickness measured using

Table 1. Baseline Characteristics, comparing eyes with Age-related Macular Degeneration (AMD-CNV) and Polypoidal Choroidal Vasculopathy (PCV).

	All (N = 167)	AMD-CNV (N = 65)	PCV (N = 102)	P
Age	69.5 (9.94)	70.47 (12.05)	68.88 (8.34)	0.08
Gender				
Men	97 (58.1%)	37 (56.9%)	60 (58.8%)	0.81
Ethnicity				
Chinese	145 (86.8%)	55 (84.6%)	90 (88.2%)	0.32
Indian	2 (1.2%)	1 (1.5%)	1 (1%)	
Malay	17 (10.2%)	9 (13.8%)	8 (7.8%)	
Others	3 (1.8%)	0 (0%)	3 (2.9%)	
Prior involvement of Fellow eye *	13 (7.8%)	8 (12.3%)	5 (4.9%)	0.08
Pseudophakia in affected eye	40 (24.1%) n = 166	20 (30.8%)	20 (19.8%) n = 101	0.11
Visual Acuity (affected eye)	0.85 (0.56),	**0.95 (0.55)**	**0.78 (0.57)**	**0.018**
% Visual Acuity 6/12 (0.3 LogMAR) or better	22 (13.2%)	6 (9.2%)	16 (15.7%)	0.23
% Visual Acuity 6/60 (1.0 LogMAR) or worse	59 (35.3%)	**29 (44.6%)**	**30 (29.4%)**	**0.045**
Visual acuity (fellow eye)	0.52 (0.64), n = 165	0.59 (0.7)	0.47 (0.59), n = 100	0.38
OCT CMT (affected eye)†	310.61 (98.51), n = 132	331.02 (106.33), n = 51	297.75 (91.61), n = 81	0.08
OCT CMT (fellow eye)	260.53 (80.05), n = 127	247.4 (65.14), n = 50	269.05 (87.75), n = 77	0.27

*Indicating whether a scar was present in the fellow eye.
†Exclude statistically outlier values of 18, 23, 785.
AMD-age-related macular degeneration, PCV- polypoidal choroidal vasculopathy, OCT- optical coherence tomography; CMT - central macular thickness.

Table 2. Initial Treatment Pattern from Baseline to Month 3, comparing eyes with Age-related Macular Degeneration (AMD-CNV) and Polypoidal Choroidal Vasculopathy (PCV).

	All (N = 167)	AMD-CNV (N = 65)	PCV (N = 102)	P value[†]
Initial treatment*				0.036
No	35 (21%)	19 (29.2%)	16 (15.7%)	
Yes	132 (79%)	46 (70.8%)	86 (84.3%)	
Eyes with initial treatment	n = 132	n = 46	n = 86	<0.001
Any anti-VEGF	97 (73.5%)	44 (95.7%)	51 (59.3%)	
Anti-VEGF monotherapy	54 (40.9%)	41 (89.1%)	13 (15.1%)	
PDT monotherapy	9 (6.8%)	2 (4.3%)	7 (8.1%)	
Laser monotherapy	25 (18.9%)	0 (0%)	25 (29.1%)	
Anti-VEGF & PDT	29 (22.0%)	0 (0%)	29 (33.7%)	
Anti-VEGF & laser	12 (9.1%)	3 (6.5%)	9 (10.5%)	
PDT & laser	1 (0.8%)	0 (0%)	1 (1.2%)	
Anti-VEGF & PDT & laser	2 (1.5%)	0 (0%)	2 (2.3%)	

* Treatment given before month 3 (inclusive).
[†]P value to test the distribution of initial treatment between AMD and PCV, Fisher's exact test.
AMD-age-related macular degeneration, PCV- polypoidal choroidal vasculopathy, anti-VEGF- anti-vascular endothelial growth factor, PDT-photodynamic therapy.

Cirrus OCT (available in 74 eyes) was significantly reduced from baseline to month 12 (300.86 μm vs 264.68 μm, $p<0.001$). The proportion of eyes with vision 0.3 (~6/12) or better increased from 15.3% to 31.5%, and the proportion of eyes with vision 1.0 (~6/60) or worse decreased from 33.3% at baseline to 22.5%. In the subgroup of 85 eyes treated with anti-VEGF, visual outcome was similar compared to the whole group, with mean gain of 7.0 letters at month 12. 32.9% (28/85) gained ≥15 letters and 12.9% (11/85) lost ≥15 letters.

Comparison of Treatment Patterns for AMD-CNV and PCV

Presenting vision was significantly worse in AMD-CNV than PCV (0.95 vs 0.78, $p = 0.018$) (**Table 1**) and more eyes with AMD-CNV had vision worse than 6/60 (44.6%) than PCV (29.4%, $p = 0.045$). However, within the group of treated eyes with at least one year follow-up (n = 113), the baseline vision was similar. There was no significant difference in age, gender, OCT thickness, proportion of previous involvement in fellow eyes and lens status. However after excluding 35 patients who did not receive treatment (29 AMD-CNV, 16 PCV), the presenting vision was similar in the remaining eyes (0.79 AMD-CNV, 0.83 PCV, $p = 0.89$) (**Table 4**).

Initial treatment choice was markedly different between AMD-CNV and PCV groups (**Table 2**, **Figure 2**). Anti-VEGF monotherapy was used in the majority of AMD-CNV (89.1%, 41/46 eyes), but only 15.1% (13/86) of PCV. Within the PCV group, the single most commonly used treatment was anti-VEGF and PDT combination (33.7%, 29/86), followed by laser monotherapy (29.1%, 25/86). Overall, 59.3% of eyes with PCV received anti-VEGF therapy alone or in combination. The mean cumulative number of anti-VEGF injections was significantly lower in PCV group (4.51 for AMD-CNV, 3.43 for PCV, $p = 0.021$).

Mean vision at month 12 was similar between AMD-CNV and PCV group (0.70 AMD-CNV, 0.67 PCV, $p = 0.94$) (**Table 3**). The mean change in vision and proportion gaining and losing ≥ 15 ETDRS letters were also similar. (**Table 3**)

Factors Influencing Treatment Patterns

Factors that influenced the choice of initial therapy were diagnosis (see above, AMD-CNV compared to PCV) and OCT CMT at baseline. Eyes treated with anti-VEGF monotherapy had thicker OCT CMT at baseline compared to eyes treated with combination. (367.62 μm vs 291.68 μm, $p = 0.001$). These two factors remained significant (diagnosis, $p<0.001$; OCT CMT $p = 0.004$) after adjusting for age, gender, baseline OCT and diagnosis Baseline VA and previous fellow eye involvement were not significantly related to treatment choice.

Factors that influenced the cumulative number of injections included diagnosis, choice of initial treatment and OCT CMT measurement at month 3. PCV eyes had significantly less injections than AMD eyes (3.43 vs 4.51 at 1 year, $p = 0.021$) This difference remained after controlling age, gender and the OCT CMT at month 3. Eyes treated with anti-VEGF combinations had significantly lower number of injections than eyes treated with anti-VEGF monotherapy only in the PCV group (3.03 vs 4.70 at 1 year, $p = 0.008$). Each 100 μm increase in OCT CMT at month 3 was associated with additional 0.925 injections after month 3 ($p = 0.029$).This remains significant after controlling for diagnosis and the baseline OCT CMT ($p = 0.025$).

Factors Influencing One-Year Visual Outcome

Using recursive partitioning and regression tree method, baseline VA, baseline OCT thickness and month 3 VA were significant predictors of VA at month 12. Eyes with baseline VA of ≥1.0 had worse vision at month 12 compared to eyes with better baseline VA (1.13 vs 0.46, $p<0.001$). However they experienced larger improvement in VA (18.5 letters vs 1 letter, $p = 0.002$) and had a larger proportion experiencing at least 15 letters gain (54.1% vs 24.3%, $p = 0.002$).

In addition, we performed a longitudinal analysis, utilizing all available data at different time points over the first year. Visual

Table 3. Cumulative number of Anti-vascular endothelial growth factor (anti-VEGF) injections and follow-up visits to month 12, comparing eyes with Age-related Macular Degeneration (AMD-CNV) and Polypoidal Choroidal Vasculopathy (PCV).

	Month 3	Month 6	Month 12
All Anti-VEGF (N=87)			
Number of injections	2.46 (1.13)	3.15 (1.47)	3.97 (2.07)
Number of visits	3.08 (1.31)	4.11 (2.00)	8.03 (1.90)
Stratified by Diagnosis & Treatment mode			
AMD-CNV (N=43)			
Number of injections	2.70 (1.19)	3.63 (1.63)	4.51 (2.25)
Number of visits	2.794 (1.41)	3.86 (2.17)	5.51 (2.76)
AMD-CNV treated with Anti-VEGF monotherapy (n=33)			
Number of injections	2.73 (1.13)	3.55 (1.6)	4.45 (2.31)
Number of visits	2.52 (1.42)	3.33 (2.16)	4.91 (2.82)
AMD-CNV treated with combination therapy (n=10)			
Number of injections	2.6 (1.43)	3.9 (1.79)	4.7 (2.21)
Number of visits	3.7 (0.95)	5.6 (0.97)	7.5 (1.27)
P value* for number of injections comparing monotherapy vs combination in AMD-CNV			
	1.000	0.536	0.511
PCV (N=44)			
Number of injections	2.23 (1.03)	2.68 (1.14)	3.43 (1.73)
Number of visits	3.36 (1.16)	4.36 (1.81)	6.20 (2.36)
PCV treated with Anti-VEGF monotherapy (n=10)			
Number of injections	3.1 (0.57)	3.8 (1.03)	4.8 (1.99)
Number of visits	3.7 (0.95)	5.2 (1.81)	7.3 (2.67)
PCV treated with combination therapy (n=34)			
Number of injections	1.97 (1)	2.35 (0.95)	3.03 (1.45)
Number of visits	3.26 (1.21)	4.12 (1.75)	5.88 (2.2)
P value* for number of injections comparing monotherapy vs combination in PCV			
	0.002	0.001	0.008
P value* for number of injections between AMD-CNV and PCV			
	0.003	**0.002**	**0.017**

*P value based on Wilcoxon rank sum test.
AMD-age-related macular degeneration, PCV- polypoidal choroidal vasculopathy, anti-VEGF- anti-vascular endothelial growth factor, PDT-photodynamic therapy.

acuity was weakly correlated with number of injections and age. For each additional injection received, there was on average an additional 1.7 letters improvement in VA at month 12 ($p=0.05$). Every year increase in age was associated with a 0.6 letter worsening of VA ($p=0.05$). OCT CMT measurement was significantly correlated with visual acuity ($p<0.001$). Each 100 μm increase in OCT CMT was correlated to a drop of 3.62 ETDRS letters in visual acuity. There was no significant difference in Month 12 VA or change in VA whether anti-VEGF therapy was alone or in combination.

Discussion

This prospective study reports the current treatment pattern and outcome for exudative maculopathy in an Asian population over a one year period. While it has been documented that anti-VEGF monotherapy is now the most common treatment for exudative AMD in the USA and Europe [11], similar data from an Asian population are limited. In addition, it is unclear how anti-VEGF usage may be affected by issues including the high prevalence of PCV in Asian populations, the apparent superior efficacy of PDT in causing polyp regression, and the uncertainty of the role of anti-VEGF monotherapy [20–29]. Recently, health authorities from some Asian countries have excluded PCV from the treatment label of anti-VEGF agents. Therefore, a clearer understanding of the management patterns and outcome of Asian eyes with exudative maculopathy is important in accurately planning eye care provision, research strategies, labelling of medications and re-imbursement of therapies.

Our study population can be compared to similar registry and insurance-based data, mostly from Western countries with largely white populations (**Table 5**). Our study population was generally younger (mean age 69.6 years), had higher male subjects (58.1%) and had lower presenting vision (44.0 ETDRS letters). Overall, 72.0% of treated eyes received at least one anti-VEGF treatment. While the widespread use of anti-VEGF is comparable to data from US [11], only 40.9% of cases received anti-VEGF as monotherapy. This pattern is remarkably different compared to reports in white people [11]. However, when stratified by diagnosis, the vast majority of AMD-CNV cases were treated with anti-VEGF monotherapy (89.1%). Therefore the lower monotherapy rate can be attributed largely to the higher

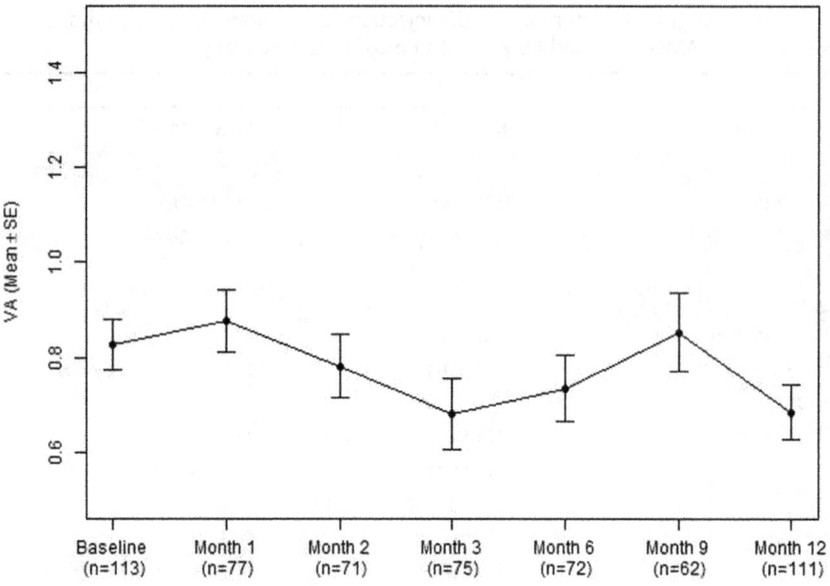

Figure 1. Mean visual acuity of all treated eyes from baseline to month 12. The number of eyes with OCT available at each timepoint is indicated by n.VA Visual acuity; SE standard error.

Table 4. Visual Acuity and Optical Coherence Tomography Central Macular Thickness at Month 3 and Month 12, stratified by Diagnosis.

	All	AMD-CNV	PCV	P
Visual acuity	N=113	N=43	N=70	
Baseline	0.82 (0.57)	0.79 (0.53)	0.83 (0.59)	0.89
Month 3	0.68 (0.65) (n=75)	0.76 (0.79) (n=25)	0.64 (0.57) (n=50)	0.94
Month 12	0.68 (0.6)	0.7 (0.64)	0.67 (0.57)	0.94
Change at month 3	−0.16 (0.47)	0.03 (0.52)	−0.26 (0.42)	0.15
Change at month 12	−0.13 (0.51)	−0.09 (0.52)	−0.16 (0.51)	0.51
Gain ≥15 letters at Month 3	25 (33.3%)	9(36.0%)	16 (32.0%)	0.73
Gain ≥15 letters at Month 12	38 (34.2%)	14 (34.1%)	24 (34.3%)	0.99
Loss ≥15 letters at month 3	7 (9.3%)	6 (24.0%)	1 (2.0%)	0.005
Loss ≥15 letters at Month 12	16 (14.4%)	6 (14.6%)	10 (14.3%)	0.96
Proportion with VA 0.3 or better				
Baseline	17 (15.3%)	7 (17.1%)	10 (14.3%)	0.69
Month 3	29 (38.7%	11 (44.0%)	18 (36.0%)	0.50
Month 12	35 (31.5%)	14 (34.1%)	21 (30%)	0.65
Proportion with VA 1.0 or worse				
Baseline	37 (33.3%)	13 (31.7%)	24 (34.3%)	0.781
Month 3	17 (22.7%)	6 (24.0%)	11 (22.0%)	0.85
Month 12	25 (22.5%)	11 (26.8%)	14 (20%)	0.406
OCT CMT	N=76	N=26	N=50	
Baseline	300.86 (98.29)	317.62 (94.79)	292.14 (99.88)	0.26
Month 12	264.68 (89.82)	272.81 (71.18)	260.46 (98.54)	0.16
Change at month 12	−36.17 (93.99)	−44.81 (79.52)	−31.68 (101.17)	0.68

P value based Wilcoxon rank sum test or Chi-square test.
AMD-age-related macular degeneration, PCV- polypoidal choroidal vasculopathy, OCT- optical coherence tomography, CMT - central macular thickness.

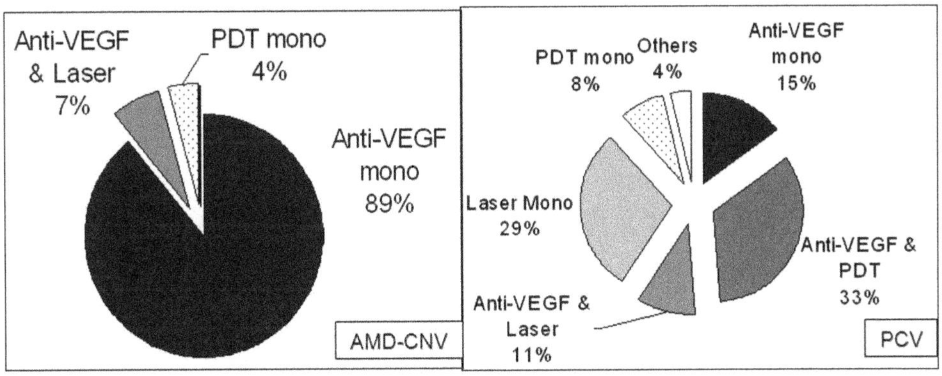

Figure 2. Distribution of Initial Treatment Modalities by diagnosis of Age-related Macular Degeneration (AMD-CNV) (left) and Polypoidal Choroidal Vasculopathy (PCV) (right).

proportion of patients needing specific PCV treatment, of which only 15.1% received anti-VEGF monotherapy. Despite the lower proportion of anti-VEGF monotherapy, a further 44.2% of PCV eyes received anti-VEGF in combination with PDT (33.7%) or laser (10.5%). Thus, an key observation of this study is that anti-VEGF therapy constitutes a significant part of treatment for PCV eyes (59.3%), although more commonly in combination with other treatments.

The overall number of injections was low at 3.97 (range 1–9) over 12 months. Even after separating PCV eyes from AMD-CNV eyes, the mean number of injections was only 4.51 injections over 12 months in AMD-CNV eyes. However, these figures are not far off published data from USA and European registries (**Table 5**) [11–18]. These data highlight the challenges in translating clinical trial results into "real life" clinical practice. As in most countries, the utilization of anti-VEGF is affected by reimbursement structure and retreatment criteria. In addition to low retreatment number, the number of follow-up visits during the first year was also low (mean 8 visits). Although only three mandatory visits were included in the study protocol (at months 1, 3 and 12), most patients attended much more frequently due to clinical need (mean 8.03 visits). However,it is likely this lack of follow-up and under-treatment contributed significantly towards the low injection numbers, as 48% of eyes still had activity on OCT at month 12, However, similar low follow-up visits (8.06 visits) had been reported from France [17], highlighting the adherence to follow-up is also a challenge in the delivery of AMD care.

We report the mean VA improved significantly by 6.5 letters, with 34.2% gaining 15 ETDRS letters and 14.4% losing ≥15 ETDRS letters. When outcome was analyzed by diagnosis of AMD-CNV versus PCV, there was no significant difference in mean VA change, or of the proportion gaining and losing 15 letters. Visual outcome from several European registries have been summarized in **Table 5** for comparison. In addition to mean change in VA, it is also important to note that patients from the current study had generally worse presenting visual acuity than those from European registries [12–18]. Despite significant mean visual gain, the vision at 1 year remained significantly lower than those from European registries [12–18]. Lower public awareness of AMD and generally later presentation in Asian setting is likely to be a significant explanation for these findings. It is also interesting to note that 35 patients did not receive treatment initially (before their month-3 visit). The most common reasons were poor prognosis (10/19 eyes in the AMD-CNV group and 6/15 eyes in the PCV group), and limited activity at presentation (3/19 in the AMD-CNV group and 8/15 in the PCV group) reason in the PCV group (8/15 eyes). The remaining patients defaulted their follow up. Of these 35 eyes, 10 eyes eventually received treatment from month 4 onwards.

In terms of predictive factors for visual outcome, we identified OCT measurement at baseline and VA at month 3 as significant predictors for both the need to continue treatment beyond month 3 and also vision at month 12. Each 100 µm increase in OCT CMT was correlated to a drop of 3.6 ETDRS letters in visual acuity ($p<0.001$). OCT CMT measurement at month 3 was also predictive of whether treatment was continued after 3 months. Each 100 µm increase in OCT CMT at month 3 was associated with 0.925 additional injections after month 3 ($p=0.025$). The number of injection was only weakly correlated with visual outcome at month 12. Each additional injection was associated with a further 1.7 letters gain in vision at month 12.

In our study, 61.1% of eyes had PCV. Apart from features on ICGA and worse baseline VA in AMD-CNV (0.95 in AMD-CNV vs 0.78 in PCV, $p=0.018$), there were no significant differences in baseline characteristics in terms of age, gender, fellow eye involvement or lens status between AMD-CNV and PCV eyes. These results highlight the importance to screen for PCV with ICGA in an Asian population. Our results showed several major findings regarding PCV treatment in our centre. First, a variety of treatment modalities are currently employed in treating PCV. Second, anti-VEGF use was common, but appears to require less injection number when used as combination therapy. Third, the visual outcome was similar in PCV and AMD-CNV eyes in the anti-VEGF era. Therefore, the role of anti-VEGF therapy in PCV, as monotherapy or as adjunct to occlusive therapies, should be further studied.

There are limitations to this study. The observational design aims to capture the current treatment pattern of exudative AMD in an Asian setting in Singapore. Variations in treatment preference between individual clinicians, between countries and regions are to be expected. Variations in reimbursement systems between countries will also influence the treatment pattern. Practice pattern, such as injection number, is likely to evolve with time and injection numbers may increase with increasing acceptance of the need for long-term therapy. We did not perform secondary grading of PCV but decided to follow the initial clinical diagnosis by the treating clinician. Therefore PCV diagnosis may be less stringent, and some of the PCV cases in this series may represent possible/probable PCV (mixed cases) in addition to definite PCV cases. Due to logistic constraints, OCT examination was performed using SD-OCT other than the Cirrus OCT in some cases. Therefore the OCT thickness measurements in these

Table 5. Comparison of Patient Characteristics and Anti-VEGF Utilization during the First Year of Treatment.

Study origin	USA (2008) [11]	Germany (2008) [12,13]	UK (2007) [14]	UK (2007) [14]	Sweden (2007) [12,15]	Belgium (2008) [12,16]	Netherlands (2008) [12,16]	France (2007) [17]	Beirut (2005) [18]	Korea (2007) [19]	Singapore, Current study (2010)	Singapore, Current study (2010)
Sample size	91,628	3,470	897 (pretreated n = 125)	897 (no pretreatment n = 772)	471	253	243	122	60	41	132 (AMD-CNV, n = 43)	132 (PCV, n = 87)
Mean age, years (SD)	81.1 (7.0)	77.6 (7.8)	75.0 (8.4)		78.1 (8.0)	78.7 (6.8)	77.9 (8.0)	78.3 (7.0)	72.2	70.3 (7.9)	69.6 (10.5)	
Female, %	63.8%	64.6%	-		66.0%	62.1%	59.3%	70.0%	43.1%	51.2%	41.9%	
Mean baseline VA ETDRS letters (SD)	NA	48.8 (18.7)	50.4	54.1	58.3 (12.2)	56.3 (14.2)	45.1 (21.5)	56.2 (14.0)	45.7	42.1	45.5	43.5
Mean VA at 1 year ETDRS letters (SD)	NA	48.0 (11.7)	53.1	57.9	59.3 (16.2)	58.8 (17.9)	50.7 (24.0)	56.9 (17.0)	53.1	46.0	50.0	51.5
Mean number of injections at 1 year (SD)			6.2 (2.6)	5.2 (2.7)							4.51 (2.25)	3.43 (1.73)

Formula of conversion from LogMAR to ETDRS letters: 85-50LogMAR.
AMD - age-related macular degeneration; PCV- polypoidal choroidal vasculopathy; SD standard deviation.

eyes were not incorporated into the current analysis. Post treatment ICGA would have been informative in all cases. However ICGA was only repeated post treatment if there is clinical suspicion (based on fundoscopy, visual acuity and OCT findings) of residual activity.

In conclusion, our prospective study showed significant variation in treatment patterns in Asian eyes with exudative maculopathy. AMD-CNV was treated predominantly with anti-VEGF monotherapy, whereas a variety of treatment modalities were used to treat PCV. Low overall injection numbers over 1 year suggest that many patients may be under-treated in the "real life" setting, a situation not dissimilar to US and European countries. Despite these variations, relatively good visual outcomes at 1 year were achieved in both AMD-CNV and PCV. Nevertheless, these data highlight the need for high quality clinical trial data to provide evidence-based guidelines to optimize the management of Asian AMD.

Acknowledgments

The authors would like to acknowledge Mr. Joseph Ho, principal ophthalmic imaging specialist, Singapore National Eye Centre, for performing the angiography for the Singapore patients.

Author Contributions

Conceived and designed the experiments: CMGC TYW. Performed the experiments: CMGC RM SYL CMC IY BKL EW DW TYW. Analyzed the data: CMGC XL RW TYW. Contributed reagents/materials/analysis tools: CMGC RM SYL CMC IY BKL RW EW DW TYW. Wrote the paper: CMGC.

References

1. Lim LS, Mitchell P, Seddon JM, Holz FG, Wong TY (2012) Age-related macular degeneration. Lancet379: 1728–38
2. Klein R, Klein BE, Knudtson MD, Wong TY, Cotch MF, et al. (2006)Prevalence of age related macular degeneration in 4 racial/ethnic groups in the Multi-ethnic Study of Atherosclerosis. Ophthalmology 113: 373–80.
3. Mitchell P, Smith W, Attebo K, Wang JJ (1995) Prevalence of age-related maculopathy in Australia. The Blue Mountains Eye Study. Ophthalmology 102: 1450–60.
4. Kawasaki R, Yasuda M, Song SJ, Cheng SJ, Jonas JB, et al (2010) The Prevalence of Age-Related Macular Degeneration in Asians. Ophthalmology 117: 921–927.
5. Rosenfeld PJ, Brown DM, Heier JS, Boyer DS, Kaiser PK, et al (2006) Ranibizumab for neovascular age-related macular degeneration. N Eng J Med 355: 1419–31.
6. Brown DM, Kaiser PK, Michels M, Soubrane G, Heier JS, et al (2006) Ranibizumab versus verteportin for neovascular age-related macular degeneration. N Eng J Med 355: 1432–44.
7. The CATT Research Group (2011) Ranibizumab and bevacizumab for neovascular age-related macular degeneration. N Eng J Med 364: 1897–908.
8. The CATT Research Group (2012) Ranibizumab and bevacizumab for neovascular age-related macular degeneration: Two-year results. Ophthalmology 119: 1388–98.
9. Chakravarthy U, Harding SP, Rogers CA, Downes SM, Lotery AJ, et al (2013) Alternative treatments to inhibit VEGF in age-related choroidal neovascularisation: tow-year findings of the IVAN randomised controlled trial. The Lancet. 382: 1258–67.
10. Heier JS, Brown DM, Chong V, Korobelnik JF, Kaiser PK, et al (2012) Intravitreal aflibercept (VEGF trap-eye) in wet age-related macular degeneration. Ophthalmology 119: 2537–48.
11. Curtis LH, Hammill BG, Qualls LG, DiMartino LD, Wang F, et al (2012) Treatment patterns for neovascular age-related macular degeneration: Analysis of 284380 Medicare Beneficiaries. Am J Ophthalmol 153: 1116–1124.
12. Holz FG, Bandello F, Gillies M, Mitchell P, Osborne A, et al (2013) Safety of ranibizumab in routine clinical practice: 1-year retrospective pooled analysis of four European neovascular AMD registries within the LUMINOUS programme. Br J Ophthalmol 97: 1161–7.
13. Finger RP, Wiedemann P, Blumhage F, Pohl K, Holz FG (2013) Treatment patterns, visual acuity and quality-of-life outcomes of the WAVE study- a noninterventional study of ranibizumab treatment for neovascular age-related macular degeneration in Germany. Acta Ophthalmologica 91: 540–6.
14. Pushpoth S, Sykakis E, Merchant K, Browning AC, Gupta R, et al (2012) Measuring the benefit of 4 years of Intravitreal Ranibizumab treatment for neovascular age-related macular degeneration. Br J Ophthalmol 96: 1469–73.
15. Hjelmqvist L, Lindberg C, Kanulf P, Dahlgren H, Johansson I, et al (2011) One-year outcomes using ranibizumab for neovascular age-related macular degeneration. J Ophthalmol 2011: 405724.
16. Rakic JM, Leys A, Brie H, Denhaerynck K, Pacheco C, et al (2013). Real-world variability in ranibizumab treatment and associated clinica, quality of life, and safety outcomes over 24 months in patients with neovascular age-related macular degeneration: the HELIOS study. Clin Ophthalmol 7: 1849–58.
17. Cohen SY, Dubois L, Tadayoni R, Fajnkuchen F, Nghiem-Buffet S, et al (2009) Results of one-year's treatment with ranibizumab for exudative age-related macular degeneration in a clinical setting. Am J Ophthalmol 148: 409–413.
18. Bashshur ZF, Haddad ZA, Schakal A, Jaafar RF, Saab M, et al (2008) Intravitreal bevacizumab for treatment of neovascular age-related macular degeneration: A one-year prospective study. Am J Ophthalmol 145: 249–256.
19. Kang S, Roh YJ (2011) Ranibizumab treatment administered as needed for occult and minimally classic neovascular membranes in age-related macular degeneration. Jpn J Ophthalmol 55: 123–7.
20. Cheung CM, Wong TY (2011) Anti-VEGF Debate: Limitation in Asia New Eng J Med 365: 2237.
21. Lamoureux EL, Mitchell P, Rees G, Cheung G, Yeo I, et al (2011) Impact of early and late age-related macular degeneration on vision-specific function. Br J Ophthalmol 95: 666–70.
22. Laude A, Cackett PD, Vithana EN, Yeo IY, Wong D, et al (2010) Polypoidal choroidal vasculopathy and neovascular age-related macular degeneration: Same or deifferent disease? Prof Ret Eye Res 29: 19–29.
23. Gomi F, Sawa M, Sakaguchi H, Tsujikawa M, Oshima Y, et al (2008) Efficacy of intravitreal bevacizumab for polypoidal choroidal vasculopathy. Br J Ophthalmol 92: 70–73.
24. Lai TY, Chan WM, Liu DT, Luk FO, Lam DS (2008) Intravitreal bevacizumab (Avastin) with or without photodynamic therapy for the treatment of polypoidal choroidal vasclopathy. Br J Ophthalmol 92: 661–666.
25. Koh A, Lee WK, Chen LJ, Chen SJ, Hashad Y, et al (2012) EVEREST STUDY: Efficacy and Safety of Verteporfin Photodynamic Therapy in Combination with Ranibizumab or Alone Versus Ranibizumab Monotherapy in Patients with Symptomatic Macular Polypoidal Choroidal Vasculopathy. Retina. 32: 1453–64
26. Chan WM, Lam DS, Lai TY, Liu DT, Li KK, et al (2004) Photodynamic therapy with verteporfin for symptomatic polypoidal choroidal vasculopathy one-year results of a prospective case series. Ophthalmology 111: 1576–1584.
27. Gomi F, Ohji M, Sayanagi K, Sawa M, Sakaguchi H, et al (2008) One-year outcomes of photodynamic therapy in age-related macular degeneration and polypoidal choroidal vasculopathy in Japanese patients. Ophthalmology 115: 141–146.
28. Kurashige Y, Otani A, Sasahara M, Yodoi Y, Tamura H, et al (2008) Two-year results of photodynamic therapy for polypoidal choroidal vasculopathy. Am J Ophthalmol 146: 513–519.
29. Koh AH, Chen LJ, Chen SJ, Chen Y, Giridhar A, et al (2013) Polypoidal choroidal vasculopathy: Evidence-based guidelines for clinical diagnosis and treatment. Retina 33: 686–716.
30. Cheung CM, Bhargava M, Li X, Mathur R, Mun CC, et al (2013) Six Month Visual Prognosis in Eyes with Submacular Hemorrhage secondary to Age-Related Macular Degeneration or Polypoidal Choroidal Vasculopathy. Graefes Arch Clin Exp Ophthalmol 251: 19–25.
31. Macular Photocoagulation Study Group (1991) Laser photocoagulation of subfoveal neovascular lesions in age-related macular degeneration: Results of a randomized clinical trial. Arch Ophthalmol 109: 1219–1230.
32. Japanese Study Group of Polypoidal Choroidal Vasculopathy (2005) Criteria for diagnosis of polypoidal choroidal vasculopathy. Nippon Ganka Gakkai Zasshi [Japanese] 109: 417–427.
33. Treatment of Age-Related Macular Degeneration with Photodynamic Therapy (TAP) Study Group (1999) Photodynamic therapy of subfoveal choroidal neovascularization in age-related macular degeneration with verteporfin. One-year results of 2 randomized clinical trials- TAP report 1. Arch Ophthalmol 117: 1329–45.

4

The 5HT$_{1a}$ Receptor Agonist 8-Oh DPAT Induces Protection from Lipofuscin Accumulation and Oxidative Stress in the Retinal Pigment Epithelium

Prajitha Thampi[1], Haripriya Vittal Rao[1], Sayak K. Mitter[1], Jun Cai[1], Haoyu Mao[2], Hong Li[2], Soojung Seo[2], Xiaoping Qi[1], Alfred S. Lewin[2], Carl Romano[3], Michael E. Boulton[1]*

1 Department of Anatomy and Cell Biology, University of Florida, Gainesville, Florida, United States of America, **2** Department of Molecular Genetics & Microbiology, University of Florida, Gainesville, Florida, United States of America, **3** Retina Research, Alcon Laboratories, Inc, Fort Worth, Texas, United States of America

Abstract

Age-related macular degeneration (AMD), a major cause of blindness in the elderly, is associated with oxidative stress, lipofuscin accumulation and retinal degeneration. The aim of this study was to determine if a 5-HT$_{1A}$ receptor agonist can reduce lipofuscin accumulation, reduce oxidative damage and prevent retinal cell loss both *in vitro* and *in vivo*. Autophagy-derived and photoreceptor outer segment (POS)-derived lipofuscin formation was assessed using FACS analysis and confocal microscopy in cultured retinal pigment epithelial (RPE) cells in the presence or absence of the 5-HT$_{1A}$ receptor agonist, 8-OH DPAT. 8-OH DPAT treatment resulted in a dose-dependent reduction in both autophagy- and POS-derived lipofuscin compared to control. Reduction in autophagy-induced lipofuscin was sustained for 4 weeks following removal of the drug. The ability of 8-OH DPAT to reduce oxidative damage following exposure to 200 μM H_2O_2 was assessed. 8-OH DPAT reduced superoxide generation and increased mitochondrial superoxide dismutase (MnSOD) levels and the ratio of reduced glutathione to the oxidized form of glutathione in H_2O_2-treated cells compared to controls and protected against H_2O_2-initiated lipid peroxidation, nitrotyrosine levels and mitochondrial damage. SOD2 knockdown mice, which have an AMD-like phenotype, received daily subcutaneous injections of either saline, 0.5 or 5.0 mg/kg 8-OH DPAT and were evaluated at monthly intervals. Systemic administration of 8-OH DPAT improved the electroretinogram response in SOD2 knockdown eyes of mice compared to knockdown eyes receiving vehicle control. There was a significant increase in the ONL thickness in mice treated with 8-OH DPAT at 4 months past the time of MnSOD knockdown compared to untreated controls together with a 60% reduction in RPE lipofuscin. The data indicate that 5-HT$_{1A}$ agonists can reduce lipofuscin accumulation and protect the retina from oxidative damage and mitochondrial dysfunction. 5-HT$_{1A}$ receptor agonists may have potential as therapeutic agents in the treatment of retinal degenerative disease.

Editor: Pedro Gonzalez, Duke University, United States of America

Funding: This work was funded by National Institutes of Health grant EY019688 (MEB) and a grant from Alcon Labs, Inc (MEB & ASL). CR is an employee of Alcon Labs, Inc. and contributed to the study design and preparation of the manuscript. The funders had no role in study design, data collection and analysis, decision to publish, or preparation of the manuscript.

Competing Interests: The authors have read the journal's policy and the authors below have the following conflicts: MEB and ASL received funding from Alcon Labs, Inc for this study. CR is an employee of Alcon Labs, Inc.

* E-mail: meboulton@ufl.edu

Introduction

Age-related macular degeneration (AMD) is the major cause of blindness in the elderly in developed countries, with more than 1.7 million Americans over age 65 having visual impairment due to AMD [1]. Although AMD has a complex etiology which is determined by a variety of environmental factors and inherent genetic susceptibilities, there is a consensus that the retinal pigment epithelium (RPE) plays a central role in its pathogenesis. Elevated levels of the age pigment lipofuscin and oxidative stress are associated with a variety of retinal degenerations including AMD, and there is considerable circumstantial evidence linking lipofuscin with the pathobiology of AMD [2,3,4,5,6]. The highest density of lipofuscin is located in the central retina where the density of rod outer segments is at its highest and where there is a preferential loss of rod cells in AMD [7]. Cumulative oxidative damage, chronic phototoxicity, lysosomotropic damage and occupation of cytoplasmic volume in RPE cells by lipofuscin throughout life will contribute to RPE dysfunction and put added stress on a highly metabolically active cell type [8,9]. Longitudinal monitoring of fundus autofluorescence demonstrates that the presence of local areas or "hot spots" of lipofuscin in the RPE layer are a risk for progression of AMD [3,4,10,11] and these areas exhibit a variable loss of retinal sensitivity [12]. Lipofuscin levels are also elevated in rodent models for AMD [13,14,15]. Lipofuscin can be observed in early drusen and these granules may serve as an immunogenic stimulus for the localized activation of dendritic cells, complement activation and the deposition of inflammatory factors [16,17]. Given the increasing evidence for lipofuscin involvement in AMD there is a growing interest in the development of therapeutic agents to both prevent lipofuscin formation and eliminate preexisting lipofuscin. These studies have primarily focused on slowing the retinoid cycle and reducing the accumulation of retinoid derivatives such as A2E in lipofuscin

[6,18,19]. However, while offering some success, these approaches have been associated with slowed dark adaptation and reduced ERG responses [19,20].

The 5-HT_{1A} receptor is a subtype of the G protein-coupled 5-HT receptor family that binds the endogenous neurotransmitter serotonin (5-hydroxytryptamine, 5-HT) [21]. The 5-HT_{1A} receptor is the most widespread of all the 5-HT receptors and is expressed in both the neural retina and the RPE [22,23,24]. 5-HT_{1A} agonists provide protection against a variety of insults, including: serum deprivation [25], staurosporine [26], anoxia [27], excitotoxicity [28] and oxidative damage [29]. Furthermore, we have recently reported that 5-HT_{1A} agonists can provide potent and complete functional and structural protection from severe blue-light induced photooxidative damage [22,23]. ERGs were significantly higher in light exposed rats treated with 5-HT_{1A} agonists and retinas were devoid of histological lesions compared to vehicle only controls. In addition, 5-HT_{1A} agonist caused a decrease in microglial activation and recruitment as well as reduced complement deposition in the outer retina.

In this study we report that the 5-HT_{1A} agonist, 8-hydroxy-2-(di-*n*-propylamino)-tetralin (8-OH DPAT), is able to reduce the accumulation of both autophagic-derived and photoreceptor outer segment-derived lipofuscin, increase antioxidant protection and reduce oxidative damage in cultured human RPE cells as well as being able to reduce lipofuscin accumulation and improve visual function in an animal model of AMD.

Results

5-HT_{1A} agonist reduces lipofuscin accumulation in cultured RPE cells

8-OH DPAT treatment resulted in a dose-dependent reduction in both autophagy- and POS-derived lipofuscin accumulation (Fig. 1). The cells showed no apparent morphological change apart from the reduction of lipofuscin. Autophagy-derived lipofuscin accumulation was reduced by 8-OH DPAT treatment over a 4 week period compared to untreated control ($p<0.01$) with approximately 50% reduction in autofluorescence at 10 and 20 μM 8-OH DPAT (Fig. 1a). Based on these observations, we elected to use 10 μM 8-OH DPAT for the majority of our subsequent experiments. We next assessed the effect of 10 μM 8-OH DPAT on the time-dependent accumulation of autophagy-derived lipofuscin over a 4 week period. We observed a significant decrease of 30% and 67% ($p<0.01$) after 3 and 4 weeks treatment respectively compared to untreated control (Fig. 1b) and that the beneficial effect of 8-OH DPAT became maximal from 3 weeks onward. The 8-OH DPAT induced decrease in lipofuscin accumulation could be visually verified using fluorescence microscopy (Fig. 1c).

8-OH DPAT was also able to reduce lipofuscin accumulation derived from phagocytosed photoreceptor outer segments (POS) by 28% over 14 days compared to untreated control ($p<0.05$) (Fig. 1d) and this reduction was visually confirmed by fluorescence microscopy (Fig. 1e). There was no significant difference between the two concentrations (1 and 10 μM) of 8-OH DPAT tested. The magnitude of autofluorescence caused by phagocytosis of POS is much greater than that caused by autophagy. (Note the scale differences in the ordinates of Fig. 1a and 1d.) Consequently, the decrease in phagocytic lipofuscin caused by 8-OH DPAT must be largely independent of its inhibition of autophagy.

To confirm that 8-OH DPAT was reducing lipofuscin by binding the $5HT_{1A}$ receptor we assessed the effect of the $5HT_{1A}$ receptor antagonist UH-301. UH-301 blocked the 8-OH DPAT-induced reduction in both autophagy- and POS-derived lipofuscin accumulation in cultured RPE (Fig. 2a,b).

To test whether reduction in lipofuscin associated with 8-OH DPAT would persist after the drug was removed, we measured autofluorescence for an additional 4 weeks after cessation of treatment. For autophagy-induced lipofuscin, this was, in fact, the case: reduction in autofluorescence was maintained for 28 days after treatment stopped (Fig. 2c). In the case of POS-derived lipofuscin, although autofluorescence accumulation remained absent for the first week after discontinuation of 8-OH DPAT, the rate of lipofuscin accumulation eventually returned to that seen in control cultures fed POS but not receiving 8-OH DPAT treatment (Fig. 2d). However, the overall decrease in lipofuscin accumulation prior to discontinuation of 8-OH DPAT was maintained. Having shown that 8-OH DPAT was able to inhibit lipofuscinogenesis we next wished to determine if 8-OH DPAT could reduce levels of prexisting lipofuscin. 8-OH DPAT did not lead to significant reduction in preformed lipofuscin that was derived from autophagy nor did it reduce autofluorescence in ARPE19 cells fed mature human lipofuscin granules (Fig. 2e,f). However, there was a small, but significant ($p<0.05$), reduction in pre-existing POS-derived lipofuscin (Fig. 2g).

5-HT_{1A} agonist reduced oxidative damage in cultured RPE cells

H_2O_2 treatment led to a 65% increase in lipid peroxidation as measured by levels of 4HNE and MDA, and to a 70% increase in the level of nitrotyrosine-modified proteins. These values were significantly reduced to control levels in cells treated with 8-OH DPAT for 24 hours (Fig. 3a,b). There was no significant difference whether 8-OH DPAT was applied pre- or post-exposure to H_2O_2.

5-HT_{1A} agonist protects against mitochondrial damage in cultured RPE cells

Since superoxide radicals are largely derived from mitochondria in the RPE we assessed if 8-OH DPAT could protect against mitochondrial damage. 8-OH DPAT alone had no effect on Complex IV activity. Pre-treatment of ARPE19 cells with 8-OH DPAT for both 3 (data not shown) and 24 hours reduced the impact of oxidative stress on the level of cytochrome *c* oxidase (Complex IV) by up to 50% (Fig. 3c). Post-treatment with 8-OH DPAT for 3 hours (data not shown) had no effect while 24 hour post-treatment did show a significant improvement of around 65%. Furthermore, both pre and post-treatment with 8-OH DPAT significantly protected cultured RPE cells from H_2O_2-induced mitochondrial DNA damage and reduced the number of lesions per 10 kb by greater than 50% (Fig. 3d).

5-HT_{1A} agonist reduces superoxide anion generation and increases antioxidant capacity in cultured RPE cells

Treatment with H_2O_2 stimulated a 102% increase in the generation of superoxide anions (Fig. 4a). 8-OH DPAT was able to reduce oxidative stressor-induced superoxide generation when given either before or after H_2O_2 treatment. However, pre-treatment appeared to be the most effective. A 3 and 24 hour 8-OH DPAT pre-treatment of H_2O_2-exposed cells resulted in a greater than 67% and 35%, respectively, reduction in superoxide anions. Post-treatment was significantly less effective compared to pre-treatment, and a significant reduction in superoxide anions was only observed for cells exposed to H_2O_2 and then treated with 8-OH DPAT for 24 hours (Fig. 4a). There was no significant difference between 1 or 10 μM 8-OH DPAT on the reduction in superoxide generation. Interestingly, although 8-OH DPAT alone

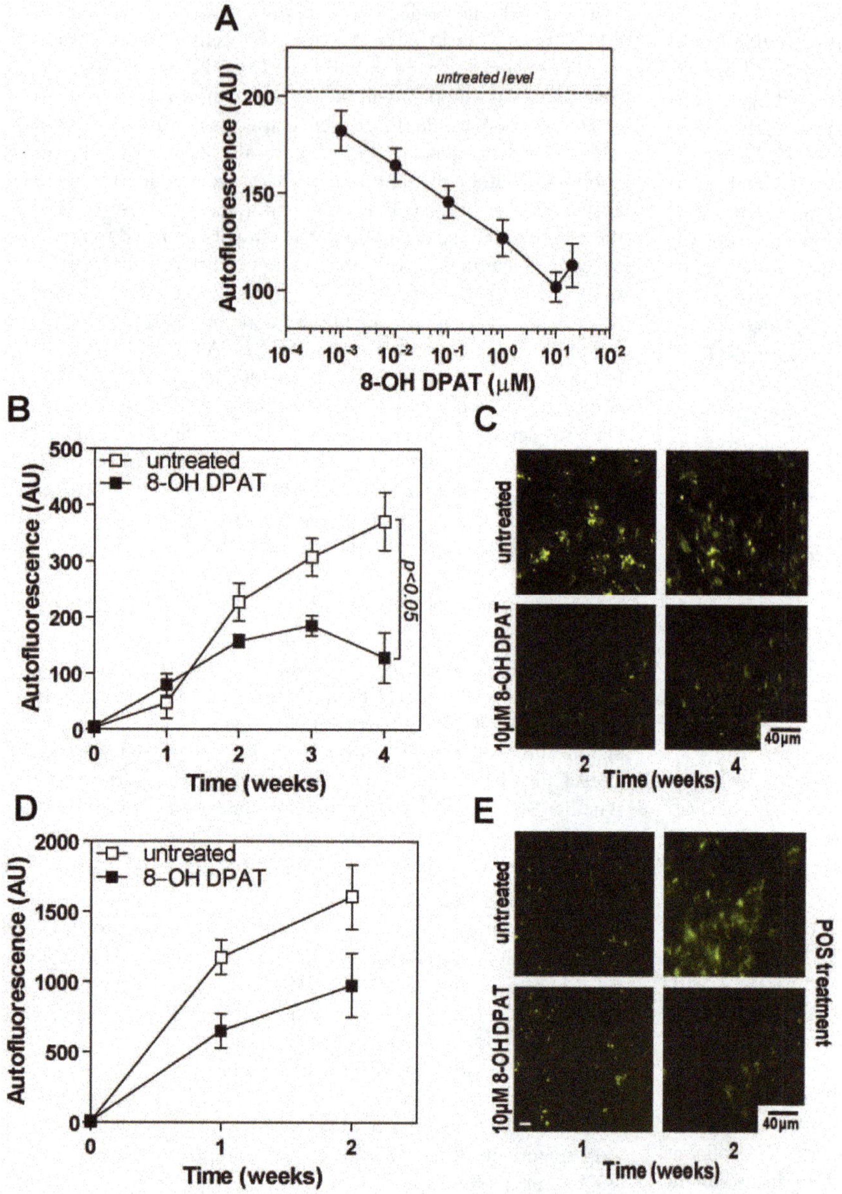

Figure 1. 8-OH DPAT reduces lipofuscin accumulation in cultured RPE cells. A - The effect of different concentrations of 8-OH DPAT on lipofuscin accumulation from autophagy in human ARPE19 cells. Cells were maintained in basal medium and received 10 μM 8-OH DPAT every two days for four weeks. **B** - Autofluorescent intensity of ARPE19 cells treated with 10 μM 8-OH DPAT every two days for up to 4 weeks. Control cells received vehicle alone. **C** - Fluorescent micrographs of ARPE19 cells as described in B showing reduced lipofuscin granules in 8-OH DPAT treated cells compared to controls. **D** - Autofluorescent intensity of ARPE19 cells fed POS treated with 10 μM 8-OH DPAT every two days for up to 14 days. Control cells received POS and saline vehicle alone. **E** - Fluorescent micrographs of ARPE19 cells described in D showing reduced lipofuscin granule accumulation in 8-OH DPAT treated cells fed POS compared to untreated controls. Fluorescence intensity was determined by flow cytometric analysis. Data represent the mean of three experiments. Bar marker is 50 μM.

had no significant effect on endogenous superoxide anion generation in the absence of oxidative stressor, in the presence of H_2O_2 it was able to reduce levels of superoxide anions to significantly less than in untreated control cultures. This effect may be due to the oxidative stressor activating one or more of the antioxidant pathways.

Treatment with 8-OH DPAT led to a 42% increase in MnSOD following H_2O_2 exposure compared with oxidatively stressed cells not receiving 8-OH DPAT (Fig. 4b). The increase in MnSOD levels were similar whether 8-OH DPAT was given before or after H_2O_2 treatment. Cells treated with both H_2O_2 and 8-OH DPAT showed a significant decrease in the GSH/GSSG ratio indicating an increase in reduced glutathione compared to untreated controls (Fig. 4c). Exposure to 8-OH DPAT for 24 hours post H_2O_2 resulted in an increase in the GSH/GSSG ratio to a level seen in untreated cells. By contrast, preexposure to 8-OH DPAT only demonstrated a small increase in the GSH/GSSG ratio compared to cells treated with H_2O_2 alone (Fig. 4c).

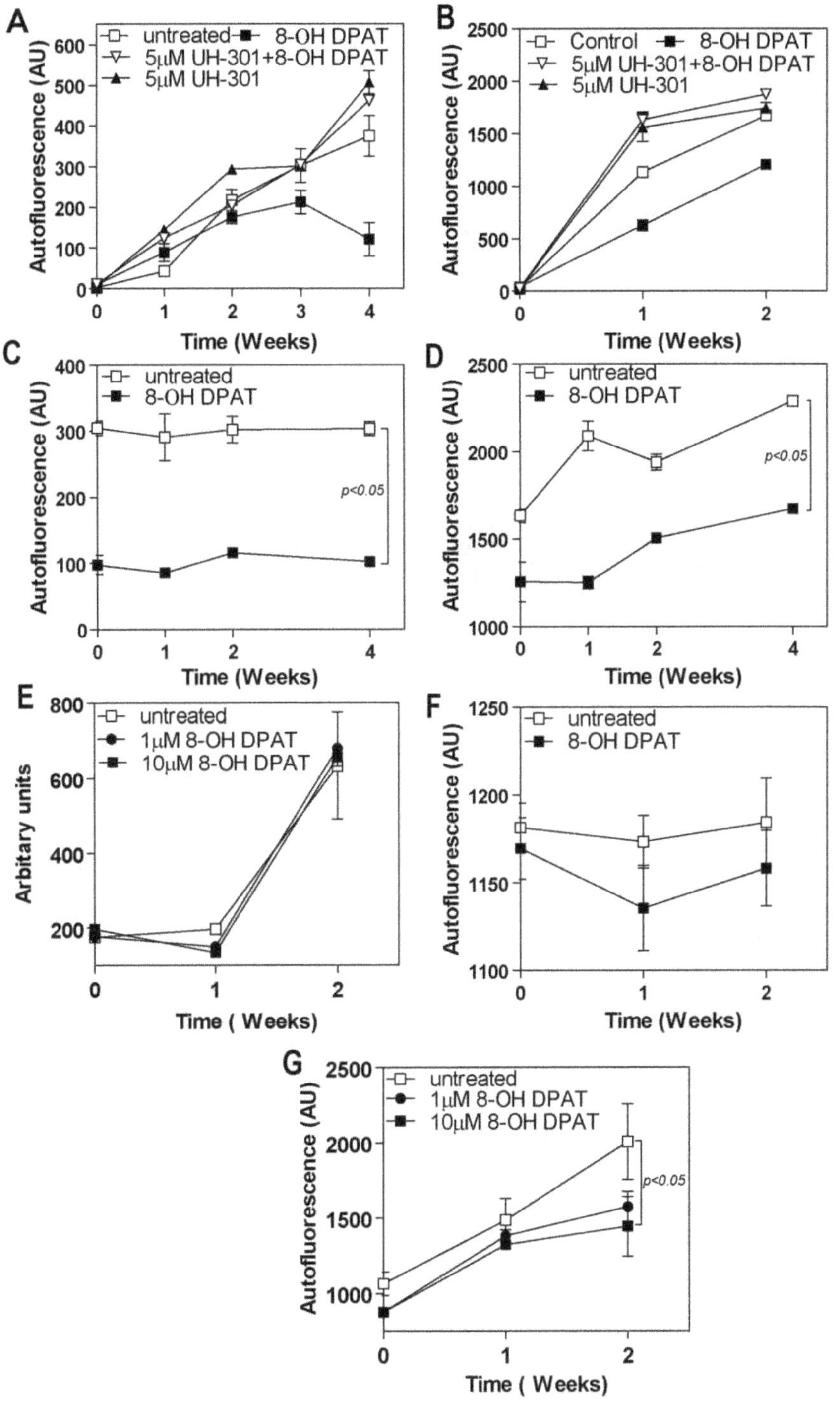

Figure 2. The effect of 8-OH DPAT is sustained following discontinuation but 8-OH DPAT has only a minimal effect on pregenerated lipofuscin. A, B - The effect of the selective 5-HT_{1A} receptor antagonist, UH-301 (5 μM) on 8-OH DPAT (10 uM) reduction in autophagy- (**A**) and POS-derived (**B**) lipofuscin accumulation in cultured RPE. **C, D** - To determine if the effect of 8-OH DPAT was sustained following discontinuation of 8-OH DPAT treatment, 8OH DPAT treatment was discontinued after 28 days and the cells maintained in basal medium (**C**) or fed POS (**D**) for a further 28 days. **E, F, G** - To assess the ability of 8-OH DPAT (10 uM) to remove pregenerated lipofuscin, 8-OH DPAT was added every second day for 28 days after: **E** – 28 days accumulation of autophagy-derived lipofuscin; **F** - cultures were fed mature lipofuscin granules; **G** - 14 days accumulation of POS-derived lipofuscin. Data represent the mean of three experiments.

5-HT_{1A} agonist mediates neuroprotection in a mouse model of AMD

The experiments in the ARPE-19 cell line indicated that 8-OH DPAT increased protection from oxidative stress and decreased the accumulation lipofuscin arising either form phagocytosis or autophagy, but would these effects have physiologic consequences in the retina? To examine possible in vivo protective actions, we employed the SOD2 knockdown model which exhibits an AMD-

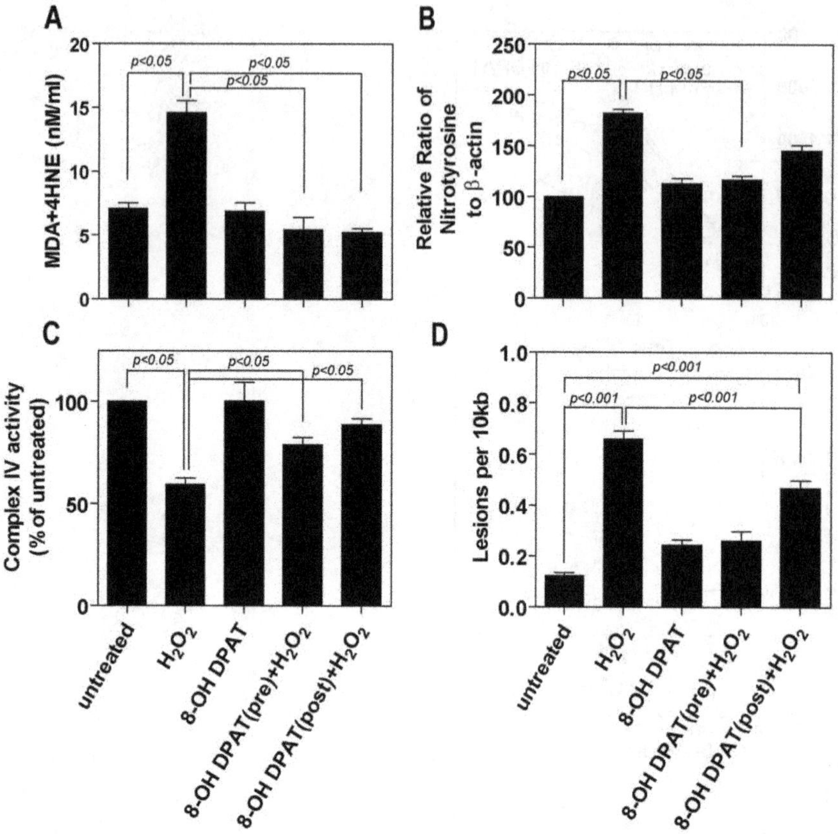

Figure 3. 8-OH DPAT reduces lipid peroxidation and peroxynitrite accumulation and protects against mitochondrial damage in cultured RPE cells exposed to H_2O_2. Cells were exposed to H_2O_2 (200 μM) for 1 hour and either pre-or post treated with 8-OH DPAT (10 μM) for 24 hours. In the case of pretreatment all measurements were made 24 hr after H_2O_2 and for post treatment 8-OH DPAT was added immediately following H_2O_2 exposure. **A** - The level of lipid peroxides (4HNE/MDA) was determined using a commercially available kit from OxisResearch. **B** – Nitrotyrosine levels were assessed by Western blotting using a polyclonal antibody and band intensities were normalized against β-actin. **C** - Cytochome *c* oxidase levels were determined using a Complex IV ELISA assay. **D** - Mitochondrial DNA damage was analyzed as previously described using the long chain PCR reaction. Data represent the mean of three experiments.

like phenotype [15]. Subretinal injection of the AAV-VMD2-*SOD2* Rz, which also contained the mCherry gene as a marker of genetic transduction routinely resulted in 60–80% transduction of the RPE which is in agreement with that previously reported [15] (Fig. 5). As a metric of neuroprotection we measured the full field scotopic ERG response at monthly intervals, beginning one month after subretinal injection of the viruses (Fig. 6a b). Subcutaneous administration of 8-OH DPAT improved the ERG response in *SOD2* knockdown eyes compared to knockdown eyes receiving vehicle control (Fig. 6a,b). In eyes injected with the control virus, AAV-VMD2-mCherry, we observed a modest decline (33%) in ERG amplitudes between the 1 month and 4 month time points. Treatment of the mice with 8-OH DPAT had no impact on the ERG response in these control-treated eyes. Injection of the AAV-VMD2-Rz432 (specific for *SOD2* mRNA) led to a 38% reduction in ERG amplitudes relative to the control treated eyes by one month post-injection. This decrease relative to control injection remained constant throughout the time course. Systemic treatment of the mice with 8-OH DPAT had a significant impact on the ERG response in eyes injected with the *SOD2* ribozyme. By one month after virus injection, a-wave amplitudes in mice treated with either the low-dose or the high dose of drug were elevated over 80% compared to saline treated mice ($P<0.01$) (Fig. 6a). By four months post injection, a-wave amplitude was increased over 100% in low-dose animals and over 130% in mice treated with the high dose of 8-OH DPAT ($P<0.001$). Results for b-wave amplitudes were not as dramatic, but by 4 months these were also elevated by over 70% in 8-OH DPAT mice at both high and low dosages (Fig. 6b).

The simplest interpretation of the ERG results is that treatment of mice with 8-OH DPAT led to increased survival of photoreceptors in the face of RPE oxidative stress. Spectral domain OCT (SD-OCT) was used to measure the thickness of the outer nuclear layer, because this dimension reflects the survival of rod photoreceptor cells. We detected a small (7–14%) but statistically significant ($p<0.01$) difference in the ONL thickness in mice treated with the high dose of 8-OH DPAT (5 mg/kg) at 1–4 months past the time of *SOD2* mRNA knockdown (Fig. 6c). Low dose (0.5 mg/kg) also led to a statistically significant improvement in ONL dimensions at 3 and 4 months past injection (data not shown). *SOD2* knockdown resulted in a significant increase in the oxidative stress marker 8OHdG in both the neural retina and RPE (Fig. 7). However, this was significantly reduced in SOD2 knockdown eyes of animals receiving high dose 8-OH DPAT and reached levels of control eyes that received AAV-VMD2-mCherry (Fig. 7).

5-HT_{1A} agonist reduces lipofuscin accumulation in vivo

In the *SOD2* knockdown model of dry AMD, loss of photoreceptors correlates with an increase in RPE autofluores-

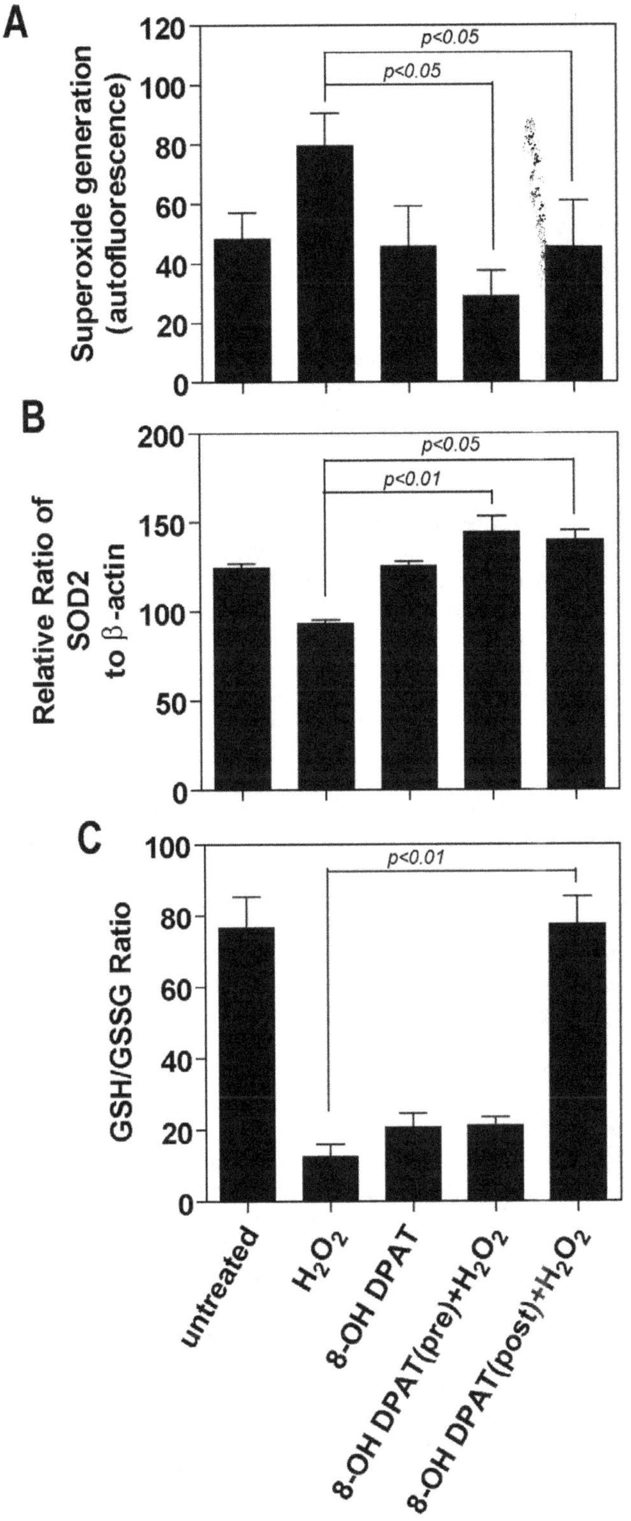

Figure 4. 8-OH DPAT reduces superoxide anion generation and increases antioxidant capacity in cultured RPE cells. Cells were exposed to H_2O_2 (200 μM) for 1 hour and either pre-or post treated with 8-OH DPAT (10 μM) for 24 hours. In the case of pretreatment all measurements were made 24 hr after H_2O_2 and for post treatment 8-OH DPAT was added immediately following H_2O_2 exposure. **A** - Superoxide generation was measured using FACS analysis following staining with MitoSOX and results are expressed as the mean fluorescence intensity. **B** - SOD2 levels were determined by Western blot analysis. **C** - The ratio of reduced glutathione (GSH) to the oxidized form of glutathione (GSSG) was measured by ELISA. Data represent the mean of three experiments.

cence [15]. To establish whether treatment with 8-OH DPAT reduced lipofuscin in ribozyme treated eyes, confocal microscroscopy was used to measure autofluorescence in the RPE layer 4 months after MnSOD knockdown (Fig. 8a). We noted a 60% reduction in autofluorescence, a measure of lipofuscin content of the RPE, in *SOD2* knockdown eyes treated with either the high or the low dose of 8-OH DPAT compared to eyes receiving vehicle alone (Fig. 8b).

Discussion

Our results demonstrate the 5-HT_{1A} receptor agonist, 8-OH DPAT, is able to protect the retina from degeneration by reducing oxidative damage. We have shown that 8-OH DPAT can protect against oxidative stress by increasing antioxidant protection, reducing lipofuscin levels which, in turn, reduced the generation of ROS and prevented mitochondrial damage. Furthermore, 8-OH DPAT was able to confer neuroprotection in an animal model of AMD by reducing both oxidative stress and lipofuscin levels. These findings extend our previous observations in which we observed that 5-HT_{1A} receptor agonists were able to protect the retina from severe photo-oxidative stress, complement deposition and microglial activation [22,23].

We used 8-OH DPAT in this study as it is a potent, and highly specific, 5-HT_{1A} receptor agonist [21] that has been extensively used to study neuroprotection in the brain [30,31,32,33,34]. The 5-HT_{1A} receptor is expressed in both the neural retina and the RPE [22,23,24] and we have previously reported that 8-OH DPAT compares well with other 5-HT_{1A} receptor agonists in providing retinal neuroprotection [22].

Both autophagy- and POS-derived lipofuscin accumulation was reduced by the 5-HT_{1A} receptor agonist in cultured ARPE19 cells. We, and others, have previously shown that autophagy-derived lipofuscin is a significant component of RPE lipofuscin [35,36,37] and that it is largely derived from the incomplete degradation of damaged organelles such as mitochondria which are prolific in the highly metabolically active RPE [9,38,39,40].

Our data show that 8-OH DPAT is able to increase the levels of antioxidants such as MnSOD and glutathione which in turn reduce the generation of superoxide anions, diminish mitochondrial DNA damage and prevent the accumulation of oxidative endproducts such as MDA, 4HNE and nitrated protein. This increase in antioxidants improves mitochondrial function and reduces mitochondrial damage thereby reducing the autophagic turnover of these organelles. In addition, 5-HT has been shown to stimulate mTOR phosphorylation [41] and therefore 8-OH DPAT may be able to decrease autophagy induction. The 5-HT_{1A} receptor agonist was also able to induce a small, but significant reduction in POS-derived lipofuscin. The reason for this is unclear but could be due to either improved lysosomal function due to a reduction in autophagic load or reduced oxidative modification of ingested POS. Prior reduction in lipofuscin levels was maintained following removal of the 5-HT_{1A} receptor agonist from the culture system although, in the case of POS-derived lipofuscin, the rate of lipofuscin accumulation eventually recovered to that seen in untreated cultures. However, 8-OH DPAT did not lead to a major reduction in preformed lipofuscin indicating that the 5-HT_{1A} receptor agonist acts by inhibiting lipofuscinogenesis rather than reducing existing lipofuscin.

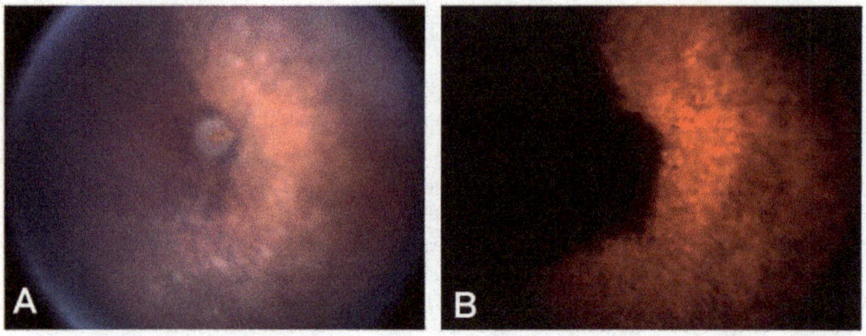

Figure 5. Extent of retinal transduction with AAV-VMD2-*SOD2* Rz. Digital fundus images were made 4 months following subretinal injection of the AAV-VMD2-*SOD2* Rz, which also contained the mCherry gene as a marker of genetic transduction. As previously reported [15] we routinely observe 60–80% transduction of the RPE. This was revealed as red-fluorescence using a long wave length filter (A) and as thinning of the retina (hypopigmentation) as a consequence of knockdown of MnSOD (B).

Activation of the 5-HT_{1A} receptor is neuroprotective in several in vitro [25,42] and in vivo [30,34,43] model systems, but the mechanisms underlying these effects are incompletely understood. 5-HT1A receptor stimulation has been shown to lead to increased expression of several components of the antioxidant defense system, including SOD and catalase [44,45,46], anti-apoptotic proteins from the prosurvival members of the BCL family (e.g., Bcl-2 and Bcl-XL) [47,48] and inhibitors of apoptosis proteins (e.g., Bax, XIAP) [47,48,49]. Similarly, we have shown that SOD2 is upregulated together with a decrease in the GSH/GSSG ratio in ARPE-19 cells by 5-HT_{1A} receptor activation. This, at least in part, explains the mechanism by which 8-OH DPAT reduced superoxide levels and protected against lipid peroxidation, nitrotyrosine levels and mitochondrial damage. The potential roles of upregulation of other endogenous defenses in RPE protection and lipofuscin inhibition remain to be explored.

Our *in vitro* observations were validated in our mouse model of atrophic AMD. We have previously shown that knockdown of SOD2 expression in the RPE leads to accumulation of lipofuscin and vacuolization and atrophy of the RPE culminating in death of overlying photoreceptor cells [15]. Systemic treatment with 8-OH DPAT sustained a- and b-wave ERG amplitudes in SOD2 knock down eyes compared to those not receiving 5-HT_{1A} receptor agonist. Furthermore, the loss in ONL thickness associated with SOD2 knock down was prevented in mice treated with 8 OH-DPAT. Taken together, these observations would suggest that systemic 5-HT_{1A} receptor agonist treatment preserves the survival of photoreceptor cells. This protection was associated with a decrease in the oxidative stress marker 8OHdG and reduced accumulation of lipofuscin in the RPE.

We conclude that 5-HT_{1A} receptor agonists offer a therapeutic option for retinal degenerations such as AMD, diabetic retinopathy or retinitis pigmentosa which involve oxidative stress and/or lipofuscin accumulation.

Materials and Methods

Cell Culture

The ARPE19 cell line was obtained from ATCC (CRL-2302). ARPE19 cells were grown to confluence as previously described [50,51] and then maintained in basal medium (Ham's F10+2% fetal bovine serum (Invitrogen, Carlsbad, CA)) for 7 days prior to experimentation.

In vitro lipofuscin formation

Lipofuscin formation in cultured RPE cells was achieved using our standard protocols [36,52]. In brief, lipofuscin formation was induced in confluent, differentiated cultures of ARPE-19 by either a) maintaining cells for up to 28 days in basal medium (a measure of autophagic-derived lipofuscin accumulation) or b) incubating with isolated bovine photoreceptor outer segments (POS, 2×10^7/ml) every two days for 14 days (a measure of phagocytic-derived lipofuscin accumulation).

Lipofuscin isolation and phagocytosis by RPE

Lipofuscin granules were isolated and from 60–80 year old human donor eyes and purified by differential sucrose gradient centrifugation as previously described [53]. Lipofuscin granules were suspended in PBS and the concentration was determined by counting granules on a hemocytometer. Cultures were fed granules at a concentration of ~300 granules/cell and maintained for 7 days prior to experimentation.

5HT_{1A} agonist treatment

To assess the ability of the 5-HT_{1A} receptor agonist, 8-OH DPAT (Sigma, St. Louis, MO, USA), to reduce lipofuscin formation in cultured RPE cells, this compound was added to the culture medium every 48 hours at concentrations ranging from 0.1 to 20 μM. All experiments were undertaken in basal medium (Ham's F10+2% FBS), and cells receiving vehicle alone (PBS) acted as negative controls. To determine if the effect of 8-OH DPAT was sustained following discontinuation of 5-HT_{1A} receptor agonist treatment, 8-OH DPAT treatment was discontinued after 28 days and the cells maintained in basal medium or fed POS for a further 28 days. To assess the ability of 8-OH DPAT to remove existing lipofuscin, autophagy-derived lipofuscin and phagocytic-derived lipofuscin were allowed to accumulate as described above and then 8-OH DPAT was added every second day for up to 28 days. To confirm that 8-OH DPAT was acting via the 5-HT_{1A} receptor agonist we included the 5-HT_{1A} receptor antagonist S(-)-UH-301 at 5 μM in some experiments. To determine the effect of timing of 8-OH DPAT treatment on oxidative stress markers, RPE cultures were either pre-treated with 8-OH DPAT (at 1 or 10 μM) for 3 or 24 hours prior to exposure to 200 μM H_2O_2 for 1 hour or treated with the 5HT_{1A} agonist for 3 or 24 hours post-exposure to H_2O_2. Cells not exposed to oxidative stressor served as a negative control, and cells exposed to oxidative stressor but not 8-OH DPAT served as a positive

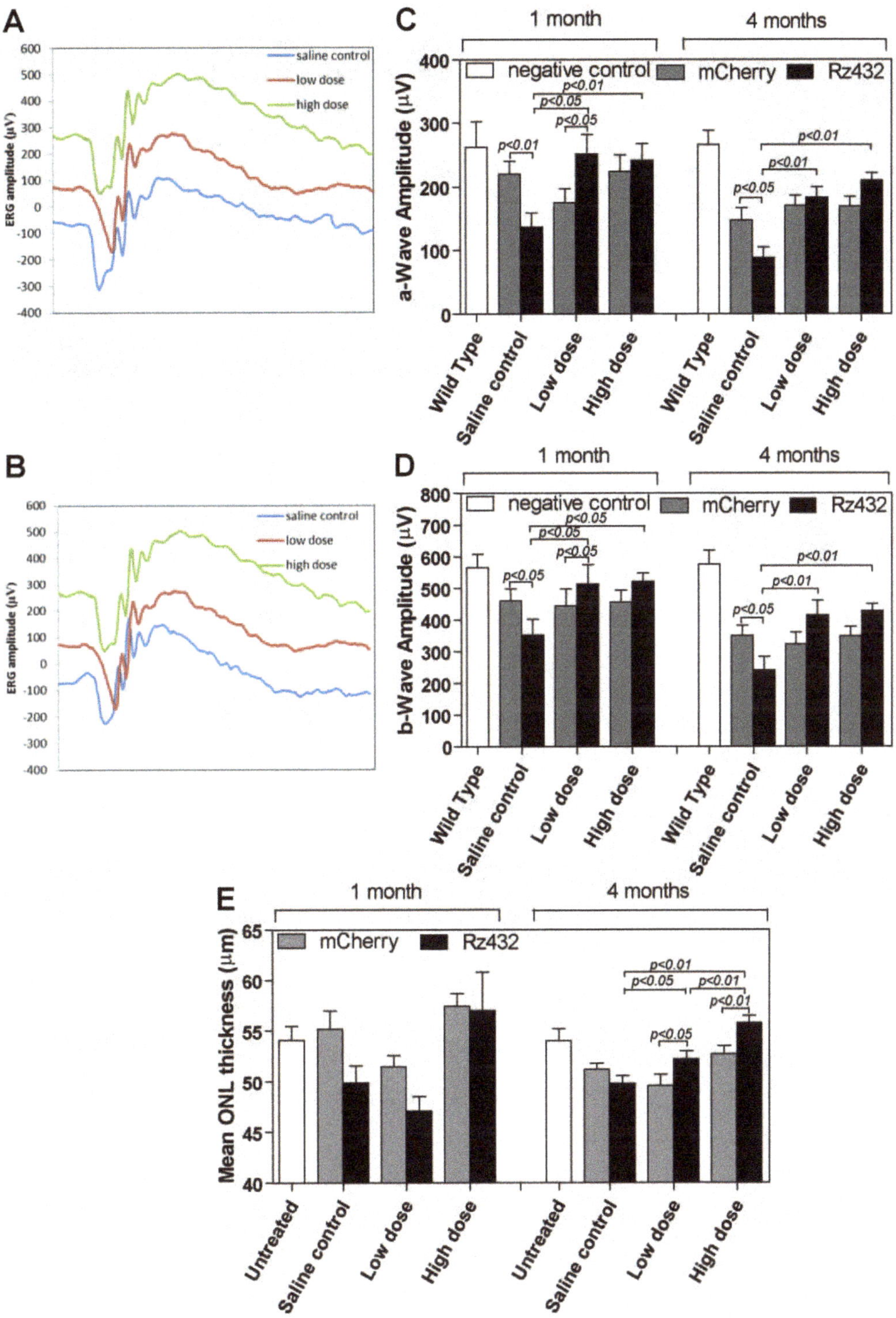

Figure 6. ERG a-wave and b-wave amplitudes and retinal thickness measured in AAV-ribozyme SOD2 knockdown eyes and control eyes treated with 8-OH DPAT. Eyes received injection of AAV-*SOD2* ribozyme or AAV-mCherry and animals received subcutaneous 8-OH DPAT or saline control for up to 4 months. ERGs were obtained at 1 and 4 months following virus injection: **A & B** - ERG wave-forms from mice treated with AAV-mCherry (**A**) or AAV-VMD2-*SOD2* Rz (**B**). Simultaneous full-field ERG measurements were recorded in dark-adapted mice four months after injection with AAV. The scale units on the ordinate are 100 microvolts. The graphs show wave forms for mice treated with saline, blue lines, low dose (0.5 mg/kg) 8-HO-DPAT, red lines, or high dose (5 mg/kg) 8-HO-DPAT, green lines. **C** – a-wave; **D** – b-wave. **E** - ONL thickness measured by SD-OCT at 1 and 4 months. Untreated wild type animals acted as the baseline control. (10 animals per group, $P \leq 0.01$ for all doses and time points).

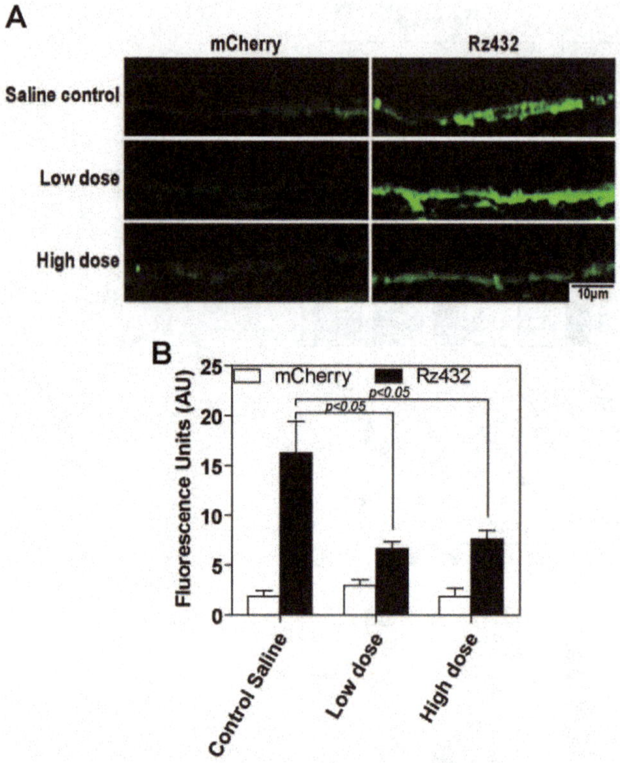

Figure 7. 8-OH DPAT decreases oxidative stress in the RPE of SOD2 knockdown eyes of mice. Eyes received injection of AAV-*SOD2* ribozyme or AAV-mCherry and animals received subcutaneous 8-OH DPAT or saline control for up to 4 months. Sections were stained for 8-hydroxydeoxyguanosine (8OHdG) (green). **A** – Representative sections of 8OHdG expression in the RPE of control and SOD2 eyes receiving different concentrations of 8-OH DPAT. **B** - Graph shows quantitation of 8OHdG fluorescence in the RPE layer.

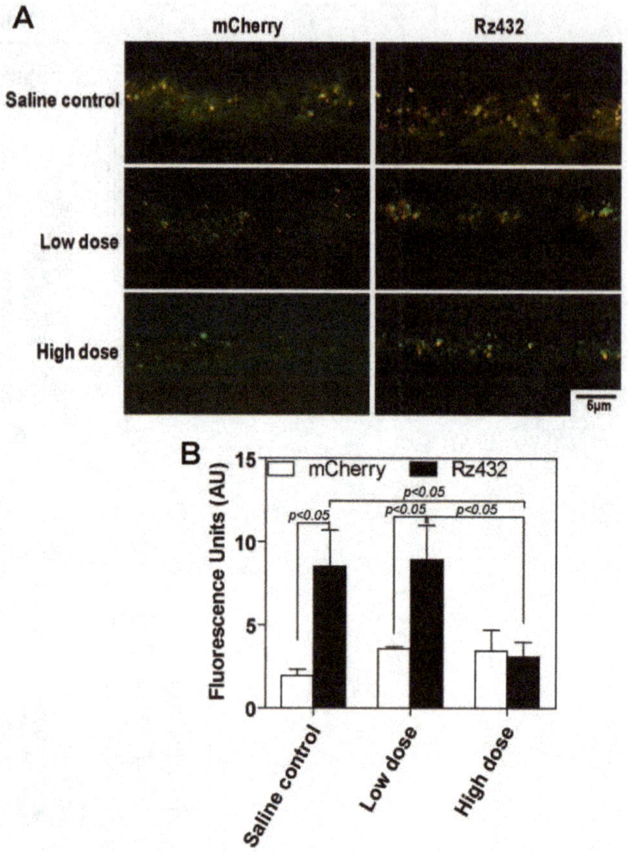

Figure 8. 8-OH DPAT decreases RPE autofluorescence in SOD2 knockdown eyes of mice. Eyes received injection of AAV-*SOD2* ribozyme or AAV-mCherry and animals received subcutaneous 8-OH DPAT or saline control for up to 4 months. **A** - Confocal fluorescence microscopy of the RPE layers from AAV-mCherry and AAV-ribozyme treated eyes treated with saline, low dose or high dose of 8-OH DPAT. **B** - Treatment with 8-OH DPAT lowered autofluorescence in oxidatively stressed RPE in mice. Mice were injected with AAV-mCherry or AAV-Rz*SOD2*-mCherry and analyzed after 4 months of daily injections of saline (no treatment) low dose or high dose of 8-OH DPAT. * $P<0.05$, ** $P<0.01$ (compared to AAV-RzSOD2 control).

control. Cells exposed to 8-OH DPAT only acted as an additional control.

Analysis of lipofuscin accumulation in cultured RPE cells

Lipofuscin levels in cultured cells were assessed by fluorescence microscopy and quantified by both FACS and image analysis at time 0 and weekly thereafter as previously described [36,52]. For FACS analysis, cells were resuspended in phosphate-buffered saline (PBS) at 1×10^5 cells/ml. The mean autofluorescence per 10,000 RPE cells was determined using a fluorophotometric flow cytometer, excitation at 488 nm and emission at 600 nm. Fluorescence microscopy images of cultured cells were obtained using an inverted microscope equipped with 450 nm to 490 nm excitation and 520-nm barrier filters. Fluorescence intensity of the intracellular, autofluorescent granules was assessed by ImageJ program available at: http://rsbweb.nih.gov/.

Superoxide anion assay

Superoxide generation was measured using FACS analysis following staining with MitoSOX (Molecular Probes, Invitrogen, Carlsbad, CA) and results are expressed as the mean fluorescence intensity.

Cytochrome Oxidase, 4HNE/MDA and nitrosylation assays

Cytochome *c* oxidase levels were measured using a Complex IV ELISA assay (MitoSciences, Eugene, Oregon, USA). The level of the lipid peroxides 4 hydroxynonenal (4HNE) and malonaldehyde (MDA) were determined using a commercially available kit from OxisResearch (Burlinghame, CA, USA). The LPO-586 method is based on the reaction of the chromogenic reagent N-methyl-2-phenyindole with MDA and 4HNE. Protein nitration was assessed by Western blotting using the polyclonal α-nitrotyrosine antibody from Millipore (Billerica, MA, USA) and normalized against β-actin.

MnSOD and Glutathione assays

MnSOD levels were determined by Western blot analysis and the ratio of reduced glutathione (GSH) to the oxidized form of glutathione (GSSG) was measured by ELISA using a kit from OxisResearch (Burlinghame, CA, USA).

Mitochondrial DNA damage assay

Mitochondrial DNA (mtDNA) damage was analyzed as previously described using the long chain PCR reaction [51]. In brief, genomic DNA was extracted and qPCR was performed to determine the average oxidative lesion frequency. The PCR conditions used in this study were based on published data using previously reported sequences for mtDNA primers [51,54]. qPCR was carried out with all reactions being a total of 100 µl containing 15 ng of total genomic DNA, 1 unit of XL r*Tth* polymerase, 3.3 XL PCR buffer II (containing potassium acetate, glycerol, and DMSO), and final concentrations of 200 µM dNTPs, 1.2 mM $Mg(AOC)_2$ and 0.1 µM primers. The gene fragments were amplified and resolved on a 1% agarose gel. The intensity of the PCR product bands was quantified with Scion Image analysis software (Scion Corp., version Beta 4.0.2).

Animals and injections

All animal studies were performed under a protocol approved by the Institutional Animal Care and Use Committee at the University of Florida , (IACUC Study #201005197), and in accordance with the NIH Guide for Care and Use of Laboratory Animals and ARVO Statement for the Use of Animals in Ophthalmic and Vision Research. We used the previously described *SOD2* knockdown model that exhibits an AMD-like phenotype including electroretinogram changes, basal deposits, elevated lipofuscin accumulation, thickening of Bruch's membrane and patchy regions of RPE atrophy overlying photoreceptor degeneration [15]. The right eyes of C57Bl/6 mice were injected with Adeno-associated virus (AAV) expressing a ribozyme that cleaves the mRNA for mitochondrial superoxide dismutase (MnSOD encoded by the *SOD2* gene). Expression of the ribozyme was restricted to the RPE using the *VMD2* (bestrophin) promoter and by subretinal injection with AAV serotype 1. This virus also expressed the marker gene, mCherry, to determine the extent and location of virus infection. The left eyes were injected with virus expressing only mCherry. All mice were housed in a 12 h:12 h light/dark cycle under specific pathogen-free (SPF) conditions. Subretinal AAV injections were performed as described by Timmers et al. [55]. C57Bl/6 mice were injected at postnatal day 15 (P15). For this purpose, mice were anesthetized by ketamine/xylazine injection. Pupils were dilated with 1 drop of 1% atropine sulfate and 2.5% phenylephrine. Right eyes were injected in the superior hemisphere with 1 µl AAV-*VMD2 Rz432* mCherry (2×10^9 vector genomes). Left eyes were injected with AAV-VMD2-mCherry at the same titer.

Effect of 8-OH DPAT in the SOD2 knockdown model for AMD

Mice were randomly assigned to one of three groups and received daily subcutaneous injections of either sterile saline, 0.5 mg/kg body weight 8-OH-DPAT in sterile saline (low dose), or 5.0 mg/kg 8-OH-DPAT (high dose). At monthly intervals mice were evaluated by digital fundus imaging, full-field scotopic (dark adapted) electroretinography (ERG) and spectral domain optical coherence tomography (SD-OCT). At four months, mice were euthanized and eyes were prepared for cryosectioning. Confocal microscroscopy was used to measure autofluorescence in the RPE layer of untreated eyes and virus-treated eyes with or without 8OH-DPAT. Excitation frequency was 387 nm and emission frequency was 440–684 nm and fluorescence intensity was assessed using ImageJ. Sections were also used to assess damage to retinal structure by light microscopy and immunostaining for 8-Oxo-2′-deoxyguanosine (8OHdG) (Abcam, Cambridge, MA, USA) as a measurement of oxidative stress using previously described methodology [56].

Statistics

All experiments were repeated at least three times. FACS, autofluorescence, antioxidant, ERG and SD-OCT data were compared using a Student's t test plus ANOVA with Bonferroni correction for multiple comparisons. The Mann-Whitney test was used to determine statistical significance in the Western blotting analysis, qPCR. Results are expressed as mean±SEM. $p<0.05$ is considered statistically significant.

Author Contributions

Conceived and designed the experiments: MEB CR ASL. Performed the experiments: PT HVR SKM JC HM HL SS XQ. Analyzed the data: MEB ASL PT JC XQ. Wrote the paper: MEB ASL PT.

References

1. Friedman DS, O'Colmain BJ, Munoz B, Tomany SC, McCarty C, et al. (2004) Prevalence of age-related macular degeneration in the United States. Arch Ophthalmol 122: 564–572.
2. von Ruckmann A, Fitzke FW, Bird AC (1999) Distribution of pigment epithelium autofluorescence in retinal disease state recorded in vivo and its change over time. Graefes Arch Clin Exp Ophthalmol 237: 1–9.
3. Lois N, Owens SL, Coco R, Hopkins J, Fitzke FW, et al. (2002) Fundus autofluorescence in patients with age-related macular degeneration and high risk of visual loss. Am J Ophthalmol 133: 341–349.
4. Holz FG, Bindewald-Wittich A, Fleckenstein M, Dreyhaupt J, Scholl HP, et al. (2007) Progression of geographic atrophy and impact of fundus autofluorescence patterns in age-related macular degeneration. Am J Ophthalmol 143: 463–472.
5. von Ruckmann A, Fitzke FW, Bird AC (1997) In vivo fundus autofluorescence in macular dystrophies. Arch Ophthalmol 115: 609–615.
6. Boulton ME (2009) Lipofuscin of the RPE. In: Lois N, Forrester JV, eds. Fundus Autofluorescence: Wolters Kluwer/Lippincott Williams and Wilkins. pp 14–26.
7. Curcio CA, Medeiros NE, Millican CL (1996) Photoreceptor loss in age-related macular degeneration. Invest Ophthalmol Vis Sci 37: 1236–1249.
8. Boulton M, Rozanowska M, Rozanowski B, Wess T (2004) The photoreactivity of ocular lipofuscin. Photochem Photobiol Sci 3: 759–764.
9. Sparrow JR, Boulton ME (2005) RPE lipofuscin and its role in retinal pathology. Exp Eye Res 80: 595–606.
10. Holz FG, Bellman C, Staudt S, Schutt F, Volcker HE (2001) Fundus autofluorescence and development of geographic atrophy in age-related macular degeneration. Invest Ophthalmol Vis Sci 42: 1051–1056.
11. Solbach U, Keilhauer C, Knabben H, Wolf S (1997) Imaging of retinal autofluorescence in patients with age-related macular degeneration. Retina 17: 385–389.
12. Schmitz-Valckenberg S, Bultmann S, Dreyhaupt J, Bindewald A, Holz FG, et al. (2004) Fundus autofluorescence and fundus perimetry in the junctional zone of geographic atrophy in patients with age-related macular degeneration. Invest Ophthalmol Vis Sci 45: 4470–4476.
13. Ambati J, Anand A, Fernandez S, Sakurai E, Lynn BC, et al. (2003) An animal model of age-related macular degeneration in senescent Ccl-2- or Ccr-2-deficient mice. Nat Med 9: 1390–1397.
14. Malek G, Johnson LV, Mace BE, Saloupis P, Schmechel DE, et al. (2005) Apolipoprotein E allele-dependent pathogenesis: a model for age-related retinal degeneration. Proc Natl Acad Sci U S A 102: 11900–11905.
15. Justilien V, Pang JJ, Renganathan K, Zhan X, Crabb JW, et al. (2007) SOD2 knockdown mouse model of early AMD. Invest Ophthalmol Vis Sci 48: 4407–4420.
16. Hageman GS, Mullins RF (1999) Molecular composition of drusen as related to substructural phenotype. Molecular Vision 5: 28.
17. Zhou J, Cai B, Jang YP, Pachydaki S, Schmidt AM, et al. (2005) Mechanisms for the induction of HNE- MDA- and AGE-adducts, RAGE and VEGF in retinal pigment epithelial cells. Exp Eye Res 80: 567–580.
18. Radu RA, Han Y, Bui TV, Nusinowitz S, Bok D, et al. (2005) Reductions in serum vitamin A arrest accumulation of toxic retinal fluorophores: a potential therapy for treatment of lipofuscin-based retinal diseases. Invest Ophthalmol Vis Sci 46: 4393–4401.
19. Travis GH, Golczak M, Moise AR, Palczewski K (2007) Diseases caused by defects in the visual cycle: retinoids as potential therapeutic agents. Annu Rev Pharmacol Toxicol 47: 469–512.
20. Radu RA, Mata NL, Nusinowitz S, Liu X, Sieving PA, et al. (2003) Treatment with isotretinoin inhibits lipofuscin accumulation in a mouse model of recessive Stargardt's macular degeneration. Proc Natl Acad Sci U S A 100: 4742–4747.

21. Pucadyil TJ, Kalipatnapu S, Chattopadhyay A (2005) The serotonin1A receptor: a representative member of the serotonin receptor family. Cell Mol Neurobiol 25: 553–580.
22. Collier RJ, Patel Y, Martin EA, Dembinska O, Hellberg M, et al. (2011) Agonists at the Serotonin Receptor (5-HT1A) Protect the Retina from Severe Photo-Oxidative Stress. Invest Ophthalmol Vis Sci 52: 2118–2126.
23. Collier RJ, Wang Y, Smith SS, Martin EA, Ornberg R, et al. (2011) Complement deposition and microglial activation in the outer retina in light-induced retinopathy: Inhibition by a 5-HT_{1A} agonist. Invest Ophthalmol Vis Sci(in press).
24. Nash MS, Osborne NN (1997) Pharmacologic evidence for 5-HT1A receptors associated with human retinal pigment epithelial cells in culture. Invest Ophthalmol Vis Sci 38: 510–519.
25. Ahlemeyer B, Krieglstein J (1997) Stimulation of 5-HT1A receptor inhibits apoptosis induced by serum deprivation in cultured neurons from chick embryo. Brain Res 777: 179–186.
26. Suchanek B, Struppeck H, Fahrig T (1998) The 5-HT1A receptor agonist BAY x 3702 prevents staurosporine-induced apoptosis. Eur J Pharmacol 355: 95–101.
27. Adayev T, El-Sherif Y, Barua M, Penington NJ, Banerjee P (1999) Agonist stimulation of the serotonin1A receptor causes suppression of anoxia-induced apoptosis via mitogen-activated protein kinase in neuronal HN2-5 cells. J Neurochem 72: 1489–1496.
28. Semkova I, Wolz P, Krieglstein J (1998) Neuroprotective effect of 5-HT1A receptor agonist, Bay X 3702, demonstrated in vitro and in vivo. Eur J Pharmacol 359: 251–260.
29. Peruche B, Backhauss C, Prehn JH, Krieglstein J (1994) Protective effects of 5-HT1A receptor agonists against neuronal damage demonstrated in vivo and in vitro. J Neural Transm Park Dis Dement Sect 8: 73–83.
30. Kline AE, Yu J, Massucci JL, Zafonte RD, Dixon CE (2002) Protective effects of the 5-HT1A receptor agonist 8-hydroxy-2-(di-n-propylamino)tetralin against traumatic brain injury-induced cognitive deficits and neuropathology in adult male rats. Neurosci Lett 333: 179–182.
31. Oosterink BJ, Harkany T, Luiten PG (2003) Post-lesion administration of 5-HT1A receptor agonist 8-OH-DPAT protects cholinergic nucleus basalis neurons against NMDA excitotoxicity. Neuroreport 14: 57–60.
32. Piera MJ, Beaughard M, Michelin MT, Massingham R (1995) Effects of the 5-hydroxytryptamine1A receptor agonists, 8-OH-DPAT, buspirone and flesinoxan, upon brain damage induced by transient global cerebral ischaemia in gerbils. Arch Int Pharmacodyn Ther 329: 347–359.
33. Ramos AJ, Rubio MD, Defagot C, Hischberg L, Villar MJ, et al. (2004) The 5HT1A receptor agonist, 8-OH-DPAT, protects neurons and reduces astroglial reaction after ischemic damage caused by cortical devascularization. Brain Res 1030: 201–220.
34. Torup L, Moller A, Sager TN, Diemer NH (2000) Neuroprotective effect of 8-OH-DPAT in global cerebral ischemia assessed by stereological cell counting. Eur J Pharmacol 395: 137–141.
35. Burke JM, Skumatz CM (1998) Autofluorescent inclusions in long-term postconfluent cultures of retinal pigment epithelium. Invest Ophthalmol Vis Sci 39: 1478–1486.
36. Wassell J, Ellis S, Burke J, Boulton M (1998) Fluorescence properties of autofluorescent granules generated by cultured human RPE cells. Invest Ophthalmol Vis Sci 39: 1487–1492.
37. Wihlmark U, Wrigstad A, Roberg K, Brunk UT, Nilsson SE (1996) Formation of lipofuscin in cultured retinal pigment epithelial cells exposed to pre-oxidized photoreceptor outer segments. Apmis 104: 272–279.
38. Brizee K, Ordy J (1981) Age pigments, cell loss and functional implications in the brain. In: Sohal RS, ed. Age Pigments Elsevier/North Holland Biomedical Press. pp 317–334.
39. Brunk UT, Jones CB, Sohal RS (1992) A novel hypothesis of lipofuscinogenesis and cellular aging based on interactions between oxidative stress and autophagocytosis. Mutat Res 275: 395–403.
40. Lin H, Xu H, Liang FQ, Liang H, Gupta P, et al. (2011) Mitochondrial DNA Damage and Repair in RPE Associated with Aging and Age-Related Macular Degeneration. Invest Ophthalmol Vis Sci 52: 3521–3529.
41. Liu Y, Fanburg BL (2006) Serotonin-induced growth of pulmonary artery smooth muscle requires activation of phosphatidylinositol 3-kinase/serine-threonine protein kinase B/mammalian target of rapamycin/p70 ribosomal S6 kinase 1. Am J Respir Cell Mol Biol 34: 182–191.
42. Madhavan L, Freed WJ, Anantharam V, Kanthasamy AG (2003) 5-hydroxytryptamine 1A receptor activation protects against N-methyl-D-aspartate-induced apoptotic cell death in striatal and mesencephalic cultures. J Pharmacol Exp Ther 304: 913–923.
43. Bezard E, Gerlach I, Moratalla R, Gross CE, Jork R (2006) 5-HT1A receptor agonist-mediated protection from MPTP toxicity in mouse and macaque models of Parkinson's disease. Neurobiol Dis 23: 77–86.
44. de Freitas RL, Santos IM, de Souza GF, Tome Ada R, Saldanha GB, et al. (2010) Oxidative stress in rat hippocampus caused by pilocarpine-induced seizures is reversed by buspirone. Brain Res Bull 81: 505–509.
45. Rojo AI, Salinas M, Martin D, Perona R, Cuadrado A (2004) Regulation of Cu/Zn-superoxide dismutase expression via the phosphatidylinositol 3 kinase/Akt pathway and nuclear factor-kappaB. J Neurosci 24: 7324–7334.
46. Sullivan NR, Crane JW, Damjanoska KJ, Carrasco GA, D'Souza DN, et al. (2005) Tandospirone activates neuroendocrine and ERK (MAP kinase) signaling pathways specifically through 5-HT1A receptor mechanisms in vivo. Naunyn Schmiedebergs Arch Pharmacol 371: 18–26.
47. Druse MJ, Tajuddin NF, Gillespie RA, Le P (2006) The effects of ethanol and the serotonin(1A) agonist ipsapirone on the expression of the serotonin(1A) receptor and several antiapoptotic proteins in fetal rhombencephalic neurons. Brain Res 1092: 79–86.
48. Kukley M, Schaper C, Becker A, Rose K, Krieglstein J (2001) Effect of 5-hydroxytryptamine 1A receptor agonist BAY X 3702 on BCL-2 and BAX proteins level in the ipsilateral cerebral cortex of rats after transient focal ischaemia. Neuroscience 107: 405–413.
49. Hsiung SC, Tamir H, Franke TF, Liu KP (2005) Roles of extracellular signal-regulated kinase and Akt signaling in coordinating nuclear transcription factor-kappaB-dependent cell survival after serotonin 1A receptor activation. J Neurochem 95: 1653–1666.
50. Boulton ME, Marshall J, Mellerio J (1983) Retinitis pigmentosa: a preliminary report on tissue culture studies of retinal pigment epithelial cells from eight affected human eyes. Exp Eye Res 37: 307–313.
51. Jarrett SG, Boulton ME (2005) Antioxidant up-regulation and increased nuclear DNA protection play key roles in adaptation to oxidative stress in epithelial cells. Free Radic Biol Med 38: 1382–1391.
52. Boulton M, McKechnie NM, Breda J, Bayly M, Marshall J (1989) The formation of autofluorescent granules in cultured human RPE. Invest Ophthalmol Vis Sci 30: 82–89.
53. Godley BF, Shamsi FA, Liang FQ, Jarrett SG, Davies S, et al. (2005) Blue light induces mitochondrial DNA damage and free radical production in epithelial cells. J Biol Chem 280: 21061–21066.
54. Yakes FM, Van Houten B (1997) Mitochondrial DNA damage is more extensive and persists longer than nuclear DNA damage in human cells following oxidative stress. Proc Natl Acad Sci U S A 94: 514–519.
55. Timmers AM, Zhang H, Squitieri A, Gonzalez-Pola C (2001) Subretinal injections in rodent eyes: effects on electrophysiology and histology of rat retina. Mol Vis 7: 131–137.
56. Cai J, Wu L, Qi X, Shaw L, Li Calzi S, et al. (2011) Placenta growth factor-1 exerts time-dependent stabilization of adherens junctions following VEGF-induced vascular permeability. PLoS One 6: e18076.

5

Quantification of Visual Field Loss in Age-Related Macular Degeneration

Jennifer H. Acton[1,2]*, Jonathan M. Gibson[2,3], Robert P. Cubbidge[2]

1 Department of Ophthalmology, New York University, New York, New York, United States of America, **2** Ophthalmic Research Group, Optometry & Vision Sciences, School of Life and Health Sciences, Aston University, Birmingham, United Kingdom, **3** Birmingham and Midland Eye Centre, Birmingham, United Kingdom

Abstract

Background: An evaluation of standard automated perimetry (SAP) and short wavelength automated perimetry (SWAP) for the central 10–2 visual field test procedure in patients with age-related macular degeneration (AMD) is presented in order to determine methods of quantifying the central sensitivity loss in patients at various stages of AMD.

Methods: 10–2 SAP and SWAP Humphrey visual fields and stereoscopic fundus photographs were collected in 27 eyes of 27 patients with AMD and 22 eyes of 22 normal subjects.

Results: Mean Deviation and Pattern Standard Deviation (PSD) varied significantly with stage of disease in SAP (both $p<0.001$) and SWAP (both $p<0.001$), but post hoc analysis revealed overlap of functional values among stages. In SWAP, indices of focal loss were more sensitive to detecting differences in AMD from normal. SWAP defects were greater in depth and area than those in SAP. Central sensitivity (within 1°) changed by −3.9 and −4.9 dB per stage in SAP and SWAP, respectively. Based on defect maps, an AMD Severity Index was derived.

Conclusions: Global indices of focal loss were more sensitive to detecting early stage AMD from normal. The SWAP sensitivity decline with advancing stage of AMD was greater than in SAP. A new AMD Severity Index quantifies visual field defects on a continuous scale. Although not all patients are suitable for SWAP examinations, it is of value as a tool in research studies of visual loss in AMD.

Editor: Demetrios Vavvas, Massachusetts Eye & Ear Infirmary, Harvard Medical School, United States of America

Funding: The authors have no support or funding to report.

Competing Interests: The authors have declared that no competing interests exist.

* E-mail: jenniferhacton@gmail.com

Introduction

Age-related macular degeneration (AMD) is the third leading cause of blindness in the world and accounts for blindness in 8.7% of the global population [1]. Due to the increasing elderly population, it is expected that 17.8 million individuals in the US will be affected by 2050 [2]. The functional loss of central vision due to age-related macular degeneration (AMD) is well documented. However of the studies investigating visual field loss in AMD, some reported reduced threshold values [3,4,5,6,7] whilst others did not [8,9,10,11] and these discrepant findings may reflect differing methods of fundus grading and analyses. In addition no attempt has previously been made to quantify the visual field loss at each stage of severity of AMD. Such knowledge improves our understanding of the natural disease process in terms of visual function and the development of retinal changes. The early identification of patients who would benefit from treatment may help improve visual prognosis.

Past studies evaluating central visual field loss in AMD using non-standard procedures have shown foveal flicker sensitivity to be affected in early AMD [12] and greater flicker perimetry deficits [13]. A number of other techniques have also found functional deficits in AMD, including scotopic sensitivity testing [14,15,16], multifocal electroretinogram [17,18] and preferential hyperacuity perimetry [19]. However these techniques are not readily available for clinical use.

Evidence of short-wavelength sensitivity (SWS) pathway vulnerability in retinal disease suggests the usefulness of short-wavelength automated perimetry (SWAP) in monitoring AMD progression. This is supported by findings of SWS pathway deficits in AMD [20,21,22], SWAP sensitivity loss in eyes with soft drusen [6] and in eyes with diabetic retinopathy [23], and the earlier detection of glaucomatous visual field progression by SWAP [24,25]. Although the use of 30–2 and 24–2 SWAP fields is not clinically widespread due to their greater variability compared to SAP fields [26], the flatter profile of the hill of vision for the 10–2 field allows for more accurate statistical interpretation and greater capability in the detection of focal loss [27].

The aims of the study were to quantify the central visual field loss in a cross-section of AMD patients in standard automated perimetry (SAP) and SWAP. Secondary aims were to evaluate the location of visual field loss in AMD and the appropriate statistical measures that describe visual field loss.

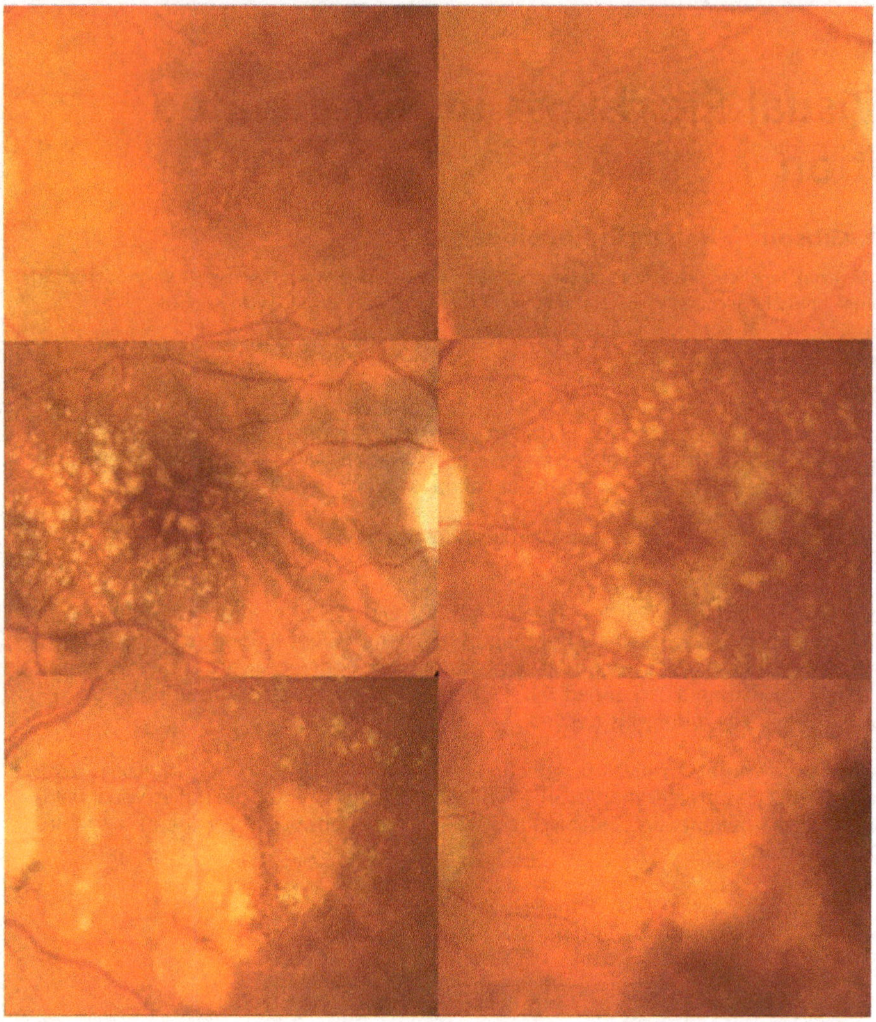

Figure 1. Stages of AMD. Example fundus images of stages of AMD. *Top left*: Stage 0, *top right*: Stage 1, *middle left*: Stage 2, *middle right*: Stage 3, *bottom left*: Stage 4 atrophic AMD, *bottom right*: Stage 4 neovascular AMD.

Methods

Subjects

Subjects were recruited from Birmingham and Midland Eye Centre and the Aston University Eye Clinic. Based on 10° SWAP variability values from the normative database and from a previous study in patients [28], a sample of 7 at each stage would give 80% confidence of detecting a difference of 1.34 dB in mean sensitivity. The sample consisted of 27 patients (mean age 68.8±7.8 years, range 46–84 years, 8 males, 19 females) with a diagnosis of AMD and 22 age-matched healthy controls (mean age 67.2±7.5 years, range 49–78 years, 13 males, 9 females). Subjects had SAP experience but were naïve to SWAP. All study eyes met the inclusion criteria of refraction less than ±5.00 DS and ±2.00 DC, clear ocular media (Lens Opacity Classification System III [29] <NC3, NO3, C1 and P1), no pseudophakia,

Table 1. Definitions of the Mutually Exclusive Stages of AMD.

Stage	Definition
Stage 0	No signs of AMD, or presence of hard drusen (<63μm) only
Stage 1	Soft distinct drusen (≥63μm) only, or pigmentary abnormalities only
Stage 2	Soft indistinct drusen (≥125μm) only, or soft distinct drusen (≥63μm) with pigmentary abnormalities
Stage 3	Soft indistinct (≥125μm) with pigmentary abnormalities
Stage 4	Atrophic or neovascular AMD

Stages of disease were derived based a longitudinal 6.5 year epidemiologic study of progression rates of AMD [31]. See example images in Figure 1.

tonometry <21 mmHg (Pulsair, Keeler, Windsor, UK), normal optic nerve head appearance (assessed by ophthalmologist, JMG), no family history of glaucoma, no history of ocular disease other than untreated AMD, no ocular trauma, no systemic disease, no systemic medication known to influence the visual field, pupil diameters >3 mm and no congenital colour vision defect. Corrected visual acuity was at least 0.1logMAR in each eye, in the normal group and ranged between 0–1logMAR in the patient group. Four patients (of 31 who initially attended) were excluded from the study for non-foveal fixation, as assessed using the ophthalmoscope cross-hair fixation target or due to inability to complete a visual field test.

Written informed consent was obtained from each subject and the study had approval from the Aston University Human Sciences Ethical Committee and the NHS West Midlands Research Ethics Committee. The study followed the Tenets of the Declaration of Helsinki.

AMD Grading

Stereoscopic 30° fundus images were acquired (EOS 10D, 6.3 megapixels, Canon, Tokyo, Japan) and stored as high quality JPEG files (3072×2048) and viewed on a 20.1″ 4is:3 monitor (1200×1600 pixel resolution), using a prismatic stereoviewer. Image grading [30] and stage of disease [31] (Table 1; Figure 1) was determined in a random order. Subjects who had any gradable features [30] were defined as belonging to the AMD patient group. All grading was determined by independent, masked graders (JMG & JHA), using custom written software (written in Liberty BASIC, Shoptalk Systems, Framingham, MA, USA), which mapped the circular grading grid to the fundus image and incorporated a measurement tool.

Perimetry

All subjects underwent visual field testing on the dominant eye, as determined by the hole-in-the-card test [32]. Each subject underwent SAP and SWAP 10–2 visual field examinations with the Humphrey Field Analyser 750 (Carl Zeiss Meditec, Dublin, CA, USA) on two occasions. For SAP, the stimulus size was 0.43° (Goldmann III) and the background luminance was 10 cd/m^2. For SWAP, blue (440 nm) 1.72° (Goldmann V) stimuli were presented on a yellow (>530 nm) 100 cd/m^2 background. SITA Standard and FASTPAC algorithms were employed for the SAP and SWAP fields, respectively, in order to mimic clinical practice as closely as possible. FASTPAC is the recommended strategy in SWAP [26] and SITA SWAP is not available for the 10–2 field. Visits were separated by 11 days, and the results from the first visit were discarded to account for the learning effect.

Before each examination, patients underwent three minutes of background adaptation. Fixation losses, false negative and false positive responses were less than 33%. Regular rest periods were given during and between examinations. The decision to include SAP (SITA standard) fields with false positives >15% and <33% was based on careful assessment of the video monitor gaze tracking function and the other parameters of fixation monitoring.

Analysis

Visual field change with stage of AMD was determined using the mean deviation (MD), pattern standard deviation (PSD), number of pattern deviation (PD) defects and local spatial variability (LSV). The LSV is a global index calculated as the root mean square of pointwise sensitivity differences between the raw and median filtered visual field [33]. All PD defects <5% were considered significant. The SAP MD and PSD were weighted indices from the HFA printout. Unweighted SWAP indices were calculated from a normal database collected previously. It consisted of 65 normal subjects (age 22–79) who performed 10–2 SWAP visual fields (FASTPAC). The normative data was analysed using univariate linear regression to give the age-corrected normal values at each stimulus location and the confidence intervals were calculated to derive probability defects.

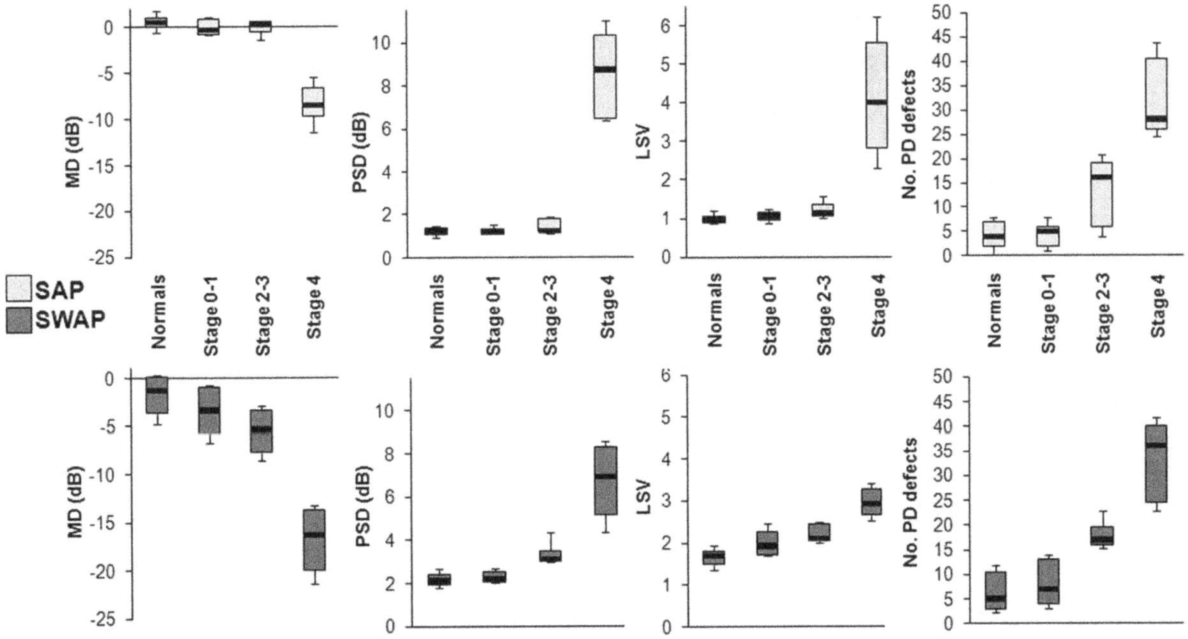

Figure 2. Boxplots representing the change in the visual field with stage of severity of disease. The change in MD (dB), PSD (dB), LSV and number of PD defects as a function of stage of severity of disease, for standard automated perimetry (SAP) and short-wavelength automated perimetry (SWAP) is shown. Boxplot limits represent the 15th, 25th, 50th, 75th and 85th percentiles.

Table 2. Summary table of global indices as a function of stage of severity of AMD.

SAP

		MS	MD	PSD	LSV	AMD Severity Index	No. PD defects
Normals	Mean	32.59	0.58	1.21	1.26	0.04	5.09
	SD	1.13	0.98	0.24	0.97	0.04	4.95
Stage 0–1	Mean	32.18	0.05	1.23	1.28	0.04	5.54
	SD	1.25	1.25	0.22	0.91	0.04	5.32
Stage 2–3	Mean	31.41	−0.45	1.39	1.46	0.16	13.86
	SD	1.92	2.10	0.47	0.84	0.15	9.21
Stage 4	Mean	22.47	−9.32	8.72	4.32	0.52	33.14
	SD	4.91	5.18	2.83	1.91	0.14	10.67

SWAP

		MS	MD	PSD	LSV	AMD Severity Index	No. PD defects
Normals	Mean	24.33	−1.66	2.22	1.71	0.05	6.55
	SD	3.06	2.75	0.40	0.32	0.03	4.42
Stage 0–1	Mean	22.14	−3.72	2.44	2.00	0.08	8.62
	SD	3.77	3.39	0.72	0.37	0.08	6.51
Stage 2–3	Mean	19.71	−5.98	4.10	2.27	0.25	19.29
	SD	4.83	4.67	2.63	0.41	0.16	9.01
Stage 4	Mean	8.64	−16.58	6.69	2.98	0.50	33.43
	SD	4.67	4.32	1.96	0.50	0.17	10.66

Mean sensitivity (MS), mean deviation (MD), pattern standard deviation (PSD), local spatial variability (LSV) and the AMD Severity Index are shown.

Table 3. Kruskal-Wallis test of significant variation in visual field measures with advancing stage of AMD.

		MD	PSD	LSV	No. PD Defects	Severity Index
SAP	Chi-square	19.630	18.605	17.597	21.032	23.038
	p	<0.001	<0.001	<0.001	<0.001	<0.001
SWAP	Chi-square	22.095	26.576	23.878	26.765	28.797
	p	<0.001	<0.001	<0.001	<0.001	<0.001

The coefficient of variation for each stimulus location was calculated. Frequency of defect maps were constructed from the PD probability maps, which were used in preference to the total deviation analysis as they were less variable and less likely to be affected by the possible presence of diffuse lenticular changes. Concentric sectors of the 10° field, based on the frequency of PD defects, were used to evaluate the unweighted MD and change in MD with stage. We then derived a new index, the AMD Severity Index, using a weighted scoring system based on the PD defects and their locations within the 10° field. The Severity Index was examined for change with stage of AMD.

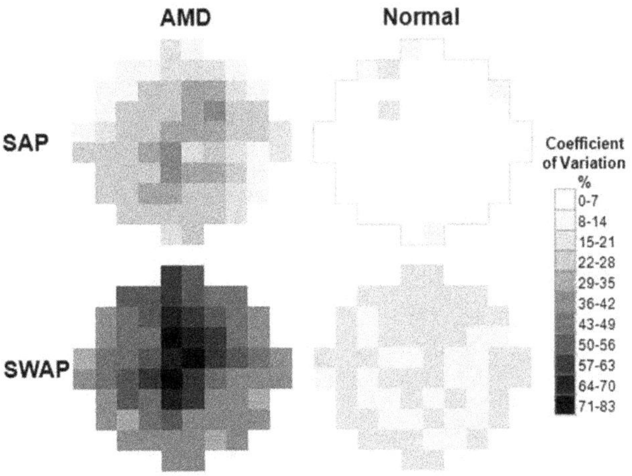

Figure 3. Coefficient of variation (%) map for SAP and SWAP. Mean coefficients of variation for the AMD patients and normal subjects are shown. Maps are displayed as a right eye.

Results

Visual field data from 27 eyes of 27 patients and 22 eyes of 22 normal subjects, were included in the analysis. There were 7 eyes

Table 4. Post hoc analyses (Mann-Whitney U test with Bonferroni adjustment) to detect significant differences in visual field measures between AMD stages and normal.

SAP MD	Stage 0–1	Stage 2–3	Stage 4		**SWAP MD**	Stage 0–1	Stage 2–3	Stage 4	
	0.129	0.221	**<0.001**	Normal		0.098	0.017	**<0.001**	Normal
		0.905	**<0.001**	Stage 0–1			0.251	**<0.001**	Stage 0–1
			0.003	Stage 2–3				**0.006**	Stage 2–3
SAP PSD	Stage 0–1	Stage 2–3	Stage 4		**SWAP PSD**	Stage 0–1	Stage 2–3	Stage 4	
	0.785	0.296	**<0.001**	Normal		0.539	**<0.001**	**<0.001**	Normal
		0.321	**<0.001**	Stage 0–1			**0.004**	**0.001**	Stage 0–1
			0.002	Stage 2–3				0.025	Stage 2–3
SAP LSV	Stage 0–1	Stage 2–3	Stage 4		**SWAP LSV**	Stage 0–1	Stage 2–3	Stage 4	
	0.384	0.039	**<0.001**	Normal		0.042	**0.001**	**<0.001**	Normal
		0.219	**0.001**	Stage 0–1			0.251	**0.001**	Stage 0–1
			0.004	Stage 2–3				0.018	Stage 2–3
SAP No. PD defects	Stage 0–1	Stage 2–3	Stage 4		**SWAP No. PD defects**	Stage 0–1	Stage 2–3	Stage 4	
	0.744	0.020	**<0.001**	Normal		0.337	**<0.001**	**<0.001**	Normal
		0.067	**<0.001**	Stage 0–1			**0.005**	**0.001**	Stage 0–1
			0.007	Stage 2–3				0.013	Stage 2–3
SAP Severity Index	Stage 0–1	Stage 2–3	Stage 4		**SWAP Severity Index**	Stage 0–1	Stage 2–3	Stage 4	
	0.313	**0.008**	**<0.001**	Normal		0.183	**<0.001**	**<0.001**	Normal
		0.032	**<0.001**	Stage 0–1			**0.003**	**<0.001**	Stage 0–1
			0.009	Stage 2–3				0.013	Stage 2–3

Results show the p-values for the mean deviation (MD), pattern standard deviation (PSD), local spatial variability (LSV), number of pattern deviation (PD) defects and AMD Severity Index. Significant differences are in bold and have a conservative Bonferroni adjustment for multiple comparisons.

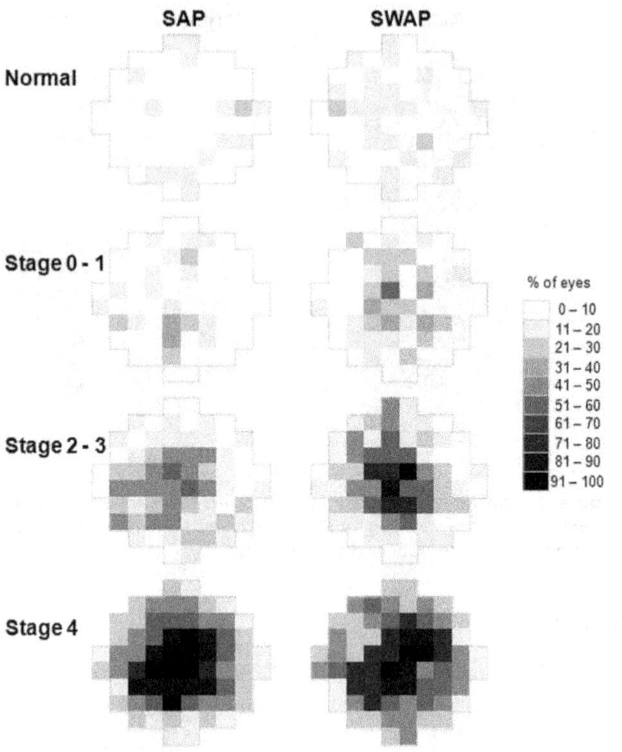

Figure 4. Frequency of defect maps. Frequency of defect maps show the % of eyes at each stimulus location which have significant defects on PD analysis for SAP and SWAP as a function of stage of disease. Maps are displayed as a right eye.

graded at stage 0, 6 at stage 1, 5 at stage 2, 2 at stage 3 and 7 at stage 4. Data from stages were combined by the following grouping: stages 0–1, stages 2–3 and stage 4.

Change in visual field measures with stage

Compared to normal subjects mean sensitivity (MS) values were decreased and SDs were increased in the AMD patients (Table 2). Figure 2 shows the measures MD, PSD, LSV and number of PD defects for normal and AMD subjects. Patients at stages 2–3 and 4 showed a greater variability than those at 0–1 and normal subjects.

All measures varied significantly (Kruskal-Wallis test) with the stage of AMD for both SAP and SWAP (Table 3). A greater number of post hoc differences (Mann-Whitney U test with Bonferroni adjustment; Table 4) were noted between subject groups for SWAP than for SAP, for the PSD and the LSV. Overall, SWAP detected more differences from normal than SAP. In SWAP, the MD had the fewest significant differences from normal. In SAP more significant differences from normal were evident for the Severity Index.

There were significant correlations between LSV and PSD for SAP (Spearman's rho = 0.455, p = 0.001) and SWAP (rho = 0.768, $p<0.001$).

Coefficient of Variation

As expected, the AMD group yielded lower MS and greater SDs than normal group for SAP and SWAP (Table 2). Variability was compared using the coefficient of variation statistic [26,27] (SD/mean, expressed as %), which represents a normalised measure of dispersion such that distributions which differ in the magnitude of their measurement scales may be compared.

SWAP consistently revealed greater coefficients of variation than SAP (Figure 3). The AMD patients had higher values than normal. At AMD stages 0–1, mean coefficients of variation were only slightly greater than normal (normals: SAP 5±3% SWAP 16±2%; Stage 0–1: SAP 6±3%, SWAP 21±5%) but at stage 4 large values were exhibited (SAP 44±20%; SWAP 105±89%).

Frequency of Defect

The frequency of defect maps (Figure 4) represent the percentage of eyes at each stimulus location with PD defects. SWAP defects occurred more frequently than SAP defects in early AMD. For late stage AMD (stage 4), for both perimetry types, 70–80% of eyes had defects within the central 5°. Enlargement of a central scotoma was noted with progressing stage of disease. The increase in frequency of defects with worsening disease stage occurred at an earlier stage in SWAP than in SAP.

Sector Analysis

Based on the frequency of defect maps, the field was divided into the following sectors: centre, middle and periphery (eccentricities: 1.4°, 3.2–7.1° and 7.1–9.1° respectively; Figure 5 *Top*). For AMD patients, central sector MD values were worse than the peripheral values for both SAP and SWAP (Figure 5 *Middle*). For the normal group, MD values remained uniform across all sectors. Figure 5 (*Bottom*) shows the regression slope of MD as a function of stage for each sector for SAP and SWAP. The most rapid sensitivity loss occurred in the centre and the slowest in the periphery.

AMD Severity Index

Based on our sector analysis and frequency of defect maps, a Severity Index of AMD visual field loss was derived (Equation 1) [34]. Visual field sectors were weighted by their location within the 10° field and multiplied by a depth defect score according to the PD probability value (Figure 6). Centrally located defects and more severe probability values carried a greater weight. The sum was then divided by the maximum possible score to give the Severity Index ranging between 0 (no field loss) and 1 (maximum defects across the entire field).

$$Severity\ Index = \frac{Spatial\ Weight \times PD\ Depth}{Weight\ Ceiling\ Score} \quad (1)$$

A larger Severity Index (Figure 6 *Bottom*) in SWAP than in SAP for each AMD group indicated deeper and more extensive sensitivity loss in SWAP. Severity scores varied significantly with stage of disease for SAP and SWAP (Table 3). Post hoc analysis (Table 4) revealed significant differences between normal subjects and AMD patients at stages 2–3 and 4, in SAP and in SWAP.

Visual Acuity

Figure 7 shows the visual acuities in the normal subjects and AMD patients. Visual acuities varied significantly with stage of AMD (Kruskall-Wallis test: Chi-square = 28.09, $p<0.001$). A greater number of post hoc differences from normal (Mann-Whitney U test with Bonferroni adjustment; Figure 7) were found than for perimetry.

Discussion

In this cross-sectional study of patients with AMD, sensitivity loss in 10–2 SAP and SWAP visual fields increased with increased

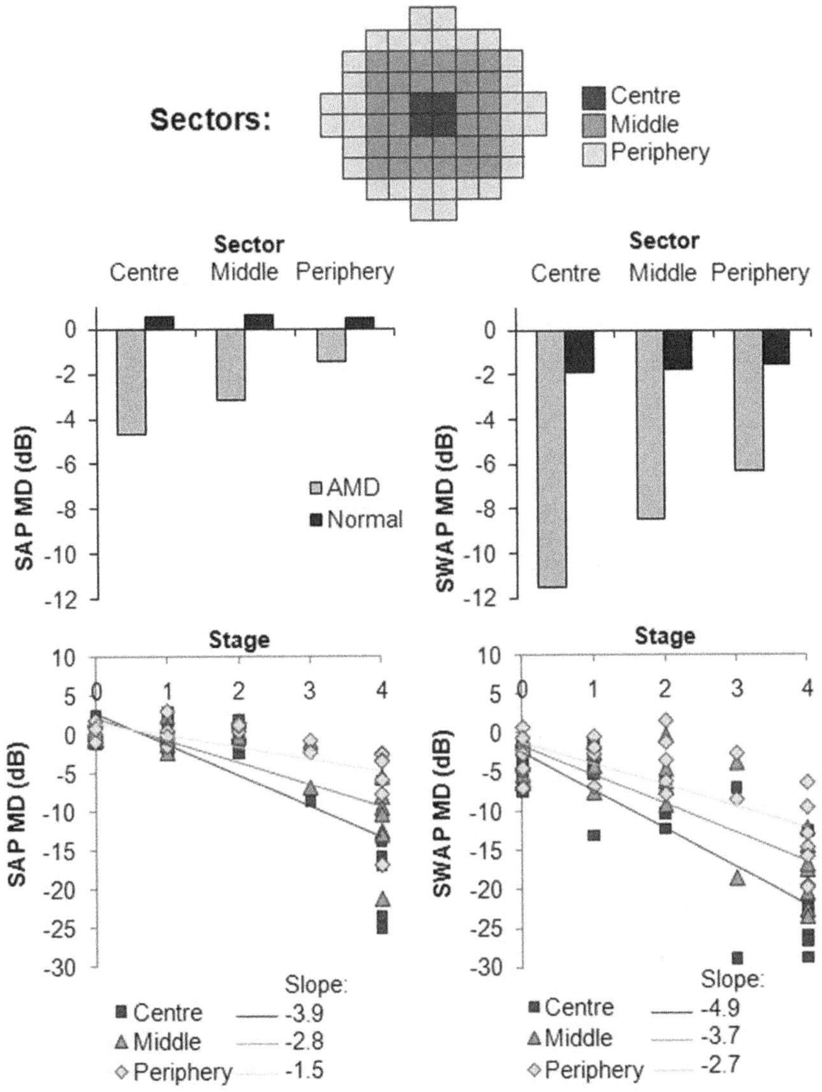

Figure 5. Sector analysis. *Top*: Sector arrangement of the 10–2 stimulus locations. *Middle*: The group mean MD in each sector for SAP and SWAP for normal and AMD subjects is displayed. *Bottom*: The scatterplot of MD as a function of stage of AMD shows the slope of univariate linear regression (dB per stage), in each sector for SAP and SWAP.

severity of disease. The finding of reduced MS and greater variability in sensitivity in the AMD patient group compared to the normal group is consistent with previous studies [3,4,5,6,9].

We quantified the visual field loss as a function of stage of AMD and found that the changes in SWAP were more significant than those in SAP. SWAP had a greater capability in detecting differences between the AMD groups and differences from normal, than SAP. Previous studies of blue-on-yellow perimetry in AMD [5,6] did not compare results to SAP, however in patients with diabetes, sensitivity loss in the 10–2 visual field, due to structural change, was better detected by SWAP than SAP [23,35,36,37]. The SWS pathway is vulnerable to a variety of retinal disease implying that SWS pathway sensitivity loss occurs at multiple sites of damage [38]. Possible explanations include reduced redundancy due to the sparse SWS system [39] and/or the smaller response range of the SWS cone system [40].

A secondary aim was to examine the location of visual field loss within the 10° field. A central scotoma within 5° was demonstrated in late stage AMD, supportive of previous findings of reduced SWS in the central compared to the peripheral 10° field in AMD [5]. Others have indicated paracentral scotoma and preservation of central vision in AMD [41,42], or no difference between central and peripheral sensitivity in the 10° SWAP field [6]. Possible explanations for these varied results include differences in instrumentation, sample sizes, classification of AMD and analyses.

In fact, we found that the most vulnerable region to AMD related sensitivity loss was the central 1°, in which the change was −3.9 dB per stage in SAP and −4.9 dB in SWAP. Our results suggested a symmetrical defect, from which the Severity Index was derived, to classify visual field defects on a continuous scale. In SAP, the Severity Index detected the most differences between groups. Thus, it may be a useful method for monitoring longitudinal progression of the visual field in AMD. From our findings, a Severity Index >0.1 in SAP and >0.2 in SWAP appeared abnormal, however a larger study is required to investigate this.

All visual field measures varied significantly with increasing stage of disease, however there was some functional overlap

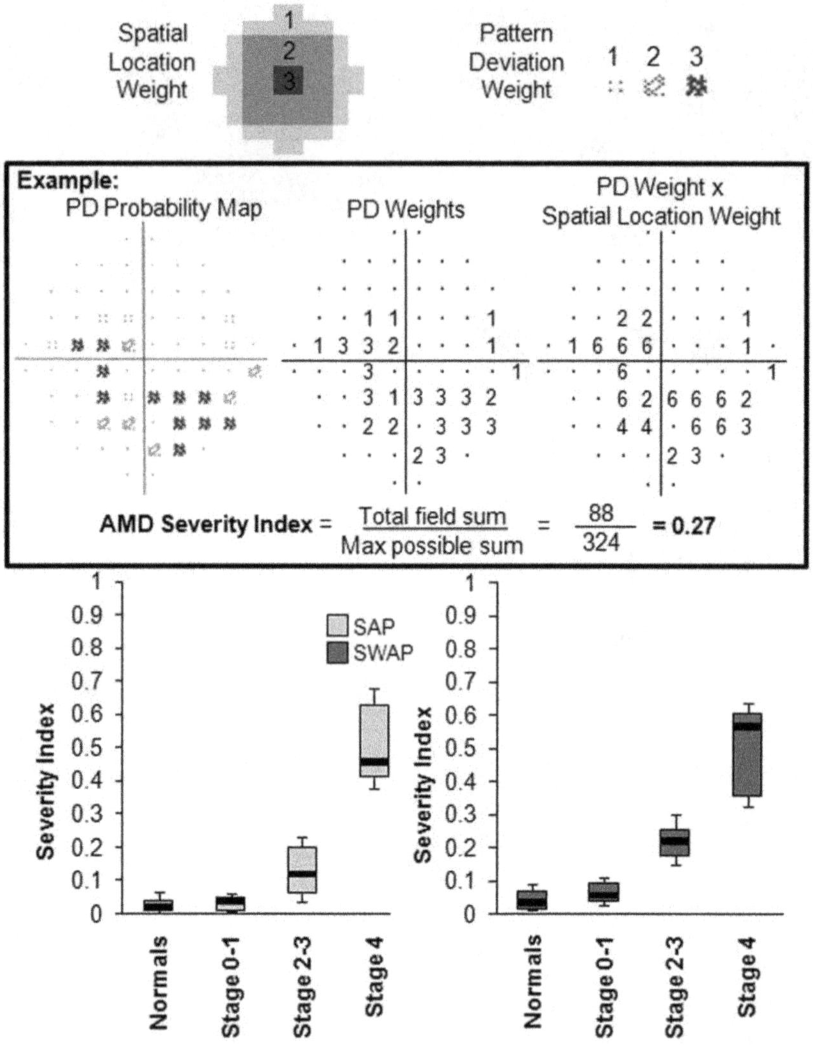

Figure 6. Calculation of Severity Index and change in Severity Index with stage of AMD. Based on Pattern Deviation (PD) maps, visual field sectors were weighted whereby the greatest weight corresponded to the central sector (Spatial Location Weight). This was then multiplied by a depth defect score according to the PD probability value (Pattern Deviation Weight). *Middle, box*: Example calculation: the sum was then divided by the maximum possible score to give the Severity Index ranging between 0 and 1, where 0 indicates no field loss and 1 indicates maximum defects across the entire field. *Bottom*: Boxplots representing the change in Severity Index as a function of stage of severity of disease, for standard perimetry (SAP) and short-wavelength automated perimetry (SWAP). Boxplot limits represent the 15th, 25th, 50th, 75th and 85th percentiles.

between stages. We found that focal measures of SWAP visual field loss, such as the PSD and number of PD defects, demonstrated greater capability in detecting AMD subjects from normal. In a previous study [23], detection of focal loss by the number of PD defects in SWAP, had a stronger relationship with diabetic retinopathy than SAP.

Of the focal indices, LSV is less common but statistically less manipulated than PSD, as well as significantly correlated with PSD. LSV is less influenced by pre-receptoral absorption, i.e. macular pigment and lenticular changes, which limit the interpretation of SWAP. Although the effect of lenticular absorption was minimised by our exclusion criteria, mild absorption and macular pigment effects may have influenced the SWAP data. However, significant attenuation of SWAP thresholds by macular pigment was not evident from normal defect maps (Figure 4), nor in our normal database. Correcting for macular pigment, which has a high within-subject variability [43], would artificially increase perimetric sensitivities and alter normal prediction limits. Since the effects of pre-receptoral absorption on SWAP are symmetrical and diffuse, a statistical approach has been recommended to separate focal loss [43,44] and our results support the conclusion that focal loss is of greater importance in AMD.

A limitation of SWAP was that overall larger coefficients of variation were found than in SAP (Figure 3), similar to previous findings [26]. However, this finding was skewed by large values at stages 3 and 4, where greater variability would be expected in scotomatous locations. In fact, coefficients of variation at earlier stages were near normal for both perimetry types, indicating SWAP as a reliable method to examine early stage AMD patients with minimal lens opacities.

In our study SWAP analysis had a high correlation with visual acuity as a means of detecting AMD and this raises the question as to what extra value SWAP measurement adds in assessing patients with AMD. It is known that central perimetry in AMD gives information about the spatial extent and depth of central visual

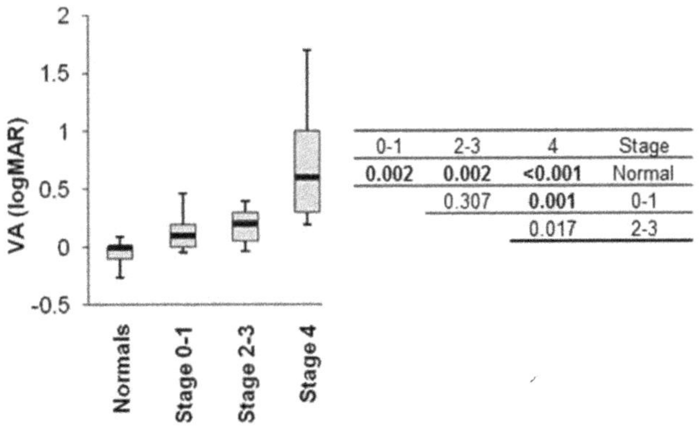

Figure 7. Boxplots representing the change in visual acuity with stage of severity of disease. The change in visual acuity (logMAR) as a function of stage of severity of disease and post hoc analyses (Mann-Whitney U test with Bonferroni adjustment) to detect significant differences in visual acuities between AMD stages and normal are shown. Boxplot limits represent the 15th, 25th, 50th, 75th and 85th percentiles. Significant differences in the posthoc analyses are the p-values in bold and have a conservative Bonferroni adjustment for multiple comparisons.

loss that visual acuity cannot measure [45], and with increasing possibilities of medical intervention available, this aspect of visual function measurement is likely to become important. In fact, visual acuity appeared to better differentiate between early stage AMD and normal, than perimetry. Therefore the value of SAP and SWAP analysis in AMD is in research, rather than as a diagnostic tool.

Limitations of the study were the small number of eyes at individual stages, which led to the grouping of stages and the cross-sectional design of the study. The difference in SAP and SWAP normative databases limits the analyses, however use of the HFA Statpac analysis is standard in clinical practice and provides greater accuracy than collection of new SAP normative data. A longitudinal study in a larger sample, following visual field progression over several years is warranted, in which the Severity Index could be used to measure field defects on a continuous scale. In a larger sample it would be possible to differentiate results between late stage patients with geographic atrophy and choroidal neovascularisation. Specific consideration in a progression study, would be necessary to account for worsening cataracts and potential involvement of fixation later in the disease, which may affect the interpretation of visual field results. Furthermore, visual field testing may be useful in assessing the effectiveness of novel treatments in either preserving or improving visual field loss in patients with AMD, enrolled in a clinical study under appropriate exclusion criteria. Due to the strict exclusion criteria of our study, our findings are limited to AMD subjects suitable to visual field testing, i.e. those who have foveal fixation and clear ocular media.

The results present evidence of a relationship between the SWAP visual field and severity of AMD, whereby sensitivity declined with advancing stage of AMD. SWAP had greater capability in detecting early AMD than SAP. The importance of early detection of functional change in AMD is clinically relevant to possible earlier intervention or lifestyle changes. Sensitivity loss in AMD was focal in nature and the central field became less uniform as stage increased. SWAP defects occurred at similar locations but were deeper and wider than corresponding SAP defects. Although not all patients are suitable for SWAP examinations, our findings support it as a useful tool in research studies of visual loss in AMD.

Acknowledgments

Presented in part at the 2009 annual meeting of the Association for Research in Vision and Ophthalmology, Florida, for which the College of Optometrists provided a travel grant to J Acton.

Thanks to Vivienne Greenstein for scientific advice, Miriam Conway for providing the SWAP 10–2 normative database and Richard Armstrong for statistical advice.

Author Contributions

Conceived and designed the experiments: JHA JMG RPC. Performed the experiments: JHA. Analyzed the data: JHA JMG RPC. Contributed reagents/materials/analysis tools: JHA JMG RPC. Wrote the paper: JHA JMG RPC.

References

1. Resnikoff S, Pascolini D, Etya'ale D, Kocur I, Pararajasegaram R, et al. (2004) Global data on visual impairment in the year 2002. Bull World Health Organ 82: 844–851.
2. Rein DB, Wittenborn JS, Zhang X, Honeycutt AA, Lesesne SB, et al. (2009) Forecasting age-related macular degeneration through the year 2050: the potential impact of new treatments. Arch Ophthalmol 127: 533–540.
3. Midena E, Degli Angeli C, Blarzino MC, Valenti M, Segato T (1997) Macular function impairment in eyes with early age-related macular degeneration. Invest Ophthalmol Vis Sci 38: 469–477.
4. Midena E, Segato T, Blarzino MC, Degli Angeli C (1994) Macular drusen and the sensitivity of the central visual field. Doc Ophthalmol 88: 179–185.
5. Remky A, Elsner AE (2005) Blue on yellow perimetry with scanning laser ophthalmoscopy in patients with age related macular disease. Br J Ophthalmol 89: 464–469.
6. Remky A, Lichtenberg K, Elsner AE, Arend O (2001) Short wavelength automated perimetry in age related maculopathy. Br J Ophthalmol 85: 1432–1436.
7. Tolentino MJ, Miller S, Gaudio AR, Sandberg MA (1994) Visual field deficits in early age-related macular degeneration. Vision Res 34: 409–413.
8. Atchison DA, Lovie-Kitchin JE, Swann PG (1990) Investigation of central visual fields in patients with age-related macular changes. Optom Vis Sci 67: 179–183.
9. Cheng AS, Vingrys AJ (1993) Visual losses in early age-related maculopathy. Optom Vis Sci 70: 89–96.
10. Frennesson C, Nilsson UL, Nilsson SE (1995) Colour contrast sensitivity in patients with soft drusen, an early stage of ARM. Doc Ophthalmol 90: 377–386.
11. Feigl B, Brown B, Lovie-Kitchin J, Swann P (2005) Monitoring retinal function in early age-related maculopathy: visual performance after 1 year. Eye (Lond) 19: 1169–1177.
12. Mayer MJ, Spiegler SJ, Ward B, Glucs A, Kim CBY (1992) Mid-Frequency Loss of Foveal Flicker Sensitivity in Early Stages of Age-Related Maculopathy. Investigative Ophthalmology & Visual Science 33: 3136–3142.
13. Phipps JA, Dang TM, Vingrys AJ, Guymer RH (2004) Flicker perimetry losses in age-related macular degeneration. Investigative Ophthalmology & Visual Science 45: 3355–3360.
14. Owsley C, Jackson GR, Cideciyan AV, Huang YJ, Fine SL, et al. (2000) Psychophysical evidence for rod vulnerability in age-related macular degeneration. Investigative Ophthalmology & Visual Science 41: 267–273.
15. Scholl HPN, Bellmann C, Dandekar SS, Bird AC, Fitzke FW (2004) Photopic and scotopic fine matrix mapping of retinal areas of increased fundus autofluorescence in patients with age-related maculopathy. Investigative Ophthalmology & Visual Science 45: 574–583.
16. Steinmetz RL, Haimovici R, Jubb C, Fitzke FW, Bird AC (1993) Symptomatic Abnormalities of Dark-Adaptation in Patients with Age-Related Bruchs Membrane Change. Br J Ophthalmol 77: 549–554.
17. Gerth C, Hauser D, Delahunt PB, Morse LS, Werner JS (2003) Assessment of multifocal electroretinogram abnormalities and their relation to morphologic characteristics in patients with large drusen. Arch Ophthalmol 121: 1404–1414.
18. Li J, Tso MOM, Lam TT (2001) Reduced amplitude and delayed latency in foveal response of multifocal electroretinogram in early age related macular degeneration. Br J Ophthalmol 85: 287–290.
19. Goldstein M, Loewenstein A, Barak A, Baruch E, Feitt N, et al. (2005) Results of a multicenter clinical trial to evaluate the preferential hyperacuity perimeter for detection of age-related macular degeneration. Retina 25: 296–303.
20. Applegate RA, Adams AJ, Cavender JC, Zisman F (1987) Early color vision changes in age-related maculopathy. Appl Opt 26: 1458–1462.

21. Eisner A, Fleming SA, Klein ML, Mauldin WM (1987) Sensitivities in Older Eyes with Good Acuity – Eyes Whose Fellow Eye Has Exudative AMD. Invest Ophthalmol Vis Sci 28: 1832–1837.
22. Haegerstrom-Portnoy G, Brown B (1989) 2-Color Increment Thresholds in Early Age-Related Maculopathy. Clin Vis Sci 4: 165–172.
23. Bengtsson B, Heijl A, Agardh E (2005) Visual fields correlate better than visual acuity to severity of diabetic retinopathy. Diabetologia 48: 2494–2500.
24. Johnson CA, Adams AJ, Casson EJ, Brandt JD (1993) Progression of early glaucomatous visual field loss as detected by blue-on-yellow and standard white-on-white automated perimetry. Arch Ophthalmol 111: 651–656.
25. Johnson CA, Adams AJ, Casson EJ, Brandt JD (1993) Blue-on-yellow perimetry can predict the development of glaucomatous visual field loss. Arch Ophthalmol 111: 645–650.
26. Wild JM, Cubbidge RP, Pacey IE, Robinson R (1998) Statistical aspects of the normal visual field in short-wavelength automated perimetry. Invest Ophthalmol Vis Sci 39: 54–63.
27. Cubbidge RP, Hosking SL, Embleton S (2002) Statistical modelling of the central 10-degree visual field in short-wavelength automated perimetry. Graefes Arch Clin Exp Ophthalmol 240: 650–657.
28. Bengtsson B, Hellgren KJ, Agardh E (2008) Test-retest variability for standard automated perimetry and short-wavelength automated perimetry in diabetic patients. Acta Ophthalmol 86: 170–176.
29. Chylack LT Jr, Wolfe JK, Singer DM, Leske MC, Bullimore MA, et al. (1993) The Lens Opacities Classification System III. The Longitudinal Study of Cataract Study Group. Arch Ophthalmol 111: 831–836.
30. Bird AC, Bressler NM, Bressler SB, Chisholm IH, Coscas G, et al. (1995) An international classification and grading system for age-related maculopathy and age-related macular degeneration. The International ARM Epidemiological Study Group. Surv Ophthalmol 39: 367–374.
31. van Leeuwen R, Klaver CC, Vingerling JR, Hofman A, de Jong PT (2003) The risk and natural course of age-related maculopathy: follow-up at 6 1/2 years in the Rotterdam study. Arch Ophthalmol 121: 519–526.
32. Durand AC, Gould GM (1910) A method of determining ocular dominance. Journal of the American Medical Association 55: 369–370.
33. Crabb DP, Edgar DF, Fitzke FW, McNaught AI, Wynn HP (1995) New approach to estimating variability in visual field data using an image processing technique. Br J Ophthalmol 79: 213–217.
34. Conway M, Cubbidge RP, Hosking SL (2008) Visual field severity indices demonstrate dose-dependent visual loss from vigabatrin therapy. Epilepsia 49: 108–116.
35. Hudson C, Flanagan JG, Turner GS, Chen HC, Young LB, et al. (1998) Short-wavelength sensitive visual field loss in patients with clinically significant diabetic macular oedema. Diabetologia 41: 918–928.
36. Remky A, Arend O, Hendricks S (2000) Short-wavelength automated perimetry and capillary density in early diabetic maculopathy. Invest Ophthalmol Vis Sci 41: 274–281.
37. Agardh E, Stjernquist H, Heijl A, Bengtsson B (2006) Visual acuity and perimetry as measures of visual function in diabetic macular oedema. Diabetologia 49: 200–206.
38. Greenstein VC, Hood DC, Ritch R, Steinberger D, Carr RE (1989) S (blue) cone pathway vulnerability in retinitis pigmentosa, diabetes and glaucoma. Invest Ophthalmol Vis Sci 30: 1732–1737.
39. Johnson CA (1994) Selective versus nonselective losses in glaucoma. J Glaucoma 3 Suppl 1: S32–44.
40. Hood DC, Benimoff NI, Greenstein VC (1984) The Response Range of the Blue-Cone Pathways – A Source of Vulnerability to Disease. Invest Ophthalmol Vis Sci 25: 864–867.
41. Hart WM, Burde RM (1983) 3-Dimensional Topography of the Central Visual-Field – Sparing of Foveal Sensitivity in Macular Disease. Ophthalmology 90: 1028–1038.
42. Swann PG, Loviekitchin JE (1991) Age-Related Maculopathy.2. the Nature of the Central Visual-Field Loss. Ophthalmic Physiol Opt 11: 59–70.
43. Wild JM, Hudson C (1995) The Attenuation of Blue-On-Yellow Perimetry by the Macular Pigment. Ophthalmology 102: 911–917.
44. Sample PA, Martinez GA, Weinreb RN (1994) Short-Wavelength Automated Perimetry Without Lens Density Testing. Am J Ophthalmol 118: 632–641.
45. Anderson AJ, Johnson CA, Werner JS (2011) Measuring Visual Function in Age-Related Macular Degeneration with Frequency-Doubling (Matrix) Perimetry. Optom Vis Sci 88: 806–815.

6

Choroidal Haller's and Sattler's Layer Thickness Measurement Using 3-Dimensional 1060-nm Optical Coherence Tomography

Marieh Esmaeelpour[1,2]*, Vedran Kajic[2], Behrooz Zabihian[2], Richu Othara[2], Siamak Ansari-Shahrezaei[1], Lukas Kellner[1], Ilse Krebs[1], Susanne Nemetz[3], Martin F. Kraus[4], Joachim Hornegger[4], James G. Fujimoto[5], Wolfgang Drexler[2], Susanne Binder[1]

1 Ludwig Boltzmann Institute of Retinology and Biomicroscopic Laser Surgery, Department of Ophthalmology, Rudolf Foundation Clinic, Vienna, Austria, **2** Center for Medical Physics and Biomedical Engineering, Medical University of Vienna, Vienna, Austria, **3** OptikNemetz, Vienna, Austria, **4** Pattern Recognition Lab and School of Advanced Optical Technologies (SAOT), Friedrich-Alexander University Erlangen-Nuremberg, Erlangen, Bavaria, Germany, **5** Department of Electrical Engineering and Computer Science, Massachusetts Institute of Technology, Cambridge, Massachusetts, United States of America

Abstract

Objectives: To examine the feasibility of automatically segmented choroidal vessels in three-dimensional (3D) 1060-nmOCT by testing repeatability in healthy and AMD eyes and by mapping Haller's and Sattler's layer thickness in healthy eyes

Methods: Fifty-five eyes (from 45 healthy subjects and 10 with non-neovascular age-related macular degeneration (AMD) subjects) were imaged by 3D-1060-nmOCT over a 36°x36° field of view. Haller's and Sattler's layer were automatically segmented, mapped and averaged across the Early Treatment Diabetic Retinopathy Study grid. For ten AMD eyes and ten healthy eyes, imaging was repeated within the same session and on another day. Outcomes were the repeatability agreement of Haller's and Sattler's layer thicknesses in healthy and AMD eyes, the validation with ICGA and the statistical analysis of the effect of age and axial eye length (AL) on both healthy choroidalsublayers.

Results: The coefficients of repeatability for Sattler's and Haller's layers were 35% and 21% in healthy eyes and 44% and 31% in AMD eyes, respectively. The mean±SD healthy central submacular field thickness for Sattler's and Haller's was 87±56 μm and 141±50 μm, respectively, with a significant relationship for AL (P<.001).

Conclusions: Automated Sattler's and Haller's thickness segmentation generates rapid 3D measurements with a repeatability correspondingto reported manual segmentation. Sublayers in healthy eyes thinnedsignificantly with increasing AL. In the presence of the thinned Sattler's layer in AMD, careful measurement interpretation is needed. Automatic choroidal vascular layer mapping may help to explain if pathological choroidal thinning affects medium and large choroidal vasculature in addition to choriocapillaris loss.

Editor: Zsolt Ablonczy, Medical University of South Carolina, United States of America

Funding: This research was supported in part by Medical University Vienna, Macular Vision Research Foundation (MVRF, USA), European Union project FUN OCT (FP7 HEALTH, contract no. 201880) and FAMOS (FP7 ICT 317744), FWF-NFN 'Photoacoustic imaging in biology and Medicine', Oesterreichische Nationalbank Jubiläumsfondsprojekt (14294), National Institutes of Health (NIH R01-EY011289-27), Deutsche Forschungsgesellschaft (DFG-GSC80-SAOT), CARL ZEISS Meditec Inc., Femtolasers GmbH and the Christian Doppler Society (Christian Doppler Laboratory 'Laser development and their application in medicine'). German Research Foundation DFG-GSC80-SAOT, DFG-HO-1791/11-1. Optik Nemetz provided support in the form of a salary for author SN, but did not have any additional role in the study design, data collection and analysis, decision to publish, or preparation of the manuscript. The specific roles of these authors are articulated in the 'author contributions' section.

Competing Interests: This study received funding from CARL ZEISS Meditec Inc., and Femtolasers GmbH. S. Nemetz is an employee of Optik Nemetz. Relevant Financial Activities Are All Outside of the Submitted Work: W. Drexler has Consultancy with CARL ZEISS Meditec Inc. and femtolasers; S. Binder with Alcon and Thrombogenics. J. Fujimoto, J. Honegger and M. Kraus have Patent and Royalties with Optovue. J. Fujimoto has Patents and Royalty from Carl Zeiss Meditec Inc. S. Binder has equipment from Carl Zeiss Meditec Inc. There are no patents, products in development or marketed products to declare.

* E-mail: marieh.esmaeelpour@meduniwien.ac.at

Introduction

The choroid is a vascular structure that provides the outer retina with oxygen and nutrition [1,2]. Most of the choroidal space is taken by vessels differentiated in three vascular layers that are markedly defined by their location and lumen size [3–5]. In the healthy eye, the choriocapillaris are a continuous network bordering Bruch's membrane. They branch from the medium- and small-sized vessels in the Sattler's layer. Haller's layer is the outermost layer and consists of posterior ciliary arteries and large lumen veins. All three sublayers are thickest at the posterior pole with many branches and larger vessel calibers in the Sattler's and Haller's layer. Total choroidal thickness is reduced with advanced age[6–8] and in prominent outer retinal pathologies such as in age-related macular degeneration (AMD)[9,10]. Pathological choroidal alterations include the reduced choroidal vessel density associated with sub-retinal pigment epithelium (RPE) deposits[11] and the fibrosis observed in AMD and subretinal deposits (reticular pseudodrusen)[12]. The role of the subretinal deposits in relation to the choroid is still under investigation. Choroidal thinning indicating atrophy has been observed after anti-vascular endothelial growth factor treatments of neovascular AMD[13]. The choriocapillaris layer accounts only for a small proportion of the total choroidal thickness in the healthy eye.[14]Choriocapillaris density decrease in relation to aging, and AMD[11,15,16] explainsthe choroidal pathogenesis in AMD only partially. Choroidal involvement in posterior ocular disease may be further explained by thickness quantification of the medium and large choroidal vessels of the Sattler's and Haller's layers.

Optical coherence tomography (OCT) used with a long wavelength light source of 1060 nm can visualize the choroid and the vasculature of Sattler's and Haller's layers in healthy eyes and AMD eyes [17,18]. An unprecedented automated blood vessel segmentation algorithm has been developed that allows segmentation and 3-dimensional (3D) visualization of the choroidal vessels in OCT images[19]. The current study tested the repeatability of vessel segmentation in healthy and AMD eyes. The vessel segmentation was validated by comparing enface OCT vessel segmentations to indocyanine green angiography (ICGA) images in eyes with AMD. The feasibility of Haller's from Sattler's layer thickness maps was examined in healthy eyes. The clinical measurement utility was improved by introducing averaging across the Early Treatment Diabetic Retinopathy Study (ETDRS) grid.

Methods

A single-institution, prospective, cross-sectional study of Sattler's and Haller's layer thickness was conducted. Ethical approval was obtained prospectively from the local Institutional Review Board, "The Ethical Commission of Vienna." This study was in adherence to the tenets of the Declaration of Helsinki. The subjects agreed to participate after explanation of the nature and possible consequences of the study. Written informed consent was obtained for experimentation with human subjects prior to participation.

Subjects

Overall, fifty-five subjects consisting of forty-five healthy subjects and ten subjects with non-neovascular AMD were recruited to test the repeatability and validity of the segmentation algorithm and the distribution of the Haller's and Sattler's thickness measurements.

For the statistical analysis of vessel distribution, Haller's and Sattler's layer thicknesses were measured in forty-five healthy subjects (27 females, age range 23 to 84 years, mean±SD 44±16 years) with no history of retinal surgery or pathology and no cataract surgery. Subjects with myopia >6 diopters (or axial eye length>26.5 mm) and smokers were excluded. All subjects had best corrected visual acuities (BCVA) of 20/20 or better (0 LogMAR or less on the ETDRS chart),whereas two subjects with cataracts and a visual acuity of 20/32 Snellen (0.2 LogMAR) were included based on the clinical appearance of healthy retinas. Only one eye per healthy subject was included. All subjects had no history of high blood pressure nor were they taking any medications for hypertension (blood pressure was taken within the trial day to confirm health status). Five axial eye length (AL) measurements were averaged from each eye using optical biometry (IOL Master Zeiss, Jena, Germany). AL was investigated as an independent factor that may relate to vessel layer thickness. For the healthy cohort, AL had a mean±SD of 23.76±1.1 mm with a range of 22.12 to 26.15 mm.

To evaluate the repeatability of the vessel segmentation, a total of twenty eyes from twenty subjects were reimaged at the same session and on another trial day within two months of the first imaging, resulting in 60 measurements. The repeatability cohort consisted of ten randomly selected healthy subjects (age range 23–45 years, 6 females, two with long ALs and moderate myopia and two with short ALs and moderate hyperopia) and ten patients with non-neovascular AMD in the study eye and neo-vascular AMD in the fellow eye. The patients had a mean visual acuity of 20/20 on both visits (0 LogMar with a range between 0.2 and −0.16). Fundus examination was performed after pupil dilation by an experienced ophthalmologist with slit lamp biomicroscopy and a Volk lens. All included AMD subjects had no cataracts, and clinical examination of the fundus was possible. According to the current classification guidelines[20], the AMD cohort consisted of low to severe AMD stages (two eyes with pigment changes, seven eyes with drusen, and one eye with geographic atrophy, age range 67–80 years, 5 females). Three of the seven eyes with drusen had areas of subretinal deposits. This range of AMDs allowed the investigation of varying signal to noise ratios. To validate vessel segmentation and to assess its resolution,ICGA images were used. Five eyes from five subjects with no cataracts were subjected to ICGA, which was needed for their clinical routine examination.

OCT imaging

High speed, 56.000 A-scans/s, spectral domain OCT (SD-OCT) imaging at 1060 nm was performed with less than 2.5 mW at the cornea, which is well below the maximum power limit for a 10-s exposure[21,22]. 3D OCT volumes were acquired at 1060 nm with a 15–20- μm transverse resolution, approximately 7- μm axial resolution and 512 voxels per depth-scan (A-scan) (Figure 1 A). Raster scans consisting of 512 A-scans and 512 B-scans were acquired across a 36×36° field in 4.68 seconds. The data processing procedure for choroid vessel segmentation has been described elsewhere[19]. Briefly, two orthogonal volumes were used to estimate retinal motion by associating a displacement field with each volume and calculating the displacements, while optimizing similarity and penalizing motion on an A-scan basis. Motion corrected 3D OCT datasets were then merged to create a 3D dataset with improved signal and reduced speckle[23]. The "Neat Video" plugin in VirtualDub (Free Software Foundation, Inc., Cambridge, MA, USA) for denoising was applied to reduce speckle.

Total choroid and choroidal vessel segmentation

Data segmentation was performed in the following order: automatic choroid segmentation [24,25], automatic vessel segmentation within the choroid, and subsequent automatic layer segmentation. Automatic choroidal segmentation was used to define the region for choroid vessel segmentation. Accordingly, axial choroidal thickness was defined as the distance between the retinal pigment epithelium/Bruch's membrane/choriocapillaris (RBC) complex and the choroidal-scleral interface (Figure 1 A). The pixel distance was converted into optical distance using the depth sampling calibration for the 1060-nm OCT system and further to the anatomical distance. Within this region, novel automated vessel segmentation was performed[19]. This method determines vessel cores by projecting probability cones to avoid relying on the poorly defined vessel wall (Figure 1 A). The probability cones are projected in three dimensions, andusing 3D

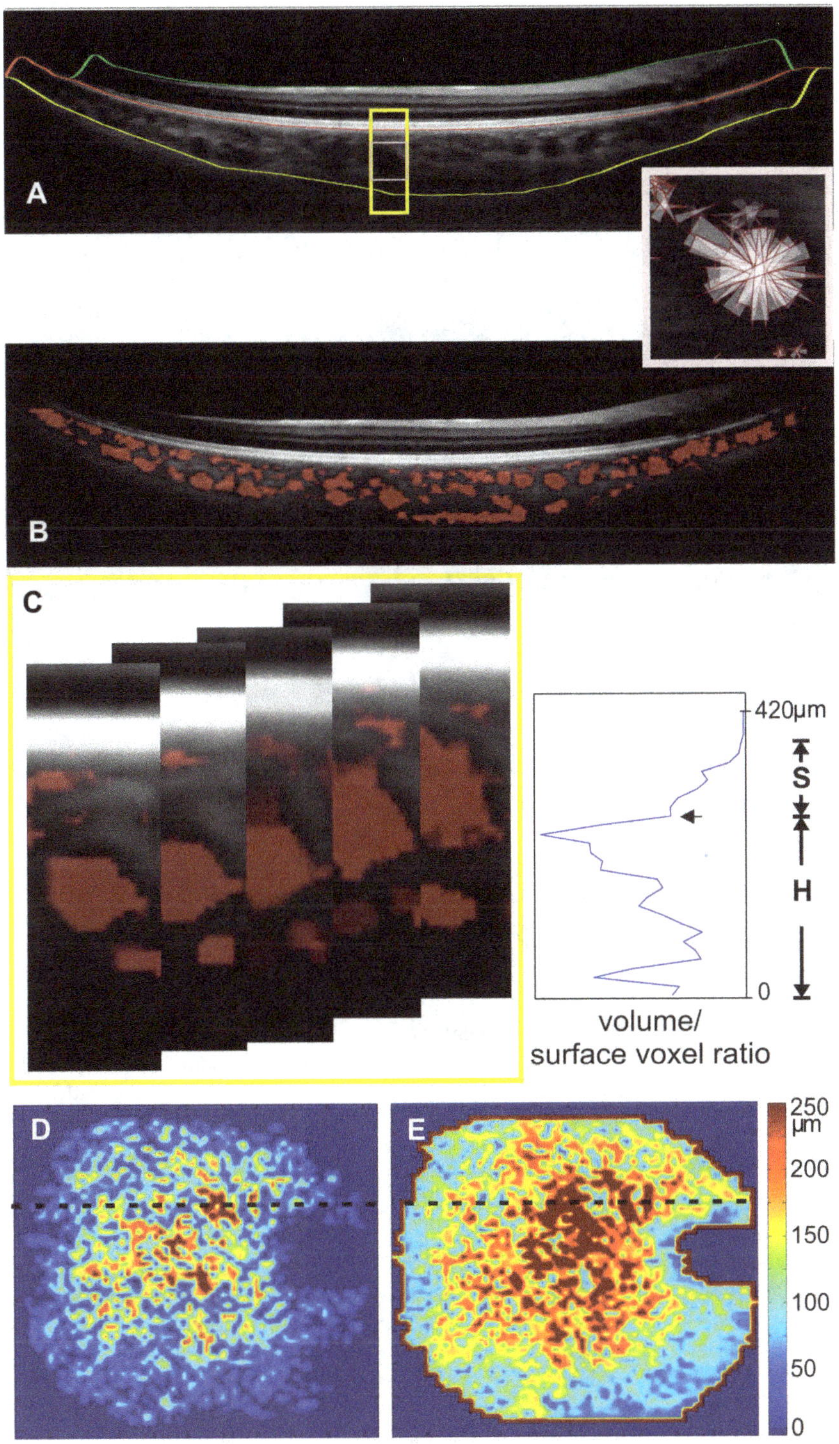

Figure 1. Automatic segmentation of Haller's and Sattler's layer for thickness mapping. OCT B-scan (A) visualizes the segmentation lines for the retina between the ILM (green line) and the RBC complex and the identified vessel voxels are visualized in red (B). The choroid is located between the RBC complex and the sclera (yellow line). Probability cones (small rectangle enlarged) were drawn to demonstrate expected vessel core position. The cone projections are in 3D, butthe concept is presented in two dimensions. The ratio of volume voxels to surface voxels that were generated was plotted for a 1×1 degree volume. This volume consists of 14 B-scans and is represented by the 5 B-scans in the yellow rectangle (C). The plot is used for determining the border between the two sublayers by detecting the largest ratio as Haller's layer vessels (H),and the local minimum is the border (arrow) to Sattler's layer (S). Plots were used to generate thickness maps for Sattler's (D) and Haller's layers (E) across the scan area.

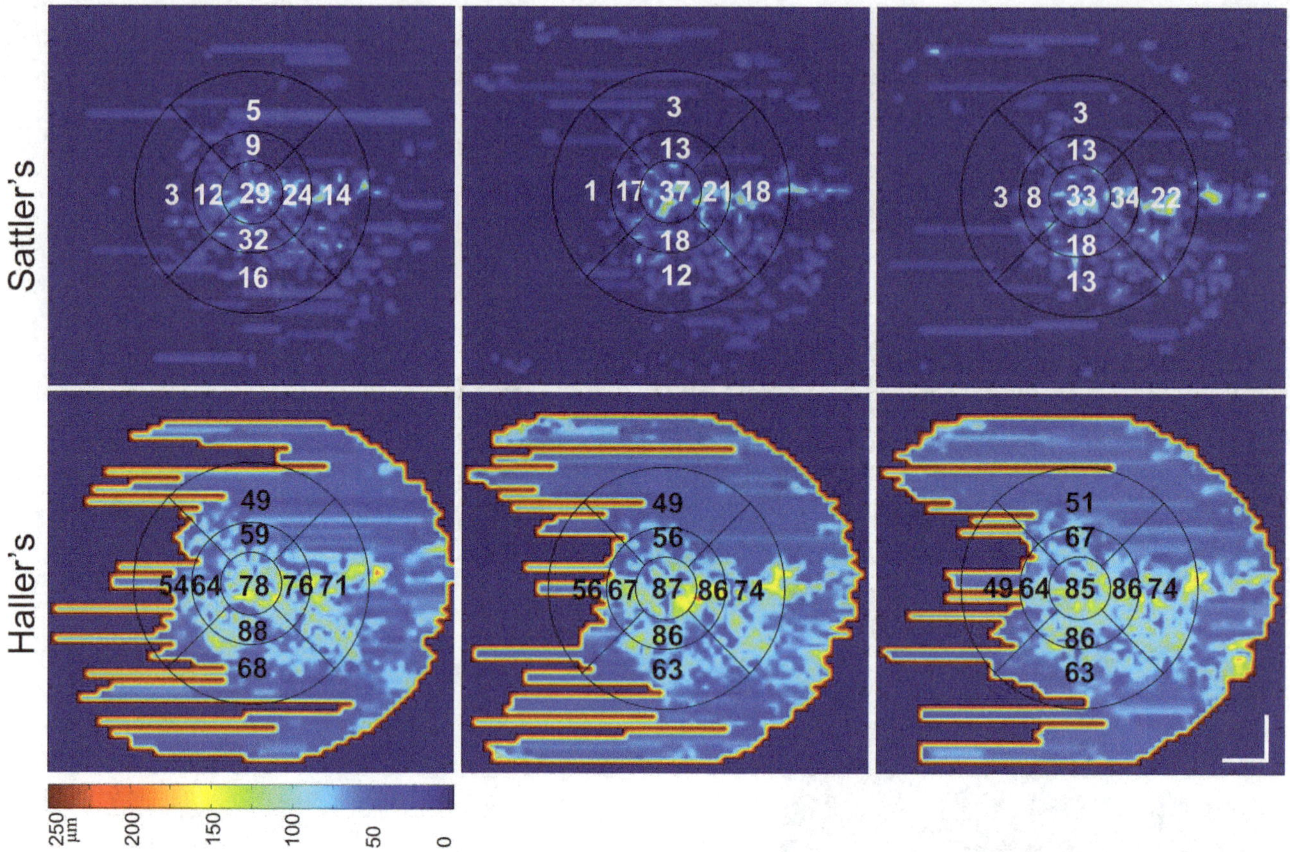

Figure 2. Repeatability of Sattler's and Haller's layer thickness mapping and ETDRS measurements in non-neovascular AMD. Sattler's layer and Haller's layer are color mapped. Imaging was performed twice at the same session (left and middle column) and on a different day (right column). The vessel segmentation and indocyanine green angiography images of this eye are depicted in Figure 3.

filtering, the estimated vessel core was dilated to approach the full vessel diameter. For the comparison of choroid vessel segmentations to ICGA images, vessel segmentations were viewed en face at different choroid depths.

Sattler's and Haller's layer segmentation

Sattler's and Haller's layers are defined as medium-size and large-size vessel layers, respectively. For determining the border between both layers, Haller's layer was defined as the layer containing the largest vessel. Vessel sizes were differentiated by using the ratio of the voxels within the vessel volume to the voxels at its surface. In general, smaller vessels have a smaller ratio than larger vessels. The ratio was plotted versus the choroidal depth and contained the ratio of a 1×1 degree volume (Figure 1 B). On the plot, Haller's layer was started from the scleral boundary, including the highest voxel ratio until the first small ratio on the plot. Therefore, this first valley after the plot's maximum marked the border between Haller's and Sattler's layer. The inner border of Sattler's layer was determined by detecting no vessels or noise, such as vessels consisting of a single voxel. Plot representations at the subfoveal choroid were qualitatively compared to actual vessel depiction by OCT and corresponded to vessel distribution in this location. Plots across the 36×36 degree field of view were used to generate Sattler's and Haller's layer thickness maps (Figures 1 D and 1 E, respectively) with Matlab software (The MathWorks, Inc., Natick, USA).

Outcome measures

The main outcome was the agreement between the repeatedly measured Sattler's and Haller's layer thicknesses in healthy and non-neovascular AMD. The secondary outcomes were the agreement of vessel segmentation with ICGA and the mean ± standard deviation of the choroidalsublayers expressed for the nine subfields of the ETDRS grid in a healthy eye cohort.

Statistical evaluation

The central submacular field (CSM) and the total macular field, with a diameter of 1.5 and 6 mm, respectively, were statistically analyzed for the repeatability testing. The difference was calculated between the same session and different day imaging and their confidence intervals (CI). To assess a possible relationship of the variability with the magnitude of the mean Bland-Altman plots for each group, each sublayer was plotted at the CSM and total macular field.[26] The 95% limits of agreement for small groups were found by multiplying the ±standard deviations by 2. To assess reliability, intraclass correlations (ICC) with measures of absolute agreement and their CIs were calculated. The coefficient of repeatability was calculated for the absolute and relative differences of repeated imaging.[27] Maps were qualitatively compared for repeatability between the three measurements (Figure 2).

The statistics software IBM SPSS Statistics for Windows, Version 20.0 (IBM Corp., Armonk, NY) was used for conducting normality testing, repeatability testing, ANOVA testing and a

Table 1. Average repeated choroidalsublayer thickness measurements for the central submacular field (CSM) and the total macular field (μm).

Layer	R1 (range)	R2 (range)	R3 (range)	*P* value	Δ R1-R2 (CI, LoA)	Δ R1-R3 (CI, LoA)
Healthy						
Sattler's (CSM)	116±66(10–217)	114±69(10–218)	123±68(6–225)	.17	2 (−8–13, 59)	−7(−18–5, 64)
Sattler's (total)	98±52(8–196)	94±508–176)	102±58(14–220)	.6	2 (−2–8, 32)	−4 (−12-2, 39)
Haller's (CSM)	226±80 (89–348)	228±86(87–361)	216±85 (86–382)	.54	1(−6–7, 31)	−4(−24–16, 66)
Haller's (total)	180±46(79–241)	184±51(78–253)	173±38 (63–228)	.2	−4 (−12-4, 45)	9(−13–30, 49)
Eyes with non-neovascular AMD						
Sattler's (CSM)	20±4(4–99)	20±4(2–88)	22±4 (5–133)	.61	−1 (−0.8-1.4, 17)	−1 (−1.5–1, 6)
Sattler's (total)	10±3(2–46)	9±3(2–40)	12±3(4–50)	.62	−1 (−0.9–1.4, 6)	0 (0−1, 5)
Haller's (CSM)	139±45 (80–234)	144±33 (82–233)	149±38 (82–219)	.37	−3(−14–9, 65)	−6 (−14–3, 50)
Haller's (total)	95±27(61–147)	93±27(57–151)	90±21(62–133)	.37	2(−3–8, 31)	3 (−5–10, 43)

R1 and R2 represent imaging at the same session. R3 was performed on a different day. P values are stated for the difference between measurements by repeated measures ANOVA. Δ represents the difference. CI is the 95% confidence interval. LoA represents 95% limits of agreement. Data are expressed as the mean ± standard deviation.

multiregression analysis of the possible contribution of independent variables (age, AL, refraction and gender) to choroidalsublayer thickness. Central measurements for statistical analysis were performed beneath the foveola.

Results

Repeatability of vessel segmentation

The average sublayer thickness measurements and their differences for the two groups obtained at each session are presented in Table 1. Intraclass correlations and coefficients of repeatability are presented in Table 2 and should be interpreted with respect to the mean measurements in Table 1.

The measurement of the total macular field repeatability was similar to measuring repeatability in the CSM field alone. The coefficients of repeatability were 35% and 21% in healthy eyes and 44% and 31% in AMD eyes for Sattler's and Haller's layers, respectively. The Sattler's layer was very thin in five of the ten AMD eyes. These eyes had a Sattler's layer thickness of <20 μm for the CSM subfield and <10 μm for the total macular field. In this small range of thickness measurements, the absolute differences yielded a high coefficient of repeatability. Sattler's and Haller's maps displayed similar thickness values and thickness distributionswhen eachrepeated imaging resultwas compared (Figure 2).

No significant difference was detected between repeated imaging (*P* values in Table 1), and no significant association between the thickness difference and the thickness mean in each group and in each choroidalsublayer was observed on the Bland-Altman plots. The ICCs indicated a strongagreement between the repeated measurements.

Validation of vessel segmentation with indocyanine green angiography

ICGA images of the non-neovascular AMD eyes (Figure 3) display a segmental vessel pattern with many large watershed zones in both phases. The enface OCT images (Figures 3 bottom row) visualize the same vessels with a comparably similar resolution to the ICGA images.

Table 2. Intraclass correlations (ICC) and coefficients of repeatability (CR).

Layer	ICC R1-R2 (CI)	ICC R1-R3 (CI)	CR R1-R2	CR R1-R3
Healthy				
Sattler's (CSM)	0.99 (0.96–1)	0.95 (0.94–1)	40 (35%)	32 (27%)
Sattler's (total)	0.96 (0.84–0.99)	0.99 (0.96–1)	22 (23%)	26 (26%)
Haller's (CSM)	0.99 (0.98–1)	0.97 (0.88–0.99)	22 (10%)	46 (21%)
Haller's (total)	0.99 (0.96–1)	0.98 (0.89–0.99)	32 (18%)	33 (19%)
Non-neovascular AMD				
Sattler's (CSM)	0.98 (0.93–0.99)	0.86 (0.44–0.97)	4 (20%)	4 (20%)
Sattler's (total)	0.95 (0.82–0.99)	0.96 (0.86–0.99)	4 (44%)	4 (34%)
Haller's (CSM)	0.9 (0.59-0-98)	0.92 (0.69–0.98)	44 (31%)	34 (23%)
Haller's (total)	0.97 (0.9–0.99)	0.95 (0.80–0.99)	21 (22%)	19 (21%)

R1 and R2 represent imaging at the same session. R3 was performed on a different day. CI is the 95% confidence interval. CR represents the coefficient of repeatability, expressed in parenthesis as the percentage of the mean difference.

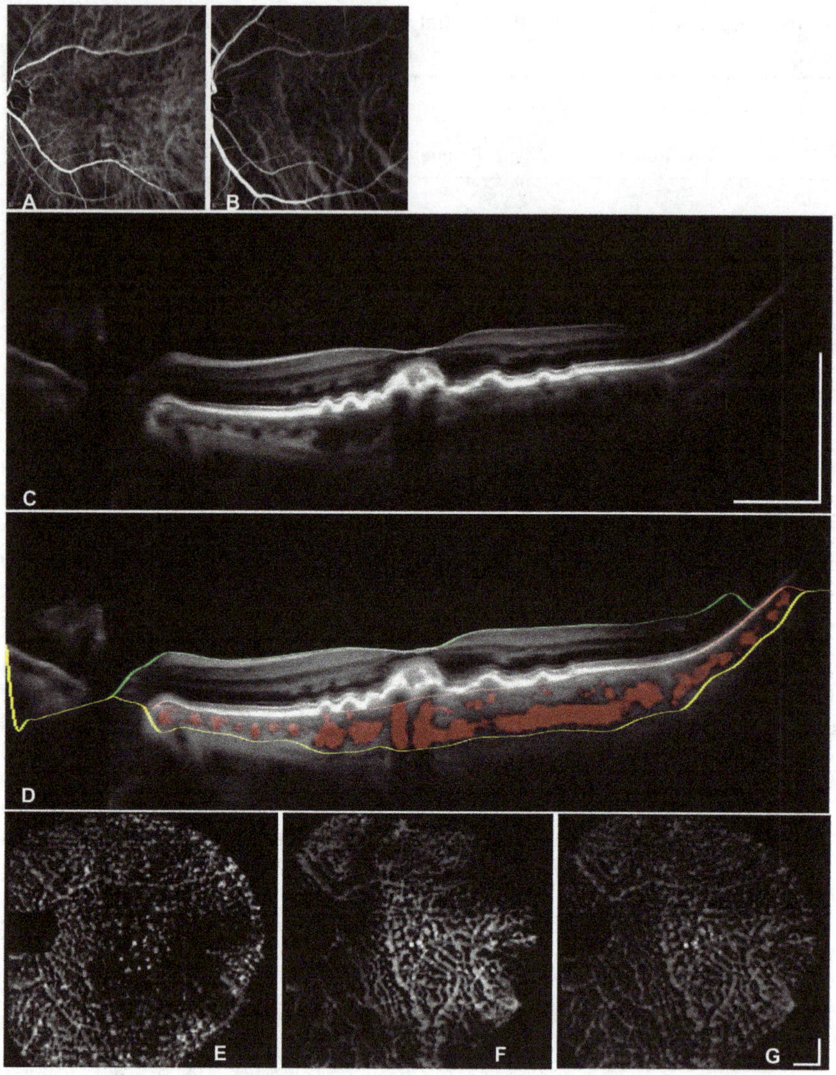

Figure 3. Segmentation validation in a non-neovascular AMD eye via a comparison of the segmented vasculature with indocyanine green angiography (ICGA). Early phase (A) and middle phase (B) angiography images show the ICGAresolution for choroidal vascular imaging. OCT B-scan centered on the fovea (C), and segmented areasare marked in red (D) to visualize vessel segmentation. The OCT B-scan (D) shows the segmentation lines for the retina between the ILM (green line) and the RBC complex. The choroid is located between the RBC complex and the sclera (yellow line). En face views are locatedat the inner choroid (E), the outer choroid (F) and the entire choroid (G) to demonstrate captured vessels and depth information. The bars represent 1 mm.

Healthy choroidal vessel segmentation and layer thicknesses

The mean layer thicknesses for each ETDRS macular subfields of Haller's and Sattler's layer for the healthy eye cohort are stated in Table 3. Multiregression analysis indicated a significant statistical relationship for each Haller's and Sattler's layer central subfield with age and AL (Sattler's layer: $R^2 = 0.24$, $P = .003$, AL: Beta = −48 $P < .001$, age Beta = −28 $P = .05$ and Haller's layer: $R^2 = 0.39$, $P < .001$, AL: Beta = −62 $P < .001$, age Beta = −30 $P = .02$). The two independent factors AL and refraction displayed a linear association with each other (collinearitydiagnostics testing of multiregression analysis). Refraction had a weaker effect than AL on Sattler's and Haller's layers (Beta = −38 and −44, respectively) and was excluded from the analysis. Therefore, despite the high variability, the relationship between AL and Sattler's and Haller's layer in the healthy cohort of 45 eyes was statistically significant, and the relationship-related variation exceededthe imprecision inherent to the methodology (Table 3).

Discussion

Different approaches to *in vivo*choroidal vessel analysis have been suggested in the literature. Choroidal vessel visualization using angiography has shown the segmental vessel structure and their respective watershed zones[28,29]. Watershed zones are highly affected by ageing and ischemia and may offer a more sensitive measure of pathological changes than choroidal thickness change alone [30]. Choroidal OCT imaging offers noninvasive vessel visualization. OCT pixel intensitymeasurementshave been suggested for the analysis of choroidal vessels in AMD eyes [31]. However, this method has been used without determining the border between Sattler's and Haller's layers and may be unfeasible when the OCT images are affected by retinal and RPE lesions.

Table 3. Automated calculated mean for healthy Sattler's and Haller's layer thickness across the Early Treatment Diabetic Retinopathy Study grid (μm).

Subfield	Sattler's layer	Haller's layer
central submacular	87±56 (3–264)	141±50 (57–237)
superior inner	77±51 (13–268)	144±44 (65–251)
temporal inner	71±52 (3–233)	131±53 (48–255)
inferior inner	77±55 (4–246)	133±47 (48–225)
nasal inner	81±60 (1–240)	133±38 (58–211)
superior outer	74±45 (10–243)	121±33 (70–195)
temporal outer	50±45 (4–213)	103±40 (50–181)
inferior outer	65±49 (5–215)	117±37 (64–180)
nasal outer	64±50 (3–203)	110±35 (66–166)
Grouped by axial eye length for statistical analysis for the CSM subfield[a]		
Hyperope n=15	114±64 (3–264)	168±43 (57–236)
Emmetrope n=18	79±45 (19–165)	133±46 (70–230)
Myope n=12	48±35 (3–99)	104±49 (50–236)
P value[b]	.006 (.004)	.003 (.002)
Grouped by age (years) for the CSM subfield		
< 45 n=27	91±51	144±50
>45 n=18	70±59	125±52

Data are expressed in μm and as the mean ± standard deviation (range).
a. Eyes were grouped based on the normal AL variation with refraction and age by myopia: AL≥24.5 mm, emmetropic: 24.5>AL≥23.4 mm or hyperopic:AL<23.4 mm)
b. univariate ANOVA (post-hoc test Tukey for hyperopic and myopic eyes)

Motaghiannezam et al. demonstrated an algorithm for automated OCT vessel segmentation in three healthy eyes [32], whereas Zhang et al. investigated a cohort of twenty-four healthy eyes, but they could not successfully reproduce repeat automated segmentation in all eyes[33]. In this study, the segmentation of vessels and Sattler's and Haller's layer was successfully applied in all healthy and pathological eyes. Furthermore, the automatic vessel segmentation was validated against ICGA and captured most choroidal vessels despite non-neovascular AMD lesions.

This study found a significant relationship with AL, and the relationship-related variationexceeded the segmentation variability. Healthy sublayer thinning with age was significant,but the level of thinning was below the measurement variability. For every 10 years of ageing,14 to 15 μm of choroidal thinning has been reported [6,8], and choroidal thinning is further increased in the presence of AMD phenotypes, such as in eyes with subretinal deposits[12] or with geographic atrophy[34]. Future research is needed to explore if pathological choroidal thinning is related to Sattler's and Haller's layers with a larger thickness difference than the coefficient of repeatability of this study.

Automatic segmentation precision is defined by measurement repeatability and is dependent on the visualization quality of the interfaces. For choroidal thickness measurements, the quality is determined by the signal to noise ratio of the OCT image. The signal is reduced with increasing depth or by image degradation below a retinal lesion,whereas depth has a stronger effect on the measurement variability [35]. Healthy eyes have commonly thick choroids, and the current study demonstrated that automatic vessel segmentation was not deteriorated in these eyes. A further source for imprecision is the noise caused by the inconsistency of positioning. In the AMD cohort, the signal may have been further reduced by unstable fixation. Some AMD eyes had a very thin Sattler's layer; therefore,small deviations resulted in high coefficients of repeatability. As such, the coefficients of repeatability need to be viewed in relation to the absolute measurements, and a large AMD cohort is needed to evaluate if a thin Sattler's layer correlates to the clinical appearance.

The choroid displays a high variability, which is reflected in large standard deviations when compared to the retina and its sublayers[25,36]. The choroidal vasculature is even more challenging. When a vessel's course is parallel to the OCT scan, the cross-section of the vessel does not appear round. This complexity reduces manual vessel segmentation precision, which is performed in two-dimensional scans. To improve manual segmentation repeatability, training is needed ideally [37] whereas there is no training or expertise needed for automatic segmentation after the initial validation. Manual segmentation in diabetic eyes has demonstrated 26% and 32% repeatability for Sattler's layer and 30% and 32% for Haller's layer for the central submacular field and total macular field, respectively [37]. The automatic segmentation in this paper displayed a comparably good variability for healthy and diseased eyes with a range of different choroidal thicknesses and noise distributions.

In conclusion, this study utilized a rapid and clinically feasible method to obtain the spatial distribution of choroidalsublayers with 3D 1060-nm OCT mapping and with the widely used ETDRS grid subfields. Sublayer variation with AL was greater thanthe imprecision of the methodology, and mapping allowed for the observation of the sublayer's thicknessover the scanning field. To the best of our knowledge, the present choroidalsublayer segmentation offers the most repeatable and reliable automated qualitative and quantitative analysis method for clinical use and the investigation of pathological choroidal thinning. For future studies of Sattler's and Haller's layers and for the clinical application of vessel segmentation in AMD eyes, the variability caused by noise and the morphological complexity of choroidal vessels need to be considered.

Acknowledgments

The authors wish to thank Dr. Michael Hagmann (Institute for Medical Statistics, Medical University Vienna, Austria) for his statistical support.

Author Contributions

Conceived and designed the experiments: ME VK BZ RO SA LK IK SN MK JH JF WD SB. Performed the experiments: ME VK BZ RO SA LK IK SN. Analyzed the data: ME VK BZ RO. Contributed reagents/materials/analysis tools: ME VK BZ RO SA LK IK SN MK JH JF WD SB. Wrote the paper: ME VK BZ RO SA LK IK SN MK JH JF WD SB.

References

1. Bill A, Sperber G, Ujiie K (1983) Physiology of the choroidal vascular bed. Int Ophthalmol 6: 101–107.
2. Linsenmeier RA, Padnick-Silver L (2000) Metabolic dependence of photoreceptors on the choroid in the normal and detached retina. Invest Ophthalmol Vis Sci 41: 3117–3123.
3. Hayreh SS (1974) The choriocapillaris. Albrecht von Graefes Arch Klin Ophthalmol 192: 165–179.
4. Zhang HR (1994) Scanning electron-microscopic study of corrosion casts on retinal and choroidal angioarchitecture in man and animals. Progress in Retinal and Eye Research 13: 243–270.
5. Nickla DL, Wallman J (2010) The multifunctional choroid. Prog Retin Eye Res 29: 144–168.
6. Margolis R, Spaide RF (2009) A pilot study of enhanced depth imaging optical coherence tomography of the choroid in normal eyes. Am J Ophthalmol147: 811–815.
7. Spaide RF (2009) Age-related choroidal atrophy. Am J Ophthalmol147: 801-810.
8. Ikuno Y, Kawaguchi K, Yasuno Y, Nouchi T (2009) Choroidal Thickness in Healthy Japanese Subjects. Invest Ophthalmol Vis Sci51: 2173–2176.
9. Manjunath V, Goren J, Fujimoto JG, Duker JS (2011) Analysis of choroidal thickness in age-related macular degeneration using spectral-domain optical coherence tomography. Am J Ophthalmol 152: 663–668.
10. Koizumi H, Yamagishi T, Yamazaki T, Kawasaki R, Kinoshita S (2011) Subfoveal choroidal thickness in typical age-related macular degeneration and polypoidal choroidal vasculopathy. Graefes Arch Clin Exp Ophthalmol 249: 1123–1128.
11. Mullins RF, Johnson MN, Faidley EA, Skeie JM, Huang J (2011) Choriocapillaris vascular dropout related to density of drusen in human eyes with early age-related macular degeneration. Invest Ophthalmol Vis Sci 52: 1606–1612.
12. Querques G, Querques L, Forte R, Massamba N, Coscas F, et al. (2012) Choroidal changes associated with reticular pseudodrusen. Invest Ophthalmol Vis Sci 53: 1258–1263.
13. Young M, Chui L, Fallah N, Or C, Merkur AB, et al. (2014) Exacerbation of choroidal and retinal pigment epithelial atrophy after anti-vascular endothelial growth factor treatment in neovascular age-related macular degeneration. Retina. doi:10.1097/IAE.0000000000000081.
14. Hogan MJ, Alvarado JA, Weddell JE (1971) Histology of the human eye: an atlas and textbook. Hogan MJ, Alvarado JA, Weddell JE, editors. Saunders. pp 322–371.
15. Ramrattan RS, van der Schaft TL, Mooy CM, de Bruijn WC, Mulder PG, et al. (1994) Morphometric analysis of Bruch's membrane, the choriocapillaris, and the choroid in aging. IOVS 35: 2857–2864.
16. McLeod DS, Taomoto M, Otsuji T, Green WR, Sunness JS, et al. (2002) Quantifying changes in RPE and choroidal vasculature in eyes with age-related macular degeneration. Invest Ophthalmol Vis Sci 43: 1986–1993.
17. Unterhuber A, Považay B, Hermann B, Sattmann H, Chavez-Pirson A, et al. (2005) In vivo retinal optical coherence tomography at 1040 nm-enhanced penetration into the choroid. Opt Express 13: 3252–3258.
18. De Bruin DM, Burnes DL, Loewenstein J, Chen Y, Chang S, et al. (2008) In vivo three-dimensional imaging of neovascular age-related macular degeneration using optical frequency domain imaging at 1050 nm. Invest Ophthalmol Vis Sci 49: 4545–4552.
19. Kajic V, Esmaeelpour M, Glittenberg C, Kraus MF, Honegger J, et al. (2013) Automated three-dimensional choroidal vessel segmentation of 3D 1060 nm OCT retinal data. Biomed Opt Express 4: 134–150.
20. Ferris FL 3rd, Wilkinson CP, Bird A, Chakravarthy U, Chew E, et al. (2013) Clinical classification of age-related macular degeneration. Ophthalmology 120: 844–851.
21. ANSI (2000) Safe Use of Lasers & Safe Use of Optical Fiber Communications. American National Standard Institute - Z136 Committee. 168 p.
22. ICNIRP (2000) Revision of the Guidelines on Limits of Exposure to Laser radiation of wavelengths between 400nm and 1.4 µm. International Commission on Non-Ionizing Radiation Protection. 431–440 p.
23. Kraus MF, Potsaid B, Mayer MA, Bock R, Baumann B, et al. (2012) Motion correction in optical coherence tomography volumes on a per A-scan basis using orthogonal scan patterns. Biomed Opt Express 3: 1182–1199.
24. Kajic V, Esmaeelpour M, Považay B, Marshall D, Rosin PL, et al. (2011) Automated choroidal segmentation of 1060 nm OCT in healthy and pathologic eyes using a statistical model. Biomed Opt Express 3: 86–103.
25. Esmaeelpour M, Povazay B, Hermann B, Hofer B, Kajic V, et al. (2010) Three-dimensional 1060nm OCT: Choroidal thickness maps in normals and improved posterior segment visualization in cataract patients. Invest Ophthalmol Vis Sci 51: 5260–6.
26. Bland JM, Altman DG (1986) Statistical methods for assessing agreement between two methods of clinical measurement. Lancet 1: 307–310.
27. Bland JM, Altman DG (1996) Statistical methods for assessing agreement between two methods of clinical measurement. Lancet 1: 307–310.
28. Hayreh SS (1990) In vivo choroidal circulation and its watershed zones. Eye (Lond) 4 (Pt 2): 273–289.
29. Hayreh SS (2004) Posterior Ciliary Artery Circulation in Health and Disease The Weisenfeld Lecture. Invest Ophthalmol Vis Sci 45: 749–757.
30. Ito YN, Mori K, Young-Duvall J, Yoneya S (2001) Aging changes of the choroidal dye filling pattern in indocyanine green angiography of normal subjects. Retina 21: 237–242.
31. Sohrab M, Wu K, Fawzi AA (2012) A Pilot Study of Morphometric Analysis of Choroidal Vasculature In Vivo, Using En Face Optical Coherence Tomography. PLoS ONE 7: e48631. doi:10.1371/journal.pone.0048631.
32. Motaghiannezam R, Schwartz DM, Fraser SE (2012) In Vivo Human Choroidal Vascular Pattern Visualization Using High-Speed Swept-Source Optical Coherence Tomography at 1060 nm. Invest Ophthalmol Vis Sci 53: 2337–2348.
33. Zhang L, Lee K, Niemeijer M, Mullins RF, Sonka M, et al. (2012) Automated segmentation of the choroid from clinical SD-OCT. Invest Ophthalmol Vis Sci 53: 7510–7519.
34. Lee JY, Lee DH, Lee JY, Yoon YH (2013) Correlation between subfoveal choroidal thickness and the severity or progression of nonexudative age-related macular degeneration. Invest Ophthalmol Vis Sci 54: 7812–7818. doi:10.1167/iovs.13–12284.
35. Kim JH, Kang SW, Kim JR, Kim SJ (2013) Variability of subfoveal choroidal thickness measurements in patients with age-related macular degeneration and central serous chorioretinopathy. Eye (Lond) 27: 809–815.
36. Ikuno Y, Maruko I, Yasuno Y, Miura M, Sekiryu T, et al. (2011) Reproducibility of Retinal and Choroidal Thickness Measurements in Enhanced Depth Imaging and High-Penetration Optical Coherence Tomography. Invest Ophthalmol Vis Sci 52: 5536–5540.
37. Sim DA, Keane PA, Mehta H, Fung S, Zarranz-Ventura J, et al. (2013) Repeatability and Reproducibility of Choroidal Vessel Layer Measurements in Diabetic Retinopathy Using Enhanced Depth Optical Coherence Tomography. Investigative Ophthalmology & Visual Science 54: 2893–2901.

7

Interleukin 27 Induces the Expression of Complement Factor H (CFH) in the Retina

Ahjoku Amadi-Obi, Cheng-Rong Yu, Ivy Dambuza, Sung-Hye Kim, Bernadette Marrero, Charles E. Egwuagu*

Molecular Immunology Section, National Eye Institute, National Institutes of Health, Bethesda, Maryland, United States of America

Abstract

Complement factor H (CFH) is a central regulator of the complement system and has been implicated in the etiology of age-related macular degeneration (AMD), a leading cause of blindness in the elderly. In view of previous studies showing that reduced expression of CFH in the retina is a risk factor for developing AMD, there is significant interest in understanding how CFH expression is regulated in the retina. In this study, we have shown that the anti-inflammatory cytokine, IL-27, induced CFH expression in mouse retinal cells and human retinal pigmented epithelial cells (RPE) through STAT1-mediated up-regulation of Interferon Regulatory Factor-1 (IRF-1) and IRF-8. We further show that cells in the ganglion and inner-nuclear layers of the retina constitutively express IRF-1 and IRF-8 and enhanced CFH expression in the retina during ocular inflammation correlated with significant increase in the expression of IRF-1, IRF-8 and IL-27 (IL-27p28 and Ebi3). Our data thus reveal a novel role of IL-27 in regulating complement activation through up-regulation of CFH and suggest that defects in IL-27 signaling or expression may contribute to the reduction of CFH expression in the retina of patients with AMD.

Editor: Prosper N. Boyaka, The Ohio State University, United States of America

Funding: The Intramural Research Programs of the National Eye Institute and National Institutes of Health provided funding for this research. The funders had no role in study design, data collection and analysis, decision to publish, or preparation of the manuscript.

Competing Interests: The authors have declared that no competing interests exist.

* E-mail: egwuaguc@nei.nih.gov

Introduction

The vertebrate eye is comprised of highly specialized tissues of the retina, cornea, lens, iris, ciliary body, choroid, sclera, aqueous humor and vitreous body and its primary function is to receive and convert incident light rays into visual images. To ensure the fidelity of the visual image, the optical axis (cornea, anterior chamber, lens and vitreous body) through which the light is transmitted, must be transparent and devoid of lymphoreticular cells [1]. Intraocular inflammation, characterized by influx of inflammatory cells into the retina, is therefore highly undesirable because it compromises the requisite transparency of the optical axis. Moreover, inflammatory mediators secreted by the inflammatory cells promote undesirable angiogenesis, fibrosis and tissue destruction [1]. Thus, ocular immunity is predicated on the paramount need to preserve vision while neutralizing pathogenic stimuli with minimal collateral damage to ocular structures. The complement system plays a central role in conferring innate immunity against microbes in the eye and it functions through sequential activation of cascades of proteases and a cell-killing membrane attack complex that generate cleavage fragments which amplify the inflammatory response. The uncontrolled activation of the complement pathway in the eye is therefore dangerous as it is potentially injurious to terminally differentiated photoreceptors and neurons of the neuroretina. This calamity is obviated by the production of a family of complement control proteins of which complement factor H (CFH) is a prominent member.

CFH is a multifunctional protein that acts as a central regulator of the complement system [2]. It regulates the levels of newly generated C3b molecules by serving as a cofactor for complement factor I in degrading C3b [2] and destabilizing the alternative complement C3 convertase, C3bBb (decay-accelerating activity). *CFH* is one of several genes identified in genome-wide association studies [3,4,5,6,7,8] to be implicated in age-related macular degeneration (AMD), the leading cause of irreversible blindness in the elderly [9,10,11]. Although the pathophysiology of AMD is not well understood, recent reports suggest that defects in mechanisms that control chronic inflammation or down-regulate complement activation play crucial roles [9,10,11]. *CFH* variants that express reduced amounts of CFH or have low complement-modulating activity have been suggested as risk factors for developing AMD [12].

CFH is constitutively expressed in the liver and the liver produces the highest level of CFH in the body [2]. Significant amounts of CFH are also produced in the eye, with the highest levels detected in the retinal pigment epithelia (RPE), choroid and the retina [13]. The pro-inflammatory cytokine, IFN-g has been shown to up-regulate the expression of CFH in hepatocytes, astrocytes, lung cells and astroglioma cell lines [14,15] and these observations are consistent with the presence of two IFN-g activation sites (GAS) within the *CFH* proximal promoter [16,17,18]. With the knowledge that defects in CFH production may contribute to the development of AMD, it is remarkable that less is known about mechanisms involved in the regulation of CFH production in the normal retina. The transcription factor, STAT1 (signal transducer and activator of transcription 1), has been shown to activate the transcription of *CFH* in the human retinal pigment epithelia (RPE) cell line, ARPE-19 following stimulation by IFN-g

[12,19]. On the other hand, oxidative stress reduced the ability of IFN-g to increase CFH expression in ARPE-19 by enhancing FOXO3a binding to the CFH promoter and inhibiting interaction of STAT1 with the CFH promoter [12,19]. These studies established the central role of STAT1 in the regulation of CFH in RPE. However, IFN-g is not present in the normal retina nor is it secreted by retinal cells and could therefore not be responsible for activating STAT1 required for constitutive expression of CFH in the retina. We therefore posited that other cytokines such as IL-27 or growth factors produced by retinal cells may be the source of the activated STAT1 needed to induce transcription of the *CFH* gene.

Interleukin-27 (IL-27) is an anti-inflammatory heterodimeric cytokine comprised of IL-27p40 and EBI3 (Epstein-Barr virus (EBV)-induced gene 3) subunits [20]. It is constitutively secreted by retinal microglia and in a previous study we showed that IL-27 suppressed intraocular inflammation through activation of STAT1 [21,22]. In this study, we have investigated whether IL-27 can up-regulate the expression of CFH in retinal cells. We show here that IL-27 induces CFH expression in freshly isolated primary mouse retinal cells and human retinal epithelial cells through activation of STAT1 and up-regulation of the STAT1 target genes, Interferon Regulatory Factor-1 (IRF-1) and IRF-8.

Methods

Mice

C57BL/6 mice (6–8 weeks old) were from Jackson Laboratory (Bar Harbor, ME). STAT1-deficient mice were a gift from Dr D. Levy New York University NY. We generated STAT3 conditional deletion in the retina by breeding $STAT3^{F/F}$ mice with a-Cre transgenic mice, which express Cre-recombinase only in the retina (generously provided by Dr. Gruss) [23]. Generation and characterization of transgenic mice with targeted over-expression of SOCS1 in the retina (SOCS1-Tg) has previously been described [24]. All mice were housed in clean animal rooms operated under barrier conditions. Animal care and use was in compliance with Association for Assessment and Accreditation of Laboratory Animal Care, International (AAALAC) and the NIH Intramural Animal Care & Use Program guidelines. This study was approved by the National Eye Institute/NIH Animal Care and Use Committee under the Animal Study Proposal (ASP) # NEI-597 approved on October 25, 2010).

Induction of EAU and Imaging Mouse Fundus

We induced EAU by active immunization with bovine interphotoreceptor retinoid-binding protein (IRBP, 150 μg for C57BL/6 mice, 50 μg for B10.A mice) and human IRBP peptide (amino acid residues 1–20; 150 μg for C57BL/6 mice), in a 0.2 ml emulsion (1:1) v/v with complete Freund's adjuvant (CFA) containing Mycobacterium tuberculosis strain H37Ra (2.5 mg/ml). Mice also received *Bordetella pertussis* toxin (0.2 μg/mouse) concurrent with immunization. Clinical disease was established and scored by funduscopy as described [24,25]. Briefly, following ip injection of ketamine (1.4 mg/mouse) and xylazine (0.12 mg/mouse), pupils were dilated by topical administration of 1% tropicamide ophthalmic solution (Alcon Inc, Fort Worth, Texas). To avoid a subjective bias, evaluation of the fundus photographs was conducted without knowledge of the mouse identity by a masked observer. At least six images (2 posterior central retinal view, 4 peripheral retinal views) were taken from each eye by positioning the endoscope and viewing from superior, inferior, lateral and medial fields and each individual lesion was identified, mapped and recorded. The clinical grading system for retinal inflammation was as previously established [26].

Isolation of Retinal Cells

Primary retinal cells were isolated as previously described [22]. Briefly, retinas were dissected out from enucleated eyes and briefly rinsed in sterile PBS. Retinas were then diced in small pieces and incubated in Hanks balanced salt solution (HBSS), containing activated papain 120 U (Worthington, Lakewood NJ) and DNase 2000 U (Worthington), for 1 hour. To make single cell suspension retinas were gently triturated with pipette and then passed through a 40 μm cell strainer and centrifuged at 200 g for 5 min. The pellet was resuspended in 1% ovalbumin (Worthington) in HBSS containing 500 U of DNase and layered on 5% ovalbumin solution in HBSS and centrifuged for 10 min at 500×g. The pellet was resuspended in medium [1:1] mixture of Dulbecco's modified Eagle's medium and F12 medium containing 2.5% heat-inactivated horse serum, B27 medium supplement (Invitrogen, Carlsbad, CA), 5 mg/ml D-glucose, 2 mM L-glutamine, 20 mM HEPES, 2.5 mg/ml bovine insulin (Sigma, ST Louis, MO), and 0.1 mg/ml human transferrin (Sigma; 15 000 cells/ml)]. Cell viability was consistently >90% as assessed by Trypan blue exclusion and the Vi-CELL Cell Viability Analyzer (Beckman Coulter).

Cell Culture and Interleukin 27 (IL-27) Treatment

The human RPE cell line (ARPE-19) was purchased from the American Type Culture Collection (Manannas, VA). The ARPE-19 cells were grown to confluence in minimum essential medium (MEM) supplemented with 10% fetal bovine serum (FBS), 100 U/ml penicillin, 100 μg/ml streptomycin, and 50 ng/ml amphotericin B. The cells were washed twice in serum-free medium (SFM) (HyClone, Logan, UT) and incubated in SFM containing human recombinant IL-27 (10 ng/ml) (R&D) for varying amounts of time at 37°C in 5% CO2. The protein synthesis inhibitor, cycloheximide (CHX) (Sigma, St. Louis, MO), was used at 35 μg/ml and added 30 minutes before addition of IL-27. Treatment with CHX allows for discrimination between immediate effects of STAT1 and effects requiring de novo protein synthesis.

Small Interfering RNA (siRNA)–mediated Silencing of CFH Expression

Cells were cultured to 60–70% confluence and transfected with siRNA oligonucleotides (Santa Cruz). Cells were replated in six-well plates and stimulated with IL-27 for varying amounts of time. Complete knockdown of CFH occurred at 72 hour-time point and was confirmed by RT-PCR analysis.

Western Blot Analysis

Whole cell lysates were prepared as previously described [27]. Briefly, extracts were fractionated on a 4–12% gradient SDS-PAGE and proteins were then transferred to a PVDF membrane. Antibodies used were: STAT1, pSTAT1, STAT3, pSTAT3 (Cell signaling Technology), CFH, IRF-1, IRF-8, (Santa Cruz Biotechnology). Pre-immune serum was used in parallel as controls and signals were detected with HRP conjugated-secondary F(ab')2 Abs (Zymed Labs, San Francisco, CA) using the ECL Plus Kit (Amersham, Arlington Heights, IL).

Immunohistochemistry

Enucleated eyes were fixed in 4% paraformaldehyde and embedded in Ameraffin tissue embedding medium (Baxter). Tissue sections (5 mm) were deparaffinized in xylene, rehydrated through a graded alcohol series. For detection of IRF-8, immunostaining was performed by the avidin-biotin-peroxidase complex method (Vector Laboratories, Burlingame, CA.). Sections were pre-incubation for 2 h with 5% blocking serum and then incubated overnight at 4°C with antibodies (0.02 mg/ml) specific to mouse IRF-8 (Santa Cruz). Control sections received the appropriate normal serum. All sections were subsequently incubated with biotinylated secondary antibody for 30 min at room temperature, and signal was visualized with diaminobenzidine-H_2O_2 as recommended (Vector). Sections were counterstained with hematoxylin. For detection of CFH expression, sections were blocked with 5% normal goat serum and then incubated with CFH antibody (Santa Cruz Biotechnology) overnight at 4°C. After washing with ICC Buffer (PBS containing 0.5% BSA, 0.2%, Tween 20 and 0.05% sodium Azide) sections were incubated with donkey anti-goat Alexa-Fluor© 488 and DAPI for 1 hr and washed with ICC Buffer. Slides were mounted with Vectashield Mounting medium for fluorescence (Vector Labs) and images taken with a confocal microscope. Gain/offset settings were set at the same level for all slides.

Quantitative and Semi-quantitative PCR Analyses

Total RNA was extracted from primary retinal cells or ARPE-19 cells using the TriZol reagent according to the procedures recommended by the manufacturer (Life Technologies, Gaithersburg, MD). All RNA samples were digested with RNase-free DNase 1 (Life Technologies) for 30 min, purified by phenol/chloroform extractions and precipitated in 0.4 M LiCl. RNA (10 µg), SuperScript III Reverse Transcriptase (Life Technologies, Gaithersburg, MD), and oligo $(dT)_{12-18}$ were used for first-strand synthesis as previously described [27]. Samples were subjected to hot-start RT-PCR with gene-specific primers and AmpliTaq Gold DNA polymerase (Applied Biosystems, Foster City, CA). First-strand synthesis containing each mRNA sample but no reverse transcriptase was performed to control for possible DNA contamination of mRNAs used as target for PCR amplification; failure to obtain RT-PCR products with any of the PCR amplimers confirmed the absence of contaminating DNA templates. PCR-amplified fragments were fractionated on agarose gels. All cDNA preparations used were suitable substrates for PCR amplification on the basis of efficient amplification of a ß-actin sequence. Real-time PCR was performed on an ABI 7500 and PCR parameters were as recommended for the TaqMan Universal PCR kit (Applied Biosystems). Primers and probes were purchased from Applied Biosystems).

Statistical Analysis

Statistical analyses were performed by independent two-tailed Student's t test. Probability values of ≤ 0.05 were considered statistically significant.

Results

IL-27 Up-regulates the Expression of CFH in Retinal Cells

CFH expression has been detected in the retina, ciliary body, sclera and the ocular lens [13]. To confirm these findings, we performed immunohistochemical analysis of 8 weeks old C57BL/6 mouse eyes and the highest level of CFH expression was detected in the RPE layer, photoreceptors, plexiform and ganglion cell layers (Fig. 1A). We also confirmed the expression of CFH in the retina of the C57BL/6 mouse by Western blot analysis. However the level expressed by retinal cells was substantially lower than the level detected in the liver (Fig. 1B). To investigate whether IL-27 induces CFH expression by the RPE, we cultured ARPE-19 cells in medium containing IL-27 and RNA analysis of CFH expression by quantitative PCR (qRT-PCR) revealed that ARPE-19 cells constitutively expressed CFH and that IL-27 significantly up-regulated the transcription of CFH (Fig. 1C) in a dose-dependent manner (Fig. 1D). These results were confirmed at the protein level by Western blotting analysis showing substantial induction of CFH protein expression by IL-27 (Fig. 1E). We further show that IL-27 induced the increase of CFH expression in ARPE-19 through activation of STAT1 and STAT3 pathways (Fig. 1F).

CFH Expression in the Mouse Retina Requires STAT1 and is Up-regulated by IL-27

IL-27 induced the expression of CFH in ARPE-19 cells through the activation of both STAT1 and STAT3 (Fig. 1E, 1F). It was therefore of interest to determine whether both STAT1 and STAT3 are required for IL-27-mediated increase of CFH by analyzing CFH levels in retina of STAT1- or STAT3-deficient mice. However, because STAT3 deficiency is embryonic lethal, we used a Cre-loxP system to generate STAT3 conditional knockout mice in which STAT3 gene was disrupted only in the retina. Cre-recombinase expression was directed under control of a retina-specific regulatory element of murine Pax6 (a-Cre) [23]. Western blot analysis of whole cell extracts of the retina-STAT3 knockout mouse strain (Ret-STAT3$^{-/-}$) indicates markedly decreased STAT3 in the retina (Fig. 2A). To address the role of STAT1 and/or STAT3 in IL-27-mediated induction of CFH, we analyzed the expression of CFH in the retina of wild type C57BL/6 (WT), STAT1-deficient (STAT1$^{-/-}$) [28] mice or mice with targeted over-expression of SOCS1 in the retina under direction of opsin promoter (SOCS1-Tg) [24]. Western blot analysis of whole cell extracts prepared from freshly isolated retinal cells revealed equivalent levels of CFH expression in the retinas of the WT and STAT3-deficient mice (Fig. 2B), indicating that STAT3 expression and/or activation is dispensable for the expression of CFH in the retina. In contrast, we observed substantial decrease in CFH levels in the retina of the STAT1$^{-/-}$ and SOCS1-Tg mice (Fig. 2B). It is of note that the SOCS1-Tg mice are deficient in STAT1 activation [24], underscoring the requirement of STAT1 for optimal expression of CFH in the normal retina. To confirm that STAT1 is indeed required for IL-27-mediated induction of CFH gene expression in the retina, we established retinal organ cultures from freshly isolate retinas of WT or STAT1-deficient mice and stimulated them overnight in medium containing IL-27. Results of RT-PCR analysis of the RNA (Fig. 2C) or Western blot analysis of whole cell extracts derived from the retinal cells (Fig. 2D) revealed marked increase in CFH expression by WT retinal cells cultured in medium containing IL-27. On the other hand, addition of IL-27 to STAT1-deficient retina cultures could not induce the up-regulation of CFH expression. Together, these results confirm the requirement of STAT1 for IL-27-mediated induction of CFH in the retina and underscore the physiological relevance of IL-27 in promoting the expression of CFH in the mammalian retina.

IRF-1 and IRF-8 Contribute to Transcriptional Activation of CFH Gene in the Retina

Interferon Regulatory Factor (IRF) family of transcription factors play important roles in gene-regulatory networks that control cell growth, differentiation and host immunity [29]. IRF-1 and IRF-8 transcription factors are induced by IFN-g through activation of STAT1 and in a previous study we showed that IFN-g signaling in human RPE is mediated by STAT1, IRF-1 and IRF-8 [30]. We therefore investigated whether the up-regulation of CFH in the retina or ARPE-19 cells by IL-27 derived from activation of *IRF-1*, *IRF-8* and/or *STAT1* genes. We starved

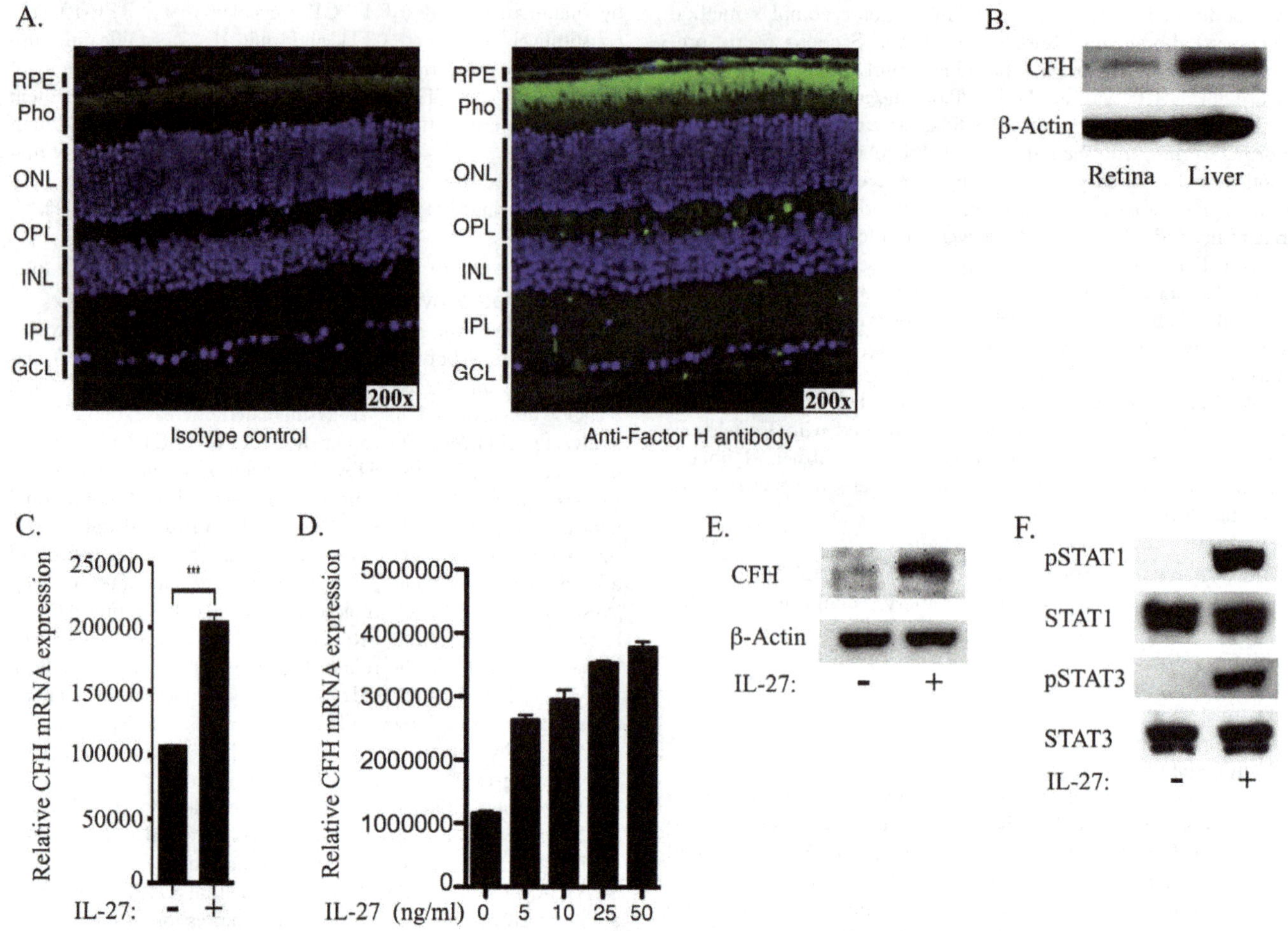

Figure 1. CFH is constitutively expressed in the retina and up-regulated in RPE cells by IL-27 through STAT1-dependent mechanism. (A) Immunohistochemical localization of CFH expression in the mouse retina. Retina pigmented epithelium (RPE); Photoreceptors (pho); outer nuclear layer (ONL); outer plexiform layer (OPL); inner plexiform layer (IPL). (B) Whole cell extracts prepared from the retina or liver of C57BL/6 mice were analyzed for expression of CFH by Western blot assay. (C) ARPE-19 cells were stimulated for 24 hours in medium containing human IL-27 (10 ng/ml). ARPE-19 cells were cultured overnight in complete medium, washed and starved in serum free medium (SFM) for 2 hours and then stimulated in SFM containing human recombinant IL-27 (10 ng/ml) for 24 hours (C, D, E) or 30 minutes (F). (C) RNA was isolated and analyzed by qRT-PCR. (D) The ARPE-19 cells were stimulated with several concentrations of human IL-27 and then subjected to qRT-PCR analysis. (E, F) Whole cell extracts were analyzed by Western blot assay.

ARPE-19 cells for 2 hours in SFM, treated the cells with IL-27 for varying amounts of time (30 minutes to 24 hours) and examined time-dependent effects of IL-27 on STAT1 activation and the expression of CFH, IRF-1 or IRF-8. Western blot analysis revealed that pSTAT1 was no longer detectable by the inception of CFH expression (Fig. 3A), suggesting that the activation of STAT1 pathway precedes CFH expression. On the other hand, the kinetics of IL-27-mediated induction of CFH protein expression correlated temporally with the expression IRF-1 and IRF-8 expression (Fig. 3A). To further discern the roles of STAT1, IRF-1 and IRF-8 in the induction of CFH expression, we blocked *de novo* protein synthesis in some cultures by adding the protein synthesis inhibitor, cycloheximide (CHX). This allowed discrimination between the immediate effects of STAT1 activation on CFH expression from secondary effects deriving from STAT1-induced expression of IRF-1 and IRF-8. The stimulation of the ARPE-19 cells with IL-27 induced robust activation of STAT1 and STAT3 pathways (pSTAT1 and pSTAT3) and was unaffected by the blockade of protein synthesis (Fig. 3B). Western blot analysis also revealed that the induction of CFH expression by IL-27 correlated temporally with the expression of IRF-1 and IRF-8 (Fig. 3C). However, blocking protein synthesis with CHX abrogated the expression of IRF-1 and significantly reduced IL-27 induction of CFH expression but had no effect on IRF-8 level (Fig. 3C). qPCR analysis revealed significant suppression of CFH mRNA transcription by cells treated with CHX despite robust STAT1 activation, indicating that de novo synthesis of IRF-1 may be required for optimal expression of *CFH* (Fig. 3D). Interestingly, the expression of CFH RNA in the CHX treated cells was still higher than untreated cells (Fig. 3D), suggesting that this increase in CFH mRNA derived from the IRF-8 still present in these cells (see Fig. 3C). To directly investigate the role of IRF-1 and IRF-8 in IL-27-mediated induction of CFH protein expression, we stimulated ARPE-19 cells with IL-27 for varying amounts of time in the presence or absence of control siRNA, IRF-1 siRNA or IRF-8 siRNA. Complete knockdown of IRF-1 or IRF-8 was observed at 72 hours and confirmed by RT-PCR analysis (data not shown). As shown siRNA-mediated knockdown of IRF-1 or IRF-8 abrogated CFH protein expression, indicating the involvement of IRF-1 and IRF-8 in CFH expression in ARPE-19 cells (Fig. 4).

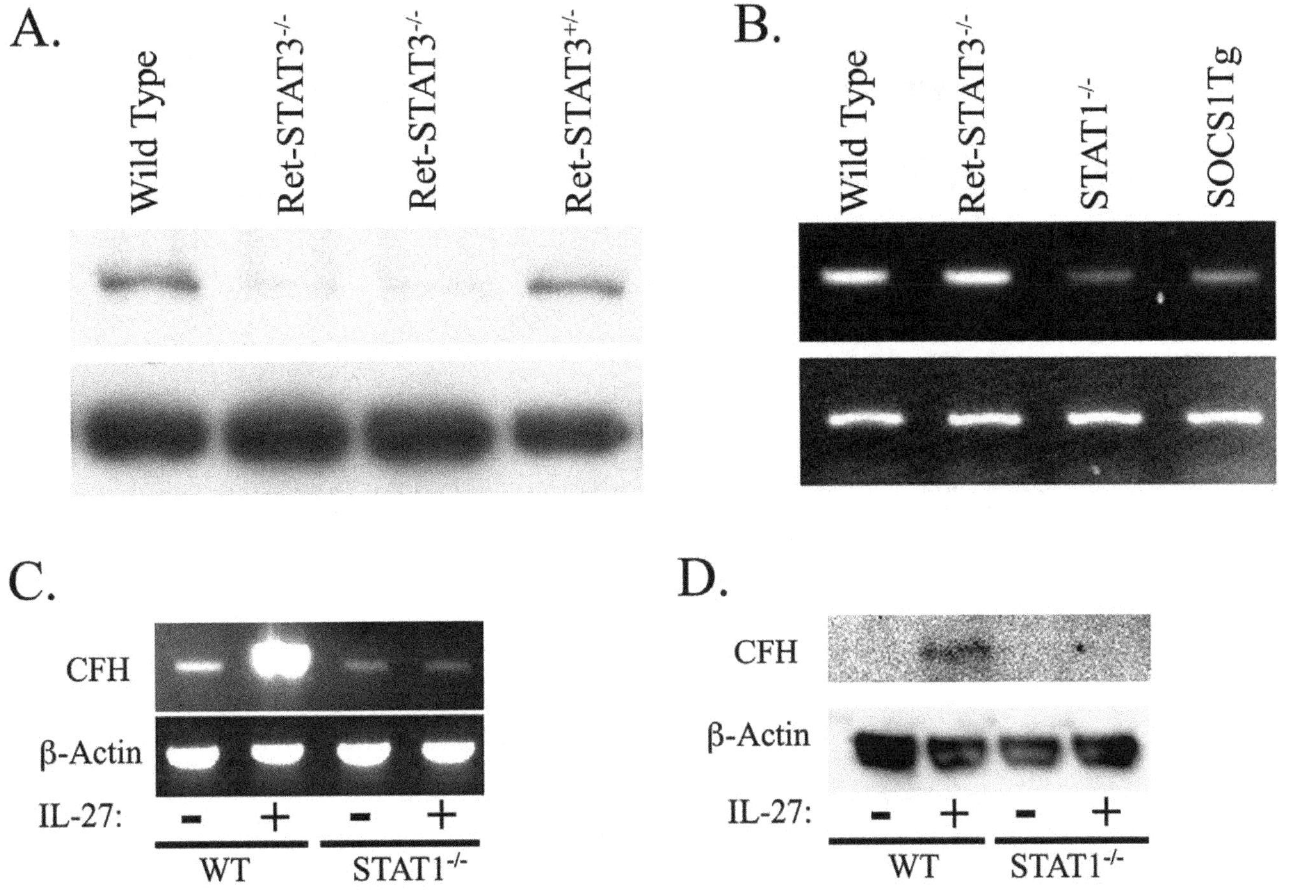

Figure 2. IL-27 induces CFH expression in the retina through STAT1-dependent mechanism. (A) Characterization of retina from mice with specific deletion of STAT3 in the retina (Ret-STAT3$^{-/-}$). (B) Freshly isolated retinas from wild type (WT), STAT1 knockout (STAT1$^{-/-}$), (Ret-STAT3$^{-/-}$), or from mice with targeted over-expression of SOCS1 in the retina (SOCS1Tg) were analyzed by RT-PCR. (C, D) Freshly isolated retinal cells from WT or STAT1$^{-/-}$ mice were cultured overnight, washed, starved for 2 hours in serum-free medium and then cultured for an additional 22 hours in medium containing IL-27 (10 ng/ml). We analyzed RNA and total cell extracts from the cells by RT-PCR (C) or Western blotting (D).

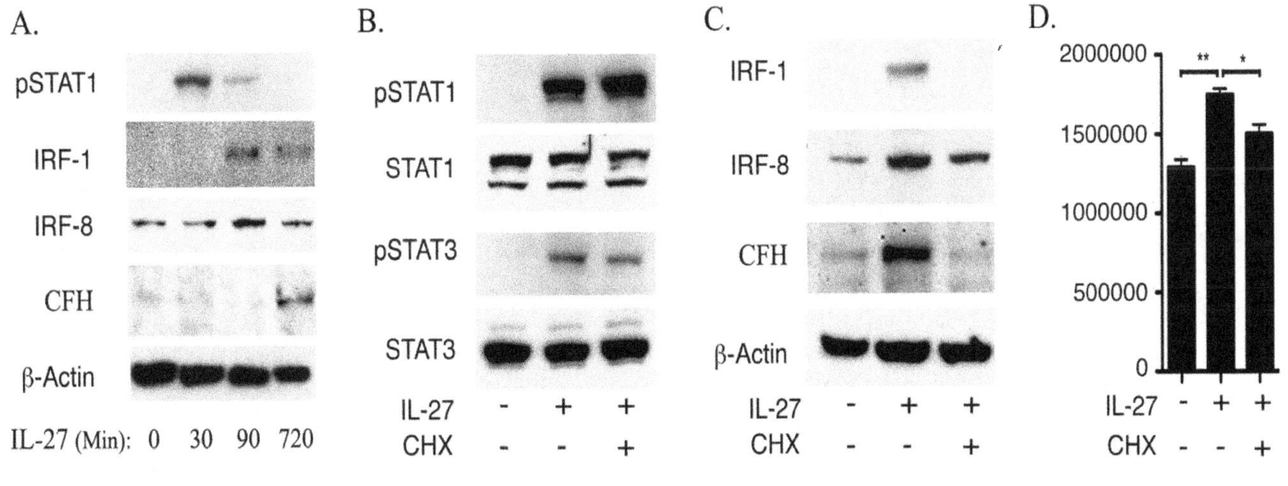

Figure 3. IL-27 induces expression of CFH through STAT1-mediated up-regulation of IRF-1 and IRF-8. (A–C) ARPE-19 cells were starved for 2 hours in serum free medium and cultures were then stimulated with IL-27 (10 ng/ml) for 30, 90 or 720 min. (B–D) In other cultures, cells were treated with CHX (35 ug/ml) for 30 min prior treatment with IL-27 for 30 min (B) or 24 h (C, D). Whole cell extracts were analyzed by Western blot assay and the antibodies used are indicated. (D) CFH mRNA transcripts were detected and quantified by qRT-PCR.

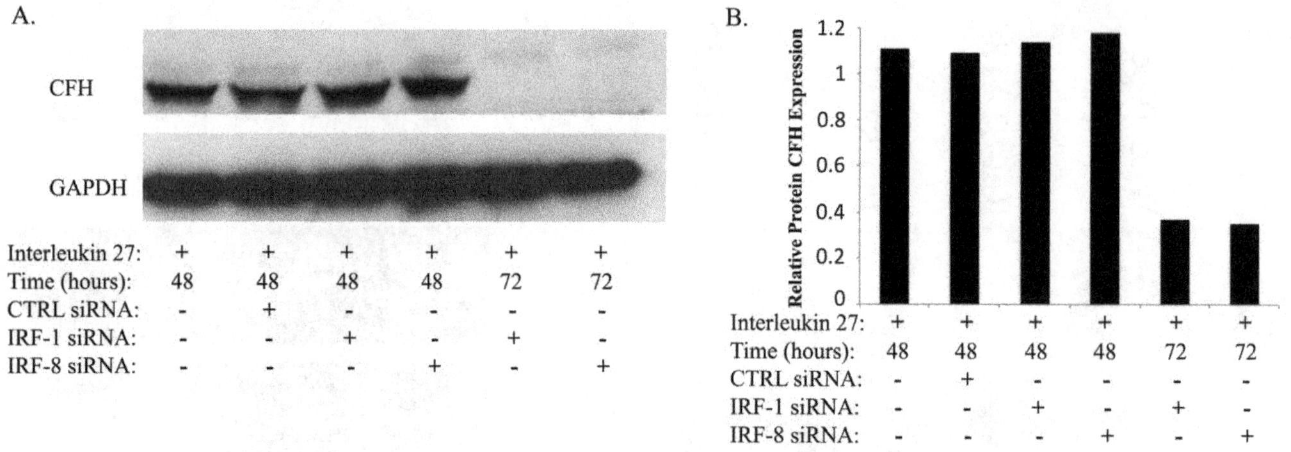

Figure 4. siRNA-mediated silencing of IRF-1 or IRF-8 abrogated the induction of CFH by IL-27. ARPE-19 cells were stimulated with human IL-27 in the presence or absence of control siRNA, IRF-1 siRNA or IRF-8 siRNA. (A) Detection of CFH expression by Western blot analysis. (B) Blots were analyzed and relative levels of CFH protein were quantified by densitometry; samples were normalized to the GAPDH expression level.

IRF-8/IRF-1 are Constitutively Expressed in Retina and Up-regulated during Ocular Inflammation

Data presented thus far suggest the involvement of IRF-1 and IRF-8 in the regulation of CFH expression in ARPE-19 cells. It was therefore of interest to investigate whether IRF-1 and IRF-8 are expressed in the mouse retina and if their levels increase during intraocular inflammation. We addressed these points in experimental autoimmune uveitis (EAU), a mouse model of intraocular inflammation or uveitis [31,32]. We induced EAU in C57BL/6 mice by immunization with the retinal autoantigen, interphotoreceptor retinoid binding protein (IRBP) [32,33]. Fundus photographs showing papillitis (black arrow), retinal vasculitis (red diamond) with cuffing (blue arrows) and brownish/whitish retinal and choroidal infiltrates (white arrows) taken at day-21 post-immunization confirmed the development of EAU (Fig. 5). Retina was isolated from un-immunized or IRBP-immunized mice and RNA analysis by qRT-PCR indicates that the increase in CFH expression in the retina during inflammation (Fig. 5B) was accompanied by a corresponding increase in the transcription of genes coding for *IRF-1, IRF-8* and IL-27 (*IL27p28* and *EBI3*) (Fig. 5C).

Detection of IRF-8 Protein in the Retina in the Ganglion and Inner Nuclear Layers of the Retina

In contrast to other members of the IRF family, IRF-8 expression has been detected mainly in myeloid cells and cells in the ocular lens [29,34]. Although IRF-1 and IRF-8 mRNA transcripts were detected in the normal retina and up-regulated during EAU (Fig. 5C), it was important to demonstrate that the proteins were also present in the retina. Consistent with our RNA data, Western blot analysis revealed that IRF-1 and IRF-8 proteins are constitutively expressed in the normal mouse retina and their levels increased dramatically during EAU (Fig. 6A, 6B). Because cells of the myeloid/hematopoietic lineage such as microglia are resident cells of the mammalian retina [22,35,36], we examined whether these cells are the source of IRF-8 detected in the retina. Immunohistochememical analysis of paraffin-mixed sections using IRF-8-specific Abs detected intense immunoreactivity within the ganglion cell layer of normal mouse retina (Fig. 6C). Consistent with increase of IRF-8 mRNA and protein in the retina during EAU, we observed marked elevation of the level of IRF-8 in ganglion and outer nuclear layers of mice with EAU (Fig. 6; right panel). Unfortunately, similar analysis using IRF-1 Abs from several commercial sources gave un-reproducible results.

Discussion

The complement system is a critical component of innate immunity in the eye and CFH is constitutively expressed by retinal cells to protect terminally differentiated photoreceptors and retinal neurons from prolonged or inappropriate activation of the complement system in the neuroretina. Although recent studies using the ARPE-19 cell line suggest that IFN-g regulates CFH expression in RPE cells through activation of STAT1 [12,19], factors that activate the STAT1 required for *CFH* transcription in the retina are unknown since retinal cells do not produce the pro-inflammatory cytokine, IFN-g.

In this study, we have shown that STAT1-deficient mice express much lower level of CFH in the retina compared to WT mice (Fig. 2B), suggesting that STAT1 is not only essential for activation of the transcription of *CFH* gene in ARPE-19 cells but also by resident cells of the mammalian retina. We further show that the anti-inflammatory cytokine, IL-27, induces the expression of CFH in retina (Fig. 2C, 2D) and ARPE-19 cells (Fig. 1C, 1D, 1E) in a dose dependent manner. Whereas IL-27 induced CFH in WT retinal cells, it could not up-regulate CFH expression in STAT1-deficient retinal cells indicating a requirement of STAT1-dependent mechanisms. In this context, it is interesting that STAT1 directly interacts with the IL-27p28 promoter and induces production of IL-27 by RPE cells, indicating the central role of STAT1 in regulating CFH and IL-27 [21,22]. The requirement of STAT1 for expression of CFH and IL-27 suggests that production of the two proteins in the retina may be linked or coordinately regulated. The physiological relevance of IL-27 in the retina and RPE is further underscored by recent reports showing that the RPE, photoreceptors and retinal ganglion cells expression IL-27 as well as IL-27 receptors [21,22]. It is particularly intriguing that the RPE and these layers of the retina express high levels of CFH [13]. Taken together, the constitutive production of IL-27 in the retina, its signaling through STAT1 and its up-regulation of CFH in ARPE-19 and mouse retinal cells, make a compelling case that IL-27 may play important roles as a physiological inducer of CFH in the mouse retina.

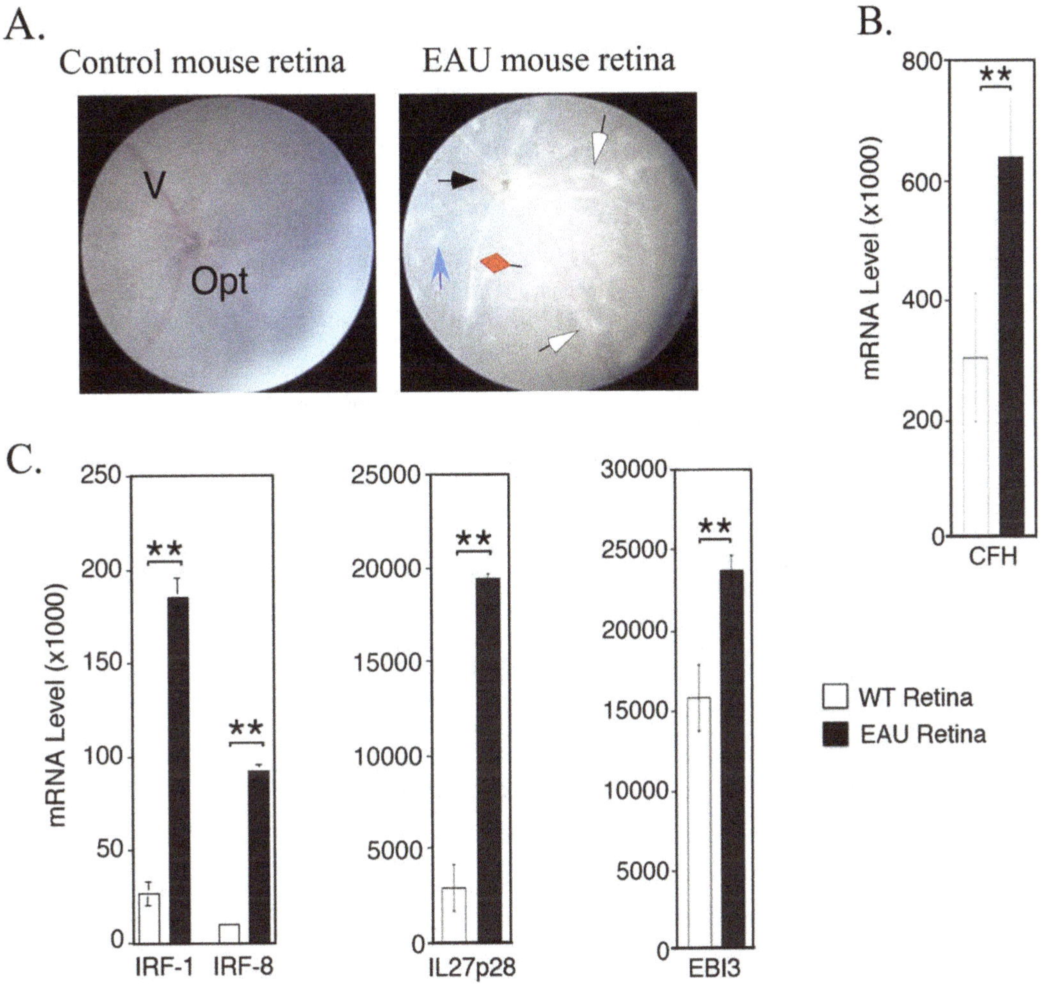

Figure 5. Expression of IRF-1, IRF-8 and IL-27 (IL27p28/EBi3) by retinal cells was up-regulated during experimental autoimmune uveitis (EAU). (A) Fundus images of the retina of un-immunized mouse and mouse with EAU. (B, C) Retinas were isolated from control or EAU mice and analyzed for IRF-1, IRF-8, CFH, IL27p28 or EBi3 expression by qRT-PCR.

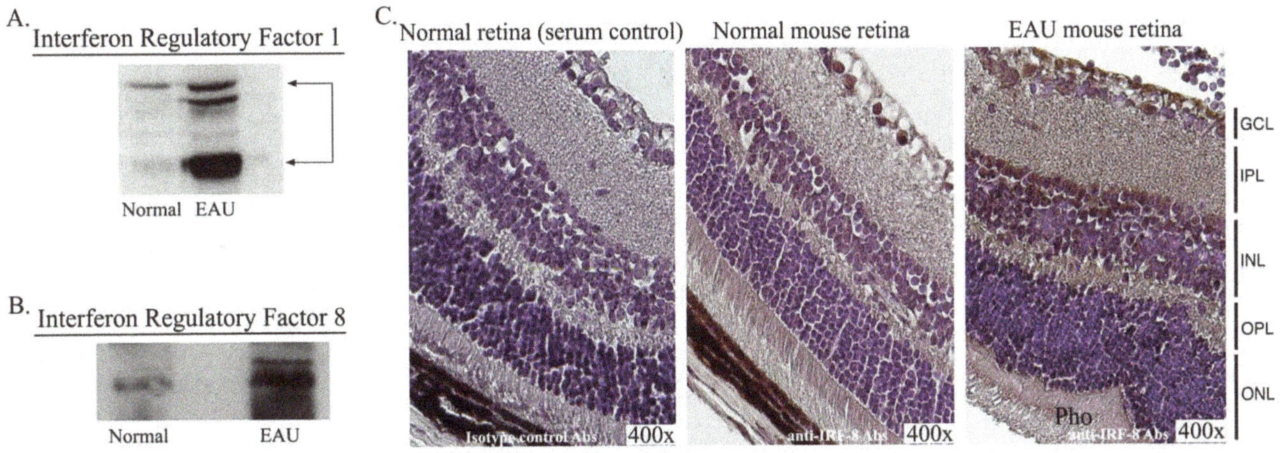

Figure 6. Detection and localization of IRF-1 and IRF-8 proteins in the retina. Retinas were isolated from control or EAU mice and whole cell extracts were analyzed for IRF-1 (A) or IRF-8 expression by Western blot analysis. (C) Immunohistochemical localization of IRF-8 expression was detected in the normal mouse retina or retina of mice with EAU using an IRF-8-specific antibody as described in Methods section. Retina pigmented epithelium (RPE); Photoreceptors (pho); outer nuclear layer (ONL); outer plexiform layer (OPL); inner plexiform layer (IPL).

Blocking protein synthesis with CHX did not inhibit STAT1 activation but abrogated the IL-27-induced expression of CFH (Fig. 3C), suggesting that *de novo* protein synthesis is required for IL-27-mediated increase in CFH expression. Although previous studies have emphasized the role of STAT1 in CFH expression, our results suggest that while STAT1 is clearly required for optimal expression of CFH (Fig. 2), its role may merely be to induce expression of additional transcriptional factors that may be the direct inducers of *CFH* transcription. We have shown that the induction of CFH expression by IL-27 was dose dependent and temporally correlated with the expression of IRF-1 and IRF-8 (Fig. 3A, 3C). In addition, both IRF-1 and IRF-8 are expressed in ARPE-19 cells and mouse retina, suggesting that they may play a role in maintaining physiological levels of CFH in the retina. IRF-1 is the best characterized of the 10-member IRF family and is thought to regulate immunological responses [29,37,38]. Constitutive expression of IRF-1 by resident retinal cells is not particularly surprising in view of the fact that IRF-1 is ubiquitously expressed in many tissues and cell types. On the other hand, with the exception of the ocular lens [34,39], the expression of IRF-8 has thus far been detected in cells of hematopoietic lineage [40,41,42]. During EAU, expression of IRF-8 and IRF-1 was dramatically increased (Fig. 6A, 6B) and we show that IRF-8 is marked elevated in ganglion and outer nuclear layers (Fig. 6C). Nonetheless, while our data indicate that IL-27 induces expression of IRF-1 and IRF-8 in the retina, a recent report indicates that IL-27p28 expression is decreased in IRF-8 knockout mice [43]. Moreover, over-expression of both IRF-8 and IRF-1 cooperatively activated IL-27p28 promoter [43], suggesting a positive regulatory mechanism for increasing IL-27, IRF-1 and IRF-8. It is therefore tempting to speculate that existence of such a feed-forward loop would undoubtedly contribute to mechanisms that sustain requisite levels of CFH in the retina.

In summary, the data presented describe the role of three transcription factors (STAT1, IRF-1, IRF-8) that converge to induce and/or enhance the expression of CFH in the retina and we have shown that they are all induced by the anti-inflammatory cytokine, IL-27. We further show that while STAT1 is required for optimal expression of CFH, its role appears to be for inducing IRF-1 and IRF-8 or other transcription factors that enhance the expression of CFH in RPE and retina. While the temporal patterns of expression suggest that IRF-1 and IRF-8 may be required for increasing CFH expression in response to IL-27 signaling, the constitutive expression of IRF-8 and IL-27 in the retina is consistent with their involvement in expression of CFH in the retina under normal physiological condition. Collectively, our data showing that IL-27 induced expression of CFH by retinal cells extends its anti-inflammatory functions in the retina and suggest that IL-27 might contribute to mechanisms of ocular immune-privilege by mitigating deleterious effects of complement proteins in retina during inflammation through activation of STAT1 and up-regulation of IRF-1 and IRF-8. Thus, it is conceivable that defects in IL-27 signaling or regulation of IRF-1/IRF-8 expression may contribute to the reduced amounts of CFH observed in retina of patients with AMD.

Acknowledgments

We thank Dr. Li Zhang (NEI, National Institutes of Health) for critical reading of the manuscript.

Author Contributions

Conceived and designed the experiments: CEE. Performed the experiments: AAO CRY ID SHK. Analyzed the data: AAO CRY ID SHK BM. Wrote the paper: CEE.

References

1. Gery I, Egwuagu CE (2002) Central tolerance mechanisms in control of susceptibility to autoimmune uveitic disease. Int Rev Immunol 21: 89–100.
2. Zipfel PF (2001) Complement factor H: physiology and pathophysiology. Semin Thromb Hemost 27: 191–199.
3. Klein RJ, Zeiss C, Chew EY, Tsai JY, Sackler RS, et al. (2005) Complement factor H polymorphism in age-related macular degeneration. Science 308: 385–389.
4. Hageman GS, Anderson DH, Johnson LV, Hancox LS, Taiber AJ, et al. (2005) A common haplotype in the complement regulatory gene factor H (HF1/CFH) predisposes individuals to age-related macular degeneration. Proc Natl Acad Sci U S A 102: 7227–7232.
5. Haines JL, Hauser MA, Schmidt S, Scott WK, Olson LM, et al. (2005) Complement factor H variant increases the risk of age-related macular degeneration. Science 308: 419–421.
6. Edwards AO, Ritter R, 3rd, Abel KJ, Manning A, Panhuysen C, et al. (2005) Complement factor H polymorphism and age-related macular degeneration. Science 308: 421–424.
7. Tuo J, Ning B, Bojanowski CM, Lin ZN, Ross RJ, et al. (2006) Synergic effect of polymorphisms in ERCC6 5' flanking region and complement factor H on age-related macular degeneration predisposition. Proc Natl Acad Sci U S A 103: 9256–9261.
8. Yang Z, Camp NJ, Sun H, Tong Z, Gibbs D, et al. (2006) A variant of the HTRA1 gene increases susceptibility to age-related macular degeneration. Science 314: 992–993.
9. Ambati J, Ambati BK, Yoo SH, Ianchulev S, Adamis AP (2003) Age-related macular degeneration: etiology, pathogenesis, and therapeutic strategies. Surv Ophthalmol 48: 257–293.
10. Augustin AJ, Kirchhof J (2009) Inflammation and the pathogenesis of age-related macular degeneration. Expert Opin Ther Targets 13: 641–651.
11. Jager RD, Mieler WF, Miller JW (2008) Age-related macular degeneration. N Engl J Med 358: 2606–2617.
12. Wu Z, Lauer TW, Sick A, Hackett SF, Campochiaro PA (2007) Oxidative stress modulates complement factor H expression in retinal pigmented epithelial cells by acetylation of FOXO3. J Biol Chem 282: 22414–22425.
13. Mandal MN, Ayyagari R (2006) Complement factor H: spatial and temporal expression and localization in the eye. Invest Ophthalmol Vis Sci 47: 4091–4097.
14. Gasque P, Julen N, Ischenko AM, Picot C, Mauger C, et al. (1992) Expression of complement components of the alternative pathway by glioma cell lines. J Immunol 149: 1381–1387.
15. Williams SA, Vik DP (1997) Characterization of the 5' flanking region of the human complement factor H gene. Scand J Immunol 45: 7–15.
16. Munoz-Canoves P, Vik DP, Tack BF (1990) Mapping of a retinoic acid-responsive element in the promoter region of the complement factor H gene. J Biol Chem 265: 20065–20068.
17. Fraczek LA, Martin BK (2010) Transcriptional control of genes for soluble complement cascade regulatory proteins. Mol Immunol 48: 9–13.
18. Fraczek LA, Martin CB, Martin BK (2011) c-Jun and c-Fos regulate the complement factor H promoter in murine astrocytes. Mol Immunol 49: 201–210.
19. Lau LI, Chiou SH, Liu CJ, Yen MY, Wei YH (2011) The effect of photo-oxidative stress and inflammatory cytokine on complement factor H expression in retinal pigment epithelial cells. Invest Ophthalmol Vis Sci 52: 6832–6841.
20. Pflanz S, Timans JC, Cheung J, Rosales R, Kanzler H, et al. (2002) IL-27, a heterodimeric cytokine composed of EBI3 and p28 protein, induces proliferation of naive CD4(+) T cells. Immunity 16: 779–790.
21. Amadi-Obi A, Yu CR, Liu X, Mahdi RM, Clarke GL, et al. (2007) T(H)17 cells contribute to uveitis and scleritis and are expanded by IL-2 and inhibited by IL-27/STAT1. Nat Med 13: 711–718.
22. Lee YS, Amadi-Obi A, Yu CR, Egwuagu CE (2011) Retinal cells suppress intraocular inflammation (uveitis) through production of interleukin-27 and interleukin-10. Immunology 132: 492–502.
23. Marquardt T, Ashery-Padan R, Andrejewski N, Scardigli R, Guillemot F, et al. (2001) Pax6 is required for the multipotent state of retinal progenitor cells. Cell 105: 43–55.
24. Yu CR, Mahdi RR, Oh HM, Amadi-Obi A, Levy-Clarke G, et al. (2011) Suppressor of cytokine signaling-1 (SOCS1) inhibits lymphocyte recruitment into the retina and protects SOCS1 transgenic rats and mice from ocular inflammation. Invest Ophthalmol Vis Sci 52: 6978–6986.
25. Oh HM, Yu CR, Lee Y, Chan CC, Maminishkis A, et al. (2011) Autoreactive memory CD4+ T lymphocytes that mediate chronic uveitis reside in the bone marrow through STAT3-dependent mechanisms. J Immunol 187: 3338–3346.
26. Xu H, Koch P, Chen M, Lau A, Reid DM, et al. (2008) A clinical grading system for retinal inflammation in the chronic model of experimental

autoimmune uveoretinitis using digital fundus images. Exp Eye Res 87: 319–326.
27. Egwuagu CE, Yu CR, Zhang M, Mahdi RM, Kim SJ, et al. (2002) Suppressors of cytokine signaling proteins are differentially expressed in Th1 and Th2 cells: implications for Th cell lineage commitment and maintenance. J Immunol 168: 3181–3187.
28. Durbin JE, Hackenmiller R, Simon MC, Levy DE (1996) Targeted disruption of the mouse Stat1 gene results in compromised innate immunity to viral disease. Cell 84: 443–450.
29. Lohoff M, Mak TW (2005) Roles of interferon-regulatory factors in T-helper-cell differentiation. Nat Rev Immunol 5: 125–135.
30. Li W, Nagineni CN, Hooks JJ, Chepelinsky AB, Egwuagu CE (1999) Interferon-gamma signaling in human retinal pigment epithelial cells mediated by STAT1, ICSBP, and IRF-1 transcription factors. Invest Ophthalmol Vis Sci 40: 976–982.
31. Nussenblatt RB (1991) Proctor Lecture. Experimental autoimmune uveitis: mechanisms of disease and clinical therapeutic indications. Invest Ophthalmol Vis Sci 32: 3131–3141.
32. Caspi RR (2010) A look at autoimmunity and inflammation in the eye. J Clin Invest 120: 3073–3083.
33. Caspi RR (2003) Experimental autoimmune uveoretinitis in the rat and mouse. Curr Protoc Immunol Chapter 15: Unit 15 16.
34. Li W, Nagineni CN, Ge H, Efiok B, Chepelinsky AB, et al. (1999) Interferon consensus sequence-binding protein is constitutively expressed and differentially regulated in the ocular lens. J Biol Chem 274: 9686–9691.
35. Dick AD, Carter D, Robertson M, Broderick C, Hughes E, et al. (2003) Control of myeloid activity during retinal inflammation. J Leukoc Biol 74: 161–166.
36. Karlstetter M, Ebert S, Langmann T (2010) Microglia in the healthy and degenerating retina: insights from novel mouse models. Immunobiology 215: 685–691.
37. Zhu J, Yamane H, Paul WE (2010) Differentiation of effector CD4 T cell populations (*). Annu Rev Immunol 28: 445–489.
38. Taniguchi T (1997) Transcription factors IRF-1 and IRF-2: linking the immune responses and tumor suppression. J Cell Physiol 173: 128–130.
39. Li W, Nagineni CN, Efiok B, Chepelinsky AB, Egwuagu CE (1999) Interferon regulatory transcription factors are constitutively expressed and spatially regulated in the mouse lens. Dev Biol 210: 44–55.
40. Qi CF, Li Z, Raffeld M, Wang H, Kovalchuk AL, et al. (2009) Differential expression of IRF8 in subsets of macrophages and dendritic cells and effects of IRF8 deficiency on splenic B cell and macrophage compartments. Immunol Res 45: 62–74.
41. Wang H, Lee CH, Qi C, Tailor P, Feng J, et al. (2008) IRF8 regulates B-cell lineage specification, commitment, and differentiation. Blood 112: 4028–4038.
42. Wang H, Morse HC, 3rd (2009) IRF8 regulates myeloid and B lymphoid lineage diversification. Immunol Res 43: 109–117.
43. Zhang J, Qian X, Ning H, Yang J, Xiong H, et al. (2010) Activation of IL-27 p28 gene transcription by interferon regulatory factor 8 in cooperation with interferon regulatory factor 1. J Biol Chem 285: 21269–21281.

8

Is Asthma Related to Choroidal Neovascularization?

Yaoyao Sun[1,2], Wenzhen Yu[1,2], Lvzhen Huang[1,2], Jing Hou[1,2], Peihua Gong[3], Yi Zheng[4], Mingwei Zhao[1,2], Peng Zhou[1,2,5], Xiaoxin Li[1,2]*

1 Department of Ophthalmology, Peking University People's Hospital, Beijing, China, **2** Key Laboratory of Vision Loss and Restoration, Ministry of Education, Beijing, China, **3** Department of Respiration, Peking University People's Hospital, Beijing, China, **4** Department of Immunology, School of Basic Medical Sciences, Peking University, Beijing, China, **5** Department of Ophthalmology, Eye and ENT, Hospital Affiliated to Fudan University, Shanghai, China

Abstract

Background: Age-related degeneration(AMD) and asthma are both diseases that are related to the activation of the complement system. The association between AMD and asthma has been debated in previous studies. The authors investigated the relationship between AMD and asthma systemically.

Principal Findings: The epidemiological study showed that asthma was related to choroidal neovascularization(CNV) subtype($OR = 1.721$, $P = 0.023$). However, the meta-analysis showed there was no association between AMD and asthma. In an animal model, we found more fluoresce in leakage of CNV lesions by FA analysis and more angiogenesis by histological analysis in rats with asthma. Western blot demonstrated an elevated level of C3α-chain, C3α′-chain and VEGF. After compstatin was intravitreally injected, CNV leakage decreased according to FA analysis, with the level of C3 and VEGF protein decreasing at the same time.

Significance: This study first investigated the relationship between AMD and asthma systematically, and it was found that asthma could be a risk factor for the development of AMD. The study may provide a better understanding of the disease, which may advance the potential for screening asthma patients in clinical practice.

Editor: Alvaro Rendon, Institut de la Vision, France

Funding: This work was supported by a grant from the National Basic Research Program of China (973 Program 2011CB510200, http://www.973.gov.cn/AreaAppl.aspx) and the National Natural Science Foundation of China (Grant No. 81070740, http://www.nsfc.gov.cn/). The funders had no role in study design, data collection and analysis, decision to publish, or preparation of the manuscript.

Competing Interests: The authors have declared that no competing interests exist.

* E-mail: dr_lixiaoxin@126.com

These authors contributed equally to this work.

Introduction

Age-related macular degeneration (AMD), the most common cause of irreversible blindness in the elderly population in many countries, affects the macular area of the retina [1,2]. There are two major clinical phenotypes of AMD–a nonexudative type(dry AMD) and an exudative type (wet AMD) [3]. During the development of AMD, choroidal neovascularization (CNV), or the development of new pathological blood vessels, is the major cause of vision loss [4]. The pathogenesis of CNV is poorly understood. As a complex disease, multiple environmental and genetic risk factors for CNV have been identified [5–9]. Studies recently indicated that inflammation, especially the alternative complement pathway, plays a fundamental role in the development of CNV [10]. Additionally, genetic evidence has identified variations in multiple genes involved in the complement cascade, including complement factor 3 (C3), complement factor H (CFH), complement factor Band complement factor 2 (C2), associated with AMD [11–13]. Apart from the complement system, other angiogenic stimuli have been reported to take part in the development of CNV, with the most important one being vascular endothelial growth factor [14].

Bronchial asthma (BA) is an inflammatory disorder of the airways characterized by airway hyper responsiveness and reversible airway obstruction [15]. Like CNV, BA is a multifunctional disorder with both environmental and genetic factors contributing to its development. Recent studies reveal that the complement system plays a crucial role in the development of immunological responses in BA by initiating and/or amplifying airway inflammation [16,17]. Variations of genes in the complement system have been shown to confer susceptibility to BA, including complement factor 3(C3) and complement factor 4(C4).

Because the mechanisms of development for both CNV and asthma are alike, we hypothesize that there is a relationship between these two diseases. During the past decade, several population-based studies reported that a history of asthma is associated with a high risk of developing CNV. However, other studies have also shown no association between asthma and CNV. Therefore, the association between these two diseases remains unknown.

In this study, we examined the cross-sectional relationship between asthma and CNV in a population-based sample of the mongoloid race in China. We then carried out a meta-analysis on all currently available studies to estimate the strength of a history of asthma being associated with CNV. Furthermore, a rat model of CNV induced by laser was developed in rats with asthma to investigate whether asthma is a risk factor for CNV and the potential mechanism of association.

Results

An Epidemiological Study Demonstrating the Association between CNV and Asthma

An epidemiological study was performed to determine if there is a correlation between a history of asthma and CNV. Of the 462 AMD patients, asthma was present in 47(10.17%) patients, whereas out of the 502 healthy controls, 31(6.18%) had asthma. The association of asthma and CNV was statistically significant (OR = 1.721, P = 0.023). As a result, asthma was found to be related to CNV (Tab.1).

Meta-analysis Showing no Association between CNV and Asthma

To obtain more information about the results of other epidemiological studies, a meta-analysis was performed. Seven epidemiological studies were identified that provided information regarding the potential association of CNV and asthma. All of the studies analyzed were written in English [18–23]. There were two articles that included multiple studies [20,23], and we treated each study separately. 4054 CNV cases and 109006 healthy controls, for a total of 113060 subjects, were included in the study. When we pooled all seven studies into this meta-analysis, we found no significant association between the risk of AMD and asthma (OR: 0.98; 95% CI:0.82–1.06) (Fig. 1). We also performed Egger's test to check whether there was publication bias, and it confirmed that in the dominant model, there was an absence of publication bias (Fig. S1).

An Asthma Rat Model Shows More Fluorescein Leakage from Laser Induced Choroidal Neovascularization Lesions on FA Analysis and More Neovascularization on Histological Analysis than in Rats without Asthma

The results of our epidemiological study and meta-analysis were inconclusive. Therefore, an animal model was established to provide further analysis. According to the epidemiological study we performed, CNV was related to asthma. Thus, a CNV model was developed in rats with asthma and in rats without asthma as a control. CNV leakage in rats with and without asthma was assessed by fluorescein angiography to see whether rats with asthma were more likely to develop CNV. Using FA performed on day 7 after laser-induced CNV, very few patches of hyper-fluorescence leakage were observed at the lesion site of rats without asthma, but leakage could be seen in rats with asthma, and there was a significant difference (P = 0.001). The leakage distribution at day 14 increased when compared to day 7. There were a total of 33 CNVs in five rats with asthma, while the number of CNV patches in the groups without asthma was 16(P = 0.002) (Fig. 2).

Two weeks after laser photocoagulation, histopathology performed on hematoxylin and eosin stains obtained from paraffin cross-sections confirmed that there was increased invasion in the retina around the laser scars in rats with asthma compared to rats without asthma. There were significant differences in the B/C ratio between the groups with asthma and the control (P = 0.001) (Fig. 3).

Table 1. The epidemiological study among Chinese people.

	Asthma (%)	Non-asthma(%)	$\chi 2$	P	OR	95%CI
CNV	47 (10.17)	415 (89.83)	5.171	0.023*	1.721	(1.073,2.759)
Non-CNV	31 (6.18)	471 (93.82)				

Patients with a history of asthma that developed CNV compared with controls in our epidemiological study.

Meta-analysis Demonstrating an Association between C3 and CNV

The relationship between C3 and CNV has been previously reported. However, to obtain a systematic review, a meta-analysis of C3 R102G and CNV was performed. 16 genetic epidemiological studies were previously preformed to analyze the association of CNV and the C3 R102G polymorphism (4 studies were overlapped) [7,24–26], and all of them were written in English. There were 14 articles published regarding the association between R102G and AMD risk. Because 3 studies were overlapping, we selected the articles with the largest sample size. There were 2 articles that included more than one study [24,25], and we treated them as separate studies.

The genotype effects for GC and GG versus CC genotypes were 1.459 (95% CI: 1.278, 1.667) and 1.471 (95% CI: 1.016, 2.130), respectively. This meant that patients who had GG and GC genotypes were roughly 1.5 times more likely to have AMD than patients with the CC genotype. These results suggested a codominant genetic model in which C3 R102G polymorphism plays an important role in the pathogenesis of AMD (Fig. 4).

Increased Expression of C3 and VEGF Could Affect the Development of CNV in Rats with Asthma

We next investigated the possible mechanism why rats with asthma developed more CNV than rats without asthma. As mentioned above, C3 and VEGF play fundamental roles in the development of both CNV and asthma. Western blot analysis of C3 and VEGF was performed, with β-actin serving as an internal loading control. We found an increase in the levels of the C3 split products (113 kDa for C3α-chain and 106 kDa for C3α'-chain) and VEGF (51 kDa) in rats with asthma compared to rats without asthma. C3α-chain levels were significantly increased by 2.59 fold (P = 0.006), with C3α'-chain levels increasing 3.00 fold (P = 0.023) and VEGF level increasing 2.87 fold (P = 0.031) (Fig. 5).

Inhibitory Effect of Compstatin on CNV-associated Down Regulation of C3 and VEGF

Given that the result has shown that CNV growth is associated with C3 and VEGF, either of the following scenarios is plausible: 1) elevated C3 levels induce an increase in VEGF, 2) elevated VEGF levels induce an increase in C3, or 3) C3 and VEGF levels are elevated independently.

To gain further insight into the relationship between VEGF and C3 and their effects on CNV in asthma, we investigated the use of compstatin to test the effect of C3 activation in the retina. 7 days after intravitreal injection of compstatin, fluorescein angiography was performed and CNV leakage was analyzed. The number of CNV patches in the rats receiving intravitreal injection was 10 compared with 33 CNV patches in rats that had not received intravitreal injection. Pathologic leakage was significantly reduced after treatment with compstatin (P = 0.03) (Fig. 6). Western blot analysis revealed a significant down regulation in the levels of C3α-

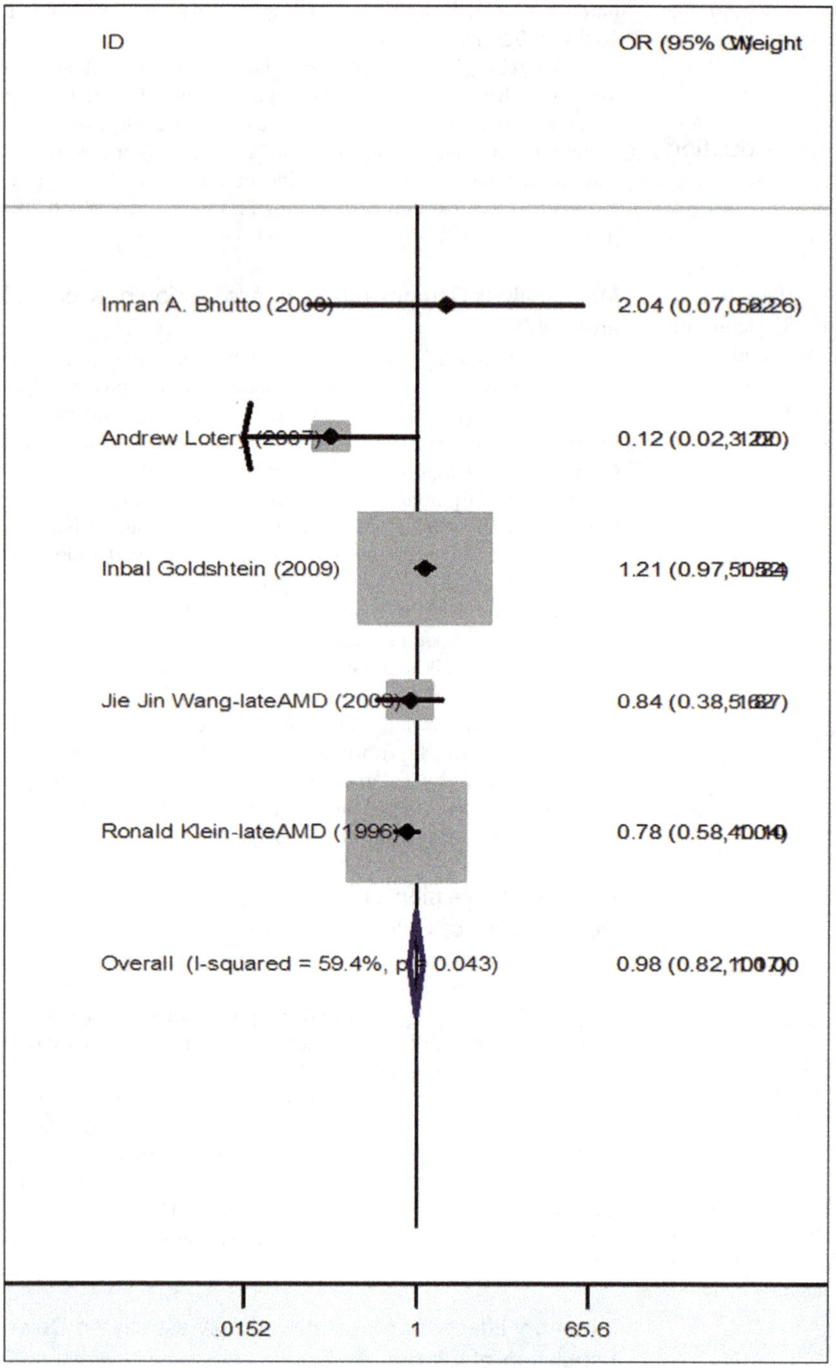

Figure 1. Forest plot showing the results of our meta-analysis. Each study is shown by the point estimate of the OR(the size of the square is proportional to the weight of each study) and 95% CI for the OR(extending lines).

chain, C3α'-chain and VEGF by 1.35 ($P = 0.001$), 1.78 ($P = 0.012$) and 1.82 ($P = 0.044$) fold, respectively, in RPE/choroid samples from CNV rats (Fig. 5). Thus, having asthma may provide a source of C3, raising the probability that locally produced C3 may precipitate VEGF release and CNV development [10].

Discussion

Our epidemiological study demonstrated that CNV was related to asthma. However, the meta-analysis showed a summary OR of 0.98(95%CI: 0.82–1. 06), which was contrary to our results. Further experiments found that in an animal model, rats with asthma had earlier and more extensive neovascularization compared with rats without asthma and C3 and VEGF may have played a fundamental role in this difference.

The association between CNV and asthma was controversial in previous studies. In our epidemiological study, asthma was associated with CNV with a 95% CI of 1.721. Among relevant studies searched, Inbal Goldshtein found a history of asthma was a risk factor for CNV. However, Jie Jin Wang and Ronald Klein

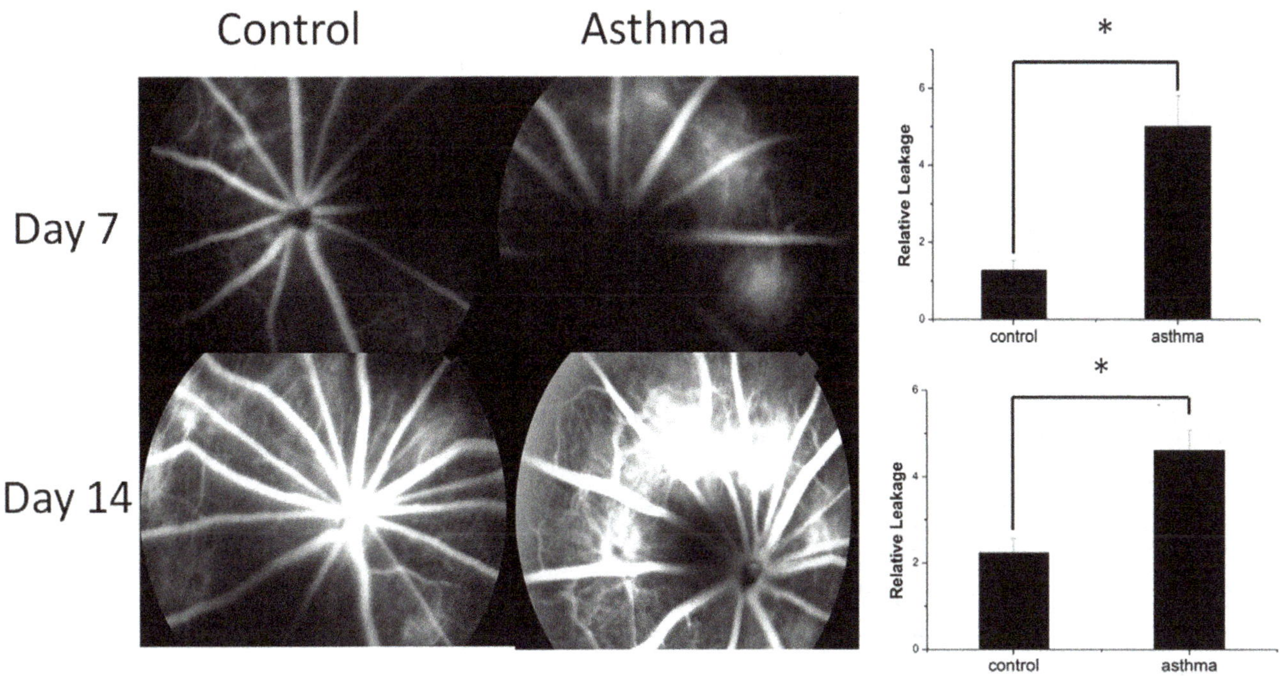

Figure 2. CNV leakage on FA. Angiographic analysis of CNV leakage 7 and 14 days after laser photocoagulation in 5rats with asthma and the control group 5 rats. Rats with asthma developed more CNV leakage on both day 7 (A, B) and day 14 than the rats in the control group (C, D).

were unable to replicate Goldshtein's findings [20,23]. After integrating the accumulating evidence, our meta-analysis demonstrated that asthma was not associated with CNV. This result was convinced because no potential publication bias was found. Thus, the results of our epidemiological study and meta-analysis were not consistent. There are several possible explanations for the inconsistency we found. First, there were a limited number of publications available, which included a total of only 7 studies. Therefore, the small sample size used for our meta-analysis could be a reason for the discrepancy. Second, because different studies were carried out in different regions and in different ethnic groups (Imran A. Bhutto in USA, Andrew Lotery in UK, Inbal Goldshtein in Israel, Jie Jin Wang in Australia and Ronald Klein in USA), there could be significant differences in both the environment and inheritance of genes that could potentially bias the results. Different regions and ethnic groups also have variability in the frequency and severity of asthma attacks, which could lead to deviations. Third, according to our epidemiological study, asthma was related to CNV but not to dry AMD. However, in the studies we searched for our meta-analysis, the subgroups CNV and dry AMD were not distinguished. The absence of subgroups, therefore, may be a factor in why different results were obtained.

Our animal model study demonstrated that asthma is a risk factor for the development of CNV, which we speculated could be a consequence of systemic inflammation associated with asthma.

Systemic inflammation induced by asthma and the ocular inflammation that results may explain the relationship between CNV and asthma. An inflammatory response is involved in the development of CNV in both rats and humans [10]. There is strong evidence suggesting that in the pathogenesis of choroidal angiogenesis both systemic and ocular inflammation are involved

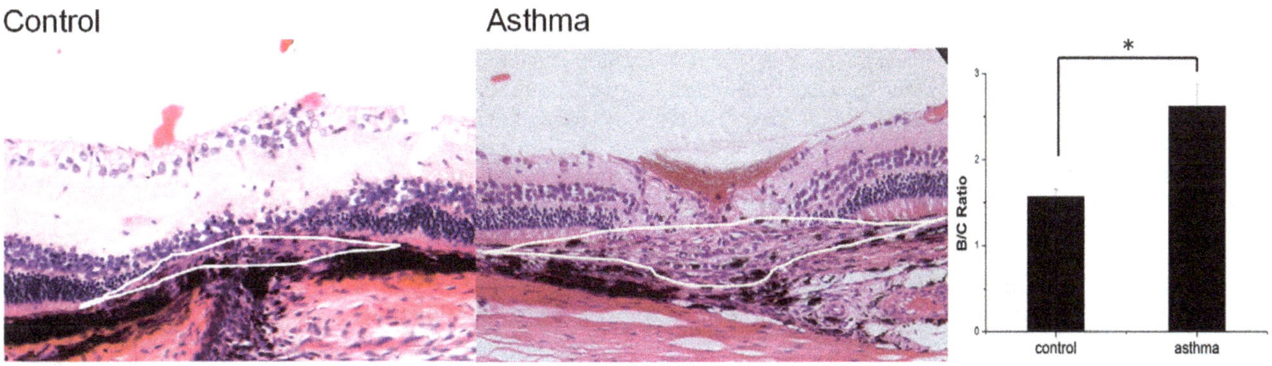

Figure 3. H&E staining of representative areas of CNV. H&E staining of representative areas of CNV at the sites of laser-induced lesions in 5 rats with asthma (A) and the 5 control group (B).Eyes were removed 14 days after laser photocoagulation. Note the presence of laser-induced CNV in each group.

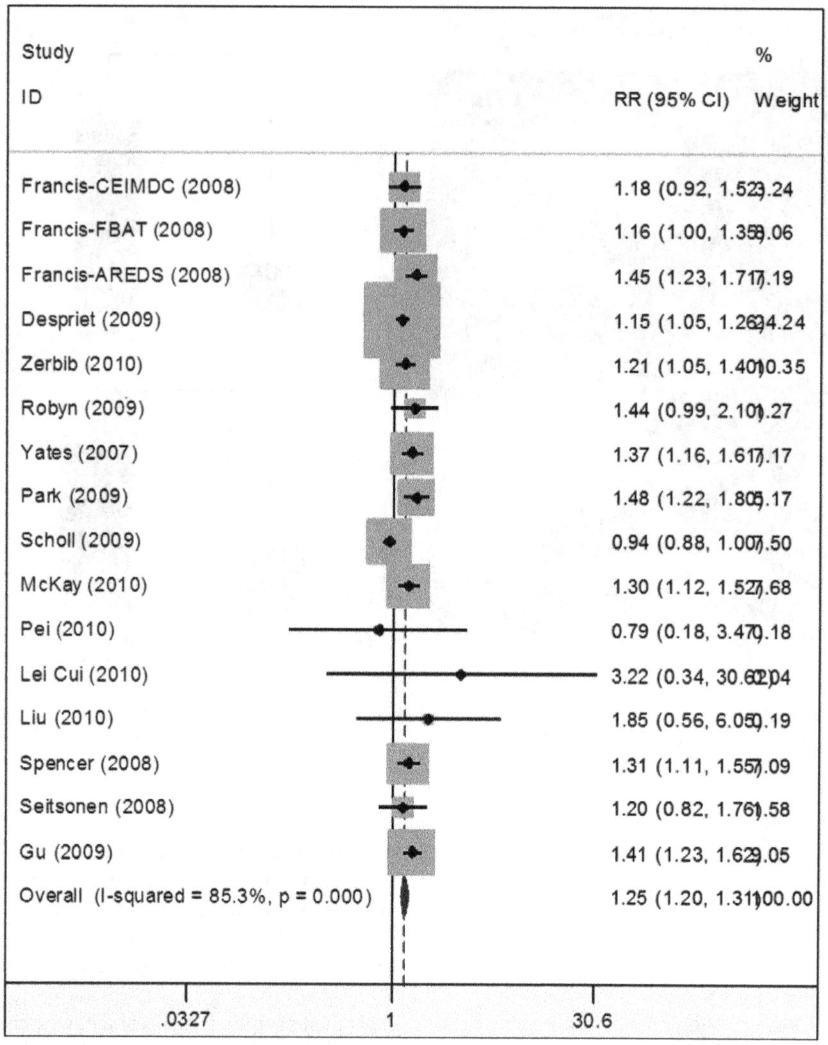

Figure 4. Meta-analysis of C3 R102G and AMD. Forest plot for meta-analysis of association between R102G and AMD risk. Each study is shown by the point estimate of the odds ratio (OR)(the size of the square is proportional to the weight of each study) and 95% confidence interval(CI) for the OR(extending lines).

[20]. In patients with asthma or animal models of asthma, allergens are known to drive allergic airway inflammation and activation of the inflammatory corpuscle resulting in systemic cytokine release.

Activation of the AP has been well documented in the development of CNV. As a point of convergence of the AP, C3 plays an important role in the control of the innate immune system and the inflammatory reaction that has been suggested to contribute in the pathogenesis of CNV. In patients with asthma, increased levels of serum C3 have been described [17]. As a result of systemic C3 elevation, local C3 levels are elevated accordingly resulting in local activation of the complement pathway.

Our study showed higher levels of C3 and VEGF in rats with asthma compared to rats without asthma. To determine whether the accumulation of C3 induced VEGF or if the opposite is true, a C3 inhibitor–compstatin was used. We found that C3 and VEGF protein levels decreased at the same time. According to Puran S. Bora, C3 activity is critical for the formation and deposition of the terminal membrane attack complex (MAC) on RPE and choroid cells, which leads to transient changes in the permeability of cell membrane. Changes in the permeability of the cell membrane lead to induction and release of VEGF, which eventually leads to the development of CNV [3] (Fig. 7).

Compstatin is a potent inhibitor of the complement system which inhibits cleavage of complement protein C3 [27]. Although it was tested to be inactive against C3 from lower mammals in a Surface Plasmon Resonance (SPR) chips measurement experiment [28], we believe in its functions intravitreally, still. As SPR only analyzes the binding process, its affinity for compstatin could be affected in vivo by other small molecules. And because of its specificity of the detection is not high enough, further studies such as IP are needed to test their result. In vivo studies are needed, too.

According to our study, asthma is a risk factor in the development of CNV because people with asthma are more likely to have CNV. This information could potentially lead to earlier screening for CNV in patients with asthma.

In conclusion, CNV is associated with asthma in our epidemiological study. However, previous studies show conflicting conclusions. We also found that asthma may affect the development of CNV, by increasing the protein levels of C3 and VEGF in the RPE/choroid layers, as observed in a rat model of allergic asthma. This study was the first to systematically investigate the

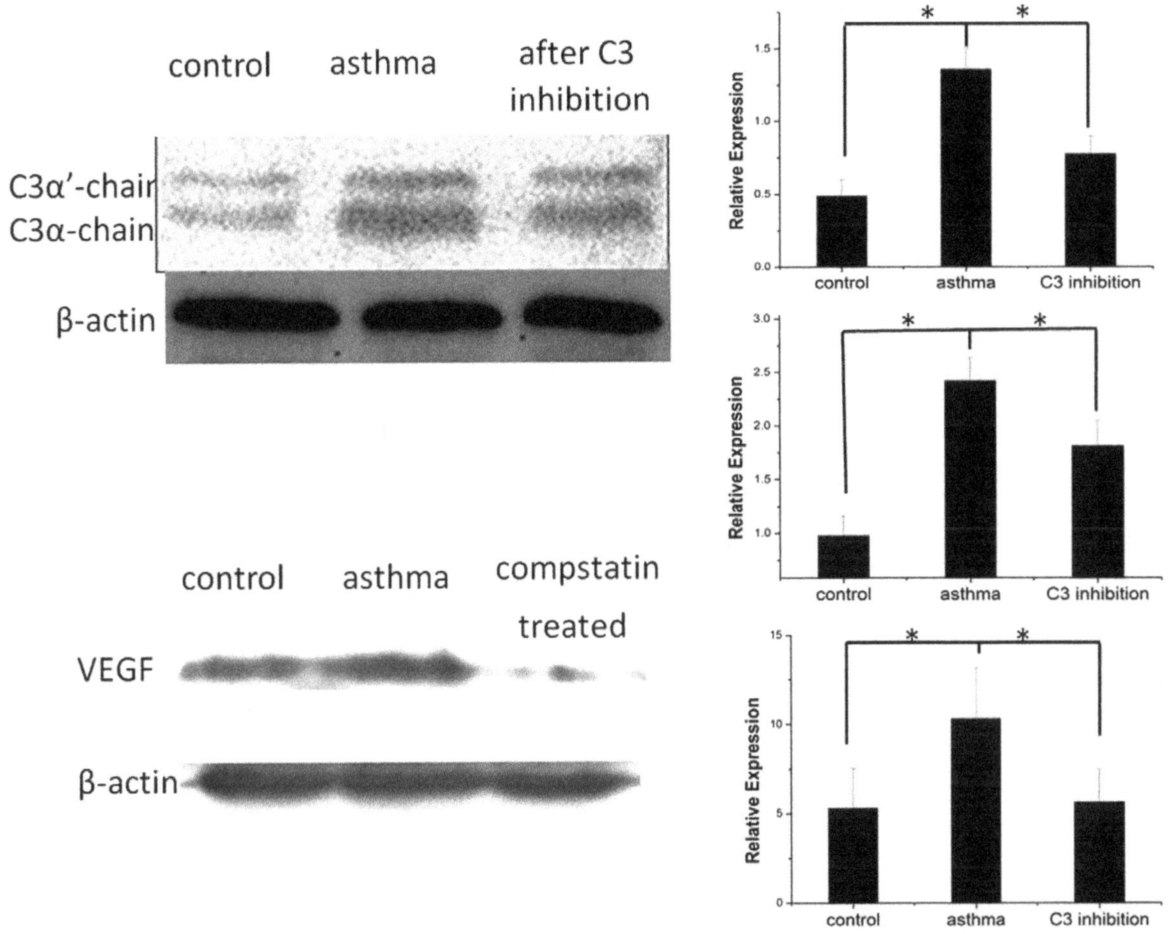

Figure 5. Western blot of C3 and VEGF. Western blot showing C3α'-chain, C3α-chain and VEGF expression in the RPE/choroid layer of rats without asthma, rats with asthma and rats with asthma treated with compstatin 14 days after laser photocoagulation. This experiment was repeated three times.

relationship between CNV and asthma and may provide a better understanding of the disease. This knowledge may help to advance the potential for screening among asthma patients in clinical practice.

Materials and Methods

Epidemiological Study

17 hospitals located in 9 different provinces in China enrolled 545 patients and 509 healthy controls from May 2010 to March

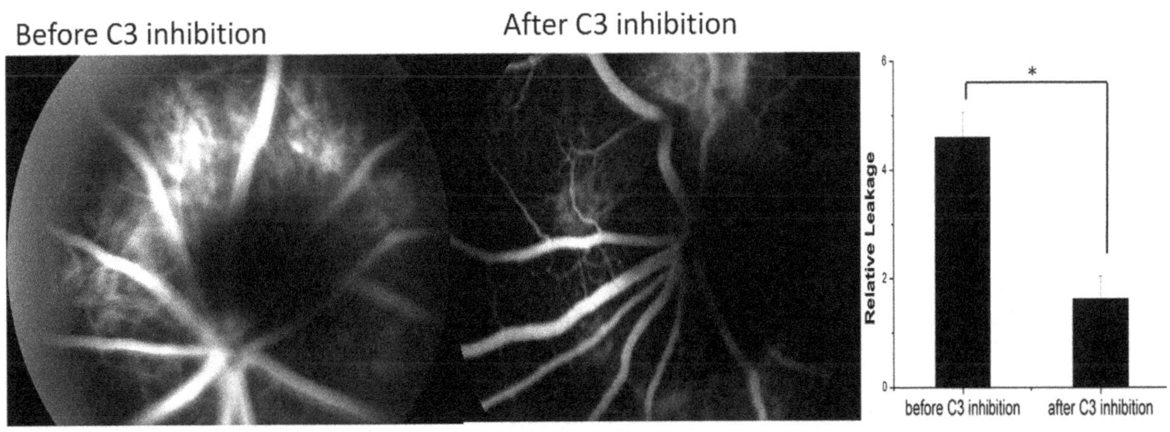

Figure 6. CNV leakage on FA after compstatin injection intravitreally. Angiographic analysis of CNV leakage 7 days after intravitreal compstatin injection. The pathologic leakage in rats with asthma was reduced after treatment.

2011. Patients over the age of 50 and diagnosed with AMD according to Fluorescein angiography (FFA) and/or Optical Coherence Tomography (OCT) were included as long as they had no other retinal diseases. Patients with pathological myopia, macular dystrophy, central serous chorioretinopathy, retinal vein occlusion, diabetic retinopathy or uveitis were excluded. All healthy patients were examined by FA and/or OCT to exclude CNV. A history of asthma was surveyed and the diagnoses were made by respiration experts according the Global Initiative for Asthma Guidelines 2007.

Meta-analysis

Publication search. Meta-analysis was performed as previously described [29]. Relevant studies were found by searching the following keywords: "asthma" and "AMD" or "CNV" in Pub Med, Medline and Web of Science databases (updated to Oct 18, 2011). All of the selected studies were retrieved, with their references checked for other relevant publications as well. No minimum number of patients was required for meta-analysis. Different sub-studies in the same article were treated as separate studies. In this meta-analysis, we selected only those studies published in English and only when the full text articles were available. For each paper, we extracted the following information into a table: first author, year of publication, number of cases and controls, and crude odds ratio (OR). Two authors (Yaoyao Sun and Peng Zhou) read the identified articles carefully and assessed them independently. For any discrepancies in their eligibility, they were adjudicated by Xiaoxin Li.

Statistical methods. The OR with 95% confidence intervals (CI) was calculated to evaluate the association strength between a history of asthma and CNV risk. Both fixed-effects (the Mantel-Hzenszel method) and random-effects (Der Simonian and Laird method) models were chosen. Cochran's Q statistic was used for determining the statistical significance of heterogeneity. If the p-value was less than 0.10, we selected the random-effects model otherwise the fixed-effects model was used. We used forest plots to describe the results from separate studies as well as for a summary containing all of the results. We used Egger's tests to test the potential for publication bias, and if $P<0.05$, the publication bias was considered to be statistically significant. Forest plots were produced to graphically present significant findings. Funnel plots were used to explore the potential for publication bias (PRISMA checklist) [30].

Because few studies investigating the association between C3 SNPs and asthma were found, we analyzed only the association between C3 SNPs R102G polymorphisms and AMD because this SNP has been the most commonly studied one. In order to obtain additional results, the following four different types of OR were calculated: (1) CG versus CC genotype, (2) GG versus CC genotype, (3) CG plus GG versus CC genotype (which was the dominant model) and (4) GG versus CG plus CC genotype (which was the recessive model).

All of the statistical calculations were conducted using Stata/Se version 11.0 software (Stata Corporation, College Station, TX).

Animals

Specific, pathogen-free female Brown Norway (BN) rats weighing 150±10 g were purchased from the Laboratory Animal Center, Peking University People's Hospital. Animal care and experiments were conducted under institutional guidelines and food and tap water were given ad libitum.

Establishment of an asthmatic rat model. On days 0 and 5, 10 rats in the asthma group were actively sensitized by intraperitoneal (i.p.) injection of 1mg ovalbumin (OVA, Sigma-Aldrich, St. Louis, MO, USA) emulsified with 40 mg Imject Alum (Pierce, Rockford, IL USA) in a total volume of 1ml. In order to elicit an airway allergic response, these rats were placed in a chamber made of plastic and challenged with an OVA aerosol (1% (w/v) in 0.9% NaCl) nebulized by an ultrasonic nebulizer (PARI BOY, PARI GmbH, Sternberg, Germany) twice a day for 1hour from days 6 to 14.10 rats in the negative control group were sham immunized with 0.9% NaCl and then challenged with an aerosol of 0.9% NaCl at the same frequency as the asthma group [31,32]. HE staining of lung in asthma was carried out (Fig. S2), and the status asthmaticus in asthma rats was recorded by video (Video S1, Video S2).

Induction of CNV. CNV was induced by laser photocoagulation (532 nm, 150 mW, 100 ms, 100 μm).

(Coherent 130SL, Coherent, Santa Clara, CA, USA) performed on day 15 when the asthma model was thought to have already been established. 8 lesions were made on one eye of each rat, and the other eye was used as the control.

Intravitreally injection of compstatin. To test the effect of suppressing complement activation in the retina of rats with asthma, 20 μg compstatin, a small cyclic synthetic peptide (Tocris Bioscience, Ellisville, Missouri, USA), was intravitreally injected into 5 rats 7 days after CNV was induced. Compstatin was dissolved in 1ml of 0.9% NaCl solution per 100 μg, filtered and intravitreally injected with a micro injector while the rats were anesthetized with 0.5 ml 10% chloral hydrate injected i.p.

The Measurement of CNV

Fluorescein angiography. Fluorescein angiography (FA) was performed on day of 7 and 14 after laser photocoagulation using a digital imaging system (TOPCON 50DX, Topcon, Tokyo, Japan) as described previously [33]. 0.2 ml of 5% fluorescein was given by i.p. after the rats were anaesthetized using the method described above and FA was done with pupil dilation. Both early-phase (1 minute after injection) and late-phase (5 minutes after injection) fundus angiograms were analyzed [34]. Fluorescein angiograms were evaluated quantitatively and the leakage area for each lesion was measured using ImageJ software, a custom programmed macro provided by the National Institutes of Health (NIH).

Histological analysis and CNV size measurement. 14 days after laser photocoagulation, the eyeballs of the experimental eye were removed and were fixed in eyeball fixing solution for 24 hours at room temperature. After removal of the anterior segments, the posterior eyecups were embedded in paraffin. Sagittal sections of 6μm were cut through the center of the eye at the site of laser photocoagulation. The sections were stained by hematoxylin and eosin and assessed by light microscopy (LEICA DFC 300FX, Leica, Solms, Germany). A computer-assisted image analysis system was used to estimate neovascularization based on the B/C ratio (B stands for the thickness between the bottom of the pigmented choroidal layer and the top of the neovascular membrane, while C stands for the thickness of the intact-pigmented choroid next to the lesion [35]. Measurements were performed on four sections from each laser photocoagulation site.

Western Blot

Fourteen days after laser photocoagulation, we removed the experimental eyeballs and extracted protein. Total protein was extracted from the pooled RPE/choroid layers and protein concentration was measured using the Bio-Rad assay kit (Bio-Rad, Hercules, CA, USA). Equal amounts of protein (30–60 μg) were resolved on 12% (for C3 antibody) or 6% (for VEGF and β-actin antibodies) Tris-HCl polyacrylamide gels and then transferred to a PVDF blotting membrane (Millipore, Billerica, MA, USA). After blocking, membranes were incubated with specific antibodies for C3 (Santa Cruz, CA, USA), VEGF (Abcam, Cambridge, MA, USA) and β-actin (Abcam, Cambridge, MA, USA). After incubation with peroxidase-conjugated goat anti-rabbit or anti-mouse secondary antibodies (ZSGB-Bio, Beijing, China), protein bands were visualized by chemiluminescence (Pierce, Rockford, IL, USA). This experiment was repeated three times, and similar results were obtained each time [36,37].

Statistical Analysis

All of the experiments were repeated three times and the data were presented as mean±SEM. Data were analyzed using Student's T test. $p<0.05$ was considered statistically significant. All data analyses were performed with SPSS 17.0 (Chicago, IL, USA).

Supporting Information

Figure S1 Publication bias of the meta-analysis. The Begg's funnel plot of studies included in the meta-analysis between asthma and AMD(A) and between C3 R102G and AMD(dominant model,B). The vertical axis represents log[OR] and the horizontal axis means the standard error of log[OR]. Horizontal line and sloping lines in funnel plot represent random effect summary OR and expected 95%CI for a given standard error, respectively. Area of each circle represents the contribution of each study to the pooled OR.

Figure S2 HE stainings of lung in asthma group and control group. Remarkble infiltration of inflammatory cells (including eosinophils and neutrophils) around the bronchioles with the destruction of epithelium, accumulation of inflammatory debris could be seen in asthma rats(A) but not in control rats(B).

Video S1 showed the status asthmaticus in asthma rats.

Video S2 showed the normal performance in the control group.

Acknowledgments

The authors thank Dr. Ronald Klein, Dr. Chelsea Myers, Dr. Gabriel Chodick and Dr. Jie Jin Wang for kindly providing the data for the meta-analysis.

Author Contributions

Conceived and designed the experiments: XL PZ YS. Performed the experiments: YS WY LH. Analyzed the data: XL YS PZ JH MZ. Contributed reagents/materials/analysis tools: PG YZ. Wrote the paper: YS.

References

1. Jager RD, Mieler WF, Miller JW (2008) Age-related macular degeneration. N Engl J Med 358: 2606–2617.
2. Bressler NM (2004) Age-related macular degeneration is the leading cause of blindness. JAMA. pp 1900–1901.
3. Bora PS, Sohn JS, Cruz JMC, P Jha, Nishihori H, et al. (2005) Role of Complement and Complement Membrane Attack Complex in Laser-Induced Choroidal Neovascularization1. J Immunol 174: 491–497.
4. Nozaki M, Raisler BJ, Sakurai E, Sarma JV, Barnum SR, et al. (2006) Drusen complement components C3a and C5apromote choroidal neovascularization. PNAS 103: 2328–2333.
5. Lee YL, Lee KF, Xu JS, He QY, Chiu JF, et al. (2004) The Embryotrophic Activity of Oviductal Cell-derived Complement C3b and iC3b, a Novel Function of Complement Protein in Reproduction. THE JOURNAL OF BIOLOGICAL CHEMISTRY 279: 12763–12768.
6. Seddon JM, Chen CA (2004) The epidemiology of age-related macular degeneration. Int Ophthalmol Clin 44.
7. Rakic JM (2006) Multifactorial influences on age-related macular degeneration. Bull Soc Belge Ophtalmol 301: 9–11.
8. Montezuma SR, Sobrin L, Seddon JM (2007) Review of genetics in age related macular degeneration. Semin Ophthalmo 22: 229–240.
9. Scholl HPN, Fleckenstein M, Issa PC, Keilhauer C, Holz FG, et al. (2007) An update on the genetics of age-related macular degeneration. Mol Vis 13: 196–205.
10. Rohrer B, Long Q, Coughlin B, Wilson RB, Huang Y, et al. (2009) A Targeted Inhibitor of the Alternative ComplementPathway Reduces Angiogenesis in a Mouse Model ofAge-Related Macular Degeneration. Investigative Ophthalmology & Visual Science 50: 3056–3064.
11. Xu L, Wang Y, Li Y, Wang Y, Cui T, et al. (2006) Causes of blindness and visual impairment in urban and rural areas in Beijing: the Beijing Eye Study. Ophthalmology 113: 1134.e1131–1111.
12. Vingerling JR, Dielemans I, Hofman A, Grobbee DE, Hijmering M, et al. (1995) The prevalence of agerelated maculopathy in the Rotterdam Study. Ophthalmology 102: 205–210.
13. Vinding T (1990) Visual impairment of age-related macular degeneration. An epidemiological study of 1000 aged individuals. Acta Ophthalmol (Copenh) 68: 162–167.
14. Ida H, Tobe T, Nambu H, Madsumura M, Uyama M, et al. (2003) RPE Cells Modulate Subretinal Neovascularization, but Do Not Cause Regression in Mice with Sustained Expression of VEGF. Investigative Ophthalmology & Visual Science 44: 5430–5438.
15. Mizutani N, Nabe T, Yoshino S (2009) Complement C3a Regulates Late Asthmatic Response and Airway Hyperresponsiveness in Mice. J Immunol 183: 4039–4046.
16. Inoue H, Mashimo Y, Funamizu M, Shimojo N, Hasegawa K, et al. (2008) Association study of the C3 gene with adult and childhood asthma. J Hum Genet 53: 728–738.
17. Abdel Fattah M, El Baz M, Sherif A, Adel A (2010) Complement Components (C3, C4) as Inflammatory Markers in Asthma. Indian Journal of Pediatrics Volume 77: 771–773.
18. Moorthy S, Cheung N, Klein R, Shahar E, Wong TY (2011) Are Lung Disease and Function Related to Age-Related Macular Degeneration? AMERICAN JOURNAL OF OPHTHALMOLOGY 151: 375–379.
19. Wysong A, Lee PP, Sloan FA (2009) Longitudinal Incidence of Adverse Outcomes of Age-Related Macular Degeneration. ARCH OPHTHALMOL 127: 320–327.
20. Klein R, Klein BK, Linton KL (1992) Prevalence of age-related maculopathy. The Beaver Dam Eye Study. Ophthalmology 99: 933–943.
21. Klein R, Knudtson MD, Klein BE (2008) Pulmonary Disease and Age-Related Macular Degeneration: The Beaver Dam Eye Study. ARCH OPHTHALMOL 126: 840–846.
22. Shalev V, Sror M, Goldshtein I, Kokia E, Chodick G (2011) Statin Use and the Risk of Age Related Macular Degeneration in a Large Health Organization in Israel. Ophthalmic Epidemiology 18: 83–90.
23. Wang JJ, Rochtchina E, Lee AJ, Chia EM, Smith W, et al. (2007) Ten-Year Incidence and Progression of Age-Related Maculopathy: The Blue Mountains Eye Study. Ophthalmology 114: 92–98.
24. Park KH, Fridley BL, Ryu E, Tosakulwong N, Edwards AO (2009) Complement component 3 (C3) haplotypes and risk of advanced age-related macular degeneration. Invest Ophthalmol Vis Sci 50: 3386–3393.
25. Francis PJ, Hamon SC, Ott J, Weleber RG, Klein ML (2009) Polymorphisms in C2, CFB and C3 are associated with progression to advanced age related macular degeneration associated with visual loss. J Med Genet 46: 300–307.
26. Seddon JM, Reynolds R, Maller J, Fagerness JA, Daly MJ, et al. (2009) Prediction Model for Prevalence and Incidence of Advanced Age-Related Macular Degeneration Based onGenetic, Demographic, and Environmental Variables. Investigative Ophthalmology & Visual Science, December 2003 50: 2050.
27. de Victoria AL, Gorham Jr. RD, Bellows-Peterson ML, Ling J, Lo DD, et al. (2011) A New Generation of Potent Complement Inhibitors of the Compstatin Family. Chem Biol Drug Des 77: 431–440.
28. Sahu A, Morikis D, Lambris JD (2003) Compstatin, a peptide inhibitor of complement, exhibits species-specific binding to complement component C3. Molecular Immunology 39: 557–566.
29. Yu KD, Yang C, Fan L, Chen AX, Shao ZM (2011) RAD51 135G>C does not modify breast cancer risk in non-BRCA1/2 mutation carriers: evidence from a meta-analysis of 12 studies. Breast Cancer Res Trea 126: 365–371.

30. Chakravarthy U, Wong TY, Fletcher A, Piault E, Evans C, et al. (2010) Clinical risk factors for age-related macular degeneration: a systematic review and meta-analysis. BMC Ophthalmol doi: 10.1186/1471–2415–10–31.
31. Chen SD, Wen ZH, Chang WK, Chan KH, Tsou MT, et al. (2008) Acute effect of methylprednisolone on the brain in a rat model of allergic asthma. Neuroscience Letter440: 89–91.
32. Werner-Klein M, Göggel R, Westhof A, Erb KJ (2008) Development and characterisation of a novel and rapid lung eosinophil influx model in the rat. Pulmonary Pharmacology & Therapeutics 21: 648–656.
33. Berdugo M, Bejjani RA, Valamanesh F, Savoldelli M, Jeanny JC, et al. (2008) Evaluation of the New Photosensitizer Stakel (WST-11) for Photodynamic Choroidal Vessel Occlusion in Rabbit and Rat Eyes. Investigative Ophthalmology & Visual Science 49: 1633–1644.
34. Sheets KG, Zhou Y, Ertel MK, Knott EJ, Regan CE Jr., et al. (2010) Neuroprotectin D1 Attenuates Laser-induced ChoroidalNeovascularization in Mouse. Molecular Vision 16: 320–329.
35. Kim C, Yu HG, Sohn J (2010) The Anti-angiogenic Effect of Chlorogenic Acid on Choroidal Neovascularization. Korean J Ophthalmol 24(3): 163–168.
36. Lyzogubov VV, Tytarenko RG, Liu J, Bora NS, Bora PS (2011) Polyethylene Glycol (PEG)-induced Mouse Model of Choroidal Neovascularization. THE JOURNAL OF BIOLOGICAL CHEMISTRY 286: 16229–16237.
37. Zhou P, Fan L, Yu KD, Zhao MW, Li XX (2011) Toll-like receptor 3 C1234T may protect againstgeographic atrophy through decreased dsRNAbinding capacity. The FASEB Journal doi: 10.1096/fj.11–189258.

9

Effect of the Gas6 c.834+7G>A Polymorphism and the Interaction of Known Risk Factors on AMD Pathogenesis in Hungarian Patients

Gergely Losonczy[1]*, Attila Vajas[1], Lili Takács[1], Erika Dzsudzsák[2], Ágnes Fekete[3], Éva Márhoffer[1], László Kardos[4], Éva Ajzner[5], Begoña Hurtado[6], Pablo Garcia de Frutos[6], András Berta[1]¶, István Balogh[2]¶

1 Department of Ophthalmology, University of Debrecen, Debrecen, Hungary, 2 Department of Laboratory Medicine, University of Debrecen, Debrecen, Hungary, 3 Department of Anesthesiology and Intensive Care, University of Debrecen, Debrecen, Hungary, 4 Hygiene and Infection Control Services, Kenézy Gyula County Hospital, Debrecen, Hungary, 5 Central Laboratory, Jósa András Teaching Hospital, Nyíregyháza, Hungary, 6 Department of Cell Death and Proliferation, Institute of Biomedical Research of Barcelona (IIBB-CSIC, IDIBAPS), Barcelona, Spain

Abstract

Age-related macular degeneration (AMD) is the leading cause of blindness in the elderly in the developed world. Numerous genetic factors contribute to the development of the multifactorial disease. We performed a case-control study to assess the risk conferred by known and candidate genetic polymorphisms on the development of AMD. We searched for genetic interactions and for differences in dry and wet AMD etiology. We enrolled 213 patients with exudative, 67 patients with dry AMD and 106 age and ethnically matched controls. Altogether 12 polymorphisms in Apolipoprotein E, complement factor H, complement factor I, complement component 3, blood coagulation factor XIII, HTRA1, LOC387715, Gas6 and MerTK genes were tested. No association was found between either the exudative or the dry form and the polymorphisms in the Apolipoprotein E, complement factor I, FXIII and MerTK genes. Gas6 c.834+7G>A polymorphism was found to be significantly protective irrespective of other genotypes, reducing the odds of wet type AMD by a half (OR = 0.50, 95%CI: 0.26–0.97, p = 0.04). Multiple regression models revealed an interesting genetic interaction in the dry AMD subgroup. In the absence of C3 risk allele, mutant genotypes of both CFH and HTRA1 behaved as strongly significant risk factors (OR = 7.96, 95%CI: 2.39 = 26.50, p = 0.0007, and OR = 36.02, 95%CI: 3.30–393.02, p = 0.0033, respectively), but reduced to neutrality otherwise. The risk allele of C3 was observed to carry a significant risk in the simultaneous absence of homozygous CFH and HTRA1 polymorphisms only, in which case it was associated with a near-five-fold relative increase in the odds of dry type AMD (OR = 4.93, 95%CI: 1.98–12.25, p = 0.0006). Our results suggest a protective role of Gas6 c.834+7G>A polymorphism in exudative AMD development. In addition, novel genetic interactions were revealed between CFH, HTRA1 and C3 polymorphisms that might contribute to the pathogenesis of dry AMD.

Editor: Katriina Aalto-Setala, University of Tampere, Finland

Funding: This study was supported by by the Hungarian Research Fund OTKA K68616 (to A.B.) and by the Social Renewal Operational Programme TAMOP 4.2.1./B-091/1/KONV-2010-0007 project (to A.B. and I.B.). The funders had no role in study design, data collection and analysis, decision to publish, or preparation of the manuscript.

Competing Interests: The authors have declared that no competing interests exist.

* E-mail: losigeri@gmail.com

¶ These authors contributed equally to this work.

Introduction

Age-related macular degeneration (AMD) is the leading cause of visual impairment in the elderly in developed countries, most prominently in white populations [1,2]. The prevalence of the disease increases with age reaching as much as 15% above the age of 80 [3]. AMD is a multifactorial disease characterized by progressive degeneration of the central retina leading to visual deterioration. Early stages of AMD are characterized by retinal pigment abnormalities and accumulation of small deposits called drusen under the macular area of the retina. Two advanced forms of the disease are distinguished: extensive pigment epithelium atrophy also referred to as geographic atrophy (GA) leading to irreversible and untreatable visual deterioration or subretinal neovascular membrane (SRNVM) formation characterized by intra- or subretinal invasion of new vessels arising from the choroid. Multiple methods have been developed to determine the severity of the disease and to estimate the risk of progression from early to late stages. The neovascular form is referred to as exudative or wet type, while AMD without any neovascular component is considered non-exudative or dry type AMD [4]. Although the etiology of the disease is still largely unclear, several risk factors have been unequivocally linked to AMD, including advanced age, European origin and smoking. Other factors including high cholesterol level, sunlight exposure, blue iris, oxidative damage, hypertension, obesity and inflammation have also been linked to AMD development, however, with inconsistent results [5,6]. Cataract surgery has been shown to increase risk exclusively of dry late AMD, however carriers of two complement factor H (CFH) risk alleles are prone to develop all types of AMD [7].

In recent years a growing number of evidence has supported the role of genetic risk factors in AMD pathogenesis. The most widely studied and strongest genetic risk factors map to genes of the alternative complement pathway and its regulators, and are most likely responsible for an imbalance in the complement activation. Additionally, there is a wide range of chromosome regions and genes with different functions implicated in AMD pathogenesis. Because in most studies sharp clinical difference between cases and controls is ascertained by recruiting cases with unequivocally advanced phenotype, little is known about the genetic background of intermediate dry AMD. It is still an open question what makes the difference in the genetic etiology of exudative and non-exudative AMD [8].

After the initial reports [9,10,11], numerous case-control studies have provided supportive evidence for a strong association between AMD and the p.Tyr402His (rs1061170) polymorphism of the CFH gene in different populations. According to a very recent meta-analysis of 24 case-control studies the p.Tyr402His variant confers a 2-fold higher risk of late-AMD per copy in individuals of European descent [12].

Other components of the complement system have also been implicated in AMD pathogenesis. The initial report demonstrated that the p.Arg102Gly (rs2230199) polymorphism in the Complement factor 3 (C3) gene confers statistically significant risk to AMD with an odds ratio of 1.7 for heterozygotes and 2.6 for homozygotes in comparison to wild type subjects [13]. Later similar odds ratios were reported equally contributing to early and late AMD. The risk was independent of CFH p.Tyr402His and LOC387715 p.Ala69Ser polymorphisms [14,15].

The rs10033900 polymorphism of Complement factor I (CFI), a proteolytic regulatory enzyme inactivating C3b has been shown to be associated with AMD [16,17], however a recent paper failed to confirm this association [18].

Strong association has been confirmed between AMD and the p.Ala69Ser (rs10490924) polymorphism in LOC387715 coding a protein of unknown function [19,20] or a promoter SNP of the HTRA serine peptidase 1 (HTRA1) gene (rs11200638) [21,22,23,24]. These two polymorphisms are located in close vicinity and it is still a subject of debate which of the two plays a role in the pathomechanism of the disease.

Although lipids are major components of drusen, proteins involved in lipid transportation have been linked to AMD pathogenesis only recently [25]. Apolipoprotein E (ApoE), a polymorphic gene with three common allelic variants (E2, E3 and E4) has also been connected to the pathogenesis of AMD. E3 is the major allele among whites. E4 allele has been reported to decrease AMD risk, or at least delay the occurrence of the disease. In contrast, the presence of the E2 allele is associated with increased risk and younger age at diagnosis [26,27,28]. ApoE E4 proved to be protective with an odds ratio of 0.5 (95%CI: 0.29–0.86) in a study comprising of 3137 individuals [29]. Another study demonstrated a protective effect of the E4 allele only in the neovascular AMD patient group with an OR of 0.61 (95%CI: 0.38–0.97) [30]. In contrast with these findings, a Spanish study reported an increased risk for AMD due to the ApoE E4 allele, with an OR of 5.6 [31]. Previously we could not demonstrate statistically significant association between ApoE alleles and AMD in a Hungarian population. However, the potential risk factor E2 allele was less frequent in patients than in controls (0.066 and 0.1, respectively) while the E4 allele was more frequent in the patient group than in controls (0.108 versus 0.084, respectively), interestingly [32]. The somewhat inconsistent findings on the association of AMD and ApoE called for a recently published pooled analysis (n = 21.160) demonstrating that the E2 allele in homozygous form confers risk (OR = 1.83, 95%CI: 1.04–3.23) and the E4 allele is protective (OR = 0.72 per haplotype; 95%CI: 0.65–0.74) in late AMD [33]. A recent well powered case-control study (including 2187 cases and 2187 age and ethnically matched controls) demonstrated disease risk of the E2 allele compared to the E3/E3 genotype (OR = 1.32, 95%CI: 1.11–1.58). However, the E2 allele only conferred risk to early AMD in the never smoker and previously smoker group, while the E4 allele was protective against early AMD exclusively in the current smoker population [34].

The growth arrest–specific gene 6 (Gas6) product is a vitamin K dependent protein secreted by leukocytes and endothelial cells in response to injury. Gas6 has a high structural homology with the natural anticoagulant protein S. It has not been implicated in AMD pathogenesis so far, however there are certain functions of the protein that make it a possible candidate for AMD. It has growth factor-like properties through its interaction with receptor tyrosine kinases of the TAM family; Tyro3, Axl and MerTK, this way it contributes to the regulation of angiogenesis, cell survival, proliferation, migration and adhesion, making it a relevant participant of biological processes like atherogenesis and thrombosis [35,36,37,38]. Recently, we found that Gas6 is present in the human circulation [39]. A Gas6 polymorphism (c.834+7AA genotype) was identified as a common SNP in the general population and gave the strongest association with stroke [40]. Others found similar association with acute coronary syndrome, and type 2 diabetes [36,40,41]. TAM receptor tyrosine kinases and their ligands Gas6 and Protein S are essential for the phagocytosis of apoptotic cells and membranes in the immune, nervous, and reproductive systems [42]. Moreover, MerTK receptor is the key player involved in photoreceptor outer segment phagocytosis by RPE cells. MerTK knock-out mice develop almost total degeneration of the retinal photoreceptor layer by 10 weeks of age [43,44,45]. MerTK SNPs were selected because of their tagging properties after Haploview analysis of the genotypes downloaded from the HapMap database for CEU population (Rel20/phase II Jan06, on NCBI B35 assembly, dbSNP b125). Haplotype (defined as a group of closely linked polymorphic alleles in a chromosomal region) tagging SNPs were selected according to the following parameters: MAF>0.05 in Caucasians, $r2>0.8$ between each pair of tagged and tagging SNPs in pairwise tagging and haplotypes coverage down to 5% of their frequency in the HapMap CEU population for each analysed gene. The 4 tagSNPs selected belong to a haplotype block and were sufficient to cover the whole gene [46].

The aim of our present case-control study was to refine the association of the known polymorphisms and AMD subtypes in the Hungarian population and to explore the interplay of different polymorphisms. We considered MerTK and its ligand Gas6 as candidate genes to play a role in AMD pathogenesis and searched for association between their polymorphisms and the disease.

Patients and Methods

Ethics Statement

The study was approved by the Institutional Ethics Committee of the University of Debrecen and the procedures strictly adhered to the tenets of the declaration of Helsinki.

Patients

In total, 386 subjects were enrolled in the case-control study: 213 patients with exudative AMD, 67 patients with dry AMD and 106 unrelated ethnically matched healthy controls were ascertained in Eastern-Hungary at the Department of Ophthalmology,

University of Debrecen between 2005 and 2011. The control group consisted of individuals attending to the Outpatient Clinic because of refractive disorders, or post-cataract follow-up visits. To maximize the reliability of our study, we deliberately selected controls to be somewhat older than patients. Written informed consent was obtained from all participants. Detailed patient history was recorded with the use of a questionnaire focusing on known or suspected non-genetic risk factors of AMD such as cigarette smoking, exposure to blue light, medical history of acute myocardial infarction, ischemic heart disease and deep venous thrombosis. Cigarette smoking was determined in packyears. Smoking of one pack of cigarettes daily for a period of one year was considered one packyear. Body mass index (BMI) was calculated on the actual body height and weight values when ascertained that no considerable change in body weight occurred in the past 10 years. An average BMI was calculated in patients with significant loss or increase of body weight based on body weight values of the previous 10 years period. Color fundus photographs were taken of patients and controls. Fluorescein angiography was used to investigate patients with exudative AMD. Grading of the severity of the disease was based on the clinical age-related maculopathy staging system (CARMS) [4]. There were 5,3,18,6 and 35 patients in the dry AMD group characterized as CARMS grade 2b, 2c, 3a, 3b and 4, respectively.

For statistical analysis, patients were classified according to the more severely affected eye into two groups corresponding to either dry or wet AMD. No signs of AMD, such as abnormal pigmentation or drusen were observed in controls. Color fundus photographs and fluorescein angiograms were evaluated by two experienced ophthalmologist (T.L. and L.G.). Patients or controls with other ocular diseases interfering with reliable evaluation of AMD were not included in the study.

Molecular genetic methods

Molecular genetic methods for the detection of the common ApoE alleles, CFH p.Tyr402His polymorphism, LOC387715 rs10490924 (p.A69S) and HTRA1 rs11200638 polymorphisms were used as described earlier [32]. Factor XIII Val34Leu polymorphism was detected using fluorescent PCR and hybridization probes [47]. Similar methodology was used for the genotyping of Gas6 rs8191974 (c.834+7G>A) polymorphism and for the MerTK rs86016 (g.2920G>A) polymorphism, as described earlier [46]. Complement C3 rs2230199 (p.Arg102Gly) polymorphism was tested using a PCR-RFLP method. Amplification was performed using the primers: C3R102F: 5′- CAG GGA GTT CAA GTC AGA AAA GG -3′ and C3R102R: TCT TGT CTG TCT GGA TGA AGA GG -3′. The 131 bp PCR product was then subjected to the digestion with *Cfo*I restriction endonuclease. The sole restriction site of the enzyme in the PCR product is lost when the mutation is present. The candidate, most likely a tag SNP, that has been shown to be associated with AMD, rs10033900 in the complement factor I (CFI) gene was tested using TaqMan SNP Genotyping assay. TaqMan assays were also used for the detection of the MerTK I1b rs17835605 (g.4916C>T), MerTK I1c rs10496440 (g.8809A>C) and MerTK I4 rs7573344 (g.60127A>G), as described earlier [46]. Over 98% of controls and 96% of patients were genotyped in each test. For the verification of all in-house mutation detection methods described above, randomly selected samples were sequenced with the same primers that were used for PCR amplification. No discrepancy was found in any of the tested samples.

Statistical methods

Biallelic polymorphisms were tested using the chi-square test for the deviation of Hardy-Weinberg equilibrium in the control group. Continuous and categorical variables were described in terms of mean (SD) and frequency (%), respectively, in AMD subtype groups and in controls. Unadjusted between-group comparisons were made using ANOVA or Kruskal–Wallis tests subject to normality and homoscedasticity assumptions (continuous variables), and Fisher's exact test (categorical variables). Unadjusted effects of explanatory variables were estimated using simple logistic regression and expressed as odds ratios and 95% confidence intervals (CI). Continuous variables were transformed with the formula providing the best achievable fit. Categorical variables were regrouped by pooling groups with close to identical effects if applicable. Models were fitted for the total sample and for subsamples formed by restricting cases to dry or wet AMD variants. Adjusted effects were estimated using multiple logistic regression. The significance criterion was set at $\alpha = 0.05$ for all tests, i.e. with no formal adjustment for multiple testing. Categorical variables were regrouped by pooling groups with close to identical effects if applicable. Age and cataract surgery were included as a priori adjustment covariates without effect interpretations, due to their association with study group inherent in the control recruitment methods used. Further variable selection was based on an iterative procedure where models were started by including all explanatory variables with significant unadjusted effects, adding each of the rest one by one and keeping if meaningful, and were made parsimonious by eliminating those of neutral behavior. Possible interactions between explanatory variables of models thus developed were systematically evaluated and kept if found significant. For comparability between dry and wet AMD variant models, genetic interactions included in any subtype model were also used in the other. Model fit was checked using Hosmer–Lemeshow tests for all three final models. As HTRA1 rs11200638 and LOC rs10490924 are in linkage disequilibrium, for the analysis HTRA1 rs11200638 was selected.

Results

Characteristics of the study population

In total, 280 patients and 106 controls were enrolled in the present study. Basic characteristics of the study population are summarized in Table 1. Patients were divided into two subgroups according to disease phenotype involving 213 patients in the wet and 67 patients in the dry AMD subgroups. There was a slight female predominance among wet AMD patients which is in line with European data on gender distribution in neovascular AMD [48].

There was no significant difference between the ages of the dry and wet subgroups of patients, however, controls were significantly older than patients as a result of intentionally older control selection. Cataract surgery was also more common in the control group because of controls selection methods and probably because the older age of the controls. There was no statistically significant difference between patients and controls in terms of frequency of hypertension, deep venous thrombosis, myocardial infarct, smoking and body mass index. Interestingly, outdoor profession was significantly more frequent among controls than patients.

Genotype distribution and unadjusted odds ratios of the analyzed polymorphisms

The genotype distributions in controls and patients are shown in Table S1. Actual sample number is provided for each test. Small differences are due to the shortage of DNA sample quantity

Table 1. Characteristics of the study population.

Attributions	Dry AMD	Wet AMD	Controls	p
	N = 67	N = 213	N = 106	
Female N (%)	34 (50.7)	125 (58.7)	53 (50.0)	0.26
Male N (%)	33 (49.3)	88 (41.3)	53 (50.0)	0.26
Age (year, mean±SD)	75.4 (11.5)	76.0 (7.3)	79.1 (6.1)	0.005
Smoking (packyear, mean± SD)	12.0 (20.1)	11.2 (19.8)	11.4 (21.9)	0.76
BMI (mean±SD)	27.3 (4.5)	27.3 (4.4)	27.6 (4.7)	0.83
Hypertension N (%)	45 (67.2)	159 (75.0)	81 (79.4)	0.21
DVT N (%)	7 (10.4)	15 (7.1)	15 (14.9)	0.09
AMI N (%)	6 (9.0)	19 (9.0)	7 (7.4)	0.90
Outdoor profession N (%)	22 (32.8)	39 (18.5)	38 (38.4)	0.0004
Cataract surgery N (%)	21 (31.3)	48 (22.6)	73 (70.2)	<0.0001

BMI: body mass index, DVT: deep vein thrombosis, AMI: acute myocardial infarction.

available. The control group showed no statistical difference from Hardy-Weinberg equilibrium in the case of the tested polymorphisms. Minor alleles of genes unequivocally linked to AMD were more frequent in patients than in controls. Except I1a, MerTK receptor polymorphisms showed a very low minor allele frequency and no notable difference between cases and controls. In case of ApoE the most common E3 allele was slightly more frequent in patients than in controls while the potential risk factor E2 allele was less frequent in patients than in controls. The ApoE E4 allele had similar frequency in all the three groups. Unadjusted odds ratios, and corresponding p values for each genotype comparison are shown in Table 2.

Multiple regression models

The model of pooled dry and wet AMD variants revealed strongly significant adjusted risks in case of the presence of homozygous polymorphisms in the CFH and HTRA1 genes, increasing the odds of AMD by more than five and nearly ten times (OR = 5.3, 95%CI: 2.5–11.5, $p<0.0001$, and OR = 9.8, 95%CI: 3.3–29.5, $p<0.0001$), respectively. No significant interactions were found between any pairs of these variables.

Factors showing significant adjusted associations with dry type AMD are shown in Table 3. and Figure 1. These are genes C3, CFH, and HTRA1, with interactions between both C3 and CFH ($p = 0.020$) and C3 and HTRA1 ($p = 0.024$). The heterozygous/homozygous genotype of C3 carried a significant risk over wild type genotype in the simultaneous absence of homozygous CFH and HTRA1 polymorphisms only. In this case it was associated with a near-five-fold relative increase in the odds of dry type AMD. The stratum of subjects with homozygous mutated HTRA1 and CFH genes contained an insufficient number and distribution of observations for C3 effect estimation. In the case of wild type C3 genotype, mutated alleles of both CFH and HTRA1 behaved as strongly significant risk factors, but reduced to neutrality otherwise.

Factors found to have remarkable associations with wet type AMD included the genes Gas6, CFH, and HTRA1 (Table 4, Figure 1). Gas6 was protective irrespective of other genotypes ($p = 0.04$), reducing the odds of wet type AMD by a half. There was no evidence for the effect of C3 (left in the model for comparability with the dry variant), and although C3's odds ratios specific for different combinations of CFH and HTRA1 genotypes showed a fairly varied pattern, the interaction was technically not significant, unlike in the case of the dry AMD. However, there was some indication that the effect of HTRA1 (homozygous vs. wild type or heterozygous genotype) was modified by the C3 genotype, with estimated odds ratios of 45.04 ($p = 0.0005$) and 4.34 ($p = 0.04$) in C3 wild type and hetero/homozygous mutated genotypes, respectively. Homozygous CFH polymorphism was observed to be a highly significant risk factor for wet type AMD, with odds ratios slightly varying around 7.5 depending on whether mutations in C3 were present or not. All models had a sufficient goodness-of-fit by Hosmer–Lemeshow tests.

Discussion

Our understanding about the genetic causes and therefore pathological pathways involved in the development of AMD has increased substantially in the last few years. The p.Tyr402His polymorphisms of the CFH gene, the rs11200638 polymorphism of the serine peptidase HTRA1 and the p.Ala69Ser polymorphism of the LOC387715 gene are unequivocally associated to AMD in different populations with robust risks. Our results further support these observations and demonstrate robust and highly significant adjusted risk conferred by these polymorphisms as shown by the analysis of the pooled AMD population. After dividing the patient group to exudative (wet) and non-exudative (dry) subgroups, other associations and an interesting genetic interplay was revealed. The rs2230199 polymorphism of the C3 gene contributed significant disease risk to non-exudative AMD in the simultaneous absence of homozygous CFH and HTRA1 polymorphisms. Alternative complement activation is the major biological process linked to AMD development so far. C3 plays a central role in the alternative pathway and its role in AMD pathogenesis is supported by epidemiological and experimental observations. The C3 polymorphism had no significant effect on the development of wet AMD in our study population.

Epidemiological reports on the p.Arg102Gly C3 polymorphism are usually limited to advanced cases including neovascular AMD and geographic atrophy. This approach, however, falls short of detecting any difference between the etiology of dry and wet AMD. Despite the fact that CFH and C3 are members of the same biological pathway, no evidence of a genetic interplay between these two has been demonstrated so far [49]. Carriers of two risk alleles of the rs2230199 polymorphism of the C3 gene are at

Table 2. Unadjusted ORs of the examined polymorphisms.

Polymorphism	Genotypes compared	Dry AMD		Wet AMD	
		OR	p value	OR	p value
CFH rs1061170	TC+CC vs. TT	1.30	0.43	3.27	<0.0001
CFH rs1061170	TC vs. TT	0.86	0.67	2.09	0.0104
CFH rs1061170	CC vs. TC	3.86	0.003	4.17	0.0001
CFH rs1061170	CC vs. TT	3.32	0.01	8.73	<0.0001
CFH rs1061170	CC vs. TT+TC	3.60	0.002	5.45	<0.0001
LOC387715 rs10490924	GT+TT vs. GG	1.50	0.20	3.29	<0.0001
LOC387715 rs10490924	GT vs. GG	1.22	0.56	2.07	0.01
LOC387715 rs10490924	TT vs. GT	3.55	0.03	7.47	<0.0001
LOC387715 rs10490924	TT vs. GG	4.31	0.01	15.5	<0.0001
LOC387715 rs10490924	TT vs. GG+GT	3.89	0.01	10.0	<0.0001
HTRA1 rs11200638	TC+CC vs.TT	1.52	0.19	3.21	<0.0001
HTRA1 rs11200638	TC vs. CC	1.24	0.52	2.00	0.01
HTRA1 rs11200638	CC vs. TC	4.03	0.03	9.18	<0.0001
HTRA1 rs11200638	CC vs. TT	5.00	0.01	18.4	<0.0001
HTRA1 rs11200638	CC vs. TT+TC	4.46	0.01	12.2	<0.0001
Gas6 rs8191974	AA vs. GA	1.51	0.39	1.00	0.99
Gas6 rs8191974	AA vs. GG	1.03	0.96	0.61	0.21
Gas6 rs8191974	AA vs. GG+GA	1.27	0.60	0.79	0.54
Gas6 rs8191974	GA vs. GG	0.68	0.26	0.61	0.05
Gas6 rs8191974	GA+AA vs. GG	0.75	0.37	0.61	0.04
C3 rs2230199	CG+GG vs. CC	1.55	0.17	1.27	0.3237
C3 rs2230199	CG vs. CC	1.47	0.24	1.22	0.4198
C3 rs2230199	GG vs. CG	1.76	0.48	1.52	0.5409
C3 rs2230199	GG vs. CC	2.59	0.23	1.86	0.3568
C3 rs2230199	GG vs. CC+GC	2.22	0.31	1.73	0.41
CFI rs10033900	CC vs. TC	1.47	0.34	1.21	0.55
CFI rs10033900	CC vs. TT	1.54	0.34	1.31	0.44
CFI rs10033900	TC vs. TT	1.04	0.91	1.09	0.76
FXIII rs5985	GT+TT vs. GG	0.59	0.10	0.66	0.08
FXIII rs5985	GT vs. GG	0.65	0.20	0.64	0.08
FXIII rs5985	TT vs. GT	0.51	0.34	1.15	0.73
FXIII rs5985	TT vs. GG	0.34	0.11	0.74	0.46
FXIII rs5985	TT vs. GG+GT	0.40	0.18	0.90	0.78
Apo-E	3/4+4 vs. 2+2/3	1.67	0.3897	1.51	0.3512
Apo-E	3/4+4 vs. 3/3	1.00	0.9929	1.02	0.9543
Apo-E	2+2/3 vs. 3/3	0.60	0.2879	0.68	0.2632
Mertk I1a	AA vs. GA	0.96	0.9251	1.08	0.8171
Mertk I1a	AA vs. GG	0.83	0.7086	1.00	0.9910
Mertk I1a	GA vs. GG	0.87	0.6891	0.93	0.7714
Mertk I1b	CT vs. CC	0.58	0.1329	0.76	0.2919
Mertk I1b	TT vs. CC	2.50	0.0989	1.16	0.7664
Mertk I1b	TT vs. CT	4.33	0.0144	1.52	0.4218
Mertk I1c	AC vs. AA	0.54	0.2623	1.13	0.7328
Mertk I4	AG vs. AA	0.88	0.7186	0.79	0.3602
Mertk I4	GG vs. AA	*	*	0.62	0.5352
Mertk I4	GG vs. AG	*	*	0.79	0.7615

*Missing data are due to insufficient minor allele frequency.

moderate risk to develop AMD compared to wild type subjects (OR: 1.88, 95%CI: 1.59–2.23) according to a recent meta-analysis [15]. Besides that, it is well known that, drusen, the hallmark of dry AMD contains complement factors 3a and 5a among other inflammatory proteins, which therefore could play a role in drusen formation and might even have an effect on neovascularisation [50,51,52,53,54]. Experimental evidence showed that suppression of the complement cascade in the retina delayed and reversed the onset of AMD in a monkey model of dry AMD [55]. The effect of CFH and C3 polymorphisms are mutually exclusive on the risk of dry AMD in our study population. On the other hand, CFH has a robust effect on neovascular AMD independent of the C3 status. Since the two proteins are located in the same biological pathway, our results can be explained with the stronger effect overriding the other. Interestingly, the interaction between C3 and HTRA1 is very similar, which indicates that C3 and HTRA1 are also competing in dry AMD development. This finding underscores previous reports on the role of HTRA1 in complement regulation [56]. Taken together our findings indicate a central role of C3 in dry AMD formation, however, CFH and HTRA1 genotype have an influence on the effect of the C3 p.Arg102Gly polymorphism most likely explained by their complement regulatory activity. CFI has been associated to AMD development with conflicting results. Fagerness et al. reported an OR of 0.7 for the lower risk C allele ($p = 6.46 \times 10^{-8}$) of the rs10033900 polymorphism within the CFI gene in a large population of European descent [16]. Chen et al found a statistically significant association of the rs2285714 risk allele and AMD with a moderate OR of 1.31 (95%CI: 1.18–1.45, $p = 3.4 \times 10^{-7}$) [57]. Seddon et al. demonstrated that the protective effect of the hepatic lipase (LIPC) rs10468017 polymorphism on AMD pathogenesis was stronger in the presence of double wild type rs10033900 compared to the homozygous polymorphism [58]. The findings of the original article by Fagerness were reflected in three case-controls studies. A report on a Japanese population demonstrated an OR of 0.28 (95%CI: 0.11–0.69, $p = 0.0035$) for the rare homozygous CC genotype [59]. The work of Ennis et al. supports the involvement of the CFI gene in AMD development by demonstrating four SNP's in the CFI gene associating to AMD, however the effect of the rs10033900 polymorphism, which had the strongest association signal in the original work of Fagerness, was not statistically significant in their cohort ($p = 0.135$). Interestingly, the haplotype including rs10033900 polymorphism and another non-significant polymorphism together conferred statistically significant disease risk ($OR = 2.15$, $p = 0.02$) [17]. A very well powered case-control study based on independent samples from England and Scotland failed to detect any statistically significant effect of the rs10033900 polymorphism on AMD ($OR = 0.95$, 95%CI: 0.83–1.09, $p = 0.47$) [18]. Similarly to that, in the present study we could not provide any additional support for the association of the rs10033900 polymorphism and AMD. Although our sample size is not as large as some of the cited works, it is large enough to detect strong or even weak but significant associations with other well established

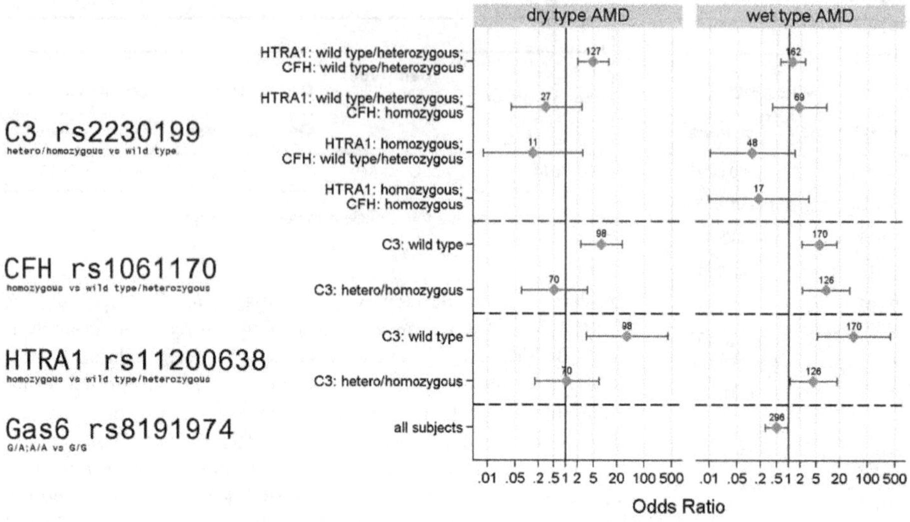

Figure 1. The effect of GAS6 c.834+7G>A polymorphism and genetic interactions on the risk of AMD. Polymorphisms with the compared genotypes are shown on the left side. Stratum of subjects involved in the corresponding analysis are on the vertical axis. Figures above markers indicate number of observations for the given stratum Adjusted odds ratios and 95% confidence intervals are represented by dots and lines, respectively. In the dry AMD group the effect of C3 polymorphism in case of double CFH/HTRA1 homozygousity could not be estimated due to low observation number. GAS6 was not included as an explanatory variable in the model for dry AMD.

risk factors of AMD as demonstrated by our findings on the CFH, LOC387715, HTRA1 and C3 polymorphisms. Our results are in line with studies showing no effect of the rs10033900 polymorphism. Although one cannot exclude such an association based on a single negative result, there are a growing number of publications falling short of detecting any effect of the polymorphism which clearly indicates that the association is not unequivocal and calls for further epidemiological and functional analysis to clarify the link between CFI and AMD.

No evidence of association with AMD could be demonstrated in the case of ApoE alleles. We neither could confirm previous reports on the protective effect of the E4 allele, nor could we show any risk related to the E2 allele. Two recent very-well powered epidemiological studies [33,34] concluded on the disease causing effect of the E2 allele and the protective role of the E4 allele. Albeit these convincing studies, our results still do not fit in the line. Interestingly, we could not observe any statistically significant disease association with any of the ApoE alleles, moreover the frequency of the E2 risk allele was higher in controls than in patients, while the protective E4 allele showed similar frequencies in the wet AMD and the control group. These data indicate that ApoE is not a key player in AMD pathogenesis in the Hungarian population. This can either be explained by a geographical difference, or by other different environmental factors, probably the different smoking habits of the Hungarian population.

Candidate gene approach is widely used to identify biological pathways and genes involved in pathological processes. Based on their biological functions, we directly tested for disease association of common polymorphisms in the FXIII, Gas6 and in one of the Gas6 receptor genes, MerTK. Blood coagulation factor XIII is a plasma transglutaminase that cross links adjacent fibrin chains in the final step of the coagulation cascade. In addition, FXIII is known to participate in wound healing, tissue remodeling and embryo implantation at least partially through its proangiogenic effect [60]. The cardioprotective p.Val34Leu polymorphism of the blood coagulation factor XIII has been associated with accelerated thrombin activation, recurrent subconjunctival haemorrhage, intracerebral haemorrhage, and a decreased immune reaction in humans [61,62,63]. Most importantly, since angiogenesis plays a crucial role in neovascular AMD, we found it reasonable to investigate if the polymorphism had any effect on AMD formation. However, we failed to detect any association of AMD and the polymorphism in our present study, indicating a neutral polymorphism in relation to both dry and wet AMD development.

Gas6, a Protein S structural homologue, has important functions in the regulation of angiogenesis, cell migration and proliferation. Its common polymorphism Gas6 c.834+7G>A is

Table 3. Polymorphisms showing significant association with dry AMD using multiple logistic regression.

Polymorphism	Genotypes compared	Stratum of subjects	OR	95% CI	p value
C3 rs2230199	CG+GG vs. CC	**HTRA1**: TT+TC **CFH**: TT+TC	4.93	1.98–12.25	0.0006
CFH rs1061170	CC vs. TT+TC	**C3**: CC	7.96	2.39–26.50	0.0007
HTRA1 rs11200638	TC+CC vs.TT	**C3**: CC	36.02	3.30–393.02	0.0033

Stratum represents genotype of subjects involved in the analysis.

Table 4. Polymorphisms showing significant association with wet AMD using multiple logistic regression.

Polymorphism	Genotypes compared	Stratum of subjects	OR	95% CI	p value
CFH rs1061170	CC vs. TT+TC	**C3**: CC	6.08	2.17–17.04	0.0006
CFH rs1061170	CC vs. TT+TC	**C3**: CT+TT	8.96	2.24–35.79	0.002
HTRA1 rs11200638	TC+CC vs.TT	**C3**: CC	45.04	5.30–382.83	0.0005
HTRA1 rs11200638	TC vs. CC	**C3**: CT+TT	4.34	1.09–17.28	0.04
Gas6 rs8191974	GA+AA vs. GG	n.a.	0.5	0.26–0.97	0.04

Stratum represents genotype of subjects involved in the analysis.

associated with decreased risk of cardiovascular diseases. Its receptors (TAM) play a crucial role in phagocytosis of apoptotic cells in the immune, nervous, and reproductive systems. These functions make Gas6 and its receptors a potential candidate involved in both dry and wet AMD development. In the pooled early and late AMD population the Gas6 polymorphism showed no statistically significant association to AMD. When analyzing dry and wet subgroups separately, no association with the dry AMD could be demonstrated; however a protective effect was detected in the wet AMD subgroup ($p = 0.04$). As formation of new vessels is a hallmark of wet AMD, it is likely that it is this function of Gas6 that is important in the context of the disease. Gas6 is able to inhibit VEGF-A signaling through Axl activation of SHP-2 phosphatases [38]. Recently, a similar inhibitory effect has been shown in metastasis induced angiogenesis [64]. This finding suggests a role of Gas6 in controlling pathological angiogenesis, and that c.834+7G>A polymorphism of the GAS6 gene, which has been linked to disease repeatedly [36,40,41], could have a direct effect on the function of the gene through an unknown mechanism. Future epidemiological and functional studies are required to further evaluate the effect of the GAS6 polymorphism on AMD development. It is to be noted, that no formal correction for multiple testing was applied in the multiple logistic regression analysis, however, this does not invalidate the conclusion that the suggested effect of the GAS6 polymorphism is worthy of further investigations.

In our case-control study we confirmed previous findings on the association of AMD and genetic polymorphisms in the CFH, LOC387715 and HTRA1 genes, however could not demonstrate any association with the CFI gene. More interestingly, we found a genetic interplay of CFH, HTRA1 and C3 genes, showing that the C3 polymorphism is a major contributor of dry AMD in the absence of the other polymorphisms, while has no effect on wet AMD development in our population. This result indicates that C3 plays a critical role in dry AMD rather than wet AMD pathogenesis, and its effect can be overdriven by other known genetic risk factors in the CFH and HTRA1 genes. We detected a protective effect of a common Gas6 c.834+7G>A polymorphism on wet AMD formation. Our results suggest a possible new player and novel genetic interactions in AMD pathogenesis, however our data should be confirmed in other populations, especially in the case of the Gas6 polymorphism.

Author Contributions

Conceived and designed the experiments: GL LT IB AB EM EA AF. Performed the experiments: GL AV EM AF ED IB LT BH PGdF LK. Analyzed the data: GL LK IB EA AB. Contributed reagents/materials/analysis tools: GL AB IB ED LK EA BH PGdF. Wrote the paper: GL LK IB AB.

References

1. Klein R, Peto T, Bird A, Vannewkirk MR (2004) The epidemiology of age-related macular degeneration. Am J Ophthalmol 137: 486–495.
2. Friedman DS, Katz J, Bressler NM, Rahmani B, Tielsch JM (1999) Racial differences in the prevalence of age-related macular degeneration: the Baltimore Eye Survey. Ophthalmology 106: 1049–1055.
3. Friedman DS, O'Colmain BJ, Munoz B, Tomany SC, McCarty C, et al. (2004) Prevalence of age-related macular degeneration in the United States. Arch Ophthalmol 122: 564–572.
4. Seddon JM, Sharma S, Adelman RA (2006) Evaluation of the clinical age-related maculopathy staging system. Ophthalmology 113: 260–266.
5. Coleman HR, Chan CC, Ferris FL 3rd, Chew EY (2008) Age-related macular degeneration. Lancet 372: 1835–1845.
6. Chakravarthy U, Wong TY, Fletcher A, Piault E, Evans C, et al. (2010) Clinical risk factors for age-related macular degeneration: a systematic review and meta-analysis. BMC Ophthalmol 10: 31.
7. Ho L, Boekhoorn SS, Liana, van Duijn CM, Uitterlinden AG, et al. (2008) Cataract surgery and the risk of aging macula disorder: the rotterdam study. Invest Ophthalmol Vis Sci 49: 4795–4800.
8. Francis PJ, Klein ML (2011) Update on the role of genetics in the onset of age-related macular degeneration. Clin Ophthalmol 5: 1127–1133.
9. Klein RJ, Zeiss C, Chew EY, Tsai JY, Sackler RS, et al. (2005) Complement factor H polymorphism in age-related macular degeneration. Science 308: 385–389.
10. Edwards AO, Ritter R 3rd, Abel KJ, Manning A, Panhuysen C, et al. (2005) Complement factor H polymorphism and age-related macular degeneration. Science 308: 421–424.
11. Haines JL, Hauser MA, Schmidt S, Scott WK, Olson LM, et al. (2005) Complement factor H variant increases the risk of age-related macular degeneration. Science 308: 419–421.
12. Sofat R, Casas JP, Webster AR, Bird AC, Mann SS, et al. (2012) Complement factor H genetic variant and age-related macular degeneration: effect size, modifiers and relationship to disease subtype. Int J Epidemiol 41: 250–262.
13. Yates JR, Sepp T, Matharu BK, Khan JC, Thurlby DA, et al. (2007) Complement C3 variant and the risk of age-related macular degeneration. N Engl J Med 357: 553–561.
14. Despriet DD, van Duijn CM, Oostra BA, Uitterlinden AG, Hofman A, et al. (2009) Complement component C3 and risk of age-related macular degeneration. Ophthalmology 116: 474–480 e472.
15. Thakkinstian A, McKay GJ, McEvoy M, Chakravarthy U, Chakrabarti S, et al. (2011) Systematic review and meta-analysis of the association between complement component 3 and age-related macular degeneration: a HuGE review and meta-analysis. Am J Epidemiol 173: 1365–1379.
16. Fagerness JA, Maller JB, Neale BM, Reynolds RC, Daly MJ, et al. (2009) Variation near complement factor I is associated with risk of advanced AMD. Eur J Hum Genet 17: 100–104.
17. Ennis S, Gibson J, Cree AJ, Collins A, Lotery AJ (2010) Support for the involvement of complement factor I in age-related macular degeneration. Eur J Hum Genet 18: 15–16.

18. Cipriani V, Matharu BK, Khan JC, Shahid H, Hayward C, et al. (2012) No evidence of association between complement factor I genetic variant rs10033900 and age-related macular degeneration. Eur J Hum Genet 20: 1–2; author reply 3.
19. Jakobsdottir J, Conley YP, Weeks DE, Mah TS, Ferrell RE, et al. (2005) Susceptibility genes for age-related maculopathy on chromosome 10q26. Am J Hum Genet 77: 389–407.
20. Rivera A, Fisher SA, Fritsche LG, Keilhauer CN, Lichtner P, et al. (2005) Hypothetical LOC387715 is a second major susceptibility gene for age-related macular degeneration, contributing independently of complement factor H to disease risk. Hum Mol Genet 14: 3227–3236.
21. Yang Z, Camp NJ, Sun H, Tong Z, Gibbs D, et al. (2006) A variant of the HTRA1 gene increases susceptibility to age-related macular degeneration. Science 314: 992–993.
22. Dewan A, Liu M, Hartman S, Zhang SS, Liu DT, et al. (2006) HTRA1 promoter polymorphism in wet age-related macular degeneration. Science 314: 989–992.
23. Yoshida T, DeWan A, Zhang H, Sakamoto R, Okamoto H, et al. (2007) HTRA1 promoter polymorphism predisposes Japanese to age-related macular degeneration. Mol Vis 13: 545–548.
24. Cameron DJ, Yang Z, Gibbs D, Chen H, Kaminoh Y, et al. (2007) HTRA1 variant confers similar risks to geographic atrophy and neovascular age-related macular degeneration. Cell Cycle 6: 1122–1125.
25. Wang L, Clark ME, Crossman DK, Kojima K, Messinger JD, et al. (2010) Abundant lipid and protein components of drusen. PLoS One 5: e10329.
26. Souied EH, Benlian P, Amouyel P, Feingold J, Lagarde JP, et al. (1998) The epsilon4 allele of the apolipoprotein E gene as a potential protective factor for exudative age-related macular degeneration. Am J Ophthalmol 125: 353–359.
27. Baird PN, Guida E, Chu DT, Vu HT, Guymer RH (2004) The epsilon2 and epsilon4 alleles of the apolipoprotein gene are associated with age-related macular degeneration. Invest Ophthalmol Vis Sci 45: 1311–1315.
28. Baird PN, Richardson AJ, Robman LD, Dimitrov PN, Tikellis G, et al. (2006) Apolipoprotein (APOE) gene is associated with progression of age-related macular degeneration (AMD). Hum Mutat 27: 337–342.
29. Francis PJ, Hamon SC, Ott J, Weleber RG, Klein ML (2009) Polymorphisms in C2, CFB and C3 are associated with progression to advanced age related macular degeneration associated with visual loss. J Med Genet 46: 300–307.
30. Yu Y, Reynolds R, Fagerness J, Rosner B, Daly MJ, et al. (2011) Association of variants in the LIPC and ABCA1 genes with intermediate and large drusen and advanced age-related macular degeneration. Invest Ophthalmol Vis Sci 52: 4663–4670.
31. Asensio-Sanchez VM, Rodriguez-Martin T, Gala-Molina I, Rodriguez-Fernandez I (2006) [Age-related macular degeneration: its association with the epsilon4 allele of the apolipoprotein E gene]. Arch Soc Esp Oftalmol 81: 9–12.
32. Losonczy G, Fekete A, Voko Z, Takacs L, Kaldi I, et al. (2011) Analysis of complement factor H Y402H, LOC387715, HTRA1 polymorphisms and ApoE alleles with susceptibility to age-related macular degeneration in Hungarian patients. Acta Ophthalmol 89: 255–262.
33. McKay GJ, Patterson CC, Chakravarthy U, Dasari S, Klaver CC, et al. (2011) Evidence of association of APOE with age-related macular degeneration: a pooled analysis of 15 studies. Hum Mutat 32: 1407–1416.
34. Adams MK, Simpson JA, Richardson AJ, English DR, Aung KZ, et al. (2012) Apolipoprotein E gene associations in age-related macular degeneration: the Melbourne Collaborative Cohort Study. Am J Epidemiol 175: 511–518.
35. Fernandez-Fernandez L, Bellido-Martin L, Garcia de Frutos P (2008) Growth arrest-specific gene 6 (GAS6). An outline of its role in haemostasis and inflammation. Thromb Haemost 100: 604–610.
36. Jiang L, Liu CY, Yang QF, Wang P, Zhang W (2009) Plasma level of growth arrest-specific 6 (GAS6) protein and genetic variations in the GAS6 gene in patients with acute coronary syndrome. Am J Clin Pathol 131: 738–743.
37. Lutgens E, Tjwa M, Garcia de Frutos P, Wijnands E, Beckers L, et al. (2008) Genetic loss of Gas6 induces plaque stability in experimental atherosclerosis. J Pathol 216: 55–63.
38. Gallicchio M, Mitola S, Valdembri D, Fantozzi R, Varnum B, et al. (2005) Inhibition of vascular endothelial growth factor receptor 2-mediated endothelial cell activation by Axl tyrosine kinase receptor. Blood 105: 1970–1976.
39. Balogh I, Hafizi S, Stenhoff J, Hansson K, Dahlback B (2005) Analysis of Gas6 in human platelets and plasma. Arterioscler Thromb Vasc Biol 25: 1280–1286.
40. Munoz X, Obach V, Hurtado B, de Frutos PG, Chamorro A, et al. (2007) Association of specific haplotypes of GAS6 gene with stroke. Thromb Haemost 98: 406–412.
41. Lee CH, Chu NF, Shieh YS, Hung YJ (2012) The growth arrest-specific 6 (Gas6) gene polymorphism c.834+7G>A is associated with type 2 diabetes. Diabetes Res Clin Pract 95: 201–206.
42. Rothlin CV, Lemke G (2010) TAM receptor signaling and autoimmune disease. Curr Opin Immunol 22: 740–746.
43. Duncan JL, LaVail MM, Yasumura D, Matthes MT, Yang H, et al. (2003) An RCS-like retinal dystrophy phenotype in mer knockout mice. Invest Ophthalmol Vis Sci 44: 826–838.
44. Hall MO, Obin MS, Heeb MJ, Burgess BL, Abrams TA (2005) Both protein S and Gas6 stimulate outer segment phagocytosis by cultured rat retinal pigment epithelial cells. Exp Eye Res 81: 581–591.
45. Chen YY, Lu QJ, Lu QX, Wang NL (2011) Gene expression profile changes caused by the dysfunction of Mer during retinal pigment epithelium phagocytosis. Chin Med J (Engl) 124: 1145–1155.
46. Hurtado B, Abasolo N, Munoz X, Garcia N, Benavente Y, et al. (2010) Association study between polymorphisms in GAS6-TAM genes and carotid atherosclerosis. Thromb Haemost 104: 592–598.
47. Shemirani AH, Muszbek L (2004) Rapid detection of the factor XIII Val34Leu (163 G→T) polymorphism by real-time PCR using fluorescence resonance energy transfer detection and melting curve analysis. Clin Chem Lab Med 42: 877–879.
48. Rudnicka AR, Jarrar Z, Wormald R, Cook DG, Fletcher A, et al. (2012) Age and gender variations in age-related macular degeneration prevalence in populations of European ancestry: a meta-analysis. Ophthalmology 119: 571–580.
49. Spencer KL, Olson LM, Anderson BM, Schnetz-Boutaud N, Scott WK, et al. (2008) C3 R102G polymorphism increases risk of age-related macular degeneration. Hum Mol Genet 17: 1821–1824.
50. Mullins RF, Russell SR, Anderson DH, Hageman GS (2000) Drusen associated with aging and age-related macular degeneration contain proteins common to extracellular deposits associated with atherosclerosis, elastosis, amyloidosis, and dense deposit disease. FASEB J 14: 835–846.
51. Johnson LV, Ozaki S, Staples MK, Erickson PA, Anderson DH (2000) A potential role for immune complex pathogenesis in drusen formation. Exp Eye Res 70: 441–449.
52. Anderson DH, Mullins RF, Hageman GS, Johnson LV (2002) A role for local inflammation in the formation of drusen in the aging eye. Am J Ophthalmol 134: 411–431.
53. Johnson LV, Leitner WP, Staples MK, Anderson DH (2001) Complement activation and inflammatory processes in Drusen formation and age related macular degeneration. Exp Eye Res 73: 887–896.
54. Nozaki M, Raisler BJ, Sakurai E, Sarma JV, Barnum SR, et al. (2006) Drusen complement components C3a and C5a promote choroidal neovascularization. Proc Natl Acad Sci U S A 103: 2328–2333.
55. Chi ZL, Yoshida T, Lambris JD, Iwata T (2010) Suppression of drusen formation by compstatin, a peptide inhibitor of complement C3 activation, on cynomolgus monkey with early-onset macular degeneration. Adv Exp Med Biol 703: 127–135.
56. An E, Sen S, Park SK, Gordish-Dressman H, Hathout Y (2010) Identification of novel substrates for the serine protease HTRA1 in the human RPE secretome. Invest Ophthalmol Vis Sci 51: 3379–3386.
57. Chen W, Stambolian D, Edwards AO, Branham KE, Othman M, et al. (2010) Genetic variants near TIMP3 and high-density lipoprotein-associated loci influence susceptibility to age-related macular degeneration. Proc Natl Acad Sci U S A 107: 7401–7406.
58. Seddon JM, Reynolds R, Rosner B (2010) Associations of smoking, body mass index, dietary lutein, and the LIPC gene variant rs10468017 with advanced age-related macular degeneration. Mol Vis 16: 2412–2424.
59. Kondo N, Bessho H, Honda S, Negi A (2010) Additional evidence to support the role of a common variant near the complement factor I gene in susceptibility to age-related macular degeneration. Eur J Hum Genet 18: 634–635.
60. Dardik R, Loscalzo J, Inbal A (2006) Factor XIII (FXIII) and angiogenesis. J Thromb Haemost 4: 19–25.
61. Kovar FM, Marsik CL, Jilma B, Mannhalter C, Joukhadar C, et al. (2009) The inflammatory response is influenced by FXIII VAL 34 LEU polymorphism in a human LPS model. Wien Klin Wochenschr 121: 515–519.
62. Balogh I, Szoke G, Karpati L, Wartiovaara U, Katona E, et al. (2000) Val34Leu polymorphism of plasma factor XIII: biochemistry and epidemiology in familial thrombophilia. Blood 96: 2479–2486.
63. Ariens RA, Philippou H, Nagaswami C, Weisel JW, Lane DA, et al. (2000) The factor XIII V34L polymorphism accelerates thrombin activation of factor XIII and affects cross-linked fibrin structure. Blood 96: 988–995.
64. Png KJ, Halberg N, Yoshida M, Tavazoie SF (2011) A microRNA regulon that mediates endothelial recruitment and metastasis by cancer cells. Nature 481: 190–194.

Ranibizumab versus Bevacizumab for Ophthalmic Diseases Related to Neovascularisation

Bin Wu[1]◎, Haixiang Wu[2]◎, Xiaoyan Liu[1], Houwen Lin[1], Jin Li[3]*

1 Department of Pharmacy, Ren Ji Hospital, affiliated with the School of Medicine, Shanghai Jiao tong University, Shanghai, China, 2 Department of Ophthalmology, and Visual Science, Eye, and ENT Hospital, Shanghai Medical College, Fudan University, Shanghai, China, 3 Department of Ophthalmology, Ren Ji Hospital, affiliated with the School of Medicine, Shanghai Jiao tong University, Shanghai, China

Abstract

Background: Bevacizumab is believed to be as effective and safe as ranibizumab for ophthalmic diseases; however, its magnitude of effectiveness and safety profile remain controversial. Thus, a meta-analysis and systematic review appears necessary.

Methods: PubMed and EMBASE were systematically searched with no restrictions. All relevant citations comparing ranibizumab and bevacizumab were considered for inclusion. Pooled effect estimates were obtained using a fixed- and random-effects meta-analysis.

Results: Nine independent randomised-controlled clinical trials (RCTs) involving 2,289 participants were identified. Compared with bevacizumab, the overall combined weighted mean difference (WMD) of the mean change in visual acuity for ranibizumab was 0.52 letters (95% CI −0.11–1.14). The odds ratios (ORs) of gaining ≥15, gaining 5–14, losing 5–14 and losing ≤15 letters were 1.10 (95% CI 0.90–1.33), 0.93 (95% CI 0.77–1.11), 0.89 (95% CI 0.65–1.22) and 0.95 (95% CI 0.73–1.25), respectively. The risk of serious systemic events increased by 17% (95% CI 6%–27%, $p = 0.0042$) for bevacizumab treatment in comparison with ranibizumab. No statistically significant differences between the two treatments were found for the nonfatal arterial thrombotic events, ocular serious adverse, death from vascular and all causes events.

Conclusions: Bevacizumab is not inferior to ranibizumab as a treatment for achieving visual acuity. The use of bevacizumab was associated with an increased risk of developing serious systemic events. Weighing the costs and health outcomes is necessary when selecting between bevacizumab and ranibizumab for ophthalmic diseases. Due to the limitations of the available data, further research is needed.

Editor: Torben Lykke Sørensen, Copenhagen University Hospital Roskilde and the University of Copenhagen, Denmark

Funding: This study was supported by a grant from the National Natural Science Foundation of China (NO. 71373160). The funders had no role in study design, data collection and analysis, decision to publish, or preparation of the manuscript.

Competing Interests: The authors declare no conflicts of interest.

* Email: wbwithtg@hotmail.com

◎ These authors contributed equally to this work.

Introduction

Pathological angiogenesis, a process mainly driven by vascular endothelial growth factor (VEGF), is a hallmark of cancer and various ischaemic and inflammatory diseases.[1,2] For several ophthalmic diseases involving neovascularisation or increased vascular permeability, such as neovascular age-related macular degeneration (AMD), diabetic macular oedema (DME), or diabetic retinopathy, VEGF-A is a critical regulator of ocular angiogenesis and vascular permeability.[3] These discoveries have resulted in the development of antineoplastic agents for reducing pathologic angiogenesis, such as bevacizumab and ranibizumab.[4]

Bevacizumab (Avastin, Genentech Inc., South San Francisco, California), a recombinant humanised monoclonal IgG1 antibody against all isoforms of VEGF-A, is able to block the binding between VEGF and its receptors (Flt-1 and KDR) on the surface of endothelial cells.[5] Bevacizumab has been widely prescribed in the treatment of many types of malignancy, including colorectal cancer, renal cell carcinoma, lung cancer and breast cancer. Due to its size (molecular weight of 150 kDa) and resultant weak penetration through the retinal layers after intravitreal injection, bevacizumab was thought to have limited efficacy in ophthalmic disease. However, it has been widely used outside of its licensed indications, such as for AMD.[6,7] In contrast to bevacizumab, ranibizumab (Lucentis, Genentech, Inc., South San Francisco, CA) is a 48 kDa antigen-binding fragment (Fab) form of the bevacizumab molecule. Ranibizumab was specifically developed for ocular indications.[8] With its increased potency, enhanced penetration, and lower possibility of complement-mediated or cell-dependent cytotoxicity, ranibizumab has been an effective treatment for neovascular AMD during several pivotal clinical trials.[9,10] It has been approved for the treatment of patients with neovascular AMD by the Food and Drug Administration and by the European Medicines Agency since 2006 and 2007, respectively.[11]

The interest in securing approval for bevacizumab in treating ophthalmic diseases of neovascularisation is mainly due to the potential cost savings (per-dose cost, approximately $2,000 for ranibizumab and $50 for bevacizumab), despite the resistance of the pharmaceutical companies concerned.[12,13] To determine whether bevacizumab is as effective and safe as ranibizumab, numerous randomised, controlled clinical trials (RCTs) and retrospective studies have been performed over the past five years, such as the Comparison of Age-related macular degeneration Treatments Trials (CATT), the Alternative treatments to Inhibit VEGF in Age-related choroidal Neovascularization (IVAN), the Multicenter Anti-VEGF Trial in Austria (MANTA), and the Groupe d'Etude Français Avastin versus Lucentis dans la DMLA néovasculaire (GEFAL).[14–22] Although the results of these studies indicated the two drugs to be both effective and safe, subtle differences in their comparative efficacy and safety profiles still exist, as suggested by the different trends of improved visual acuity with ranibizumab in the CATT and GEFAL studies, which should be further assessed. Our aim was to compare the clinical effectiveness and safety between ranibizumab and bevacizumab by performing a systematic review of head-to-head RCTs. Furthermore, this information could be used to address the question of whether off-label bevacizumab therapy is as effective and safe as licensed ranibizumab therapy for patients with ophthalmic diseases.

Methods

Search Strategy

This analysis was performed according to the preferred reporting items for systematic reviews and meta-analyses (PRISMA) guidelines and the methods described in the Cochrane Handbook.[23] Two investigators independently (HW and XL) searched all eligible studies in four electronic databases, including PubMed and EMBASE (Excerpta Medica Database), until August 2013; no specific restrictions on language or publication year were applied. The electronic search strategy included the terms ("macular degeneration" OR "retinal degeneration" OR "retinal neovascularisation" OR "choroidal neovascularisation" OR "macula Lutea" OR "diabetic retinopathy" OR "macular oedema") AND ("bevacizumab or avastin" OR "ranibizumab or lucentis or rhufab") combined with "randomised controlled trial". The titles and abstracts were scanned to exclude any clearly irrelevant studies. Furthermore, to identify any additional published reports, a manual search was performed by checking all the references of original reports. In addition, the cited lists of eligible studies by Google Scholar were reviewed to ensure that all appropriate studies were included. The results were compared, and any questions or discrepancies were resolved through iteration and consensus.

This study is an analysis of published data and did not require ethics committee approval.

Inclusion Criteria

To be eligible, studies had to fulfil the following inclusion criteria: (1) comparative RCT study; (2) study population with ophthalmic diseases; (3) head-to-head comparison of results between ranibizumab and bevacizumab; and (4) full text manuscript available. Exclusion criteria were the following: (1) non-RCT; (2) RCTs that enrolled less than 20 patients; (3) patients previously treated with VEGF inhibitors or patients receiving systemic anti-VEGF therapy; (4) less than six months follow-up; and (5) studies without data from a comparison group.

Outcome Measures

The primary outcome chosen was change from baseline in the best corrected visual acuity (BCVA) (Snellen equivalent) measured on Early Treatment of Diabetic Retinopathy Study (ETDRS) charts after at least six months of follow-up, including the proportions of patients whose acuity increased by ≥ 15, increased by 5–14, decreased by 5–14, or decreased by ≤ 15 letters, as well as the mean number of letters.

Secondary measures evaluated included any ocular/systemic adverse events (death from any cause, arteriothrombotic event, or serious ocular event) and assessment of CNV by fluorescein angiography or OCT.

Data Extraction and Quality Assessment

Articles were reviewed and cross-checked independently by two investigators (HW and XL), and disagreements were resolved by consensus. Data extracted included the following: the first author's last name, year of publication, study design, number of patients, age, specific ocular disease, intervention, injection times, follow-up days (Table 1), efficacy, and adverse event data. The included studies were critically evaluated using the Jadad composite scale, which scores studies' based on their descriptions of randomisation (2 points), blinding (2 points), and attrition information (1 point).[24] If the above data were not available in the published study, the authors were contacted and asked to supply the information.

Statistical Analysis

The pooled odds ratio (OR), weighted mean difference (WMD) and relative risk (RR) with 95% CI between ranibizumab and bevacizumab were used to estimate the effect and ADR sizes using the 'metafor' and 'meta' packages, respectively, in R version 2.15.1 for Windows (The R Foundation for Statistical Computing, Vienna, Austria). Statistical heterogeneity among the studies was assessed using Cochran's Q test and the I^2 statistic.[25]. A value of $I^2 > 50\%$ was considered to indicate substantial heterogeneity, and a P value<0.05 was considered to suggest significant heterogeneity.[26] Fixed effects models were employed if there was low heterogeneity ($I^2 < 30\%$); otherwise, random effects models were used. To assess whether publication bias may have impacted the statistical results, a funnel plot was created, and Egger's and Begg's tests were performed.[27,28] For Egger's and Begg's tests, $P<0.05$ was considered to be statistically significant. All statistical tests were two-sided.

Results

Study Selection

The literature search produced a total of 2,024 citations, of which 180 were considered potentially relevant (Figure 1). Of these, 37 articles were considered of interest, and their full texts were retrieved for detailed evaluation. Twenty-seven of these 36 articles were subsequently excluded, and the remaining 9 articles were included in the meta-analysis.

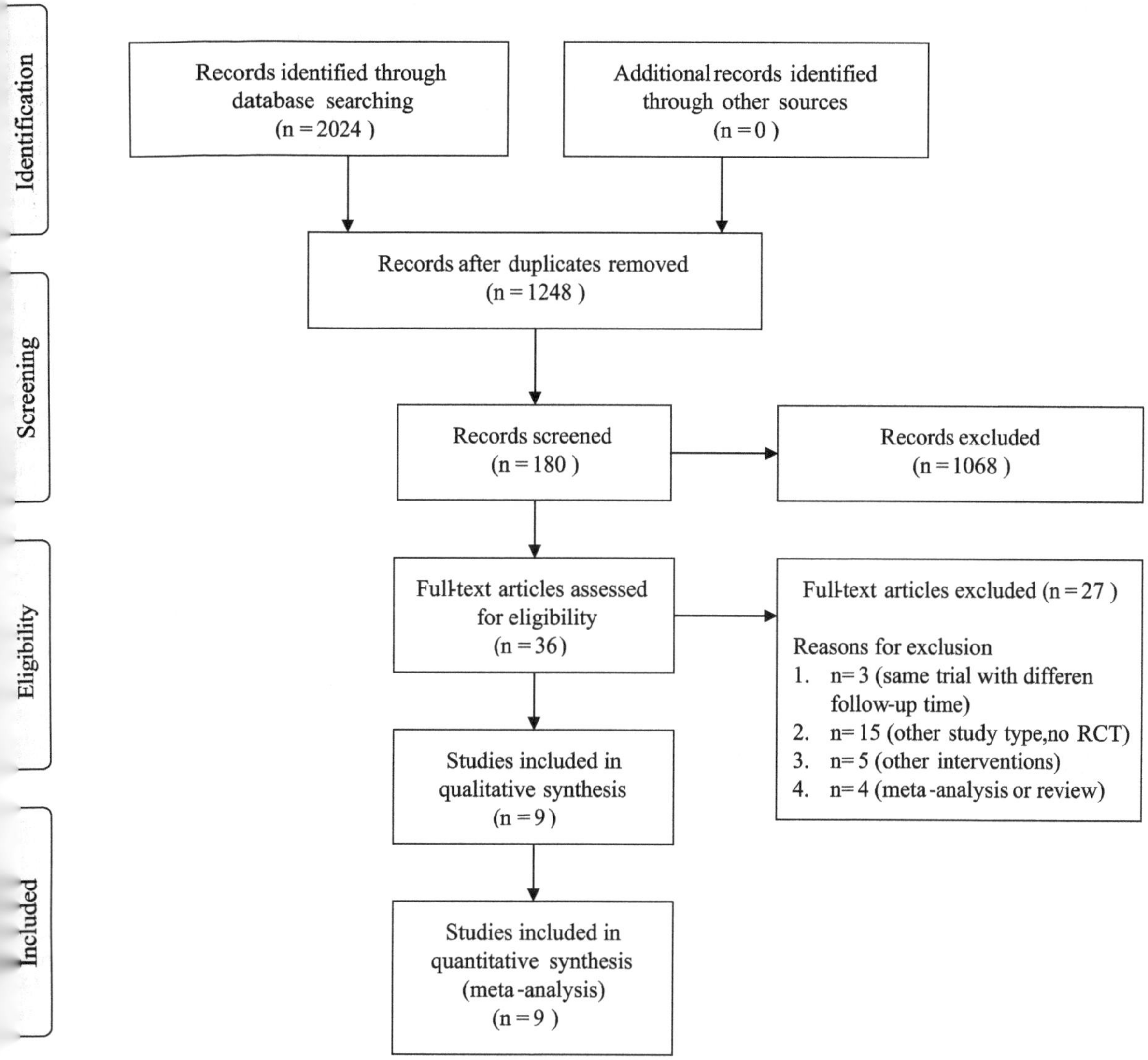

ıure 1. Selection process for randomised controlled trials on the effects of ranibizumab and bevacizumab therapy on ophthalmic ;eases.

udy	Ranibizumab Total	Mean	SD	Bevacizumab Total	Mean	SD	WMD	95%-CI	W(fixed)
ATT(monthly), 2012	134	8.80	14.60	129	7.80	17.90	1.00	[-2.96; 4.96]	2.5%
ATT(needed), 2012	264	6.70	15.90	251	5.00	15.50	1.70	[-1.01; 4.41]	5.3%
AN, 2013	271	4.90	15.00	254	4.10	13.50	0.80	[-1.64; 3.24]	6.5%
ANJU, 2010	15	7.60	13.70	7	6.30	15.30	1.30	[-12.26; 14.86]	0.2%
EFAL, 2013	183	2.93	15.09	191	4.82	14.85	-1.89	[-4.93; 1.15]	4.2%
ENTA, 2013	163	4.10	15.60	154	4.90	15.20	-0.80	[-4.19; 2.59]	3.4%
ITONIO, 2013	28	14.50	7.10	32	11.50	7.60	3.00	[-0.72; 6.72]	2.8%
AGDA, 2010	16	17.31	11.10	16	15.87	8.41	1.44	[-5.38; 8.26]	0.8%
ERLUIGI, 2012	23	9.00	1.35	25	8.50	1.25	0.50	[-0.24; 1.24]	71.4%
AURIZIO, 2013	24	8.00	6.60	26	8.00	6.90	0.00	[-3.74; 3.74]	2.8%
ked effect model							**0.52**	**[-0.11; 1.14]**	**100%**

terogeneity: I-squared=0%, tau-squared=0, p=0.7692

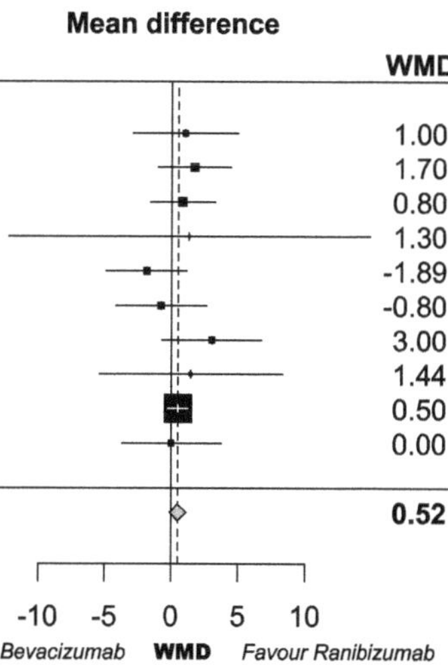

ure 2. Forest plot of WMD for visual acuity change. CI, confidence interval; WMD, weighted mean difference.

Table 1. Characteristics of randomised controlled trials included in the meta-analysis.

Study	Ocular disease	Patients for analysis		Baseline visual acuity (letters)		Follow-up (months)	Dosage (mg)		Treatment pattern	Injections per patient(mean)	
		Ranibizumab	Bevacizumab	Ranibizumab	Bevacizumab		Ranibizumab	Bevacizumab		Ranibizumab	Bevacizumab
GEFAL,2013[17]	AMD	183	191	55.78±13.99	54.62±14.07	12	0.5	1.25	As needed after the first injection	6.5	6.8
CATT,2012[14]	AMD	134	129	59.9±14.2	60.2±13.6	24	0.5	1.25	Monthly	11.7	11.9
CATT,2012[14]	AMD	264	251	61.6±13.1	60.6±13.0	24	0.5	1.25	As needed	12.6	14.1
IVAN,2013[15]	AMD	314	296	61.8±15	61.1±15.5	24	0.5	1.25	mix of monthly and as needed	18	19
MENTA,2013[16]	AMD	163	154	56.4±13.5	57±13	12	0.5	1.25	monthly for 3 month then as needed	5.8	6.1
MANJU,2010[18]	AMD	15	7	34.9±14.5	34.9±14.5	12	0.5	1.25	monthly for 3 month then as needed	3.9	7.6
MAGDA,2010[19]	PM	16	16	26.44±12.58	29.5±12.98	6	0.5	1.25	as needed after the first injection	2.81	2.44
PIERLUIGI,2012[20]	PM	23	25	29.5±16	30.5±14	18	0.5	1.25	as needed after the first injection	2.56	4.72
MAURIZIO,2013[21]	RAP	24	26	33±16.5	29.5±10.5	12	0.5	1.25	monthly for 3 month then as needed	3.9	4.6
ANTONIO,2013[22]	DME	28	32	31.5±3	30±2.5	12	0.5	1.5	monthly for 3 month then as needed	7.67	9.84

Study Characteristics

Nine independent RCT studies enrolled including 1,162 patients assigned to the ran 1,127 patients assigned to the bevacizuma qualified articles were published between November 2013, and all were in the Eng studies focused on AMD, two on pathologic m each on retinal angiomatous proliferation (macular oedema (DME). The methodolog included studies was generally good. The duration ranged from 6 to 24 months. Patien an average of over 1 year in a majority of s number of included patients in the study var with the two largest studies recruiting over 5((Table 1).[14,15]

In all of the studies, the dose was 0.50 n Eight studies administered 1.25 mg for bev: one used 1.5 mg of bevacizumab for DME.[2 compared the outcomes of monthly and as ne four arms.[14] In the IVAN study, outcomes ranibizumab and bevacizumab groups with monthly and as needed administrations.[15] . two arms on a monthly schedule for 1 or 3 m needed administrations. Change in visual baseline (letters) was available for all studies. reported data from an adverse event: seriou studies), nonfatal arterial thrombotic events from any cause (four studies), and deaths from studies). There were no differences in the acuity, and foveal thickness between th ranibizumab and bevacizumab.

Effects of interventions

The WMD in the change in the visua baseline for ranibizumab versus bevacizun (95% CI −0.11–1.14, p = 0.1046), as shown shows the results from the fixed-effects mode for the changed proportions of visual ac ranibizumab, compared with bevacizumab statistically significant improvement in the degree of ≥15 (OR: 1.10 [95% CI 0.90–1.33 letters (OR: 0.93 [95% CI 0.77–1.11, p = (ORs of visual acuity for ranibizumab relative 0.89 (95% CI 0.65–1.22, p = 0.4602) for a 5– 0.95 (95% CI 0.73–1.25, p = 0.7241) for a We did not observe heterogeneity among clear disparities in the ocular disease types a

Neither the funnel plot nor the Egge demonstrated any evidence of publication versus bevacizumab (Egger's, p = 0.8365; (Figure 4).

Adverse Events

We conducted a meta-analysis to estima ADRs associated with ranibizumab versus than serious systemic events, no statisticall neity was found among the studies included clear disparities in the ocular disease types (Figure 5). Using a fixed-effect model, the for ranibizumab versus bevacizumab were 0.94, p = 0.0035) for serious systemic event 1.46, p = 0.4845) for death from vascular 0.63–1.32, p = 0.6329) for death from all 0.65–1.72, p = 0.8226) for nonfatal arterial

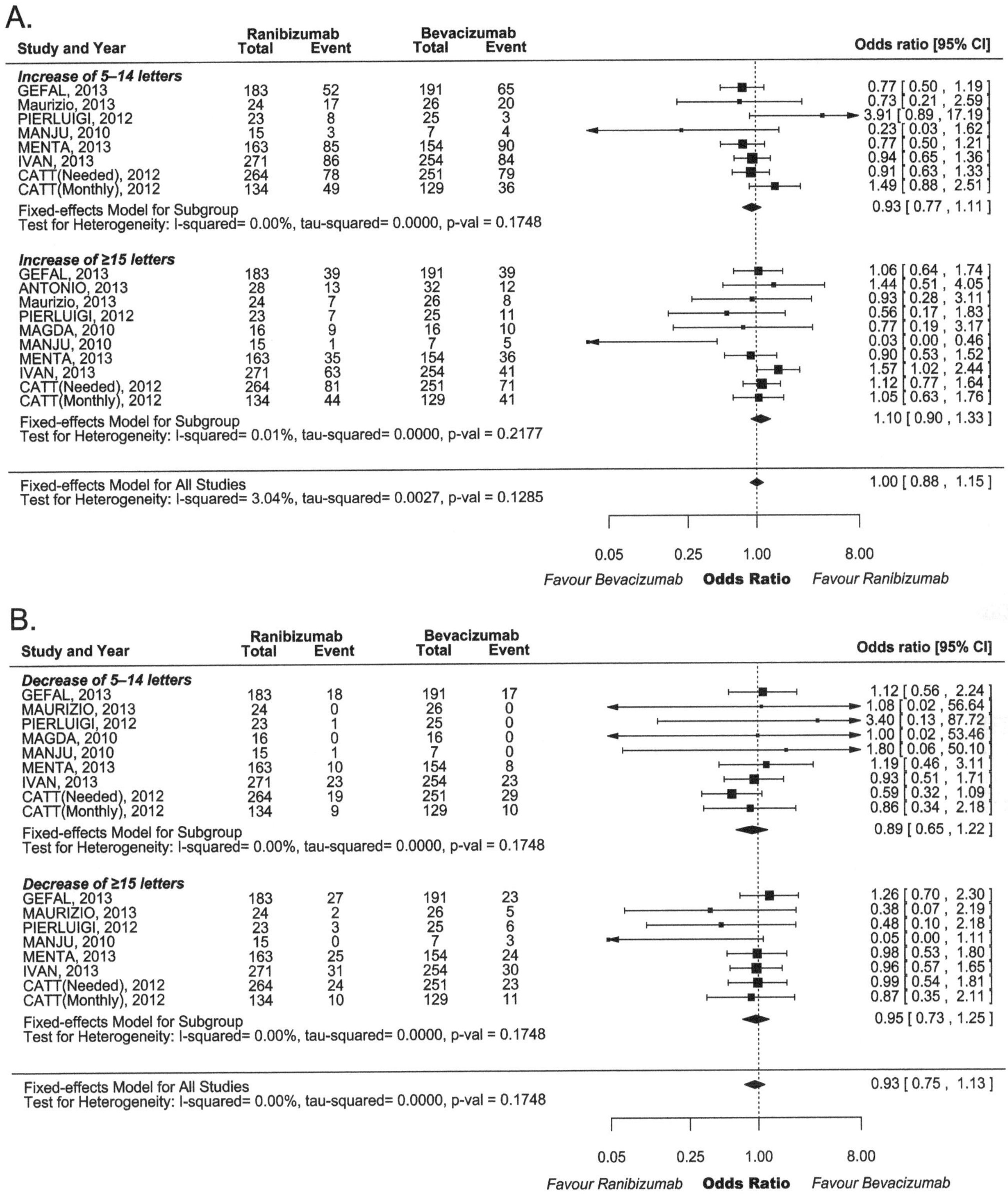

Figure 3. Forest plot of the odds ratios (OR) for visual acuity changes. (A) Gain of ≥15 letters and 5–14 letters; (B) Loss of 5–14 letters or ≥15 letters. CI, confidence interval; OR, odds ratio.

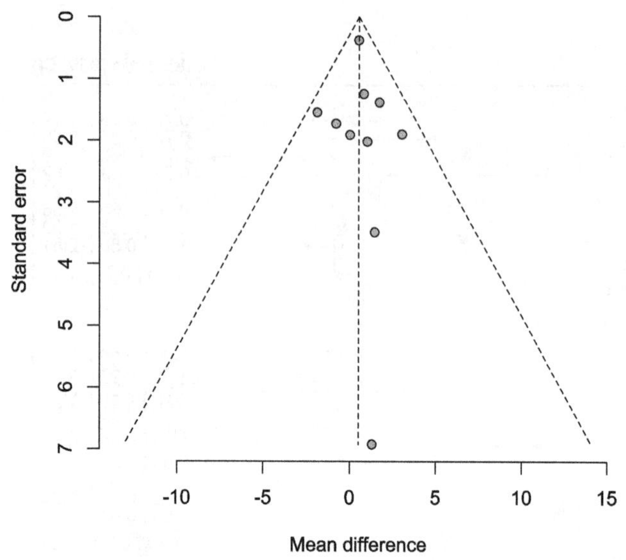

Figure 4. Funnel plot examining the effects of ranibizumab versus bevacizumab therapy.

0.67 (95% CI 0.39–1.15, p = 0.1454) for ocular serious adverse events.

Discussion

This study goes beyond prior analyses regarding the choice between ranibizumab and bevacizumab for the treatment of ophthalmic diseases. Improved confidence in the findings is obvious through the incorporation of results from 9 RCT trials representing nearly 2,300 patients. As such, the findings from this study have implications for treatment and for study interpretation and design.

Our meta-analysis demonstrated the non-inferiority of bevacizumab against ranibizumab by using the strict criteria of a non-inferior margin of 3.5 letters in the IVAN study, although the results trend favoured ranibizumab.[15] Likewise, we observed no significant differences in the specific degrees of visual acuity change, including an increase of ≥15, an increase of 5–14, a decrease of 5–14, and a decrease of ≤15 letters. The findings were consistent with the results of the study reported by Chakravarthy U and colleagues, which showed the WMD of the change between ranibizumab and bevacizumab in visual acuity to be 1.15 (95%CI: −0.51 to 2.82) by pooling IVAN and CATT data.[15] To the best of our knowledge, this meta-analysis is the first to confirm the non-inferiority of bevacizumab relative to ranibizumab for ophthalmic diseases by pooling more than two head-to-head RCT trials. The results of non-RCT and preliminary studies that directly compared the outcomes of the two drugs also indicated the efficacy of bevacizumab to be non-inferior to that of ranibizumab in patients with corneal neovascularisation, wet AMD, glaucoma, polypoidal choroidal vasculopathy, RAP or DME.[29–35] Based on an indirect comparison in a systematic review for AMD, Ford JA and colleagues found that 27% of patients treated with bevacizumab and 39% of those treated with ranibizumab experienced an improvement in their best corrected visual acuity of >2 lines [OR: 0.95 (95% credible interval 0.23 to 4.32)], which suggests no difference in the relative effectiveness of bevacizumab and ranibizumab. However, this indirect comparison had wide credibility intervals and was not able to exclude the possibility that either drug might be superior. [36]

The safety and tolerability of anti-VEGF therapy is a concern of clinicians and patients, especially regarding arterial thromboembolic events.[37,38] One meta-analysis showed that the intravitreal use of anti-VEGF antibodies was not associated with an increased risk of arterial thromboembolic events.[39] Our meta-analysis focused on the relative safety of bevacizumab and ranibizumab. We found that the bevacizumab arm, compared with the ranibizumab arm, experienced a significant 17% increased risk of developing serious systemic events, consistent with the findings reported by Chakravarthy U and colleagues[15]. In a retrospective cohort study of 146,942 Medicare beneficiaries 65 years or older with a claim for AMD, Curtis and colleagues found that the adjusted hazard ratios for ranibizumab versus bevacizumab were 0.86 (95% CI 0.75–0.98) for mortality and 0.78 (95% CI 0.64–0.96) for stroke, respectively.[40] However, in contrast to this finding, other studies have suggested that there is no sufficient evidence to conclude that there is a difference between the safety profiles of the different VEGF inhibitors.[11,41] Considering these controversies and the differential cost, cheaper bevacizumab treatments may be continued if the benefits of the drug outweigh the risk. Furthermore, the treatment patterns of bevacizumab should be taken into account because injections on an as-needed basis would have a lower risk of serious systemic events than scheduled monthly injections.[15,17] This lower risk of ischaemic events that coincides with a lower versus higher dosage of bevacizumab has been documented in cancer patients by one recently published meta-analysis.[42] Our meta-analysis also showed that death from vascular causes, death from all causes, and nonfatal or serious adverse ocular events were favourable in the ranibizumab treatment group, whereas nonfatal arterial thrombotic events favoured the ranibizumab treatment group. However, no statistically significant differences for the four adverse event endpoints were found between the two arms.

The strengths of this meta-analysis include the comprehensive literature review, strict inclusion criteria, large number of patients analysed, inclusion of the most up-to-date published RCT trial data, and robustness of the findings. By examining both the visual efficacy acuity and serious adverse events, the potential utility of bevacizumab instead of ranibizumab can be adequately evaluated. The present meta-analysis also resolved the question of the inadequate power of individual studies to compare the differences in harm between the two treatments. For example, only four studies included in this review reported any data on death from all causes for more than 100 patients.[14–17] A major strength of the current meta-analysis is that the pooled results allowed for the examination of both bevacizumab and ranibizumab for potential ophthalmic diseases related to neovascularisation.

There are also limitations that should be noted regarding this analysis. The first possible limitation of this study is the heterogeneity of the studies regarding different ophthalmic diseases, including AMD, DME, PM, and RAP, which were assumed to have equivalent therapeutic responses for anti-VEGF treatment due to the active role of neovascularisation in their pathophysiology. Furthermore, the paucity of RCT trials comparing ranibizumab and bevacizumab in patients with non-AMD ophthalmic diseases was investigated; the non-inferiority and safety profile between bevacizumab and ranibizumab in other diseases still needs to be further elucidated. The second limitation is the lack of individual-level data, which prohibited the evaluation of the associations between individual variables with study outcomes. Instead, we used between-study meta-regressions when possible. Third, our results are limited to Western populations due to the absence of the data from Eastern populations. Fourth, due to the absences of the detailed definition of serious adverse events for

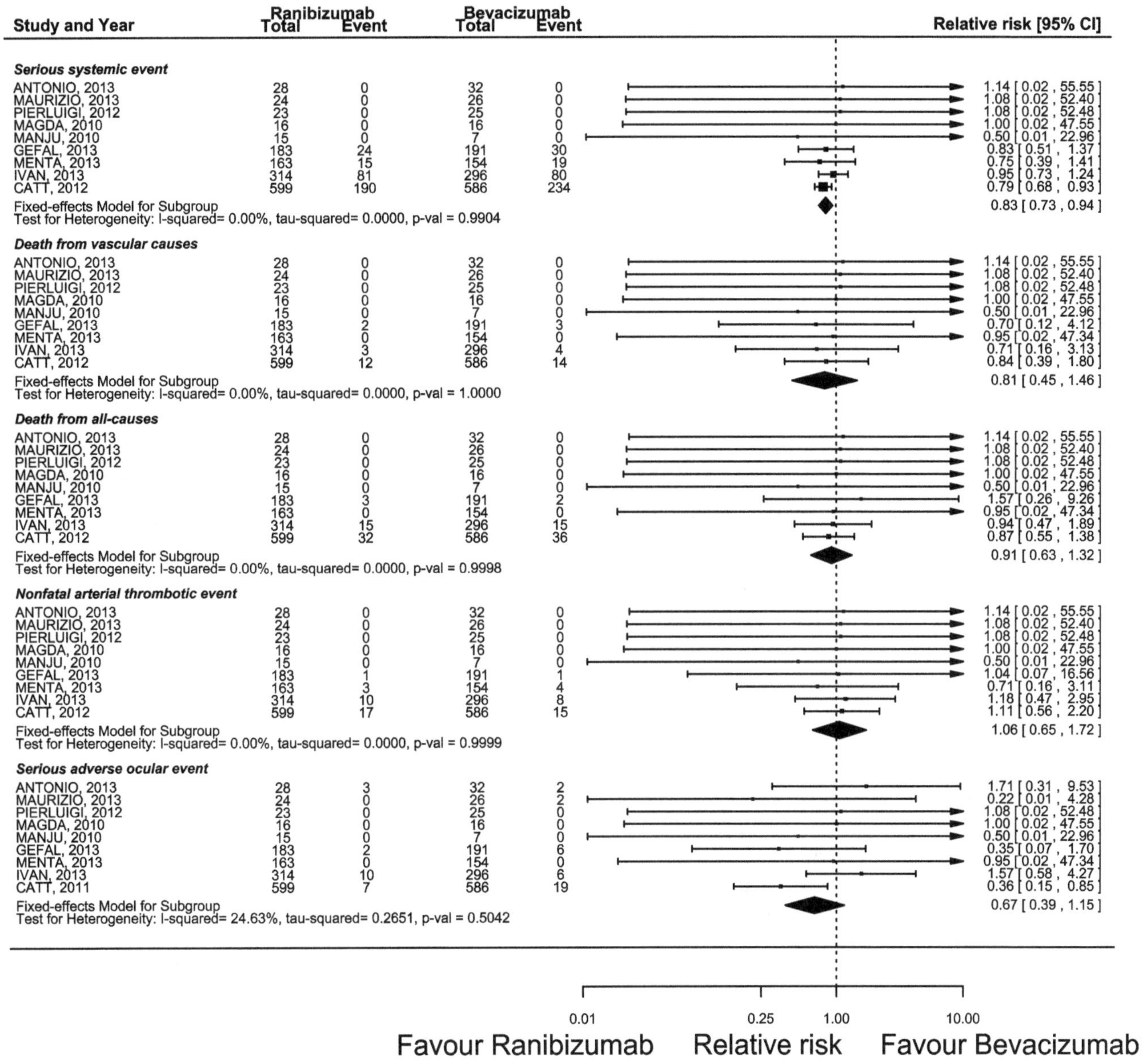

Figure 5. Forest plot of the odds ratios (OR) for adverse events. CI, confidence interval; OR, odds ratio.

each trial, we only used the adverse information judged by investigators, such as nonfatal or fatal thrombotic events. Therefore, information bias associated with the different definitions could not be excluded, if any was present. Fifth, small sample size of the trial included in the current analysis might have potential impact on detecting the rare adverse events, the bias should be taken into account. Sixth, this meta-analysis only included serious adverse events that had a potential relationship with anti-VEGF therapies.[37,38] Finally, all studies included in this meta-analysis had a short-term follow-up of less than 2 years, and five studies had a sample size of less than 100 participants. Further larger trials with long-term outcome data are needed.

In summary, ranibizumab treatment resulted in slightly more visual acuity improvement than did bevacizumab, but there were no significant differences. Safety profiles, especially regarding serious systemic events, were also more favourable for ranibizumab than for bevacizumab. The two anti-VEGF agents and their treatment patterns should be carefully chosen by weighing the costs and health benefits. Further studies are needed to compare the effective and safety outcomes between bevacizumab and ranibizumab for ophthalmic diseases, and the appropriate doses of each is an important issue that merits further evaluation by high-quality RCTs. Finally, a high priority should be placed on the need for a detailed description of adverse events, especially serious systemic events, in primary studies.

Acknowledgments

Source of financial support: This study was supported by a grant from the National Natural Science Foundation of China (NO. 71373160).

Author Contributions

Conceived and designed the experiments: JL. Performed the experiments: BW HW XL HL JL. Analyzed the data: BW HW. Contributed reagents/materials/analysis tools: BW HW XL HL. Contributed to the writing of the manuscript: BW.

References

1. Folkman J (1995) Angiogenesis in cancer, vascular, rheumatoid and other disease. Nat Med 1: 27–31.
2. Carmeliet P, Jain RK (2000) Angiogenesis in cancer and other diseases. Nature 407: 249–257.
3. Shams N, Ianchulev T (2006) Role of vascular endothelial growth factor in ocular angiogenesis. Ophthalmol Clin North Am 19: 335–344.
4. Dixon JA, Oliver SC, Olson JL, Mandava N (2009) VEGF Trap-Eye for the treatment of neovascular age-related macular degeneration. Expert Opin Investig Drugs 18: 1573–1580.
5. Presta LG, Chen H, O'Connor SJ, Chisholm V, Meng YG, et al. (1997) Humanization of an anti-vascular endothelial growth factor monoclonal antibody for the therapy of solid tumors and other disorders. Cancer Res 57: 4593–4599.
6. McCartney M (2011) Off-label prescribing in macular degeneration. BMJ 343: d6778.
7. Brechner RJ, Rosenfeld PJ, Babish JD, Caplan S (2011) Pharmacotherapy for neovascular age-related macular degeneration: an analysis of the 100% 2008 medicare fee-for-service part B claims file. Am J Ophthalmol 151: 887–895 e881.
8. Ferrara N, Damico L, Shams N, Lowman H, Kim R (2006) Development of ranibizumab, an anti-vascular endothelial growth factor antigen binding fragment, as therapy for neovascular age-related macular degeneration. Retina 26: 859–870.
9. Brown DM, Michels M, Kaiser PK, Heier JS, Sy JP, et al. (2009) Ranibizumab versus verteporfin photodynamic therapy for neovascular age-related macular degeneration: Two-year results of the ANCHOR study. Ophthalmology 116: 57–65 e55.
10. Rosenfeld PJ, Brown DM, Heier JS, Boyer DS, Kaiser PK, et al. (2006) Ranibizumab for neovascular age-related macular degeneration. N Engl J Med 355: 1419–1431.
11. Schmucker C, Ehlken C, Agostini HT, Antes G, Ruecker G, et al. (2012) A safety review and meta-analyses of bevacizumab and ranibizumab: off-label versus goldstandard. PLoS One 7: e42701.
12. Banfi R, Attanasio F, Palazzi N, Colombini S, Falai T, et al. (2013) Bevacizumab versus ranibizumab: why are we not playing the joker? Int J Clin Pharm 35: 507–509.
13. Group CR, Martin DF, Maguire MG, Ying GS, Grunwald JE, et al. 2011) Ranibizumab and bevacizumab for neovascular age-related macular degeneration. N Engl J Med 364: 1897–1908.
14. Comparison of Age-related Macular Degeneration Treatments Trials Research G, Martin DF, Maguire MG, Fine SL, Ying GS, et al. (2012) Ranibizumab and bevacizumab for treatment of neovascular age-related macular degeneration: two-year results. Ophthalmology 119: 1388–1398.
15. Chakravarthy U, Harding SP, Rogers CA, Downes SM, Lotery AJ, et al. (2013) Alternative treatments to inhibit VEGF in age-related choroidal neovascularisation: 2-year findings of the IVAN randomised controlled trial. Lancet 382: 1258–1267.
16. Krebs I, Schmetterer L, Boltz A, Told R, Vecsei-Marlovits V, et al. (2013) A randomised double-masked trial comparing the visual outcome after treatment with ranibizumab or bevacizumab in patients with neovascular age-related macular degeneration. Br J Ophthalmol 97: 266–271.
17. Kodjikian L, Souied EH, Mimoun G, Mauget-Faysse M, Behar-Cohen F, et al. (2013) Ranibizumab versus Bevacizumab for Neovascular Age-related Macular Degeneration: Results from the GEFAL Noninferiority Randomized Trial. Ophthalmology 120: 2300–2309.
18. Subramanian ML, Abedi G, Ness S, Ahmed E, Fenberg M, et al. (2010) Bevacizumab vs ranibizumab for age-related macular degeneration: 1-year outcomes of a prospective, double-masked randomised clinical trial. Eye (Lond) 24: 1708–1715.
19. Gharbiya M, Giustolisi R, Allievi F, Fantozzi N, Mazzeo L, et al. (2010) Choroidal neovascularization in pathologic myopia: intravitreal ranibizumab versus bevacizumab–a randomized controlled trial. Am J Ophthalmol 149: 458–464 e451.
20. Iacono P, Parodi MB, Papayannis A, Kontadakis S, Sheth S, et al. (2012) Intravitreal ranibizumab versus bevacizumab for treatment of myopic choroidal neovascularization. Retina 32: 1539–1546.
21. Parodi MB, Iacono P, Menchini F, Sheth S, Polini G, et al. (2013) Intravitreal bevacizumab versus ranibizumab for the treatment of retinal angiomatous proliferation. Acta Ophthalmol 91: 267–273.
22. Nepomuceno AB, Takaki E, Paes de Almeida FP, Peroni R, Cardillo JA, et al. (2013) A prospective randomized trial of intravitreal bevacizumab versus ranibizumab for the management of diabetic macular edema. Am J Ophthalmol 156: 502–510 e502.
23. Moher D, Liberati A, Tetzlaff J, Altman DG, Group P (2009) Preferred reporting items for systematic reviews and meta-analyses: the PRISMA statement. PLoS Med 6: e1000097.
24. Jadad AR, Moore RA, Carroll D, Jenkinson C, Reynolds DJ, et al. (1996) Assessing the quality of reports of randomized clinical trials: is blinding necessary? Control Clin Trials 17: 1–12.
25. Higgins JP, Thompson SG, Deeks JJ, Altman DG (2003) Measuring inconsistency in meta-analyses. BMJ 327: 557–560.
26. Higgins JP, Thompson SG (2002) Quantifying heterogeneity in a meta-analysis. Stat Med 21: 1539–1558.
27. Egger M, Smith GD (1998) Bias in location and selection of studies. BMJ 316: 61–66.
28. Begg CB, Mazumdar M (1994) Operating characteristics of a rank correlation test for publication bias. Biometrics 50: 1088–1101.
29. Kim JH, Seo HW, Han HC, Lee JH, Choi SK, et al. (2013) The effect of bevacizumab versus ranibizumab in the treatment of corneal neovascularization: a preliminary study. Korean J Ophthalmol 27: 235–242.
30. Anti-VEGF therapy for the treatment of glaucoma: a focus on ranibizumab and bevacizumabLi J, Zhang H, Sun P, Gu F, Liu ZL (2013) Bevacizumab vs ranibizumab for neovascular age-related macular degeneration in Chinese patients. Int J Ophthalmol 6: 169–173.
31. Park SC, Su D, Tello C (2012) Anti-VEGF therapy for the treatment of glaucoma: a focus on ranibizumab and bevacizumab. Expert Opin Biol Ther 12: 1641–1647.
32. Cho HJ, Baek JS, Lee DW, Kim CG, Kim JW (2012) Short-term effectiveness of intravitreal bevacizumab vs. ranibizumab injections for patients with polypoidal choroidal vasculopathy. Korean J Ophthalmol 26: 157–162.
33. Hufendiek K, Hufendiek K, Panagakis G, Helbig H, Gamulescu MA (2012) Visual and morphological outcomes of bevacizumab (Avastin(R)) versus ranibizumab (Lucentis(R)) treatment for retinal angiomatous proliferation. Int Ophthalmol 32: 259–268.
34. Cho HJ, Kim JW, Lee DW, Cho SW, Kim CG (2012) Intravitreal bevacizumab and ranibizumab injections for patients with polypoidal choroidal vasculopathy. Eye (Lond) 26: 426–433.
35. Ozturk BT, Kerimoglu H, Bozkurt B, Okudan S (2011) Comparison of intravitreal bevacizumab and ranibizumab treatment for diabetic macular edema. J Ocul Pharmacol Ther 27: 373–377.
36. Ford JA, Elders A, Shyangdan D, Royle P, Waugh N (2012) The relative clinical effectiveness of ranibizumab and bevacizumab in diabetic macular oedema: an indirect comparison in a systematic review. BMJ 345: e5182.
37. Scappaticci FA, Skillings JR, Holden SN, Gerber HP, Miller K, et al. (2007) Arterial thromboembolic events in patients with metastatic carcinoma treated with chemotherapy and bevacizumab. J Natl Cancer Inst 99: 1232–1239.
38. Nalluri SR, Chu D, Keresztes R, Zhu X, Wu S (2008) Risk of venous thromboembolism with the angiogenesis inhibitor bevacizumab in cancer patients: a meta-analysis. JAMA 300: 2277–2285.
39. Cheng JW, Cheng SW, Lu GC, Wei RL (2012) Effect of intravitreal anti-vascular endothelial growth factor therapy on the risk of arterial thromboembolic events: a meta-analysis. PLoS One 7: e41325.
40. Curtis LH, Hammill BG, Schulman KA, Cousins SW (2010) Risks of mortality, myocardial infarction, bleeding, and stroke associated with therapies for age-related macular degeneration. Arch Ophthalmol 128: 1273–1279.
41. van der Reis MI, La Heij EC, De Jong-Hesse Y, Ringens PJ, Hendrikse F, et al. (2011) A systematic review of the adverse events of intravitreal anti-vascular endothelial growth factor injections. Retina 31: 1449–1469.
42. Chen XL, Lei YH, Liu CF, Yang QF, Zuo PY, et al. (2013) Angiogenesis inhibitor bevacizumab increases the risk of ischemic heart disease associated with chemotherapy: a meta-analysis. PLoS One 8: e66721.

11

Human Retinal Transmitochondrial Cybrids with J or H mtDNA Haplogroups Respond Differently to Ultraviolet Radiation: Implications for Retinal Diseases

Deepika Malik[1], Tiffany Hsu[1], Payam Falatoonzadeh[1], Javier Cáceres-del-Carpio[1], Mohamed Tarek[1,2], Marilyn Chwa[1], Shari R. Atilano[1], Claudio Ramirez[1], Anthony B. Nesburn[1,3], David S. Boyer[4], Baruch D. Kuppermann[1], S. Michal Jazwinski[5], Michael V. Miceli[5], Douglas C. Wallace[6], Nitin Udar[1], M. Cristina Kenney[1,7]*

1 Gavin Herbert Eye Institute, University California Irvine, Irvine, California, United States of America, **2** Department of Ophthalmology, El-Minya University, El-Minya, Egypt, **3** Cedars-Sinai Medical Center, Los Angeles, California, United States of America, **4** Retina-Vitreous Associates Medical Group; Beverly Hills, California, United States of America, **5** Tulane Center for Aging, Tulane University, New Orleans, Louisiana, United States of America, **6** Center for Mitochondrial and Epigenomic Medicine, Children's Hospital of Philadelphia and Department of Pathology and Laboratory Medicine, University of Pennsylvania, Philadelphia, Pennsylvania, United States of America, **7** Department of Pathology and Laboratory Medicine, University California Irvine, Irvine, California, United States of America

Abstract

Background: It has been recognized that cells do not respond equally to ultraviolet (UV) radiation but it is not clear whether this is due to genetic, biochemical or structural differences of the cells. We have a novel cybrid (cytoplasmic hybrids) model that allows us to analyze the contribution of mitochondrial DNA (mtDNA) to cellular response after exposure to sub-lethal dose of UV. mtDNA can be classified into haplogroups as defined by accumulations of specific single nucleotide polymorphisms (SNPs). Recent studies have shown that J haplogroup is high risk for age-related macular degeneration while the H haplogroup is protective. This study investigates gene expression responses in J cybrids versus H cybrids after exposure to sub-lethal doses of UV-radiation.

Methodology/Principal Findings: Cybrids were created by fusing platelets isolated from subjects with either H ($n=3$) or J ($n=3$) haplogroups with mitochondria-free (Rho^{0}) ARPE-19 cells. The H and J cybrids were cultured for 24 hours, treated with 10 mJ of UV-radiation and cultured for an additional 120 hours. Untreated and treated cybrids were analyzed for growth rates and gene expression profiles. The UV-treated and untreated J cybrids had higher growth rates compared to H cybrids. Before treatment, J cybrids showed lower expression levels for CFH, CD55, IL-33, TGF-A, EFEMP-1, RARA, BCL2L13 and BBC3. At 120 hours after UV-treatment, the J cybrids had decreased CFH, RARA and BBC3 levels but increased CD55, IL-33 and EFEMP-1 compared to UV-treated H cybrids.

Conclusion/Significance: In cells with identical nuclei, the cellular response to sub-lethal UV-radiation is mediated in part by the mtDNA haplogroup. This supports the hypothesis that differences in growth rates and expression levels of complement, inflammation and apoptosis genes may result from population-specific, hereditary SNP variations in mtDNA. Therefore, when analyzing UV-induced damage in tissues, the mtDNA haplogroup background may be important to consider.

Editor: Neena B. Haider, Schepens Eye Research Institute/Massachusetts Eye and Ear, Department of Ophthalmology, Harvard Medical School, Boston, MA, United States of America

Funding: This work was supported by Discovery Eye Foundation, Guenther Foundation, Beckman Initiative for Macular Research, Polly and Michael Smith Foundation, Max Factor Family Foundation, Skirball Foundation, Lincy Foundation, Iris and B. Gerald Cantor Foundation, and unrestricted grant from Research to Prevent Blindness. National Institute on Aging grant (AG006168) to SMJ and MVM. The funders had no role in study design, data collection and analysis, decision to publish, or preparation of the manuscript.

Competing Interests: The authors have declared that no competing interests exist.

* E-mail: mkenney@uci.edu

Introduction

Age-related macular degeneration (AMD) is a multifactorial disease, wherein multiple genetic variants and environmental risk factors, including diet, smoking, hypertension, light exposure, ultraviolet (UV) radiation, blue light and ionizing radiation, contribute to the disease [1]. Despite new medical and surgical interventions, AMD is one of the important causes of decreased vision in the United States. According to the National Health And Nutrition Examination Survey (NHANES 2005–2008 report), the estimated prevalence of any AMD was 6.5% and of late AMD was 0.8% in the US population 40 years and older [2]. Aging and oxidative damage to retinal pigment epithelial (RPE) cells, a monolayer of cells located between the neural retina and Bruch's membrane contributes to AMD [3]. Early AMD has sub-retinal drusen, and can progress to advanced AMD, which includes dry (non-exudative, atrophic) and wet (exudative, neovascular) forms

[4]. The dry form of advanced AMD is characterized by geographic atrophy involving the macula and accounts for approximately 25% of cases with central vision loss [5]. The wet form accounts for 75% of the central loss of vision and is characterized by choroidal neovascularization and if untreated, eventually a disciform scar in the macular region [5].

Solar radiation consists of variable wavelengths: UV-C (100–280 nm), UV-B (280–315 nm), UV-A (315–400 nm) and visible spectrum (400–700 nm) [6]. Light with shorter wavelengths has higher energy and can produce intense tissue damage. The human cornea filters out most of the radiation below 295 nm [7]. The human lens in younger individuals can transmit UV-B radiation but by adulthood, the lens blocks almost all UV-A and UV-B and most of the blue light [8]. However, exposure to both UV-A and UV-B are known to produce cataract and UV-radiation imposes increased damage to both pediatric and adult retina. Damage induced by UV-radiation is cumulative and depends on the duration, wavelength and intensity of exposure.

After 3 years of age, the yellow pigment 3-hydroxykynurenine, a tryptophan metabolite, gradually develops in the human lens and absorbs UV-radiation, which provides protection to the retina. Lutein and zeaxanthin are macular pigments and along with glutathione protect the retina against inflammatory and photo-oxidative damage. Antioxidants, antioxidant enzymes, and melanin pigments within RPE cells and the choroid provide protection against light-induced ocular damage. However, with age, these pigments and antioxidants are gradually depleted, thereby making the retina more susceptible to free radical damage. Acute exposure to UV-radiation, as in sunlight reflected from snow or an eclipse, can produce inflammatory damage and interleukin responses [9,10]. Over a lifetime, chronic exposure induces accumulative photo-oxidative damage via singlet oxygen and free radical production that leads to damage of DNA, proteins and lipids.

Aging is associated with increased DNA damage, including both mitochondrial (mtDNA) and nuclear DNA (nDNA), and decreased efficacy of the DNA repair mechanisms [11]. The DNA repair process becomes less efficient in presence of risk factors such as UV exposure and environmental toxins [11]. The repair mechanisms for nDNA are more efficient than mtDNA and over time, the accumulation of DNA damage can be associated with age-related vascular dysfunctions [12], which may correlate to the wet form of AMD. Increased DNA damage can also trigger apoptosis and autophagy [13], which can contribute to degenerative retinal diseases. The production of reactive oxygen/nitrogen species (ROS/RNS), such as superoxide radicals, hydrogen peroxide and peroxynitrites, are key factors as they lead to oxidative damage and apoptosis. Mitochondria are a major site of ROS production via the electron transport chain and because of this close proximity, the mtDNA is very susceptible to oxidative damage. Mitochondria are present in large numbers in retinal tissue since photoreceptors are one of the highest consumers of oxygen in the body. In 2006, Feher et al, reported significant decreases in numbers and size of mitochondria and an increase in peroxisomes in AMD retinas [14]. Harman theorized that mtDNA mutations and production of free radicals played a large role in the aging process [15].

The human mtDNA is a circular double stranded DNA that encodes 37 genes including 13 protein subunits essential for oxidative phosphorylation, and a non-coding region mtDNA D-loop which is critical for replication and transcription. The mtDNA have been classified into various haplogroups based on variable combinations of single nucleotide polymorphisms (SNPs) that have accumulated over 150,000 years. The oldest haplogroups have been identified from Africa and with eventual migration to other continents, mtDNA SNP variations due to adaptations to different environmental conditions evolved. At this time, geographic origins of populations can be identified by their haplogroup patterns. In general, the mtDNA SNP variations in coding and non-coding regions are associated with different rates of replication, transcription and metabolic processes [16] and it has been proposed that haplogroup-related variants may lead to differential responses for cell functions.

Both haplogroups H and J represent European-Caucasian populations. However, J haplogroup originated from northern Europe and the H haplogroup was from southern Europe. Recent studies have shown that individuals with the J haplogroup have higher susceptibility to developing AMD and that the H haplogroup is protective [17]. Our work, among others, has used the cybrid (cytoplasmic hybrid) model to demonstrate that the H and J haplogroups have differences in production of ATP, ROS and lactate levels, as well as cell growth rates and expressions of genes involved in the complement pathway [18–21]. However, it is not known if the different mtDNA haplogroups might influence the responses of the cells to stress factors.

In the present study, we have used the human RPE cybrids that contain either the H or J haplogroups to investigate their responses to environmental stress using UV-radiation, a potential risk factor for AMD. After exposure to sub-lethal dose of UV-radiation, the H cybrids and J cybrids, which have identical nuclei but differ only in their mtDNA haplogroups, show different rates of cell growth and expression levels for genes involved in inflammation, cell proliferation and apoptosis. Our findings support the hypothesis that in responses UV radiation, the inherited mtDNA variants (haplogroups) influence cells to have differential responses in major molecular pathways, which are associated with many aging diseases.

Materials and Methods

Ethics Statement

All research involving human participants was approved by the Institutional Review Board of University of California, Irvine (#2003-3131). Written informed consents were obtained and all clinical investigations were conducted according to the principles expressed in the Declaration of Helsinki.

Transmitochondrial Cybrid Cultures

The preparations of transmitochondrial cybrids were performed as described in our previous manuscripts [22–24]. Cybrids were grown in DMEM/Ham's F12 1:1 (Invitrogen-Gibco, Grand Island, NY) containing 24 mM sodium bicarbonate, 10% dialyzed fetal bovine serum and 1.0 mM sodium pyruvate. Mitochondrial haplogroups of each cybrid were confirmed by using PCR, restriction enzyme digestion and sequencing of mtDNA. All experiments utilized the H and J cybrids, which were at passage 5. Cybrids that contained mitochondria with haplogroup H (n = 3 different individuals) or J (n = 3 different individuals) were studied in 2 groups, the Control (untreated) group and Study group (treated with UV-radiation). Assays to determine the growth curve and gene expression analyses were performed for the individual cybrids in the Control and Study groups.

UV-radiation Treatment

A sub-lethal dose of UV-radiation was defined as the dose sufficient to decrease the growth rate of cells but not cause irreversible damage to cell viability. Initially the cybrids were treated with 5, 10, and 20 mJ of UV-radiation using the Stratalinker 1800 (Stratagene, Santa Clara, CA) and analyzed for cell viability 48 and 96 hours later to identify the sub-threshold dose. 5 mJ UV-radiation did not have any impact on growth rate in the study group when compared to the untreated cells (data not shown). When cybrid cultures were treated with 20 mJ of UV exposure, there was significant loss of cells in both the H and J cybrids (data not shown). However, ninety-six hours after a single pulse of 10 mJ UV-radiation, we found that the growth rates of cells were temporarily reduced but they increased by 120 hours indicating that the UV radiation had a sub-lethal effect on the cells. Therefore, we chose 10 mJ UV-radiation as the dosage to treat the cybrids. Individual H or J cybrids were plated at 300,000 cells per well onto six well plates with 2 ml of culture media. Twenty-four hours after plating, the culture media were removed and the cybrids were treated with a single 10 seconds pulse of 10 mJ of UV-radiation using Stratalinker 1800. For the Control group, no treatment was given but culture media were changed at that time. Thereafter, culture media were changed every 48 hours in both groups.

Growth Curve Assay

The growth curves of three different H cybrids and three different J cybrids in both Study and Control groups were analyzed over 6 days. For each individual cybrid, cells were plated and treated with UV-radiation as described above. Cells numbers were measured with the Cell Viability Analyzer (ViCell, Beckman Coulter, Miami, FL) using the trypan blue staining technique, which counts and averages cells over 50 images. The number of cells at the time of treatment (time-point 0 hours) was designated as 100% and percentage increase in growth of each cybrid were measured at 48, 96, 120 and 144 hours. The assays were run in triplicate and experiments were repeated twice. There were biological triplicates within each experiment.

Isolation of RNA and cDNA Synthesis

RNA was isolated from both the Study and Control groups at 0 hours, 72 hours and 120 hours after UV exposure using the RNeasy Mini-Extraction kit (Qiagen, Inc.) as per the manufacturer's protocol. The RNA was quantified using NanoDrop 1000 (Thermoscientific, Inc.). RNA was reverse transcribed into cDNA using the QuantiTect Reverse Transcription Kit (Qiagen, Inc.).

Quantitative-PCR (Q-PCR) Analyses

In our previous publication, we demonstrated that CFH, C3 and EFEMP-1 genes were differentially expressed in H versus J cybrids (at 0 hours) [18]. In the present study, Q-PCR was performed using primers (QuantiTect primer assay, Qiagen) for genes associated with alternate complement pathway- Complement Factor-H (CFH), Decay Accelerating Factor for Complement (CD55/DAF), Complement Regulatory Protein (CD59), genes related to inflammation and cellular proliferation- Interleukin-33 (IL-33), Transforming Growth Factor, alpha (TGF-A), EGF containing fibulin like extracellular matrix protein 1 (EFEMP-1) and pro-apoptotic genes- Retinoic acid receptor, alpha (RARA), BCL2 binding component 3 (BBC3), BCL2-like 13 (BCL2L13) (Table 1). The Q-PCR was performed on individual H cybrids (n = 3) and J cybrids (n = 3) using a QuantiFast SYBR Green PCR kit (Qiagen) on a Bio-Rad iQ5 iCycler detection system. Gene expression levels were standardized for all primers using Hypoxanthine-guanine phosphoribosyltransferase (HPRT1, NM_000194) as a reference gene. Each sample at individual time-points was assessed in triplicate.

The selection of the genes analyzed in this study was based on our previous studies using the untreated H and J cybrids. Each of these genes were initially identified when cDNA from the H and J cybrids were analyzed by the Affymetrix Human U133 Plus 2.0 Array, which is a comprehensive human genome expression array that allows for the analyses of over 40K transcripts. Then differences between the individual H and individual J cybrids were verified by Q-PCR analyses [22,24]. The CD59 were analyzed because it is a major inhibitor of the alternative pathway.

Statistical Analysis

Data were subjected to statistical analysis by ANOVA using GraphPad Prism 5.0 version statistics program (GraphPad Software Inc., San Diego, CA). For the growth curve assays, the Control samples were normalized to 100% and then the cell count for the 48, 96, 120 and 144 hours samples were calculated accordingly. In the gene expression assays, the ΔCt was calculated as the difference between the Ct (threshold cycle) of primer and Ct of the housekeeper/reference gene. The ΔΔCt was calculated as the mean difference of ΔCts of a specific primer at a single time point between H and J cybrids or ΔCts of the primer being compared at two different time points of either H or J cybrids. The fold values were calculated using the formula $\text{Fold} = 2^{-\Delta\Delta Ct}$. Fold values were calculated relative to the readings for corresponding H cybrids at 0 hours. Data is presented as mean ± standard error of mean (SEM). Experiments were performed in triplicate. *P* values <0.05 (two-tail test) were considered statistically significant.

Results

Growth Curve Assay

The 0 hour cell counts were normalized to 100% in the both Control (untreated) and Study (UV-treated) groups (Figure 1). At each time point, J-untreated cybrids showed greater growth than H-untreated cybrids (48 hours- 141% vs. 122%, 96 hours- 183% vs. 157%, 120 hours- 254% vs. 192%, and 144 hours- 272% vs. 198%). In the UV-treated groups at time interval between 48 and 96 hours, there was initially a downslope followed by an upward trend in the growth patterns. The J-treated cybrids showed higher growth rates than H-treated cybrids (48 hours-116% vs. 98%, 96 hours- 113% vs. 72%, 120 hours- 188% vs. 156%, and 144 hours- 234% vs. 148%), but the growth rates were reduced in comparison to their corresponding untreated groups.

Expression of Genes Normalized to 0-Hour H Cybrids

Complement pathway inhibition genes. Initially we normalized the H-untreated cybrids at 0 hour value to 1 and then compared the H and J cybrid values of gene expression at 0, 72 and 120 hours (Figure 2). At 0 hours, we found that the H-untreated cybrids had significantly higher expression levels of CFH than J-untreated cybrids (1 vs. 0.69±0.05 fold, $p = 0.003$). In the H-untreated cybrids, there was an increase in CFH gene expression at 72 hours (6.9±0.19 fold, $p<0.0001$) and 120 hours (5.85±0.07 fold, $p<0.0001$) compared to the 0 hours H-untreated cybrids. The J-untreated cybrids started at a lower level of CFH expression (0.69±0.05 fold, $p<0.01$) and increased to 4.4±0.1 fold, $p<0.0001$ and 5.2±0.03 fold, $p<0.0001$ at 72 and 120 hours, respectively. Compared to the 0-hour H cybrids, the H-treated cybrids cultured 72 hours and 120 hours had increased levels of CFH expression (4.8±0.15 fold, $p<0.001$ and 5.52±0.12 fold, $p<0.0001$, respectively). At 72 hours and 120 hours, the J-treated cybrids also showed an increase expression of CFH compared to the 0-hour H-untreated cybrids (3.63±0.2 fold, $p<0.001$ and 4.31±0.13 fold, $p<0.0001$), respectively (Figure 2a).

At 0-hours, the CD55 gene expression levels were significantly higher in the H-untreated cybrids versus J-untreated cybrids

Table 1. Gene Functions and Accession Numbers.

Gene	Gene name	Gene Bank Accession No.	Function
CFH	Complement Factor H	NM_000186.	Essential in regulation of complement activation.
CD55/DAF	Decay accelerating factor for complement	NM_000574, NM_001114543, NM_001114544, NM_00111475.	Involved in regulation of complement cascade by accelerating decay of complement proteins and disrupting the cascade.
CD59	CD59 Molecule, Complement Regulatory Protein	NM_000611, NM_203329, NM_203331, NM_001127223, NM_001127225, NM_001127226, NM_001127227.	Cell surface glycoprotein that regulates complement-mediated cell lysis, inhibits complement membrane attack complex and is involved in lymphocyte signal transduction.
IL-33	Interleukin 33	NM_033439, NM_001127180, NM_001199640.	Member of IL-1 family; Critical pro-inflammatory cytokine involved in production of T helper 2 associated cytokines.
TGF-A	Transforming Growth Factor, alpha	NM_003236, NM_001099691.	Ligand for EGFR that activates signaling pathway for cell proliferation, differentiation and activation. It is also upregulated in human cancers.
EFEMP-1	EGF containing fibulin like extracellular matrix protein 1	NM_004105, NM_018894, NM_001039348, NM_001039349.	High-risk gene associated with AMD, misfolded EFEMP-1 protein accumulates within RPE cells causing altered cellular function and inflammation. High EFEMP-1 levels are associated with tumor metastasis.
RARA	Retinoic acid receptor, alpha	NM_000964, NM_001145301, NM_001033603.	Nuclear retinoic acid receptor. Regulates transcription. Involved with apoptosis and differentiation.
BBC3	BCL2 binding component 3	NM_014417, NM_00112741, NM_001127240.	Member of BCL2 family, BH3 only pro-apoptotic subclass to induce mitochondrial outer membrane permeabilization, apoptosis, mitochondrial dysfunction and caspase activation.
BLC2L13	BCL2-like 13	NM_015367	Mitochondria specific protein whose over-expression results in apoptosis.

(1.00 vs. 0.77±0.05 fold, p = 0.002), however, both H and J cybrids did not increase greatly after UV treatment (Figure 2b).

The CD59 expression levels at 0-hours were not significantly different between H-untreated and J-untreated cybrids (1 vs.

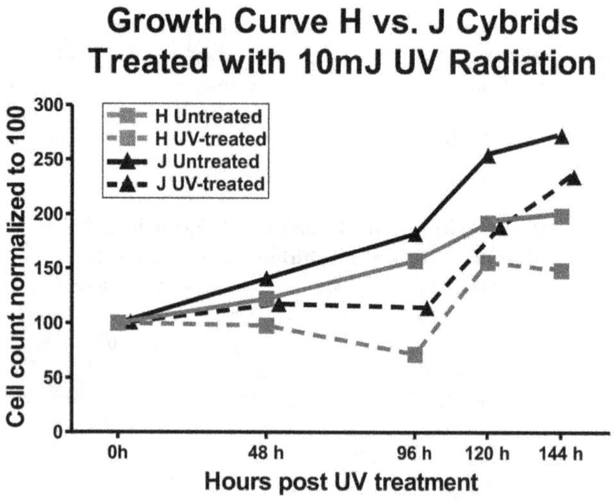

Figure 1. Differential growth patterns were observed for H cybrids versus J cybrids in UV-treated and untreated groups. Cybrids containing J haplogroup mtDNA showed a steeper slope for the growth curve than H haplogroup mtDNA in both UV-treated and untreated groups. In untreated there were constant increases in growth patterns for both H and J cybrids. In the UV-treated samples, the growth rates slowed or declined until approximately 96 hours post treatment, and then increased again. Triplicate wells were run for each sample and the experiments were repeated twice. During the growth curve assay, each sample was run in triplicate. Grey solid line, untreated H cybrids; Grey broken line, UV-treated H cybrids; Black solid line, untreated J cybrids; Black broken line, UV-treated J cybrids.

0.89±0.10 fold, p = 0.30) or after 120 hours of UV treatment (0.86±0.08 fold, p = 0.14 vs 1.12±0.04 fold, p = 0.06) (Figure 2c).

Inflammation, cellular proliferation and angiogenesis genes. With this category of genes, we again normalized the H cybrids at 0-hours to a value of 1 and then compared this against all other values (Figure 3). At 0-hours, Q-PCR analyses showed lower expression levels in J-untreated cybrids for IL-33 (0.37±0.01 fold, p<0.0001) compared to the 0-hour H cybrids. At 120 hours, the J-untreated cybrids and the H-untreated cybrids showed significantly elevated levels of IL-33 compared to the 0-hour H cybrids (4.09±0.09 fold, p<0.001 and 2.09±0.09 fold, p<0.001, respectively, Figure 3a). At 120 hours after UV treatment, the IL-33 expression in the J-treated cybrids increased to 5.01±0.1 fold (p<0.001) while the H-treated cybrids increased 2.97±0.07 fold (p<0.001).

A similar pattern was seen for the TGF-A expression levels, with the J-untreated cybrids having lower levels than the H-untreated cybrids at 0 hours (0.38±0.02 vs. 1 fold, p<0.0001, Figure 3b). At 120 hours, the J-untreated (2.26±0.08 fold, p<0.001) and H-untreated cybrids (1.97±0.08 fold, p = 0.04) showed an elevated expression levels of TGF-A compared to the 0-hour H-untreated cybrids. After UV treatment, there was an increase for TGF-A expression in the J-treated cybrids (3.71±0.14 fold, p<0.0001) and H cybrids, (2.7±0.05 fold, p<0.0001) compared to the 0-hour H cybrids.

At 0-hour, Q-PCR analyses showed lower expression levels for EFEMP-1 in J-untreated cybrids (0.26±0.02 fold, p = 0.001) compared to the 0-hour H cybrids (Figure 3c). At 120 hours, compared to the 0-hours H cybrids, the EFEMP-1 gene expression for both the J-untreated cybrids, (3.3±0.17 fold, p<0.0001) and J-treated cybrids (4.0±0.09 fold, p<0.0001) increased to a greater degree than H-untreated cybrids (1.54±0.11 fold, p< 0.0001) and H-treated cybrids (2.39±0.08 fold, p<0.0001).

Expression levels for apoptosis genes. We analyzed 3 pro-apoptotic genes and found that only RARA and BBC3

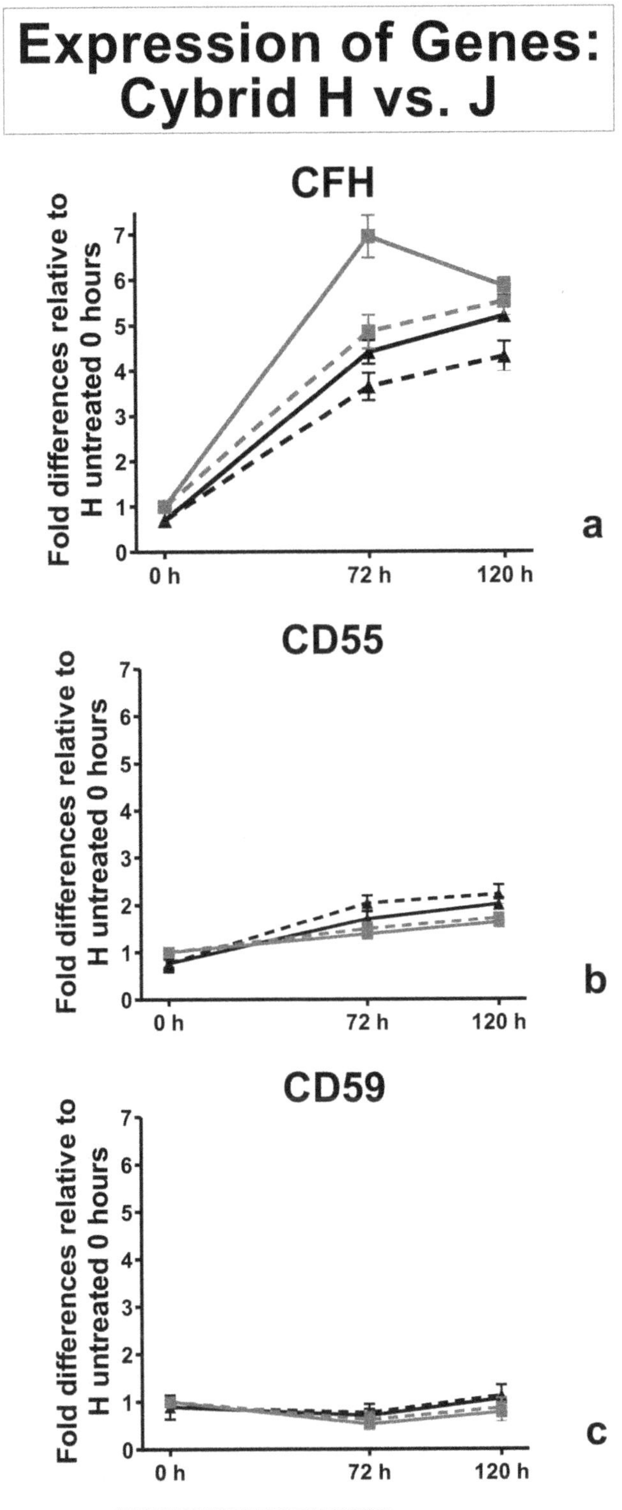

Figure 2. Expression patterns of alternate complement inhibitor genes after UV treatment. The 0-hour value for H-untreated cybrid was normalized to 1 and then compared to gene expression values at 0, 72 and 120 hours. Panel 2a: At 0-hour, the J-untreated cybrids had lower levels of CFH compared to H-untreated cybrids (p = 0.003). At 72 hours and 120 hours, the H-untreated cybrids (grey solid line) showed higher levels of CFH expression compared to the J-untreated cybrids (black solid line). After UV exposure, the H-treated cybrids (grey broken line) expressed increased CFH levels compared to the J-treated cybrids (black broken line) at both 72 and 120 hours. Panel 2b: At 0-hours the H-untreated cybrids showed higher expression levels for CH55 (grey solid line) compared to J-untreated cybrids (black solid line, p = 0.002). At 72 and 120 hours post-UV treatment, there were no significant differences in the CD55 expression levels. Panel 2c: The CD59 expression levels were similar for the untreated (grey solid and black solid lines) and UV-treated (grey broken and black broken lines) H and J cybrids. There were triplicate wells for each sample and the experiments were repeated twice. n = 3 different individuals for the H cybrids and n = 3 different individuals for the J cybrids.

showed significant increases after UV treatment (Figure 4). All samples were normalized to the H-untreated cybrid at time point 0-hours. The gene expression levels for the 0-hour J-untreated cybrids were significantly lower compared to the 0-hour H-untreated cybrids (RARA, 0.88+0.03 fold, p = 0.003, Figure 4a; BBC3, 0.71±0.2 fold, p<0.01, Figure 4b; and BCL2L13; 0.81±0.05 fold, p = 0.002, Figure 4c). At 120 hours after UV treatment, the H-treated and J-treated cybrids showed increased expression levels for RARA (1.96±0.05 fold, p<0.001 and 1.64±0.03 fold, p = 0.009, respectively); BBC3 (3.78±0.15, p< 0.001 fold and 3.21±0.09 fold, p<0.0001); and BCL2L13 (2.39±0.05 fold, p<0.001 and 2.20±0.15 fold, p<0.0001, respectively) compared to the 0-hour H-untreated cybrids.

Comparison of Gene Expression Levels from 0 to 120 Hours

The analyses performed above compared the gene expression values for all samples to the 0-hour H-untreated cybrids. However, in all cases the 0-hours J-untreated cybrids showed lower gene expression levels at baseline than the 0-hour H-untreated cybrids. Therefore, in order to measure the total expression increase of each of the genes, we needed to compare the values at the 120-hour period compared to the original 0-hour baseline for the H cybrids and J cybrids (represented as ΔΔCt values). Figure 5 shows the ΔΔCt values of the 120-hour UV-treated H cybrids compared to the 0-hour H-untreated cybrids and the UV-treated 120-hour J cybrids compared to the 0-hour J-untreated cybrids.

At 120 hours after UV treatment, there was a significant increase in CFH gene expression from their respective baseline levels in the H-treated cybrids compared to the J-treated cybrids (ΔΔCt 2.44±0.11 vs. ΔΔCt 2.09±0.07, p<0.02, Figure 5a). The ΔΔCt values for CD55 expression were decreased in the H-treated cybrids compared to the J-treated cybrids, (ΔΔCt 0.78±0.09 vs. ΔΔCt 1.12±0.11, p<0.03, Figure 5a). There were no significant differences in ΔΔCt values of CD59 expression for the H-treated cybrids compared to J-treated cybrids (ΔΔCt −0.23±0.2 vs. ΔΔCt 0.15±0.13, p = 0.064).

The mean ΔΔCt values in the H-treated cybrids were significantly lower for the IL-33 gene (1.56±0.12, p<0.001 vs. 2.29±0.1, p<0.0008) and the EFEMP-1 gene (ΔΔCt 1.34±0.004 vs. ΔΔCt 1.99±0.03, p<0.001) compared to the J-treated (Figure 5b). There were no statistically significant differences in ΔΔCt values for the TGF-A expression (H cybrids value was ΔΔCt 1.43±0.05 vs. J cybrids value of ΔΔCt 1.8±0.22, p = 0.14,). This demonstrates that when H and J cybrids were treated with the same amount of UV radiation under identical conditions, the J-treated cybrids showed significantly greater IL-33 and EFEMP1 expression levels from baseline, when compared to

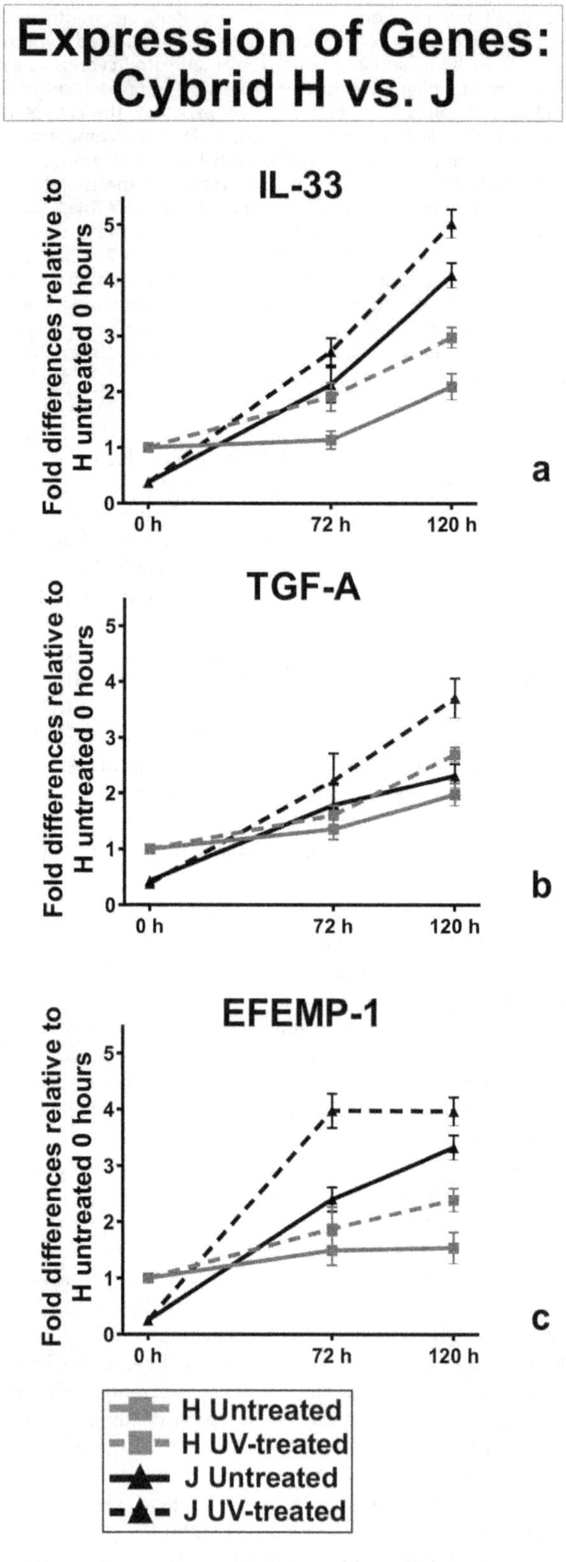

Figure 3. Expression patterns of inflammation, cellular proliferation and angiogenesis genes after UV treatment. The 0-hour values for H-untreated cybrids were normalized to 1 and then compared to gene expression values at 0, 72 and 120 hours. Panel 3a: At 0-hour, the J-untreated cybrids (black solid line) had lower expression levels of IL-33 compared to H-untreated cybrids (grey solid line, $p<0.0001$). At 120 hours, the H-untreated cybrids (grey solid line) showed higher levels of IL-33 expression compared to the J-untreated cybrids (black solid line). At both 72 and 120 hours, the J-treated cybrids showed higher levels of IL-33 expression compared to the H-treated cybrids. Panel 3b: At 0-hours, the TGF-A expression levels were lower for the J-untreated cybrids (black solid line) compared to the H-untreated cybrids (grey solid line, $p<0.0001$). At 120 hours after UV-treatment, the TGF-A levels for both H-treated (grey broken line) and J-treated (black broken line) were higher than the untreated H (grey solid line) or J (black solid line) cybrids. Panel 3c: At 0-hours, the expression levels for EFEMP1 were lower in the J-untreated (black solid lines) compared to H-untreated cybrids (grey solid lines, $p=0.0001$). By 120 hours, the J-treated cybrids (black broken line) and J-untreated cybrids (black solid line) showed greater fold increases of EFEMP1 expression compared to the H-treated (grey broken line) and H-untreated (grey solid line) cybrids. There were triplicate wells for each sample and the experiments were repeated twice. J cybrids, n = 3 different individuals; H cybrids, n = 3 different individuals.

H-treated cybrids. However, the increases in TGF-A gene expression levels from their respective baseline values were quantitatively similar in both H-treated and J-treated cybrids.

In Figure 5c, we analyzed the expression levels for the three pro-apoptosis genes comparing H-treated cybrids to J-treated cybrids at 120 hours. The J-treated cybrids consistently showed lower mean change in ΔΔCt values compared to the H-treated cybrids for the RARA (ΔΔCt 0.71±0.07 vs. ΔΔCt 1.01±0.03, $p=0.02$) and BBC3 genes (ΔΔCt 1.67±0.06 vs. ΔΔCt 1.94±0.04, $p=0.004$) but not the BCL2L13 gene (ΔΔCt 1.12±0.07 vs. ΔΔCt 1.25±0.05, $p=0.28$). This indicates that after UV radiation, the H-treated cybrids showed greater increases of expression levels of pro-apoptotic genes than J-treated cybrids.

In summary, our findings demonstrate that at different time periods after UV sub-lethal radiation, the J cybrids maintains higher rates of growth, higher expression levels for inflammation genes but lower expression levels for apoptosis-related genes (Figure 6).

Discussion

The study investigates the response of cybrids, with identical nuclei but either H haplogroup mtDNA or J haplogroup mtDNA, to sub-lethal UV-radiation, which is an oxidative stressor and a risk factor for AMD [25]. Our previous study has shown that J cybrids have higher growth rates than H cybrids when cultured in similar environmental conditions [18]. In addition, we reported that although both H and J cybrids have similar copy numbers of mtDNA, H cybrids produce higher ATP levels and utilize oxidative phosphorylation (OXPHOS) while the J cybrids utilize predominantly glycolysis [18].

In our study, we observed that J haplogroup cybrids, with or without UV treatment, had more rapid growth rates even though the J cybrids are less energy efficient [18]. After 144 hours in vitro, the J-untreated cybrids had approximately 75% higher numbers of cells than the H-untreated cybrids. After UV treatment, the J-treated cybrids showed an approximately 85% higher cell count levels compared to the H-treated cybrids. The increased growth rates may be related in part to increased expression of IL-33 and EFEMP-1 genes, which play key roles in cell proliferation. The mechanisms by which the J haplogroup mtDNA affects rapid growth rates and glycolysis are not understood. One can speculate that the phenomenon might be similar to Warburg effect, described in 1956 by Dr. Otto Warburg [26], which suggested that tumor cells with damaged respiratory mechanisms have uncontrolled proliferation. These cancer cells had adapted to hypoxic conditions by shifting to glycolysis for ATP production, and even if returned to normoxic conditions, the cells continued with glycolysis as their main source of energy production.

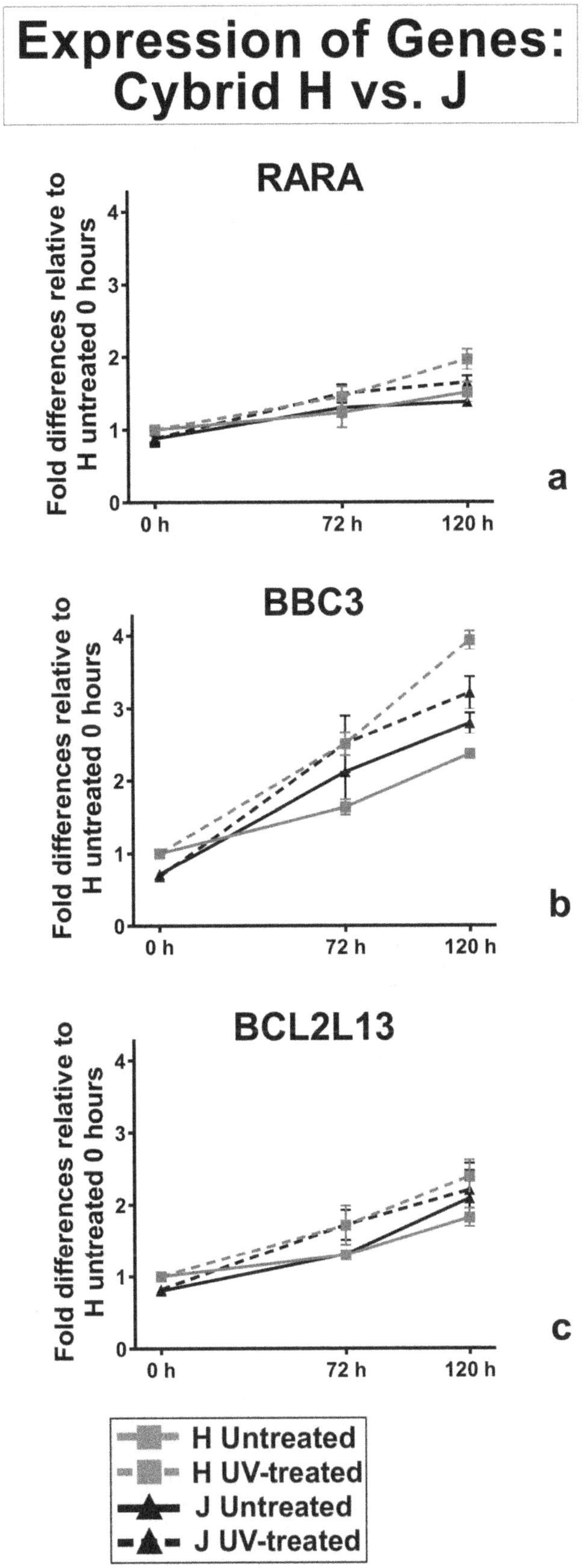

Figure 4. Expression patterns of pro-apoptosis genes after UV treatment. The 0-hour values for H-untreated cybrids were normalized to 1 and then compared to gene expression values at 0, 72 and 120 hours. Panel 4a: At 0-hour, the J-untreated cybrids (black solid line) had lower expression levels of RARA compared to H-untreated cybrids (grey solid line, $p = 0.0036$). Panel 4b: At 0-hour, the J-untreated cybrids (black solid line) had lower expression levels of BBC3 compared to H-untreated cybrids (grey solid line, $p<0.01$). At 120 hours after UV treatment, the H-treated cybrids (grey broken line) and J-treated cybrids (black broken line) showed higher expression levels of BBC3 compared to H-untreated (grey solid line) and J-untreated (black solid line). Panel 4c: At 0-hours, the J-untreated cybrids (black solid line) showed lower expression levels of BCL2L13 compared to the H-untreated cybrids (grey solid line, $p = 0.002$). After 120 hour of UV treatment, the H-treated (grey broken line) and J-treated (black broken line) cybrids showed an increase in BCL2L13 expression levels. There were triplicate wells for each sample and the experiments were repeated twice.

Similarly, the J haplogroups represent a subgroup of the Caucasian population which originated in Northern Europe, and over thousands of years, in response to extremely cold climatic conditions, may have developed adaptations within the mtDNA which preferentially uses glycolysis rather than OXPHOS. Others have shown that J haplogroups have accumulated higher levels of non-synonymous SNPs compared to other haplogroups, suggesting either a high mutation rate or a continuous selection process in the lineage [27]. We speculate these divergent energy efficiencies, as seen in the J versus H haplogroups, may influence the mitochondrial-nuclear interactions, thereby causing different expression levels of genes in major pathways. Further studies are underway to clarify the relationships between mtDNA variants and nuclear responses.

Complement system activation and inflammation are major events contributing to AMD pathogenesis [28]. Studies have reported accumulation of immunoglobulin and complement components within drusen [29–31], associations between genetic variants of CFH, C2/CFB, C3, and CFI with increased risk for AMD [32,33], and elevated serum CRP levels in AMD patients [34]. Studies of European mtDNA variants have revealed that J, T and U haplogroups are associated with AMD [17,35–38] while the H haplogroup is protective [39]. Our previous paper shows that at resting state, the J cybrids express lower levels of CFH than H cybrids. After UV-treatment, J cybrids still showed lower CFH levels at 72 and 120 hours in both the untreated and UV-treated samples. Since CFH is a negative regulator of the alternative complement pathway, the lower levels in J haplogroup subjects would likely lead to increased activation of the complement pathway and higher levels of inflammation. Alternatively, the higher CFH levels in H cybrids, as seen at all time points, may be associated with the protective effects associated between H haplogroup and AMD. In cells from the outer retinal layers, photo-oxidative stress induces complement activation and decreases the level of CFH, which results in increased inflammatory responses [40]. Interestingly, we found less than 2-fold increase of CD55 expression after UV treatment, suggesting that CFH was the major inhibitor mediated by mtDNA. This makes the CFH gene an attractive target for future therapies to treat AMD and other complement-related diseases.

RPE cells, with their high oxygen demands and metabolic rates [41], are susceptible to UV radiation, which can cause loss of cell viability, mitochondrial dysfunction, DNA damage and apoptosis [42]. UV exposure can increase ROS production in RPE cells that can trigger inflammation [43–45]. In our study, we found similar expression patterns for IL-33 and EFEMP-1 genes, whereby at resting stages, the J-untreated cybrids had levels lower than H-untreated cybrids but after UV stress, the J-treated cybrids showed increased expression levels of each gene compared to H-treated cybrids. This is important because these genes play a role in

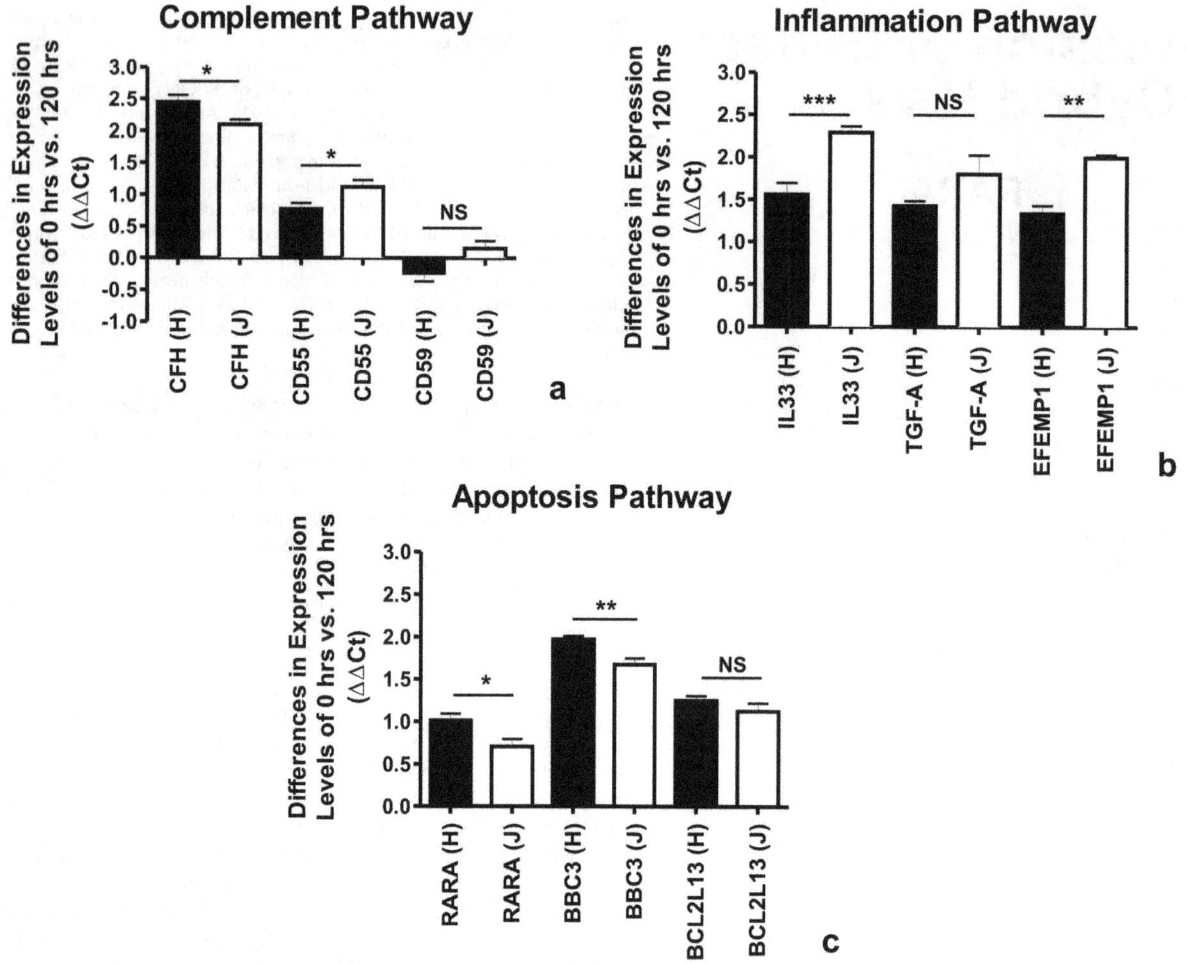

Figure 5. Comparison of gene expression levels from 0 to 120 hours after UV treatment. The solid black bars represent the ΔΔCt values of H-untreated cybrids at 0 hour compared to H-treated cybrids at 120 hours. The open bars represent the ΔΔCt values of the J-untreated cybrids at 0 hours compared to J-treated cybrids at 120 hours. Panel 5a: At 120 hours after UV treatment, the H-treated cybrids have higher expression levels for CFH compared to the J-treated cybrids ($p<0.02$) but lower expression for the CD55 gene ($p<0.03$). There was no significant difference for the CD59 levels in the H-treated versus the J-treated cybrids. Panel 5b: At 120 hours after UV treatment, the J-treated cybrids have higher expression levels for IL-33 and EFEMP1 genes compared to the H-treated cybrids ($p<0.02$) but similar expression levels for the TGF-A gene. ($p=0.14$). Panel 5c: At 120 hours after UV treatment, the H-treated cybrids have higher expression levels for RARA ($p=0.02$) and BBC3 ($p=0.004$) genes compared to the J-treated cybrids. There expression levels for the BCL2L13 gene were similar for both cybrids ($p=0.28$).

inflammation, innate immunity and/or angiogenesis, which are pathologic processes of AMD. IL-33, which can be found in RPE cells, is a cytokine belonging to the IL-1 superfamily, and can regulate inflammatory cytokines including IL-6, IL-8, IL-1B and TNF-alpha. Alipoprotein E (ApoE), a high-risk gene associated with AMD, mediates the distribution of lipids and cholesterol. Abnormal functions of ApoE can lead to hypercholesteremia [46], and increased production of amyloid, a protein associated with both AMD (geographic atrophy) and Alzheimer's disease. It has been reported that in RPE cells, beta-amyloid can stimulate IL-33 mediated inflammatory responses [47], which suggests that there may be a correlation between amyloid production, IL-33 and ApoE levels related to RPE cells responses to oxidative stressors.

TGF-A plays a role in both angiogenesis and wound healing [48]. In addition, elevated levels of TGF-A have been consistently observed in gastrointestinal cancers, breast cancers and primary epithelial ovarian cancers [49–51]. While an association between TGF-A and AMD has not been reported, it is a relatively newly described gene and little is known about its functions. It is worth noting that the TGF-A and IL-33 may interact at some level because their expression patterns closely followed each other in our experiments.

Increased expression of EFEMP-1 genes was also found in untreated and UV-treated J cybrids. EFEMP-1 is another important cancer-related gene that was differentially expressed in UV-treated J cybrids. EFEMP-1, a favorable prognostic marker for glioblastoma multiforme tumors [52], modulates the extracellular environment and influences important signaling pathways. Song and coworkers transfected EFEMP-1 into HeLa cells and observed increased VEGF expression, acceleration of angiogenesis, increased growth and proliferation of cervical carcinoma *in vivo* [53]. It is reported that misfolded EFEMP-1 accumulates within endoplasmic reticulum and up-regulates VEGF expression in pancreatic adenocarcinoma [54]. Therefore, the finding that EFEMP-1 expression is mediated by mtDNA haplogroups is exciting because it implies that the mtDNA can greatly influence this important pathway and that it is responsive to sub-lethal UV radiation.

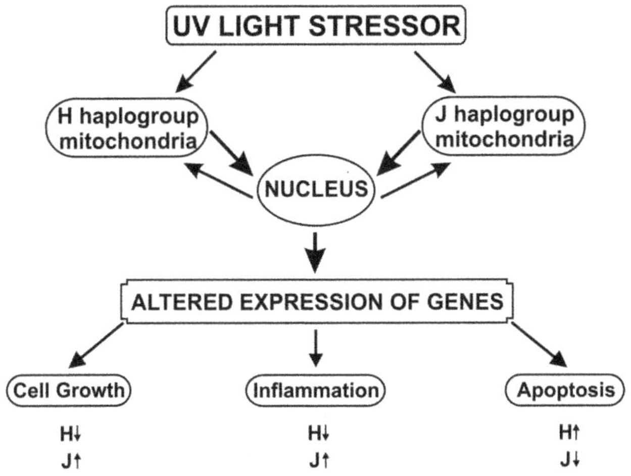

Figure 6. Schematic summary of the changes found in cybrids after UV treatment. In response to identical UV conditions, cybrids with identical nuclei but different mtDNA haplogroups (H vs. J) showed differential responses of cell growth and expression patterns genes related to inflammation and apoptosis. After UV treatment, the J-treated cybrids had increased cell growth rates but a gene expression pattern consistent with higher levels of inflammation (elevated IL-33 and EFEMP1 along with decreased expression of CFH, a complement pathway inhibitor) compared to H-treated cybrids. The pro-apoptosis genes (RARA and BBC3) were expressed at a lower level in J-treated cybrids after UV treatment.

With respect to AMD, EFEMP-1 expressed in RPE cells is a high-risk gene associated with AMD and Doyne honeycomb retinal dystrophy. Misfolded EFEMP-1 protein accumulates within RPE cells causing altered cellular function and inflammation [55]. EFEMP-1 protein is present between RPE layer and drusen [56,57]. Roybal et al. studied the response of transfected EFEMP-1 wild type and mutant EFEMP-1 R345W on VEGF expression in ARPE-19 cell line. R345W mutation in EFEMP-1 is linked to two inherited early–onset macular degenerative retinal diseases Malattia Leventinese (ML) and Doyne honeycomb retinal dystrophy (DHRD). There was an abnormal accumulation and retention of EFEMP-1 R345W in the endoplasmic reticulum that induced the unfolded protein response (UPR) activation followed by increased VEGF expression. Activation of UPR and VEGF expression may be correlated with RPE dysfunction and choroidal neovascularization in AMD patients [58]. In our study, the UV-treated J cybrids showed a 4-fold increase in EFEMP-1 levels while the UV-treated H cybrids had a 2.56-fold increase. Even though the mechanisms by which EFEMP-1 might contribute to AMD is not known, based upon the cancer studies, it is reasonable to speculate that numerous downstream pathways are activated by increased EFEMP-1 levels. Most importantly, it must be pointed out that (1) the J and H cybrids showed a differential response to the UV treatment, and (2) these cybrids differed only in their mtDNA but had identical nuclei and treatment conditions. This is important because it strongly suggests that within an individual, the mtDNA haplogroup background may provide a baseline for expression of major signaling pathways, which are then influenced to different degrees by identical stressors, depending upon which haplogroup the individual possesses. One can speculate that this may explain in part why some individuals are more susceptible to environmental stressors, such as smoking or UV light, while others are not.

In our study, we investigated expression levels for three apoptosis-related genes and found significant changes in RARA and BBC3. In general, BBC3 is involved in BAX-dependent cell death related to developing retina and brain [59] but in the adult nervous system the cell death process is mediated by BIM. BBC3 expression can be altered in response to various insults and is involved in adult retinal cell degeneration [60–62]. In a mouse model, UV exposure can increase BIM expression, which in turn can increase BBC3 expression and caspase-dependent cell death in retinal photoreceptor cells [63]. Our study demonstrates a 3.78-fold increase expression for BBC3 in UV-treated H cybrids occurring in response to UV-radiation stress. We need to be cautious because although the BBC3 expression levels are elevated, this may or may not translate into higher apoptotic activities in the UV-treated H cybrids.

A second apoptotic gene, RARA, was differentially expressed in the H versus J cybrids after UV treatment. RARA, which is present in the bipolar cells and retinal ganglion cells, is an important regulator for development [64]. In addition, RARA upregulates expression of glial cell-derived neurotrophic factors (GNDF), which inhibits vascular permeability factor-VEGF [65]. We observed increased expression of RARA in UV-treated H cybrids as compared to J cybrids. If RARA indirectly inhibits VEGF expression, then this may correlate with lower incidence of wet AMD in individuals having H haplogroup mtDNA.

The cybrid model using different Rho^0 cells as the host cell line has provided similar findings to ours by showing that the mtDNA haplogroup profiles influence cellular/molecular responses. After H_2O_2–induced oxidative stress, the SIRT3 gene was downregulated in osteosarcoma cybrids with the J haplogroup compared to H cybrids [66]. Lin and coworkers used cybrids created with Taiwanese haplogroups and showed that the B4b haplogroup had increased susceptibility to H_2O_2 compared to other ethnic Chinese backgrounds. Bellizzi and co-workers used the osteosarcoma cybrid model to demonstrate that at baseline the H cybrids had significantly lower levels of heat shock protein (HSP)60 and HSP75 but after oxidative stress, the H cybrids accumulated HSP60 within mitochondria at a much greater rate than other cybrids [67]. In another series of experiments, they showed that in basal and H_2O_2-stressed conditions, the H and J cybrids showed different levels of interleukin (IL)-6, IL-1beta and tumor necrosis factor receptor 2, which are stress–related cytokines [68]. Finally, an osteosarcoma cybrid model showed that the H cybrids differed significantly from Uk cybrids with respect to mitochondrial RNA levels, protein synthesis, membrane potential and growth capacity [69]. These findings, along with ours, strongly support our hypothesis that mtDNA haplogroups can mediate molecular pathways that influence the complement/inflammation responses of cells.

Conclusions

Our findings support the hypothesis that nuclear-mitochondrial interactions play significant roles in modulating complex phenotypic responses to sub-lethal UV radiation. We found that mtDNA variability, as represented by H versus J haplogroups, can influence genetic expressions of cells after UV stress. Increasing our understanding of nuclear-mitochondrial interactions, and their relationship to environmental stimuli, will lead to an entirely new era of disease management in which the mitochondria, with its unique DNA, will become a target for therapy.

Author Contributions

Conceived and designed the experiments: DM MCK MC NU. Performed the experiments: DM TH PF CR MT JCDC. Analyzed the data: DM MCK MC SRA PF ABN DCW. Contributed reagents/materials/analysis tools: SMJ MVM DSB BDK. Wrote the paper: DM MCK JCDC.

References

1. Sacca SC, Roszkowska AM, Izzotti A (2013) Environmental light and endogenous antioxidants as the main determinants of non-cancer ocular diseases. Mutat Res 752: 153–171.
2. Klein BE, Lee KE, Klein R (2011) Refraction in adults with diabetes. Arch Ophthalmol 129: 56–62.
3. Zarbin MA (2004) Current concepts in the pathogenesis of age-related macular degeneration. Arch Ophthalmol 122: 598–614.
4. Campisi J, d'Adda di Fagagna F (2007) Cellular senescence: when bad things happen to good cells. Nat Rev Mol Cell Biol 8: 729–740.
5. Baynes JW (2002) The Maillard hypothesis on aging: time to focus on DNA. Ann N Y Acad Sci 959: 360–367.
6. Artigas JM, Felipe A, Navea A, Artigas C, Menezo JL (2013) Ultraviolet radiation at Mediterranean latitudes and protection efficacy of intraocular lenses. J Fr Ophthalmol 36: 23–28.
7. Cullen AP (2002) Photokeratitis and other phototoxic effects on the cornea and conjunctiva. Int J Toxicol 21: 455–464.
8. Felipe A, Artigas JM, Diez-Ajenjo A, Garcia-Domene C, Peris C (2012) Modulation transfer function of a toric intraocular lens: evaluation of the changes produced by rotation and tilt. J Refract Surg 28: 335–340.
9. Sliney DH (2005) Exposure geometry and spectral environment determine photobiological effects on the human eye. Photochem Photobiol 81: 483–489.
10. Coroneo MT (1990) Albedo concentration in the anterior eye: a phenomenon that locates some solar diseases. Ophthalmic Surg 21: 60–66.
11. Blasiak J, Glowacki S, Kauppinen A, Kaarniranta K (2013) Mitochondrial and nuclear DNA damage and repair in age-related macular degeneration. Int J Mol Sci 14: 2996–3010.
12. Durik M, Kavousi M, van der Pluijm I, Isaacs A, Cheng C, et al. (2012) Nucleotide excision DNA repair is associated with age-related vascular dysfunction. Circulation 126: 468–478.
13. Harper JW, Elledge SJ (2007) The DNA damage response: Ten years after. Mol Cell 28: 739–745.
14. Feher J, Kovacs I, Artico M, Cavallotti C, Papale A, et al. (2006) Mitochondrial alterations of retinal pigment epithelium in age-related macular degeneration. Neurobiol Aging 27: 983–993.
15. Harman DG, Blanksby SJ (2006) Trapping of a tert-adamantyl peroxyl radical in the gas phase. Chem Commun (Camb): 859–861.
16. Wallace DC (2005) The mitochondrial genome in human adaptive radiation and disease: On the road to therapeutics and performance enhancement. Gene 354: 169–180.
17. Mueller EE, Schaier E, Brunner SM, Eder W, Mayr JA, et al. (2012) Mitochondrial haplogroups and control region polymorphisms in age-related macular degeneration: A case-control study. PLoS One 7: e30874.
18. Hain JH, Hampp JD, McKenney SA, Albert JA, Kenney RD (2013) Swim speed, behavior, and movement of North Atlantic right whales (Eubalaena glacialis) in coastal waters of northeastern Florida, USA. PLoS One 8: e54340.
19. Baudouin SV, Saunders D, Tiangyou W, Elson JL, Poynter J, et al. (2005) Mitochondrial DNA and survival after sepsis: A prospective study. Lancet 366: 2118–2121.
20. Vives-Bauza C, Gonzalo R, Manfredi G, Garcia-Arumi E, Andreu AL (2006) Enhanced ROS production and antioxidant defenses in cybrids harbouring mutations in mtDNA. Neurosci Lett 391: 136–141.
21. Ma YS, Wu SB, Lee WY, Cheng JS, Wei YH (2009) Response to the increase of oxidative stress and mutation of mitochondrial DNA in aging. Biochim Biophys Acta 1790: 1021–1029.
22. Kenney MC, Chwa M, Atilano SR, Pavlis JM, Falatoonzadeh P, et al. (2013) Mitochondrial DNA variants mediate energy production and expression levels for CFH, C3 and EFEMP1 genes: Implications for age-related macular degeneration. PLoS One 8: e54339.
23. Kenney MC, Chwa M, Atilano SR, Falatoonzadeh P, Ramirez C, et al. (2014) Molecular and bioenergetic differences between cells with African versus European inherited mitochondrial DNA haplogroups: Implications for population susceptibility to diseases. Biochim Biophys Acta 1842: 208–219.
24. Kenney MC, Atilano SR, Falatoonzadeh P, Ramirez C, Malik D, et al Udar N (2014) Inherited mitochondrial DNA variants can affect complement, inflammation and apoptosis pathways: Insights into mitochondrial-nuclear interactions. Hum Mol Genet In Press.
25. Aimjongjun S, Sutheerawattananonda M, Limpeanchob N (2013) Silk lutein extract and its combination with vitamin E reduce UVB-mediated oxidative damage to retinal pigment epithelial cells. J Photochem Photobiol B 124: 34–41.
26. Warburg O (1956) On the origin of cancer cells. Science 123: 309–314.
27. Pierron D, Chang I, Arachiche A, Heiske M, Thomas O, et al. (2011) Mutation rate switch inside Eurasian mitochondrial haplogroups: Impact of selection and consequences for dating settlement in Europe. PLoS One 6: e21543.
28. Charbel Issa P, Chong NV, Scholl HP (2011) The significance of the complement system for the pathogenesis of age-related macular degeneration - current evidence and translation into clinical application. Graefes Arch Clin Exp Ophthalmol 249: 163–174.
29. Anderson DH, Radeke MJ, Gallo NB, Chapin EA, Johnson PT, et al. (2010) The pivotal role of the complement system in aging and age-related macular degeneration: Hypothesis re-visited. Prog Retin Eye Res 29: 95–112.
30. Patel M, Chan CC (2008) Immunopathological aspects of age-related macular degeneration. Semin Immunopathol 30: 97–110.
31. Umeda S, Suzuki MT, Okamoto H, Ono F, Mizota A, et al. (2005) Molecular composition of drusen and possible involvement of anti-retinal autoimmunity in two different forms of macular degeneration in cynomolgus monkey (Macaca fascicularis). FASEB J 19: 1683–1685.
32. Despriet DD, Klaver CC, Witteman JC, Bergen AA, Kardys I, et al. (2006) Complement factor H polymorphism, complement activators, and risk of age-related macular degeneration. JAMA 296: 301–309.
33. Ratnapriya R, Chew EY (2013) Age-related macular degeneration-clinical review and genetics update. Clin Genet 84: 160–166.
34. Simonelli F, Frisso G, Testa F, di Fiore R, Vitale DF, et al. (2006) Polymorphism p.402Y>H in the complement factor H protein is a risk factor for age related macular degeneration in an Italian population. Br J Ophthalmol 90: 1142–1145.
35. Jones MM, Manwaring N, Wang JJ, Rochtchina E, Mitchell P, et al. (2007) Mitochondrial DNA haplogroups and age-related maculopathy. Arch Ophthalmol 125: 1235–1240.
36. Udar N, Atilano SR, Memarzadeh M, Boyer DS, Chwa M, et al. (2009) Mitochondrial DNA haplogroups associated with age-related macular degeneration. Invest Ophthalmol Vis Sci 50: 2966–2974.
37. SanGiovanni JP, Arking DE, Iyengar SK, Elashoff M, Clemons TE, et al. (2009) Mitochondrial DNA variants of respiratory complex I that uniquely characterize haplogroup T2 are associated with increased risk of age-related macular degeneration. PLoS One 4: e5508.
38. Canter JA, Olson LM, Spencer K, Schnetz-Boutaud N, Anderson B, et al. (2008) Mitochondrial DNA polymorphism A4917G is independently associated with age-related macular degeneration. PLoS One 3: e2091.
39. Kenney MC, Hertzog D, Chak G, Atilano SR, Khatibi N, et al. (2013) Mitochondrial DNA haplogroups confer differences in risk for age-related macular degeneration: A case control study. BMC Med Genet 14: 4.
40. Lau LI, Chiou SH, Liu CJ, Yen MY, Wei YH (2011) The effect of photo-oxidative stress and inflammatory cytokine on complement factor H expression in retinal pigment epithelial cells. Invest Ophthalmol Vis Sci 52: 6832–6841.
41. Sparrow JR, Boulton M (2005) RPE lipofuscin and its role in retinal pathobiology. Exp Eye Res 80: 595–606.
42. Youn HY, McCanna DJ, Sivak JG, Jones LW (2011) In vitro ultraviolet-induced damage in human corneal, lens, and retinal pigment epithelial cells. Mol Vis 17: 237–246.
43. Gill R, Tsung A, Billiar T (2010) Linking oxidative stress to inflammation: Toll-like receptors. Free Radic Biol Med 48: 1121–1132.
44. Khaper N, Bryan S, Dhingra S, Singal R, Bajaj A, et al. (2010) Targeting the vicious inflammation-oxidative stress cycle for the management of heart failure. Antioxid Redox Signal 13: 1033–1049.
45. Roduit R, Schorderet DF (2008) MAP kinase pathways in UV-induced apoptosis of retinal pigment epithelium ARPE19 cells. Apoptosis 13: 343–353.
46. Ding JD, Lin J, Mace BE, Herrmann R, Sullivan P, et al. (2008) Targeting age-related macular degeneration with Alzheimer's disease based immunotherapies: Anti-amyloid-beta antibody attenuates pathologies in an age-related macular degeneration mouse model. Vision Res 48: 339–345.
47. Liu XC, Liu XF, Jian CX, Li CJ, He SZ (2012) IL-33 is induced by amyloid-beta stimulation and regulates inflammatory cytokine production in retinal pigment epithelium cells. Inflammation 35: 776–784.
48. Pochampalli MR, Bitler BG, Schroeder JA (2007) Transforming growth factor alpha dependent cancer progression is modulated by Muc1. Cancer Res 67: 6591–6598.
49. Moskal TL, Huang S, Ellis LM, Fritsche HA Jr, Chakrabarty S (1995) Serum levels of transforming growth factor alpha in gastrointestinal cancer patients. Cancer Epidemiol Biomarkers Prev 4: 127–131.
50. Chakrabarty S, Huang S, Moskal TL, Fritsche HA Jr (1994) Elevated serum levels of transforming growth factor-alpha in breast cancer patients. Cancer Lett 79: 157–160.
51. Chien CH, Huang CC, Lin YH, Shen J, Chow SN (1997) Detection of serum transforming growth factor-alpha in patients of primary epithelial ovarian cancers by enzyme immunoassay. Gynecol Oncol 66: 405–410.
52. Wang QE, Milum K, Han C, Huang YW, Wani G, et al. (2011) Differential contributory roles of nucleotide excision and homologous recombination repair for enhancing cisplatin sensitivity in human ovarian cancer cells. Mol Cancer 10: 24.
53. Song EL, Hou YP, Yu SP, Chen SG, Huang JT, et al. (2011) EFEMP1 expression promotes angiogenesis and accelerates the growth of cervical cancer in vivo. Gynecol Oncol 121: 174–180.

54. Seeliger H, Camaj P, Ischenko I, Kleespies A, De Toni EN, et al. (2009) EFEMP1 expression promotes in vivo tumor growth in human pancreatic adenocarcinoma. Mol Cancer Res 7: 189–198.
55. Marmorstein LY, Munier FL, Arsenijevic Y, Schorderet DF, McLaughlin PJ, et al. (2002) Aberrant accumulation of EFEMP1 underlies drusen formation in Malattia Leventinese and age-related macular degeneration. Proc Natl Acad Sci U S A 99: 13067–13072.
56. Andreozzi R, Canterino M, Di Somma I, Lo Giudice R, Marotta R, et al. (2008) Effect of combined physico-chemical processes on the phytotoxicity of olive mill wastewaters. Water Res 42: 1684–1692.
57. Ramkumar HL, Zhang J, Chan CC (2010) Retinal ultrastructure of murine models of dry age-related macular degeneration (AMD). Prog Retin Eye Res 29: 169–190.
58. Roybal CN, Marmorstein LY, Vander Jagt DL, Abcouwer SF (2005) Aberrant accumulation of fibulin-3 in the endoplasmic reticulum leads to activation of the unfolded protein response and VEGF expression. Invest Ophthalmol Vis Sci 46: 3973–3979.
59. Ren D, Tu HC, Kim H, Wang GX, Bean GR, et al. (2010) BID, BIM, and PUMA are essential for activation of the BAX- and BAK-dependent cell death program. Science 330: 1390–1393.
60. Yu JS, Koujak S, Nagase S, Li CM, Su T, et al. (2008) PCDH8, the human homolog of PAPC, is a candidate tumor suppressor of breast cancer. Oncogene 27: 4657–4665.
61. Marti A, Hafezi F, Lansel N, Hegi ME, Wenzel A, et al. (1998) Light-induced cell death of retinal photoreceptors in the absence of p53. Invest Ophthalmol Vis Sci 39: 846–849.
62. Doonan F, Donovan M, Gomez-Vicente V, Bouillet P, Cotter TG (2007) Bim expression indicates the pathway to retinal cell death in development and degeneration. J Neurosci 27: 10887–10894.
63. Gomez-Vicente V, Doonan F, Donovan M, Cotter TG (2006) Induction of BIM(EL) following growth factor withdrawal is a key event in caspase-dependent apoptosis of 661W photoreceptor cells. Eur J Neurosci 24: 981–990.
64. Zhou G, Strom RC, Giguere V, Williams RW (2001) Modulation of retinal cell populations and eye size in retinoic acid receptor knockout mice. Mol Vis 7: 253–260.
65. Nishikiori N, Osanai M, Chiba H, Kojima T, Mitamura Y, et al. (2007) Glial cell-derived cytokines attenuate the breakdown of vascular integrity in diabetic retinopathy. Diabetes 56: 1333–1340.
66. D'Aquila P, Rose G, Panno ML, Passarino G, Bellizzi D (2012) SIRT3 gene expression: a link between inherited mitochondrial DNA variants and oxidative stress. Gene 497: 323–329.
67. Bellizzi D, Taverna D, D'Aquila P, De Blasi S, De Benedictis G (2009) Mitochondrial DNA variability modulates mRNA and intra-mitochondrial protein levels of HSP60 and HSP75: Experimental evidence from cybrid lines. Cell Stress Chaperones 14: 265–271.
68. Bellizzi D, Cavalcante P, Taverna D, Rose G, Passarino G, et al. (2006) Gene expression of cytokines and cytokine receptors is modulated by the common variability of the mitochondrial DNA in cybrid cell lines. Genes Cells 11: 883–891.
69. Gomez-Duran A, Pacheu-Grau D, Lopez-Gallardo E, Diez-Sanchez C, Montoya J, et al. (2010) Unmasking the causes of multifactorial disorders: OXPHOS differences between mitochondrial haplogroups. Hum Mol Genet 19: 3343–3353.

12

Dynamic Increase in Extracellular ATP Accelerates Photoreceptor Cell Apoptosis via Ligation of P2RX7 in Subretinal Hemorrhage

Shoji Notomi[1], Toshio Hisatomi[1,2]*, Yusuke Murakami[1], Hiroto Terasaki[3], Shozo Sonoda[3], Ryo Asato[1,2], Atsunobu Takeda[1], Yasuhiro Ikeda[1], Hiroshi Enaida[1], Taiji Sakamoto[3], Tatsuro Ishibashi[1]

1 Department of Ophthalmology, Graduate School of Medical Sciences, Kyushu University, Fukuoka, Japan, 2 Clinical Research Institute, National Hospital Organization Kyushu Medical Center, Fukuoka, Japan, 3 Department of Ophthalmology, Graduate School of Medical Sciences, Kagoshima University, Kagoshima, Japan

Abstract

Photoreceptor degeneration is the most critical cause of visual impairment in age-related macular degeneration (AMD). In neovascular form of AMD, severe photoreceptor loss develops with subretinal hemorrhage due to choroidal neovascularization (CNV), growth of abnormal blood vessels from choroidal circulation. However, the detailed mechanisms of this process remain elusive. Here we demonstrate that neovascular AMD with subretinal hemorrhage accompanies a significant increase in extracellular ATP, and that extracellular ATP initiates neurodegenerative processes through specific ligation of Purinergic receptor P2X, ligand-gated ion channel, 7 (P2RX7; P2X7 receptor). Increased extracellular ATP levels were found in the vitreous samples of AMD patients with subretinal hemorrhage compared to control vitreous samples. Extravascular blood induced a massive release of ATP and photoreceptor cell apoptosis in co-culture with primary retinal cells. Photoreceptor cell apoptosis accompanied mitochondrial apoptotic pathways, namely activation of caspase-9 and translocation of apoptosis-inducing factor (AIF) from mitochondria to nuclei, as well as TUNEL-detectable DNA fragmentation. These hallmarks of photoreceptor cell apoptosis were prevented by brilliant blue G (BBG), a selective P2RX7 antagonist, which is an approved adjuvant in ocular surgery. Finally, in a mouse model of subretinal hemorrhage, photoreceptor cells degenerated through BBG-inhibitable apoptosis, suggesting that ligation of P2RX7 by extracellular ATP may accelerate photoreceptor cell apoptosis in AMD with subretinal hemorrhage. Our results indicate a novel mechanism that could involve neuronal cell death not only in AMD but also in hemorrhagic disorders in the CNS and encourage the potential application of BBG as a neuroprotective therapy.

Editor: Mike O. Karl, Center for Regenerative Therapies Dresden, Germany

Funding: This study was supported by a Grant-In-Aid for Scientific Research (number 21791690) from the Ministry of Education, Culture, Sports, Science, and Technology, Japan. The funders had no role in study design, data collection and analysis, decision to publish, or preparation of the manuscript.

Competing Interests: The authors have declared that no competing interests exist.

* E-mail: hisatomi@med.kyushu-u.ac.jp

Introduction

Age-related macular degeneration (AMD) is the leading cause of irreversible vision loss in the elderly in the developed world [1]. Among Americans, the estimated prevalence of AMD is projected to increase by more than 50% by the year 2020 [2]. In the neovascular form of this disorder, severe visual loss commonly occurs as a result of the invasion of abnormal blood vessels from the choroidal circulation, namely choroidal neovascularization (CNV), which induces irreversible damage to the overlying retina [3]. CNV could be induced by focally increased inflammatory and proangiogenic factors and/or by a decrease in anti-angiogenic factors. Various clinical as well as experimental studies have shown that vascular endothelial growth factor (VEGF), a proangiogenic glycoprotein, could be the most important factor for development of CNV [4]. In recent years, pharmacological inhibition of VEGF has offered the first opportunity to improve visual outcomes in patients diagnosed with this disorder [5]. Intraocular injections of an anti-VEGF antibody, such as ranibizumab or bevacizumab, have improved visual outcomes in several clinical trials [6]. However, patients with predominant subretinal hemorrhage, a commonly encountered event in neovascular AMD, still have poor visual prognoses [7]. Pneumatic displacement or surgical evacuation of subretinal blood with the use of recombinant tissue plasminogen activator (tPA) failed to improve the visual outcomes of patients with submacular hemorrhage due to AMD in a controlled clinical trial [8].

The most crucial stage of severe visual impairment is photoreceptor loss due to development of the CNV and related events such as subretinal hemorrhage or exudative retinal detachment in neovascular AMD [3]. Several clinical and experimental studies have shown that subretinal hemorrhage induces severe photoreceptor cell apoptosis [9–10] in line with severe tissue damage due to subarachnoid or intracerebral hematoma in the central nervous system (CNS) [11–12]. Previous studies have found that several potential neurotoxic agents were released from extravascular blood, such as hemoglobin [13], iron [10] [14–15], or glutamate [16], indicating that neurotoxic agents released from extravascular blood can be potential therapeutic targets.

Photoreceptor degeneration involves the activation of several signaling pathways of regulated cell death that can constitute potential therapeutic targets. Accordingly, attempts have been made to inhibit caspases, which play major roles in the apoptotic machinery [17–18], although pharmacological pan-caspase inhibitors largely failed to preserve the structures and functions of photoreceptors [19–20]. Caspases can be activated as a result of mitochondrial outer membrane permeabilization (MOMP) and the subsequent mitochondrial release of cytochrome *c* that triggers the Apaf-1 (apoptotic protease activating factor 1) apoptosome activation. MOMP also results in the mitochondrial release of apoptosis-inducing factor (AIF), which translocates to the nucleus and participates in the caspase-independent peripheral chromatin condensation and large-scale DNA fragmentation [21]. These findings suggest the existence of redundant cell death mechanisms downstream of MOMP [19] [22–23].

An alternative strategy to inhibit the mitochondrial apoptotic pathway is to intercept the initiating upstream proapoptotic signals. Recently, adenosine-5′-triphosphate (ATP) has been discovered as a major extracellular messenger that can contribute to lethal signaling [24]. Extracellular ATP can act on purinergic receptors, which are classified into two classes, the ionotropic, ligand-gated P2X receptors and the metabotropic, G protein-coupled P2Y receptors [25]. Among the seven subtypes of mammalian P2X receptors [26], the P2X7 receptor (P2RX7) differs from other P2X receptor subtypes by its long cytoplasmic, carboxy-terminal tail (240 amino acids) and mediates cellular signals that can trigger cell death [27–28]. P2RX7 is widely expressed in various organs, including those of immune system [29] and central nervous system [30]. In the retina, P2RX7 is expressed in Müller glia [31] as well as in both inner and outer retinal neurons, including retinal ganglion cells [32] and photoreceptor cells [33–34]. Furthermore, Fletcher and her group reported that P2RX7 has physiological functions as a neurotransmitter receptor in the retina [35], while photoreceptor cells have been shown to undergo apoptosis in response to an excess of extracellular ATP [36]. Recently, we have shown that photoreceptor cell apoptosis involves P2RX7 activation with caspase-8, -9 cleavage and mitochondrio-nuclear translocation of AIF. Moreover, photoreceptor cell apoptosis can be attenuated by Brilliant Blue G (BBG), a pharmacological P2RX7 antagonist that acts by blocking the interaction between extracellular ATP and P2RX7 [37]. Indeed, BBG administration can confer neuroprotective effects in several models of Alzheimer's, Parkinson's disease, and spinal cord injury [38–40] as well as in the retina [41–42]. BBG is also known as an adjuvant approved for intraoperative use in ocular surgery. In chromovitrectomy, vital dyes are introduced to improve the visualization of intraocular tissues for specific procedures, such as internal limiting membrane (ILM) peeling during vitrectomy [43–44].

Hence, we hypothesized that ATP acting on P2RX7 is involved in the pathogenesis of photoreceptor loss in subretinal hemorrhage. To examine the clinical relevance of this hypothesis, we compared extracellular ATP concentrations in human vitreous samples from patients with retinal diseases, including AMD. Our results showed that increased extracellular ATP substantially contributes to photoreceptor loss and that BBG provides substantial neuroprotective effects in cases of subretinal hemorrhage.

Materials and Methods

Ethics Statement

Procedures using human samples were conducted in accordance with the Declaration of Helsinki and approved by the Kyushu University Institutional Review Board for Clinical Research. We obtained written informed consent from all the participants. All procedures using mice were performed in strict accordance with the guidelines for Association for Research in Vision and Ophthalmology (ARVO) and Proper Conduct of Animal Experiments (Science Council of Japan). The experimental protocol was approved by the Animal Care and Use Committee of Kyushu University. All efforts were made to minimize the number of animals used and their suffering.

Animals

Adult (8 weeks of age) male C57BL6JJcl mice (CLEA, Tokyo, Japan) and isogenic P2rx7$^{-/-}$ mice, the latter kindly provided by Pfizer Inc. (Gorton, CT), were used in this study. Recently, the rd8 (retinal degeneration 8) mutation was reported to be widely inherited across strains supplied by common commercial vendors and ES cell lines [45–46]. We confirmed that P2rx7$^{-/-}$ mice do not carry the rd8 mutation by DNA sequencing (Supporting Information S1). All procedures using mice were performed in strict accordance with the guidelines for Association for Research in Vision and Ophthalmology (ARVO) and Proper Conduct of Animal Experiments (Science Council of Japan). The experimental protocol was approved by the Animal Care and Use Committee of Kyushu University. All efforts were made to minimize the number of animals used and their suffering.

Human Vitreous Samples

Procedures using human samples were conducted in accordance with the Declaration of Helsinki and approved by the Kyushu University Institutional Review Board for Clinical Research. We obtained written informed consent from all the participants. Vitreous samples (1.0–1.2 ml) were collected from patients who underwent pars plana vitrectomy at the Vitreoretinal Center in Kyushu University Hospital and Kagoshima University Hospital, for the treatment of macular hole (MH, $n = 10$), epiretinal membrane (ERM, $n = 10$), or age-related macular degeneration (AMD) with vitreous hemorrhage (VH) ($n = 15$). The clinical characteristics of the patients are summarized in Table 1 and Supporting Information S2.

ATP Measurements

The ATP levels of collected samples (100 μl each in 96-well microplates; BD Falcon, Franklin Lakes, NJ) were immediately determined by using luciferin-luciferase reaction buffer (ATP bioluminescence assay kit, FL-AA; Sigma-Aldrich, St. Louis, MO) and a Flex Station 3 Multi-Mode Microplate Reader (Molecular

Table 1. Clinical characteristics of patients with MH, ERM, and AMD with VH.

Characteristics	MH	ERM	AMD with VH	*P*
n	10	10	15	
Age (years)				
Mean (SD)	67.9 (6.8)	70.7 (6.4)	70.7 (10.4)	NS
Gender, *n*				
Male	4	2	9	
Female	6	8	6	NS

The patients underwent pars plana vitrectomy and the collected vitreous samples were subjected to ATP measurement by luciferase assay. There were no significant differences in age or sex ratio among the three groups.

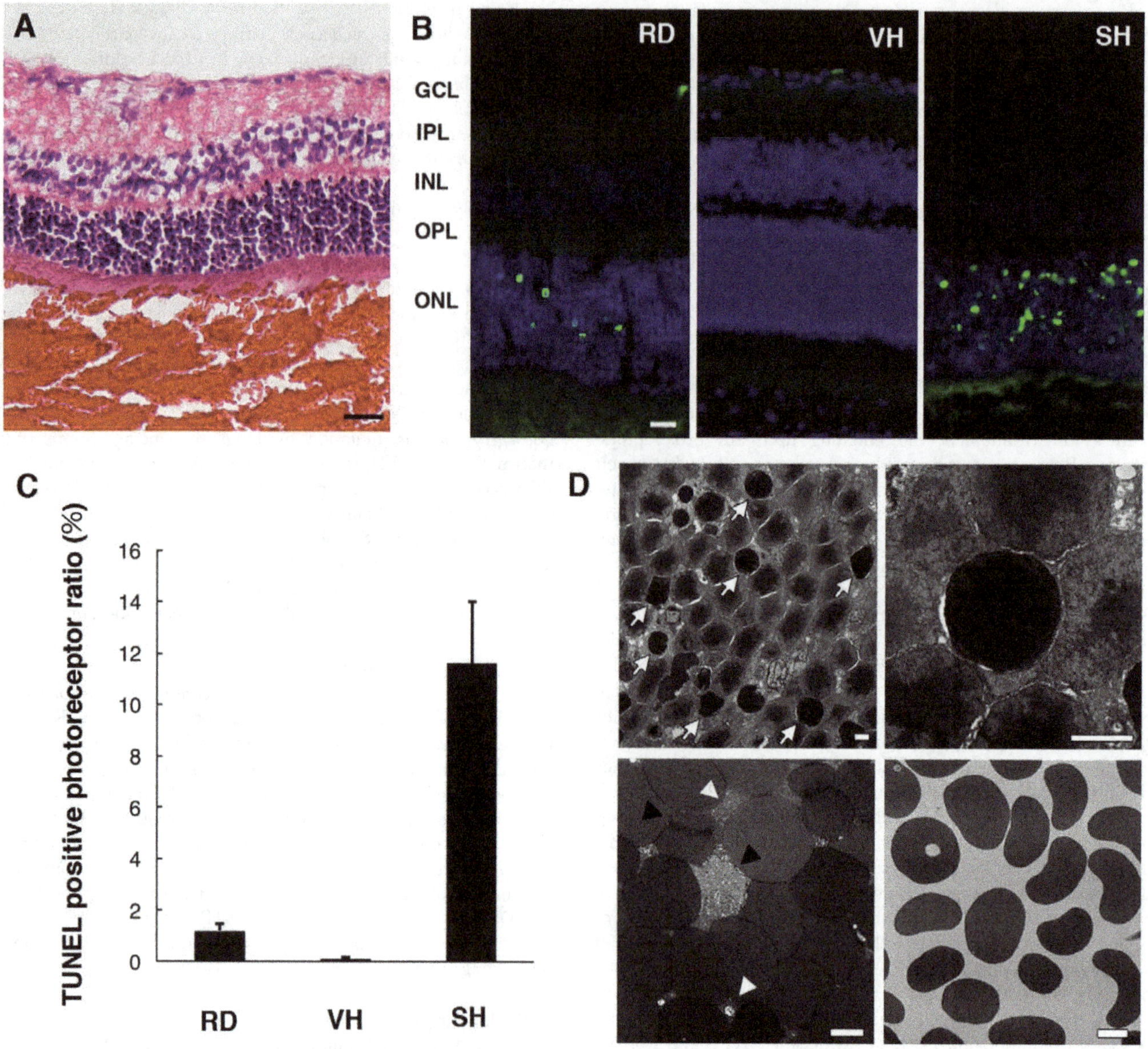

Figure 1. Abundant photoreceptor cell apoptosis in subretinal hemorrhage. Subretinal injection or vitreous injection of autologous blood was performed in C57BL6 mice. (A) A representative image of hematoxylin/eosin staining in subretinal hemorrhage is shown. Scale bar: 100 μm. (B) Some TUNEL$^+$ nuclei were detected in the outer nuclear layer (ONL) in retinal detachment (RD), while abundant TUNEL$^+$ nuclei were found in subretinal hemorrhage (SH). TUNEL$^+$ cells were less detectable in vitreous hemorrhage (VH) (TUNEL in green, propidium iodide in blue). Scale bar: 20 μm. GCL; ganglion cell layer, IPL; inner plexiform layer, INL; inner nuclear layer, OPL; outer plexiform layer, ONL; outer nuclear layer. (C) The numbers of TUNEL$^+$ photoreceptors in RD, VH, and SH. (D) Electron microscopy revealed that numerous photoreceptor cells had undergone apoptosis with chromatin condensation (arrows in the top left panel) or cellular shrinkage (top right panel). Some erythrocytes lost their plasma membranes (black arrowheads in the bottom left panel) and hemolytic debris was observed among erythrocytes (white arrowheads in the bottom left panel) in the subretinal hemorrhage. Minimal hemolytic change was observed in the vitreous hemorrhage (bottom right panel). Scale bars: 2 μm.

Devices, Sunnyvale, CA). The ATP levels detected by the luminometer were expressed in relative light units (RLU).

Mouse Blood Collection

Mice were anesthetized with an intraperitoneal injection of pentobarbital and exsanguinated via cardiac puncture into collection tubes containing heparin. For the isolation of plasma, collected whole blood was immediately centrifuged at 18000 g for 60 seconds at 4°C to isolate plasma as previously described [47]. For the isolation of erythrocytes, the plasma, platelets, and leukocytes were removed as supernatant and buffy coat after centrifugation at 900 g for 3 min. Isolated erythrocytes were resuspended in medium supplemented with 0.5% bovine serum albumin to the corresponding final hematocrit. To determine ATP levels after hemolysis, whole blood or isolated erythrocytes were lysed in distilled water and then assayed using a firefly luciferase assay (FL-AA) as described above.

Adult Mouse Primary Retinal Cell Cultures

Adult primary retinal cell cultures were prepared as previously described with minor modifications [48] [22]. Primary retinal cells were cultured in 4-well chambers (Nunc; part of Thermo Fisher

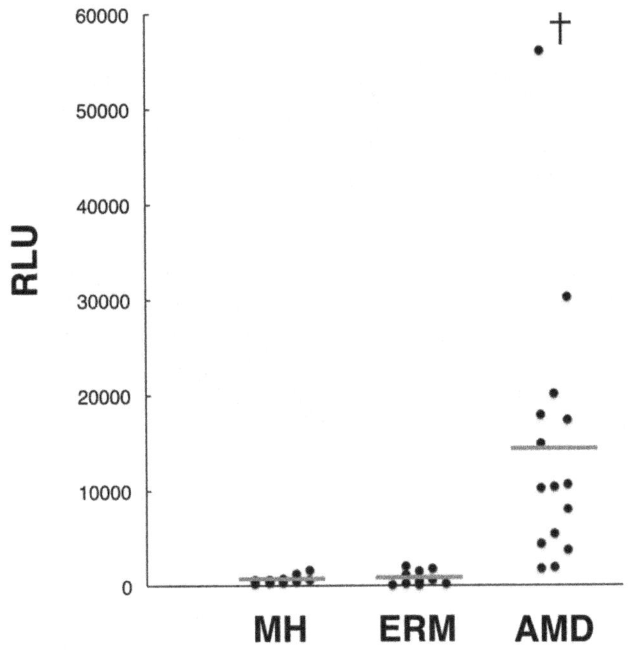

Figure 2. The ATP levels in human vitreous of retinal diseases. Human vitreous samples were collected during vitreoretinal surgery from patients with MH ($n = 10$), ERM ($n = 10$), and AMD ($n = 15$). The ATP levels of vitreous samples were determined by luciferin-luciferase assay (RLU: relative light units). †$P<0.01$.

Scientific, Bremen, Germany) with Neurobasal-A medium (Invitrogen, Carlsbad, CA) containing B27 supplement without antioxidants (NBA/B27AO–; Invitrogen), 1 µg/ml insulin, and 12 µg/ml gentamicin. To determine the number of adherent photoreceptor cells, immunofluorescent staining was performed with a rabbit anti-recoverin antibody (Millipore, Bedford, MA). For blood clot exposure, we utilized a double chamber system [49]. After 50 µl of whole blood was placed on membranes with micropores in the upper chamber (Transwell; Corning Life Sciences, Lowell, MA), 100 µl of culture medium was added to the upper chamber. Primary retinal cell cultures were prepared in the lower chamber and incubated with or without 10 U/ml apyrase (Sigma-Aldrich, St. Louis, MO) for 24 h. The culture medium was collected and centrifuged, and the ATP levels of supernatants were analyzed by the luciferin-luciferase assay. For exogenous ATP administration, 1 mM ATP (Sigma-Aldrich) was added to the culture medium, and the medium were incubated for 24 h with or without 30 min pre-incubation of BBG.

Viability Assay in Primary Retinal Cell Cultures

To assess the viability of primary retinal cells, we used calcein AM (2 µM) or MitoTracker Orange CMTMRos (200 nM; M7510; Invitrogen), added for 30 min to primary retinal cell cultures. Then, cultured cells were fixed with 4% paraformaldehyde and recoverin-labeled calcein$^+$ or CMTMRos$^+$ photoreceptor cells were counted in 10 random fields by blinded observers using ImageJ software. Values are given as the means ± SDs of 10 replicate wells.

Subretinal Injections

Experimental retinal detachment was performed as previously described [19] [22] [48] [50]. Mice were anesthetized with an intraperitoneal injection of pentobarbital, and their pupils were dilated with topical 1% tropicamide and 2.5% phenylephrine hydrochloride. Then, 2 µl of sodium hyaluronate (Opegan-Hi; Santen Pharmaceuticals, Tokyo, Japan) with a mixture of 1 mM ATP or vehicle PBS, was gently injected into the subretinal space with a 30-gauge needle through the sclera posterior to the limbus to produce focally detached retina. The injection of sodium hyaluronate reproducibly generated similar retinal detachments. Successful retinal detachment was confirmed by ophthalmoscopy and generally involved one third of the retina as previously described [51]. To establish a mouse model of subretinal hemorrhage, autologous blood with a mixture of 50 µM BBG or vehicle PBS was immediately injected into the subretinal space as previously described [10]. The height of retinal detachments was measured at the top of the detached retina in cryosections (Supporting Information S3). Subretinal injections were only performed in the right eye of each animal, and 6 eyes were examined in each group. The mice were sacrificed 24 h after treatment. Their eyes were harvested, frozen at nitrogen liquid temperature, and cryosectioned for histochemical examinations.

TdT-dUTP Terminal Nick-end Labeling (TUNEL)

TUNEL analysis and quantification of TUNEL-positive cells were performed as previously described using the ApopTag Fluorescein In Situ Apoptosis Detection Kit (Millipore) [22]. Nuclei were counter-stained with propidium iodide or Hoechst 33342. The center of the detached retina was photographed, and the TUNEL-positive cells in the outer nuclear layer (ONL) were counted by two blinded observers. The ratios of photoreceptor cell apoptosis were expressed as the percentage of TUNEL-positive nuclei among the total number of nuclei in the section, and the results are presented as the means ± SDs.

Electron Microscopy

The posterior segments of enucleated mouse eyes were fixed in PBS containing 1% glutaraldehyde and 1% paraformaldehyde, postfixed in veronal acetate buffer osmium tetroxide (2%), dehydrated in ethanol and water, and embedded in Epon. Ultrathin sections were cut from blocks and mounted on copper grids. The specimens were observed with an H-7770 transmission electron microscope (Hitachi, Tokyo, Japan).

Immunofluorescence

Immunofluorescence was performed with slight modifications to a previous method [22]. Briefly, rabbit anti-AIF (R&D Systems, Minneapolis, MN), anti-mouse cleaved caspase-9 (Cell Signaling Technology, Beverly, MA), and anti-recoverin (Millipore) were used as primary antibodies and incubated at 4°C overnight. Goat anti-rabbit IgGs conjugated to Alexa Fluor 546 or 647 (Invitrogen) were used as secondary antibodies and incubated at room temperature for 1 h.

Statistical Analysis

Statistical differences between the two groups were analyzed by means of the Mann–Whitney U-test. Multiple group comparison was performed by ANOVA followed by Tukey–Kramer adjustments. The sex ratio in each group was analyzed by Fisher's exact test. Differences were considered significant at $P<0.05$ (*) and $P<0.01$ (**). All values were expressed as the means ± SDs.

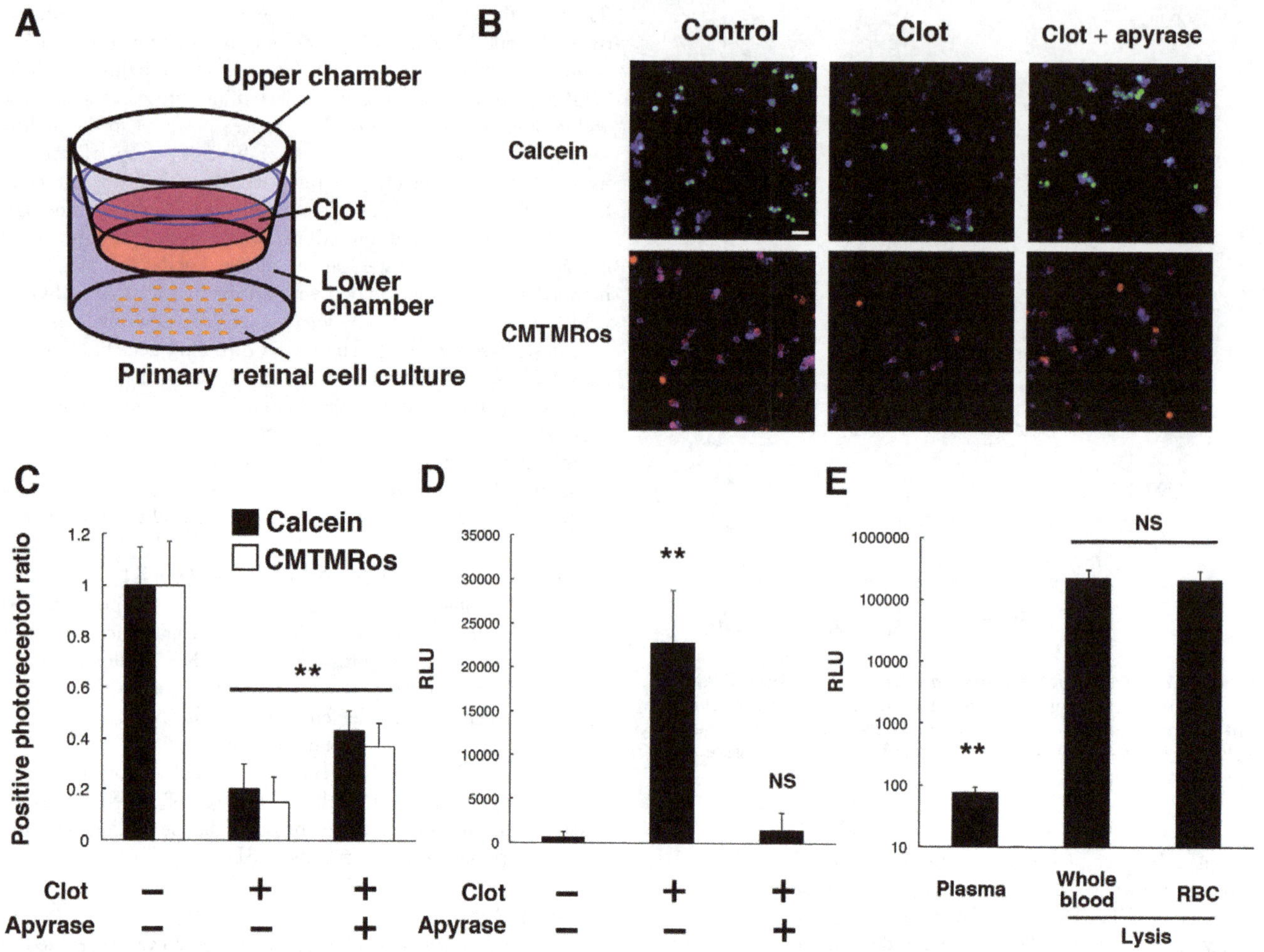

Figure 3. Photoreceptor cell apoptosis in primary retinal cell cultures with blood clots. (A) Schematic image of the double chamber co-culture system of primary retinal cells and blood clots. (B) and (C) The viability of primary retinal cells in the lower chamber was accessed by calcein AM or MitoTracker CMTMRos after 24 h of culture with addition of a clot in the upper chamber (calcein in green, CMTMRos in red, recoverin in blue). The frequency of calcein$^+$ or CMTMRos$^+$ photoreceptors significantly decreased after incubation with clots. Apyrase treatment significantly rescued photoreceptors. (D) The ATP levels of culture medium in the lower chamber were significantly increased by clot exposure, and reversed by apyrase treatment. (E) The ATP levels in plasma and blood. $n = 10$ per group; $^{**}P<0.01$. Scale bar: 20 μm.

Results

Abundant Photoreceptor Cell Apoptosis in a Mouse Model of Subretinal Hemorrhage

To investigate the clinically relevant pathology of photoreceptor cell death in neovascular AMD, we created a mouse model of subretinal hemorrhage. Autologous blood drawn from the tail vein was injected into the subretinal space (Figure 1A). Retinal cell death has also been shown to occur after detachment of neurosensory retina [19] [52]. To evaluate the toxicity of subretinal blood to the overlying retina, a control condition was established by performing the retinal detachment using subretinal injections of sodium hyaluronate in line with our previous methods [19]. We examined the height of retinal detachment after injections of sodium hyaluronate or autologous blood and found no significant difference (Supporting Information S3). Abundant TUNEL$^+$ photoreceptor cells were detected in the outer nuclear layer (ONL) 24 h after the injections of autologous blood, while quite a small number of apoptotic photoreceptor cells were detected in control retinal detachment within 24 h (Figure 1, B and C). This result indicates that subretinal blood induces massive apoptotic photoreceptor cell death within 24 h and thus would cause irreversible visual impairment in the case of subretinal hemorrhage. Next, to investigate the toxicity of vitreous hemorrhage, autologous blood was injected into the vitreous cavity. Only a few TUNEL$^+$ cells were found after this injection in contrast to the case with subretinal hemorrhage (Figure 1, B and C), suggesting that a massive hemorrhage could severely reduce the integrity of photoreceptors, if it were tightly packed into the subretinal space. Moreover, electron microscopy revealed the characteristic signs of photoreceptor cell apoptosis, such as chromatin condensation or cellular shrinkage (Figure 1D). Numerous erythrocytes were observed in the subretinal clots. Some of those erythrocytes lost their plasma membranes with hemolytic debris 24 h after the injections, while minimal hemolytic change was observed in vitreous hemorrhage (Figure 1D). These observations suggest that potential neurotoxic factors were released from the blood clots during erythrocyte hemolysis.

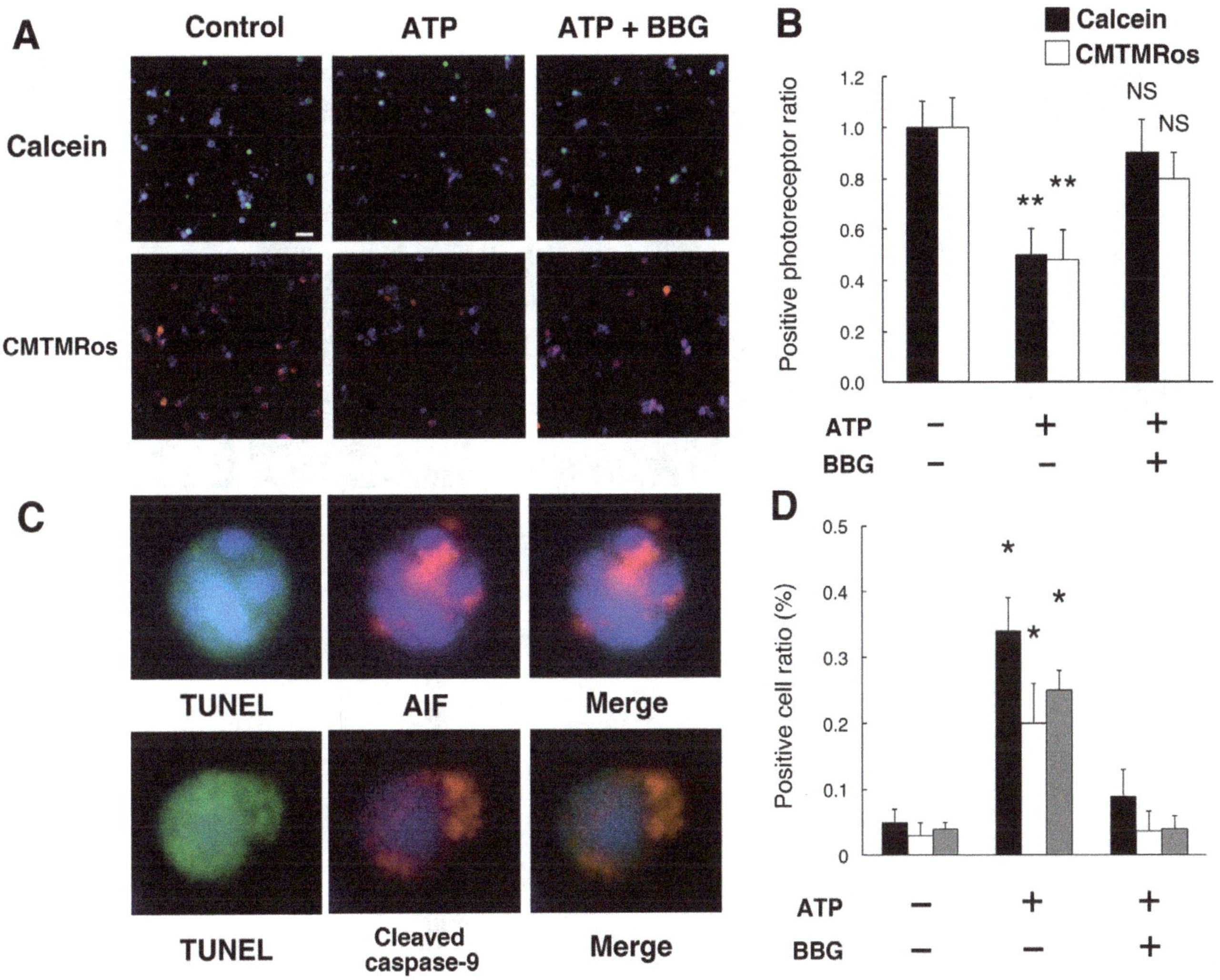

Figure 4. Photoreceptor cell apoptosis by ATP administration *in vitro.* (A) and (B) Calcein$^+$ or CMTMRos$^+$ photoreceptors were reduced by 24 h incubation of 1 mM ATP (calcein in green, CMTMRos in red, recoverin in blue). BBG notably attenuated the decline of viable photoreceptors. (C) and (D) Representative images of immuno-cytochemistry of AIF (top panels) and cleaved caspase-9 (bottom panels) in TUNEL$^+$ cells in primary retinal cell cultures (TUNEL in green, AIF or cleaved caspase-9 in red, Hoechst 33342 in blue) and the quantifications. $n = 10$ per group; *$P<0.05$. **$P<0.01$. Scale bar: 20 μm.

Increased ATP Levels in the Vitreous of Patients with Age-related Macular Degeneration

To examine the potential role of extracellular ATP in subretinal hemorrhage, we investigated the intraocular concentrations of ATP by using vitreous samples collected during vitreoretinal surgery from patients with MH, ERM, or AMD with vitreous hemorrhage (VH). There is minimal breakdown of the blood retinal barrier (BRB)–i.e., exudation or bleeding–in MH or ERM. In contrast, vitreous hemorrhage–that is, diffusion of a large amount of blood into the vitreous cavity from the subretinal hemorrhage–often occurs in AMD, and in some of these cases vitrectomy is performed for removal of the vitreous opacity [53–54]. ATP levels of vitreous samples were analyzed by luciferin-luciferase assay, which is used to quantify chemiluminescence upon ATP-dependent oxidation of luciferin. Notably, ATP concentrations were much higher in AMD with VH compared to MH or ERM (Figure 2). These results suggest that ATP levels in the subretinal space could be potentially higher than those detected in the vitreous, because extracellular ATP diffuses into the vitreous cavity from the subretinal space. Hence, the local concentration of ATP around photoreceptors might be higher than the concentration of ATP observed in vitreous samples. Moreover, the increase in extracellular ATP may be neurotoxic to the overlying retina in subretinal hemorrhage.

Extracellular ATP Induces Neurotoxicity in Primary Retinal Cell Cultures with Blood Clot

To identify potential neurotoxic factors released from the extravascular blood clots, we prepared mouse primary retinal cells in double chamber slides. Primary mouse retinal cell cultures were prepared as previously described [22] [48] in the lower chamber, while mouse blood was added to the upper chamber on membranes with micropores (Figure 3A). In this double chamber system, released soluble factors can easily diffuse between two chambers, while the blood clot itself remains in the upper chamber. Primary retinal cell cultures were incubated for 24 h with or without addition of a clot to the upper chamber. The cultures were also examined in the absence or presence of 10 U/

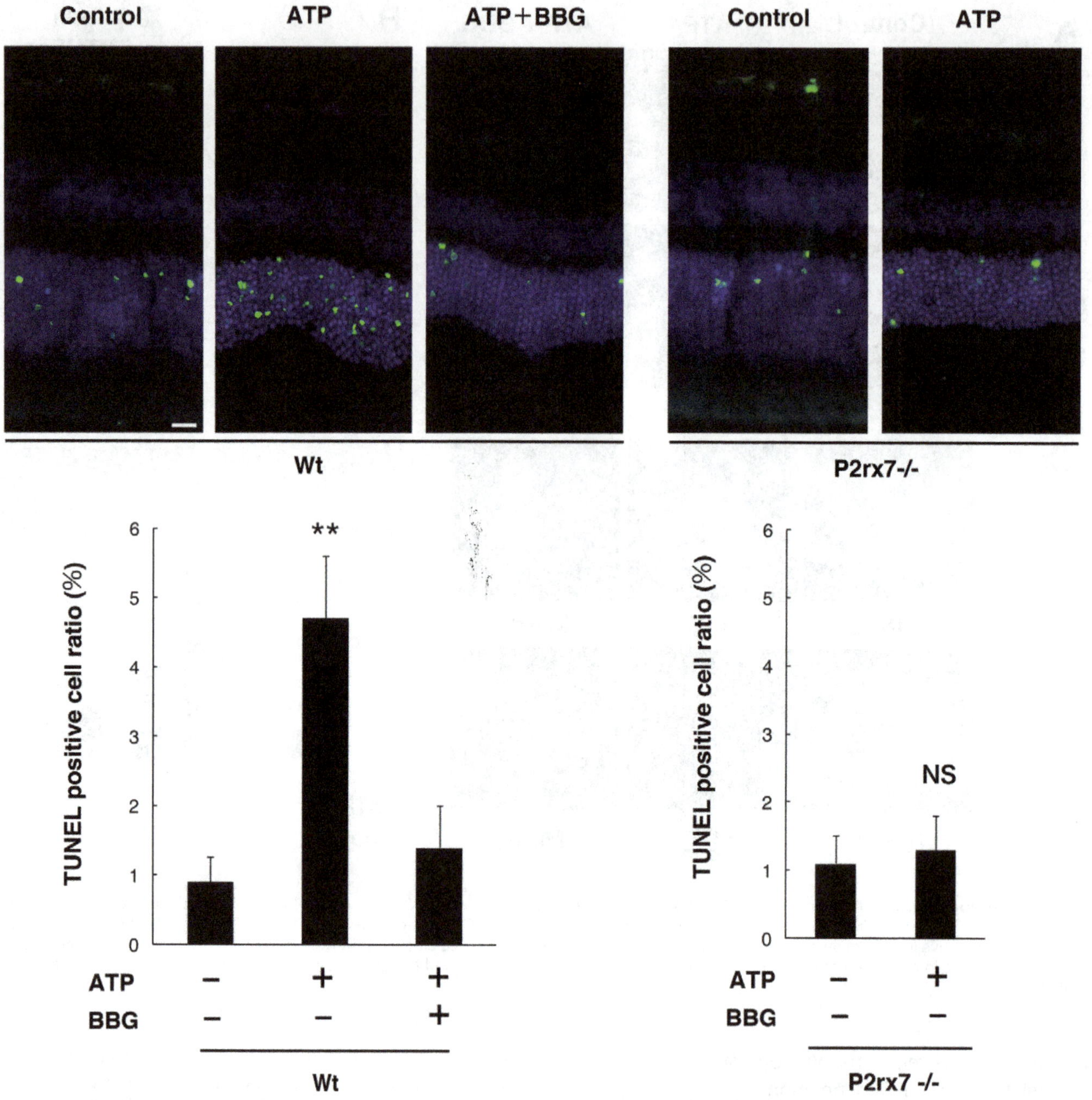

Figure 5. Photoreceptor cell apoptosis by subretinal injection of ATP. Exogenous ATP was injected into the subretinal space of Wt or P2rx7$^{-/-}$ mice. TUNEL-positive apoptotic cells developed in the ONL 24 h after the subretinal injection of 1 mM ATP (TUNEL in green and Hoechst 33342 in blue). $n=6$ per group; $^{**}P<0.01$. Scale bar: 20 μm.

ml apyrase, a soluble ATP-degrading enzyme (ecto-ATPase) in the lower chamber. At 24 h of incubation, the clot showed a significant reduction in live photoreceptor cells (Figure 3, B and C), which were identified by two fluorescent live cell sensors, calcein AM and MitoTracker CMTMRos, which only label intact, non-apoptotic cells, and metabolically active cells, respectively. Of note, addition of apyrase, an ecto-ATPase, rescued photoreceptors from blood toxicity (Figure 3, B and C), suggesting that ATP released from clots was a critical factor in reducing photoreceptor cell survival. To confirm the ATP release from the clot, ATP levels in the lower chamber were analyzed by luciferase assay. The ATP levels were markedly elevated in the culture medium in the lower chamber after the addition of a clot in the upper chamber (Figure 3D). Apyrase treatment efficiently reversed the increase in ATP levels in the lower chamber (Figure 3D), demonstrating the contribution of extracellular ATP to the clot-induced toxicity consistent with the results of the cell viability assay. To clarify the source of extracellular ATP, we examined the ATP concentrations of mouse plasma. Only a small amount of ATP was detected in collected plasma, suggesting that the ATP levels in plasma were minimal under physiological conditions. However, massive ATP release was observed after hemolysis in whole blood (Figure 3E). In addition, ATP levels did not differ significantly between whole blood and isolated erythrocytes after hemolysis (Figure 3E),

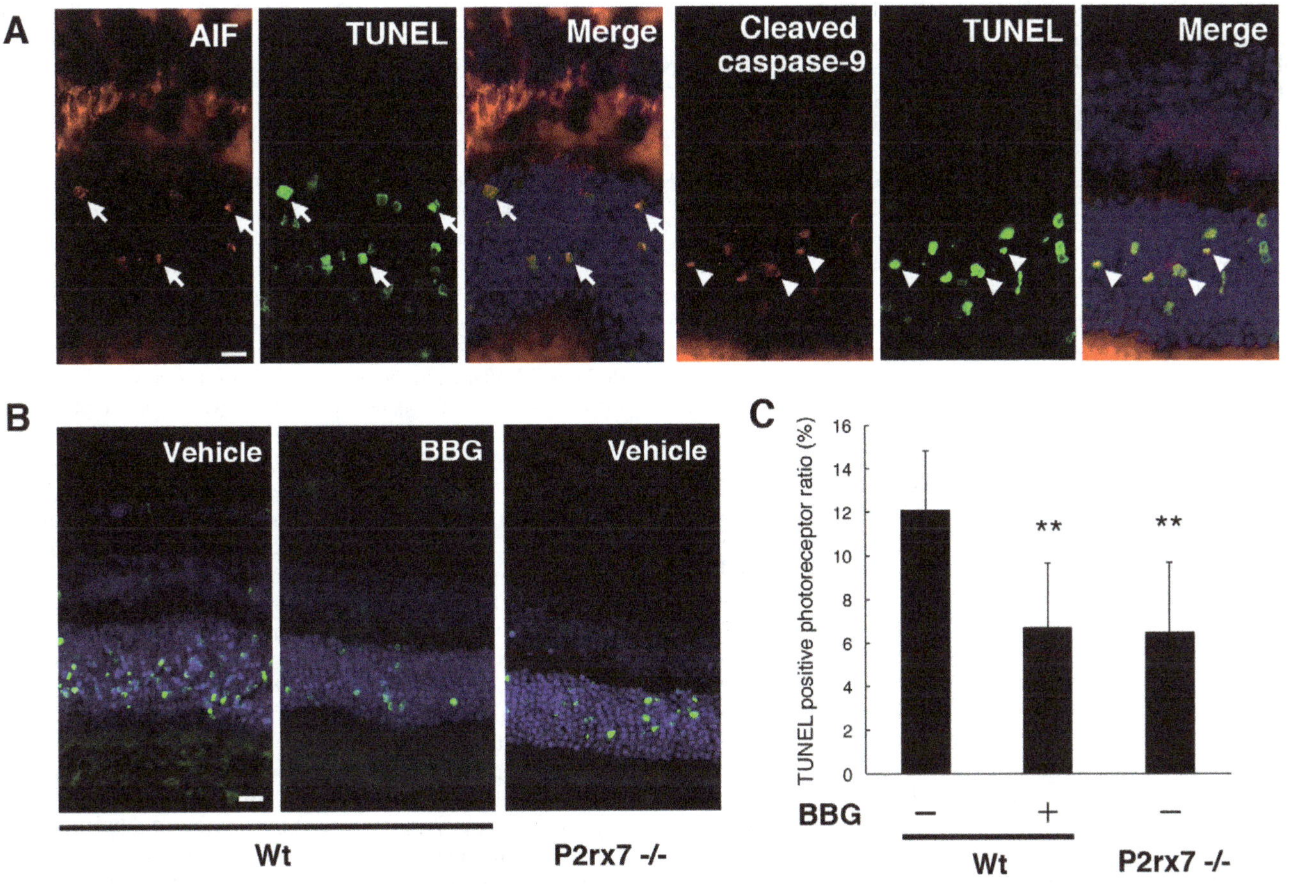

Figure 6. A P2RX7 antagonist prevents photoreceptor cell apoptosis in a mouse model of subretinal hemorrhage. (A) After the subretinal injection of autologous blood, photoreceptor cells underwent apoptotic cell death, and AIF-positive staining was observed in TUNEL$^+$ photoreceptor nuclei (arrows; AIF in red, TUNEL in green, and Hoechst 33342 in blue). Caspase-9 cleavage was also detected among TUNEL$^+$ nuclei (arrowheads; cleaved caspase-9 in red). Scale bar: 10 μm. (B) and (C) TUNEL$^+$ apoptotic cells in the absence or presence of 50 μM BBG treatment after experimental subretinal hemorrhage in Wt or P2rx7$^{-/-}$ mice. $n = 6$ per group; $^{**}P < 0.01$. Scale bar: 20 μm.

indicating that erythrocytes could be a dominant source of extracellular ATP from clots. Taken together, these results suggest that released extracellular ATP may be a potential neurotoxic factor in neovascular AMD with subretinal hemorrhage.

Extracellular ATP Induces Photoreceptor Cell Apoptosis *in vitro* and *in vivo*

To obtain the mechanistic insights into the contribution of ATP/P2RX7 to photoreceptor death, we performed ATP administrations in primary culture. The addition of exogenous ATP significantly reduced viable, calcein$^+$ or CMTMRos$^+$ photoreceptor cells, while BBG reversed the decline in live photoreceptor cells (Figure 4, A and B). Furthermore, ATP administration induced TUNEL-detectable degradation of DNA with signs of the mitochondrial apoptotic pathway, namely AIF translocation to the nucleus and caspase-9 cleavage, whereas BBG treatment significantly inhibited those effects (Figure 4, C and D). These results indicate that extracellular ATP can trigger photoreceptor cell apoptosis via P2RX7-dependent machinery.

Next, we measured retinal cell apoptosis in the presence or absence of subretinal administration of exogenous ATP to determine whether the increase of subretinal ATP could trigger photoreceptor cell death *in vivo*. Exogenous ATP was mixed with sodium hyaluronate and injected into the subretinal space of C57BL/6 mice. We confirmed that the height of retinal detachment in the presence of the ATP mixture was not significantly different from that in the absence of ATP mixture (Supporting Information S3). Subretinal injections without ATP induced only limited TUNEL-positive apoptotic events in the ONL after 24 h of injections (Figure 5), whereas TUNEL-detectable DNA degradation was significantly accelerated by the administration of 1 mM ATP in the subretinal space (Figure 5). The increased photoreceptor cell apoptosis was substantially reduced by administration of 50 μM BBG (Figure 5). Furthermore, the numbers of TUNEL$^+$ photoreceptor cells were reduced in P2rx7$^{-/-}$ mice, while there was massive loss of photoreceptors in wild-type (Wt) mice (Figure 5), indicating that the induction of apoptosis by P2RX7 activation was truly specific. Thus, ATP administration substantially mimicked the effects of ATP release from clots. Taken together, these results showed that excessive ATP facilitates photoreceptor cell apoptosis via P2RX7 activation *in vitro* and *in vivo*, indicating a pathological contribution of extracellular ATP in subretinal hemorrhage.

BBG Protects Photoreceptors in a Mouse Model of Subretinal Hemorrhage

The results obtained from clinical samples and the *in vitro* and *in vivo* experiments led us to investigate whether the pharmacological P2RX7 antagonist would have a beneficial effect on retinal damage in a more pathological setting–namely, an animal model of subretinal hemorrhage. Autologous blood was injected into the subretinal space alone or with a mixture of BBG (50 μM). Twenty-four hours after experimental subretinal hemorrhage, abundant TUNEL$^+$ photoreceptor cells were detected in the ONL with AIF translocation to the nucleus and caspase-9 cleavage (Figure 6A) in line with our previous reports that photoreceptor cells undergo apoptosis via the mitochondrial pathway as a result of MOMP [22]. These effects were notably attenuated by local injection of BBG (Figure 6, B and C). Moreover, TUNEL-detectable photoreceptor cell apoptosis was reduced in P2rx7$^{-/-}$ mice compared to Wt mice (Figure 6, B and C). Taken together, these results demonstrate that pharmacological inhibition of P2RX7 could results in neuroprotection of photoreceptors in cases of subretinal hemorrhage.

Discussion

In the present work, we have shown that severe human hemorrhagic pathologies, in particular AMD, are accompanied by a dynamic increase in extracellular ATP, which worsens photoreceptor degeneration. ATP was released from extravascular blood in primary retinal cell cultures *in vitro* and in a model of subretinal hemorrhage *in vivo*, and triggered severe photoreceptor cell apoptosis via P2RX7 ligation. We also provided mechanistic insights into exogenous ATP-induced photoreceptor cell apoptosis via mitochondrial apoptotic pathways–namely, the activation of caspase-9 and the mitochondrio-nuclear translocation of AIF. To our knowledge, this is the first report on pathogenic increase of extracellular ATP in hemorrhagic disorders in the retina as well as in the CNS. Finally, we demonstrated that BBG, a pharmacological P2RX7 antagonist, could correct photoreceptor cell death in a rodent model of subretinal hemorrhage.

The clinical application of anti-VEGF antibodies has enabled the regulation of CNV progression in patients with AMD worldwide [6]. However, patients still tend to have poor prognosis in neovascular AMD after massive subretinal hemorrhage. AMD as well as intracerebral hemorrhage causes severe tissue damage, suggesting that extravascular blood may become highly toxic to surrounding cells through the release of toxins [49]. In the current study, based on *in vitro* and *in vivo* models of blood neurotoxicity, we proposed a novel pathological pathway by which extracellular ATP could mediate mitochondrial apoptotic signaling. Moreover, we found that extracellular ATP levels can substantially increase in the presence of subretinal hemorrhage. Several potential mechanisms may account for the increase in extracellular ATP in hemophagic disorders. Acute cell lysis could be a source of ATP, in line with previous observations that ATP is released by acute stresses such as ischemia [55], hypotony [56], or oxygen/glucose deprivation [57]. In the present study, we observed that some erythrocytes underwent hemolysis under the retina and that blood clot exposure caused significant elevation of extracellular ATP *in vitro*. Hence, hemolysis could be a part of the cause of the ATP increase in subretinal hemorrhage. Moreover, the massive ATP release may be caused by usurpation of the physiological mechanism of release. Indeed, erythrocytes are sensitive to low oxygen supply and upregulate ATP efflux to modulate vascular tone via P2Y receptors on the endothelium [58]. These effluxes of ATP from erythrocytes may account for the findings that there were sustained elevation of ATP levels in the vitreous samples from AMD but not in those from MH or ERM.

Our results demonstrated that subretinal hemorrhage induced massive photoreceptor cell apoptosis, while the level of apoptosis was limited in cases of vitreous hemorrhage. The finding that vitreous hemorrhage induced minimal retinal cell apoptosis could be explained as follows. First, ATP concentrations around photoreceptors could be much higher in conditions in which blood clots are tightly packed in the subretinal space, while ATP can rapidly disperse into the vitreous space in cases of vitreous hemorrhage. In addition, subretinal injections of toxic agents have a greater risk of toxicity than vitreous injections [59–60]. The difference in the effect between intravitreous and subretinal injections was found to be more than 40-fold. This might be due to the presence of internal limiting membrane (ILM) and Müller glial cells that separate the vitreous cavity and neural retina, or the various cellular sensitivities to the specific stimulant. Another plausible explanation for the various sensitivities to extracellular ATP is localization of ecto-nucleoside triphosphate diphosphohydrolases (NTPDase) in the retina. NTPDase 1 and NTPDase 2 are mainly located in the ganglion cell layer (GCL), inner plexiform layer (IPL), and outer plexiform layer (OPL), indicating synaptic localization. In the OPL, NTPDases mainly localize in post-synaptic processes but not photoreceptor terminals [61]. In subretinal hemorrhage, ATP released from blood might be degraded by NTPDase during its diffusion through those synaptic layers, while photoreceptors could be exposed to ATP before its degradation. Hence, photoreceptors rather than ganglion cells and other inner retinal cells may tend to undergo apoptosis. Also in the case of vitreous hemorrhage, ATP might be degraded during diffusion through NTPDase-abundant inner retinal layers, which could account for why ATP had less toxic effect in vitreous hemorrhage than in subretinal hemorrhage.

Our present results also showed that subretinal injections of ATP markedly accelerated photoreceptor cell apoptosis, whereas other cells in the retina underwent limited TUNEL-detectable apoptosis. However, ganglion cells are reported to undergo cell death in response to the vitreous injection of BzATP [62]. A possible explanation for this discrepancy is that the local ATP concentration might not be sufficient to induce cell death in the inner retina. In our experiment, the highest concentration of ATP is assumed to be localized around photoreceptor cells. In addition, the retinal pigment epithelium (RPE) may have played roles in the observed photoreceptor degeneration. RPE cells also express P2RX7 [63] and may undergo cell death by subretinal hemorrhage. RPE degeneration could further worsen the photoreceptor degeneration, because RPE provides neurotrophic factors essential for photoreceptor survival. Further investigations will be needed to elucidate the role of RPE and extracellular ATP in retinal degeneration.

BBG, a selective P2RX7 antagonist, has been shown to be a potential therapeutic agent in a mouse model of spinal cord injury [40] [64]. Hence, BBG administration may have a neuroprotective effect in neurodegenerative diseases potentially linked to excessive extracellular ATP. In this context, it is worth noting that BBG is a clinically approved adjuvant for the surgical procedure of chromovitrectomy. We have introduced BBG as a safe staining dye for chromovitrectomy and an increasing number of reports support the safety and efficacy of BBG [44] [65–68]. Taken together, these findings demonstrate that BBG is biocompatible with ocular tissues, including neurosensory retina. Our results further encourage the potential application of BBG as a neuroprotective agent in degenerative disorders, especially in ATP-releasing subretinal hemorrhage. Furthermore, we have also reported that dying cells could release their own intracellular ATP into the extracellular space, resulting in a positive feed-forward loop that worsens the surrounding tissue damage [37]. Our current study further suggests that similar severe neurodegenerative pathologies, such as subarachnoid hemorrhage or intracerebral hemorrhage, could be linked to important elevations of extracellular ATP, accelerating neuronal cell death and irreversible tissue damage. P2RX7 antagonists including BBG may have a neuroprotective therapeutic effect in retinal diseases as well as in CNS diseases with excessive extracellular ATP.

Supporting Information

Supporting Information S1 Genotyping of the rd8 mutation by DNA sequencing in $P2rx7^{-/-}$ mice. Recently, the rd8 mutation has been reported to be widely inherited across strains supplied by common commercial vendors and ES cell lines [45–46]. To confirm that $P2rx7^{-/-}$ mice do not carry the rd8 mutation, we performed genotyping of the $Crb1^{rd8}$ allele carrying a single base pair deletion in exon 9 of the Crb1 gene. PCR amplification using flanking primers (5′-GCC CCT GTT TGC ATG GAG GAA ACT-3′ and 5′- GCC CCA TTT GCA CAC TGA TGA C-3′) and subsequent DNA sequencing demonstrated that the genotype of $P2rx7^{-/-}$ mice is the wild type allele ($n = 6$). Ocular fundus examination also confirmed that $P2rx7^{-/-}$ mice have no phenotype of retinal degeneration, namely drusen-like lesions, which are found in mice carrying the rd8 mutation [46].

Supporting Information S2 Characteristics and clinical data in patients with vitreous hemorrhage due to AMD. About 2,000 AMD patients are referred to our Vitreoretinal Center every year. Patients undergo ophthalmologic examinations, including visual acuity testing with standardized refraction using decimal charts and slit-lamp biomicroscopy. Decimal fractions of visual acuity were converted to the logarithm of the minimal angle of resolution (LogMAR) according to previous reports [69–70]. The mean preoperative visual acuity in AMD with VH was 0.008/2.10 (decimal/LogMAR), ranging from light perception to 0.03. At the preoperative examinations, the ocular fundi were almost invisible due to vitreous hemorrhage in AMD patients who underwent vitrectomy. After surgical removal of the vitreous opacity, the area of subretinal hemorrhage was confirmed by a postoperative review of the video records. A large area of subretinal hemorrhage ranging 4 to 30 disc diameters that involves the macula was observed in the fundus of those patients.

Supporting Information S3 The height of retinal detachment by injections of sodium hyaluronate, sodium hyaluronate with a mixture of ATP, and autologous blood. The height of retinal detachment was measured as the length between the photoreceptor outer segment and RPE in cryosections. The mean lengths in the three groups were not significantly different.

Acknowledgments

We thank Mari Imamura and Fumiyo Morikawa (Kyushu University) for technical assistance.

Author Contributions

Conceived and designed the experiments: SN TH HE TI. Performed the experiments: SN HT YM. Analyzed the data: SN AT YI. Contributed reagents/materials/analysis tools: HT SS RA TS. Wrote the paper: SN TH YI HE TI.

References

1. Ferris FL 3rd, Fine SL, Hyman L (1984) Age-related macular degeneration and blindness due to neovascular maculopathy. Arch Ophthalmol 102: 1640–1642.
2. Klein R, Rowland ML, Harris MI (1995) Racial/ethnic differences in age-related maculopathy. Third National Health and Nutrition Examination Survey. Ophthalmology 102: 371–381.
3. Grossniklaus HE, Green WR (2004) Choroidal neovascularization. Am J Ophthalmol 137: 496–503.
4. Ishibashi T, Hata Y, Yoshikawa H, Nakagawa K, Sueishi K, et al. (1997) Expression of vascular endothelial growth factor in experimental choroidal neovascularization. Graefes Arch Clin Exp Ophthalmol 235: 159–167.
5. Jager RD, Mieler WF, Miller JW (2008) Age-related macular degeneration. N Engl J Med 358: 2606–2617.
6. Rosenfeld PJ (2011) Bevacizumab versus ranibizumab for AMD. N Engl J Med 364: 1966–1967.
7. Steel DH, Sandhu SS (2011) Submacular haemorrhages associated with neovascular age-related macular degeneration. Br J Ophthalmol 95: 1051–1057.
8. Bressler NM, Bressler SB, Childs AL, Haller JA, Hawkins BS, et al. (2004) Surgery for hemorrhagic choroidal neovascular lesions of age-related macular degeneration: ophthalmic findings: SST report no. 13. Ophthalmology 111: 1993–2006.
9. Dunaief JL, Dentchev T, Ying GS, Milam AH (2002) The role of apoptosis in age-related macular degeneration. Arch Ophthalmol 120: 1435–1442.
10. Bhisitkul RB, Winn BJ, Lee OT, Wong J, Pereira Dde S, et al. (2008) Neuroprotective effect of intravitreal triamcinolone acetonide against photoreceptor apoptosis in a rabbit model of subretinal hemorrhage. Invest Ophthalmol Vis Sci 49: 4071–4077.
11. Sacco RL, Wolf PA, Bharucha NE, Meeks SL, Kannel WB, et al. (1984) Subarachnoid and intracerebral hemorrhage: natural history, prognosis, and precursive factors in the Framingham Study. Neurology 34: 847–854.
12. Hua Y, Keep RF, Hoff JT, Xi G (2007) Brain injury after intracerebral hemorrhage: the role of thrombin and iron. Stroke 38: 759–762.
13. Regan RF, Panter SS (1996) Hemoglobin potentiates excitotoxic injury in cortical cell culture. J Neurotrauma 13: 223–231.
14. Glatt H, Machemer R (1982) Experimental subretinal hemorrhage in rabbits. Am J Ophthalmol 94: 762–773.
15. Nakamura T, Keep RF, Hua Y, Schallert T, Hoff JT, et al. (2004) Deferoxamine-induced attenuation of brain edema and neurological deficits in a rat model of intracerebral hemorrhage. J Neurosurg 100: 672–678.
16. Qureshi AI, Ali Z, Suri MF, Shuaib A, Baker G, et al. (2003) Extracellular glutamate and other amino acids in experimental intracerebral hemorrhage: an in vivo microdialysis study. Crit Care Med 31: 1482–1489.
17. Ellis HM, Horvitz HR (1986) Genetic control of programmed cell death in the nematode C. elegans. Cell 44: 817–829.
18. Yuan J, Shaham S, Ledoux S, Ellis HM, Horvitz HR (1993) The C. elegans cell death gene ced-3 encodes a protein similar to mammalian interleukin-1 beta-converting enzyme. Cell 75: 641–652.
19. Hisatomi T, Sakamoto T, Murata T, Yamanaka I, Oshima Y, et al. (2001) Relocalization of apoptosis-inducing factor in photoreceptor apoptosis induced by retinal detachment in vivo. Am J Pathol 158: 1271–1278.
20. Green DR, Kroemer G (2005) Pharmacological manipulation of cell death: clinical applications in sight? J Clin Invest 115: 2610–2617.
21. Susin SA, Lorenzo HK, Zamzami N, Marzo I, Snow BE, et al. (1999) Molecular characterization of mitochondrial apoptosis-inducing factor. Nature 397: 441–446.
22. Hisatomi T, Nakazawa T, Noda K, Almulki L, Miyahara S, et al. (2008) HIV protease inhibitors provide neuroprotection through inhibition of mitochondrial apoptosis in mice. J Clin Invest 118: 2025–2038.
23. Murakami Y, Ikeda Y, Yonemitsu Y, Onimaru M, Nakagawa K, et al. (2008) Inhibition of nuclear translocation of apoptosis-inducing factor is an essential mechanism of the neuroprotective activity of pigment epithelium-derived factor in a rat model of retinal degeneration. Am J Pathol 173: 1326–1338.
24. Dubyak GR, el-Moatassim C (1993) Signal transduction via P2-purinergic receptors for extracellular ATP and other nucleotides. Am J Physiol 265: C577–606.
25. Abbracchio MP, Burnstock G (1994) Purinoceptors: are there families of P2X and P2Y purinoceptors? Pharmacol Ther 64: 445–475.
26. Ralevic V, Burnstock G (1998) Receptors for purines and pyrimidines. Pharmacol Rev 50: 413–492.
27. Surprenant A, Rassendren F, Kawashima E, North RA, Buell G (1996) The cytolytic P2Z receptor for extracellular ATP identified as a P2X receptor (P2X7). Science 272: 735–738.
28. Ferrari D, Los M, Bauer MK, Vandenabeele P, Wesselborg S, et al. (1999) P2Z purinoreceptor ligation induces activation of caspases with distinct roles in apoptotic and necrotic alterations of cell death. FEBS Lett 447: 71–75.
29. Chused TM, Apasov S, Sitkovsky M (1996) Murine T lymphocytes modulate activity of an ATP-activated P2Z-type purinoceptor during differentiation. J Immunol 157: 1371–1380.
30. Deuchars SA, Atkinson L, Brooke RE, Musa H, Milligan CJ, et al. (2001) Neuronal P2X7 receptors are targeted to presynaptic terminals in the central and peripheral nervous systems. J Neurosci 21: 7143–7152.
31. Pannicke T, Fischer W, Biedermann B, Schadlich H, Grosche J, et al. (2000) P2X7 receptors in Muller glial cells from the human retina. J Neurosci 20: 5965–5972.

32. Mitchell CH, Lu W, Hu H, Zhang X, Reigada D, et al. (2009) The P2X(7) receptor in retinal ganglion cells: A neuronal model of pressure-induced damage and protection by a shifting purinergic balance. Purinergic Signal 5: 241–249.
33. Puthussery T, Fletcher EL (2004) Synaptic localization of P2X7 receptors in the rat retina. J Comp Neurol 472: 13–23.
34. Puthussery T, Yee P, Vingrys AJ, Fletcher EL (2006) Evidence for the involvement of purinergic P2X receptors in outer retinal processing. Eur J Neurosci 24: 7–19.
35. Vessey KA, Fletcher EL (2012) Rod and cone pathway signalling is altered in the P2X7 receptor knock out mouse. PLoS One 7: e29990.
36. Puthussery T, Fletcher E (2009) Extracellular ATP induces retinal photoreceptor apoptosis through activation of purinoceptors in rodents. J Comp Neurol 513: 430–440.
37. Notomi S, Hisatomi T, Kanemaru T, Takeda A, Ikeda Y, et al. (2011) Critical involvement of extracellular ATP acting on P2RX7 purinergic receptors in photoreceptor cell death. Am J Pathol 179: 2798–2809.
38. McLarnon JG, Ryu JK, Walker DG, Choi HB (2006) Upregulated expression of purinergic P2X(7) receptor in Alzheimer disease and amyloid-beta peptide-treated microglia and in peptide-injected rat hippocampus. J Neuropathol Exp Neurol 65: 1090–1097.
39. Diaz-Hernandez M, Diez-Zaera M, Sanchez-Nogueiro J, Gomez-Villafuertes R, Canals JM, et al. (2009) Altered P2X7-receptor level and function in mouse models of Huntington's disease and therapeutic efficacy of antagonist administration. FASEB J 23: 1893–1906.
40. Peng W, Cotrina ML, Han X, Yu H, Bekar L, et al. (2009) Systemic administration of an antagonist of the ATP-sensitive receptor P2X7 improves recovery after spinal cord injury. Proc Natl Acad Sci U S A 106: 12489–12493.
41. Zhang X, Zhang M, Laties AM, Mitchell CH (2005) Stimulation of P2X7 receptors elevates Ca2+ and kills retinal ganglion cells. Invest Ophthalmol Vis Sci 46: 2183–2191.
42. Sugiyama T, Oku H, Shibata M, Fukuhara M, Yoshida H, et al. (2010) Involvement of P2X7 receptors in the hypoxia-induced death of rat retinal neurons. Invest Ophthalmol Vis Sci 51: 3236–3243.
43. Rodrigues EB, Meyer CH, Kroll P (2005) Chromovitrectomy: a new field in vitreoretinal surgery. Graefes Arch Clin Exp Ophthalmol 243: 291–293.
44. Enaida H, Hisatomi T, Hata Y, Ueno A, Goto Y, et al. (2006) Brilliant blue G selectively stains the internal limiting membrane/brilliant blue G-assisted membrane peeling. Retina 26: 631–636.
45. Mehalow AK, Kameya S, Smith RS, Hawes NL, Denegre JM, et al. (2003) CRB1 is essential for external limiting membrane integrity and photoreceptor morphogenesis in the mammalian retina. Hum Mol Genet 12: 2179–2189.
46. Mattapallil MJ, Wawrousek EF, Chan CC, Zhao H, Roychoudhury J, et al. (2012) The Rd8 mutation of the Crb1 gene is present in vendor lines of C57BL/6N mice and embryonic stem cells, and confounds ocular induced mutant phenotypes. Invest Ophthalmol Vis Sci 53: 2921–2927.
47. Wood RE, Wishart C, Walker PJ, Askew CD, Stewart IB (2009) Plasma ATP concentration and venous oxygen content in the forearm during dynamic handgrip exercise. BMC Physiol 9: 24.
48. Nakazawa T, Hisatomi T, Nakazawa C, Noda K, Maruyama K, et al. (2007) Monocyte chemoattractant protein 1 mediates retinal detachment-induced photoreceptor apoptosis. Proc Natl Acad Sci U S A 104: 2425–2430.
49. Jaremko KM, Chen-Roetling J, Chen L, Regan RF (2010) Accelerated hemolysis and neurotoxicity in neuron-glia-blood clot co-cultures. J Neurochem 114: 1063–1073.
50. Trichonas G, Murakami Y, Thanos A, Morizane Y, Kayama M, et al. (2010) Receptor interacting protein kinases mediate retinal detachment-induced photoreceptor necrosis and compensate for inhibition of apoptosis. Proc Natl Acad Sci U S A.
51. Yang L, Bula D, Arroyo JG, Chen DF (2004) Preventing retinal detachment-associated photoreceptor cell loss in Bax-deficient mice. Invest Ophthalmol Vis Sci 45: 648–654.
52. Zacks DN, Hanninen V, Pantcheva M, Ezra E, Grosskreutz C, et al. (2003) Caspase activation in an experimental model of retinal detachment. Invest Ophthalmol Vis Sci 44: 1262–1267.
53. Sakamoto T, Sheu SJ, Arimura N, Sameshima S, Shimura M, et al. (2010) Vitrectomy for exudative age-related macular degeneration with vitreous hemorrhage. Retina 30: 856–864.
54. Jung JH, Lee JK, Lee JE, Oum BS (2010) Results of vitrectomy for breakthrough vitreous hemorrhage associated with age-related macular degeneration and polypoidal choroidal vasculopathy. Retina 30: 865–873.
55. Melani A, Turchi D, Vannucchi MG, Cipriani S, Gianfriddo M, et al. (2005) ATP extracellular concentrations are increased in the rat striatum during in vivo ischemia. Neurochem Int 47: 442–448.
56. Oike M, Kimura C, Koyama T, Yoshikawa M, Ito Y (2000) Hypotonic stress-induced dual Ca(2+) responses in bovine aortic endothelial cells. Am J Physiol Heart Circ Physiol 279: H630–638.
57. Liu HT, Sabirov RZ, Okada Y (2008) Oxygen-glucose deprivation induces ATP release via maxi-anion channels in astrocytes. Purinergic Signal 4: 147–154.
58. Burnstock G (2008) Dual control of vascular tone and remodelling by ATP released from nerves and endothelial cells. Pharmacol Rep 60: 12–20.
59. Lee JE, Yoon TJ, Oum BS, Lee JS, Choi HY (2003) Toxicity of indocyanine green injected into the subretinal space: subretinal toxicity of indocyanine green. Retina 23: 675–681.
60. Ueno A, Hisatomi T, Enaida H, Kagimoto T, Mochizuki Y, et al. (2007) Biocompatibility of brilliant blue G in a rat model of subretinal injection. Retina 27: 499–504.
61. Ricatti MJ, Alfie LD, Lavoie EG, Sevigny J, Schwarzbaum PJ, et al. (2009) Immunocytochemical localization of NTPDases1 and 2 in the neural retina of mouse and zebrafish. Synapse 63: 291–307.
62. Hu H, Lu W, Zhang M, Zhang X, Argall AJ, et al. (2010) Stimulation of the P2X7 receptor kills rat retinal ganglion cells in vivo. Exp Eye Res 91: 425–432.
63. Yang D, Elner SG, Clark AJ, Hughes BA, Petty HR, et al. (2011) Activation of P2X receptors induces apoptosis in human retinal pigment epithelium. Invest Ophthalmol Vis Sci 52: 1522–1530.
64. Wang Q, Wang L, Feng YH, Li X, Zeng R, et al. (2004) P2X7 receptor-mediated apoptosis of human cervical epithelial cells. Am J Physiol Cell Physiol 287: C1349–1358.
65. Hisatomi T, Enaida H, Matsumoto H, Kagimoto T, Ueno A, et al. (2006) Staining ability and biocompatibility of brilliant blue G: preclinical study of brilliant blue G as an adjunct for capsular staining. Arch Ophthalmol 124: 514–519.
66. Enaida H, Hisatomi T, Goto Y, Hata Y, Ueno A, et al. (2006) Preclinical investigation of internal limiting membrane staining and peeling using intravitreal brilliant blue G. Retina 26: 623–630.
67. Farah ME, Maia M, Rodrigues EB (2009) Dyes in ocular surgery: principles for use in chromovitrectomy. Am J Ophthalmol 148: 332–340.
68. Rodrigues EB, Penha FM, de Paula Fiod Costa E, Maia M, Dib E, et al. (2010) Ability of new vital dyes to stain intraocular membranes and tissues in ocular surgery. Am J Ophthalmol 149: 265–277.
69. Holladay JT (1997) Proper method for calculating average visual acuity. J Refract Surg 13: 388–391.
70. Schulze-Bonsel K, Feltgen N, Burau H, Hansen L, Bach M (2006) Visual acuities "hand motion" and "counting fingers" can be quantified with the freiburg visual acuity test. Invest Ophthalmol Vis Sci 47: 1236–1240.

13

MFGE8 Does Not Influence Chorio-Retinal Homeostasis or Choroidal Neovascularization *in vivo*

William Raoul[1,2,3]*, Lucie Poupel[5,6], David-Alexandre Tregouet[9,15], Sophie Lavalette[1,2,3], Serge Camelo[8,9,10], Nicole Keller[8,9,10], Sophie Krumeich[11,12], Bertrand Calippe[1,2,3], Xavier Guillonneau[1,2,3], Francine Behar-Cohen[4,8,9,10], Salomon-Yves Cohen[14], Holger Baatz[13], Christophe Combadière[5,6,7], Clotilde Théry[11,12], Florian Sennlaub[1,2,3,4]*

1 INSERM, U968, Paris, France, **2** University Pierre and Marie Curie, Institut de la Vision, Paris, France, **3** Centre National de la Recherche Scientifique, Paris, France, **4** Assistance Publique-Hôpitaux de Paris, Hôtel Dieu, Service d'Ophtalmologie, Paris, France, **5** INSERM, UMR S945, Laboratory of Immunity and Infection, Paris, France, **6** University Pierre and Marie Curie, Laboratory of Immunity and Infection, Paris, France, **7** Assistance Publique-Hôpitaux de Paris, Groupe Hospitalier Pitié-Salpétrière, Service d'Immunologie, Paris, France, **8** INSERM, UMR S 872, Centre de Recherche des Cordeliers, Paris, France, **9** University Pierre and Marie Curie, Paris, France, **10** Université Paris Descartes, Paris, France, **11** INSERM, U932, Paris, France, **12** Institut Curie, Centre de Recherche, Paris, France, **13** Augenärztliche Gemeinschaftspraxis, Augenzentrum Recklinghausen und Zentrum der Augenheilkunde, J-W Goethe Universität Frankfurt am Main, Frankfurt, Germany, **14** Centre d'Angiographie et de Laser, Paris, France, **15** INSERM, UMR S 937, Faculté de Médecine La Pitié-Salpêtrière, Paris, France

Abstract

Purpose: Milk fat globule-epidermal growth factor-factor VIII (MFGE8) is necessary for diurnal outer segment phagocytosis and promotes VEGF-dependent neovascularization. The prevalence of two single nucleotide polymorphisms (SNP) in *MFGE8* was studied in two exsudative or "wet" Age-related Macular Degeneration (AMD) groups and two corresponding control groups. We studied the effect of MFGE8 deficiency on retinal homeostasis with age and on choroidal neovascularization (CNV) in mice.

Methods: The distribution of the SNP (rs4945 and rs1878326) of *MFGE8* was analyzed in two groups of patients with "wet" AMD and their age-matched controls from Germany and France. MFGE8-expressing cells were identified in $Mfge8^{+/-}$ mice expressing ß-galactosidase. Aged $Mfge8^{+/-}$ and $Mfge8^{-/-}$ mice were studied by funduscopy, histology, electron microscopy, scanning electron microscopy of vascular corrosion casts of the choroid, and after laser-induced CNV.

Results: rs1878326 was associated with AMD in the French and German group. The *Mfge8* promoter is highly active in photoreceptors but not in retinal pigment epithelium cells. $Mfge8^{-/-}$ mice did not differ from controls in terms of fundus appearance, photoreceptor cell layers, choroidal architecture or laser-induced CNV. In contrast, the Bruch's membrane (BM) was slightly but significantly thicker in $Mfge8^{-/-}$ mice as compared to controls.

Conclusions: Despite a reproducible minor increase of rs1878326 in AMD patients and a very modest increase in BM in $Mfge8^{-/-}$ mice, our data suggests that MFGE8 dysfunction does not play a critical role in the pathogenesis of AMD.

Editor: Alfred Lewin, University of Florida, United States of America

Funding: This work was supported by grants from INSERM, Agence Nationale pour la Recherche (ANR) "blanc" (AO5120DD), ANR "Maladies Neurologiques et Maladies Psychiatriques" (R08098DS), ANR "Genopat" (R09099DS), European Grant "Innochem" (LSHB-CT-2005-518167), ERC starting Grant (ERC-2007 St.G. 210345), and a grant from Fondation de France to C.T. F.S. a is recipient of ERC starting grant. C.C. and F.S. are recipients of a contract "Interface" from Assistance Publique-Hôpitaux de Paris. The funders had no role in study design, data collection and analysis, decision to publish, or preparation of the manuscript.

Competing Interests: The authors have declared that no competing interests exist.

* E-mail: william.raoul@inserm.fr (WR); florian.sennlaub@inserm.fr (FS)

Introduction

Milk fat globule-EGF-factor (MFGE8), also named lactadherin, PAS 6/7, SED1, BA46, p47, is a secreted glycoprotein first described in milk fat globules released in milk by mammary epithelial cells [1,2]. Secreted by different cell types, it promotes phagocytosis by linking phosphatidylserine at the surface of membrane vesicles [3] and apoptotic cells [4] to the αvβ3/β5 integrin on phagocytic cells. MFGE8 mediated phagocytosis induces a regulatory T cell response [5] and $Mfge8^{-/-}$ mice develop spontaneous late onset lupus-like disease and glomerulonephritis [6]. In humans, the association of two nucleotide polymorphisms in the coding region of *MFGE8* predisposes subjects to systemic lupus erythematosus [7], suggesting that these single nucleotide polymorphisms (SNP) lead to a dysfunctional MFGE8. Furthermore, MFGE8 binds to αvβ3/β5 of vascular endothelial cells and promotes VEGF-driven neovascularization [8].

Phagocytosis of spent outer segments (OS) is critical for the long-term maintenance of the retina [9,10] and dependent upon a tyrosine kinase receptor (Mertk) [11,12] and the αvβ5 integrin [13]. The neural retina and the retinal pigment epithelium (RPE) express MFGE8 [14], whose interaction with αvβ5 integrin of RPE cells is essential in the diurnal OS phagocytosis [15]. Furthermore, we have previously shown that OS phagocytosis by the RPE is necessary for choroidal maintenance *in vivo* [16].

Age-related macular degeneration (AMD) is a major cause of central vision loss in the elderly in Western countries [17]. AMD's most prominent pathological features are lesions involving the RPE and Bruch's membrane (BM), the degeneration of photoreceptors, [18] and VEGF-driven choroidal neovascularization (CNV) [19], that occurs approximately in 10% of patients. The causes of AMD are not well understood, but epidemiological studies [20] and murine models [21] have identified key factors in its pathogenesis such as age [17,22], family history [23] and smoking [24,25].

In summary, MFGE8 has been shown to be essential in diurnal OS phagocytosis and in angiogenesis. In the eye, its dysfunction could therefore lead both to retinal degeneration and choroidal involution as a consequence of impaired RPE phagocytosis and/or to inhibition of neovascularization. We investigated whether a SNP associated with increased prevalence of lupus in human patients [7] is associated with AMD. Furthermore, we investigated whether the deficiency of MFGE8 affects chorioretinal homeostasis and CNV *in vivo* using *Mfge8*$^{-/-}$ mice.

Materials and Methods

Ethics statement

In accordance with the Declaration of Helsinki, patients and volunteers provided written and informed consent for the studies, which were approved by the Hôtel Dieu ethics committee (CCPPRB no. 0611303) and by the ethics committee of the Ärztekammer Westfalen-Lippe and the University of Münster (no. 2007-246-f-S).

Animal experiments were approved by the Institutional Animal Care and Use Committee, "Comité d'éthique pour l'expérimentation animale Charles Darwin" (ID Ce5/2010/002), and treated in compliance with the ARVO Statement for the Use of Animals in Ophthalmic and Vision Research.

Single Nucleotide Polymorphisms analysis in AMD

Studies, including participants' assessments and ethics details of each cohort were described in Combadiere *et al.* [26] and Baatz *et al.* [27]. White Caucasian control subjects and AMD patients were recruited in Paris (France: 251 control subjects, 274 "wet" AMD patients) and in Recklinghausen (Germany: 317 control subjects, 263 "wet" AMD patients). The mean age and gender distribution are summarized in Tables 1 and 2.

Rs4945 is in open reading frame SNP and leads to Arginine replacement of a Serine in the amino acid number 3. Rs1878326 is also in open reading frame SNP of *MFGE8* and leads to Leucine replacement of Methionine in the amino acid number 76. Allelic frequencies were calculated by gene counting.

Table 1. The mean age and gender distribution in the patient and control groups.

Patients	FCTL, n (%)	FAMD, n (%)
Men	91 (36,25)	81 (29,56)
Women	160 (63,75)	193 (70,44)
Total	251	274
Mean Age	71,8+/−7,75	79,5+/−6,72
P value (χ^2 test)	0.1	

French groups (control group : FCTL; AMD group : FAMD).

Table 2. The mean age and gender distribution in the patient and control groups.

Patients	GCTL, n (%)	GAMD, n (%)
Men	115 (43,73)	126 (39,75)
Women	148 (56,27)	191 (60,25)
Total	263	317
Mean Age	77,8+/−5,38	79,2+/−5,47
P value (χ^2 test)	0.3	

German groups (control group : GCTL; AMD group : GAMD).

We used the chi-square test ($\chi^{2)}$ to compare genotype distributions and allele frequencies in participants. The Hardy-Weinberg equilibrium was tested using a χ^2 test with 1 degree of freedom. Association between SNP and "wet" AMD was assessed by use of the Cochran-Armitage's trend test [28]. Linkage disequilibrium and haplotype association analyses were performed by the use of THESIAS software [29].

Animals

Mfge8$^{-/-}$ and $^{+/-}$ mouse strains were generated as described before [8]. *Mfge8*$^{-/-}$ are functionally deficient in MFGE8 due to a gene-trap insertion of ß-galactosidase in the *Mfge8* gene (C57Bl/6 background, N8). The mice were maintained at the Institut Curie animal facility or Centre de Recherche des Cordeliers animal facility (Paris, France) under pathogen-free conditions. All animals were housed in a 12/12 hour light/dark (100–500 lux) cycle with food and water available *ad libitum*.

Fundus Photography and Laser-Photocoagulation

Mice were anesthetized by intraperitoneal injection of pentobarbital (40 mg/kg). Pupils were fully dilated with 1% tropicamide. Coverslips positioned on the mouse cornea were used as a contact glass. Fundus photographs were taken with a digital CCD camera (Nikon D3) coupled with an endoscope (Karl Storz, Guyancourt, France) as previously described [30].

Laser-photocoagulations were performed 1 to 2 disc diameters away from the papillae with an Argon laser (Viridis 532 nm, Quantel Medical, Clermont-Ferrand, France) mounted on a slit lamp (400 mW, 50 ms and 50 µm; Hagg-Streitt, BQ 900). For CNV visualization at day 14, 3 months old mice were anesthetized and perfused through their heart with phosphate buffered saline (PBS) containing fluorescein (FITC)-dextran 50 mg/ml (2.10^6 mW). Animals were sacrificed with 100% CO_2 and their eyes were removed and processed as described below. CNV was quantified on photographs with Image J analysis software. CNV was quantified as FITC positive surface.

Choroidal Flatmounts and Immunohistochemistry

The eyes were enucleated, fixed in 4% paraformaldehyde (PFA) for 20 minutes at room temperature, and sectioned at the limbus; the cornea and lens were discarded. The retinas were peeled from the RPE/choroid/sclera. Retinas and choroids were incubated with the indicated primary and secondary antibodies. The choroids and retinas were radially incised and flatmounted. The primary antibodies used were rabbit anti-IBA1 (1:400; Wako,

Neuss, Germany) and rhodamine phalloidine (1:200; Invitrogen, Cergy-Pontoise, France). Sections were counterstained with 4–6-diamino-2-phenylindole (DAPI). Choroids, retinas and sections were viewed with a fluorescence microscope (DM5500B, Leica, Nanterre, France).

For ß-galactosidase activity detection, frozen sections from eyes were fixed in 4% PFA before incubation. The samples were then incubated in the beta-galactosidase detection reagent (5 mM potassium ferricyanide, 5 mM potassium ferrocyanide, 2 mM MgCl, 0.30 mg X-gal/ml in PBS) overnight at 37°C before mounting in Immumount (Thermo Scientific, Courtaboeuf, France).

Histology and Electron Microscopy

For histology, eyes were fixed in 0.5% glutaraldehyde/4% PFA for 2 h, dehydrated and mounted in historesin. 5-µm sections were cut and stained with toluidin blue. For electron microscopy, eyes were fixed in 2.5% glutaraldehyde of cacodylate buffer (0.1 M, pH 7.4). After 1 hour, eyeballs were dissected, fixed for another 3 hours, post-fixed in 1% osmium tetroxide in cacodylate buffer, and dehydrated in graduated ethanol solution. The samples were included in epoxy resin and oriented. Semi-thin sections (1 µm), obtained with an ultramicrotome Reichert Ultracut E (Leica), were stained with toluidin blue, examined with a light microscope, and photoreceptor layer thickness was measured. Ultra-thin sections (80 nm) were contrasted by uranyl acetate and lead citrate, then observed in an electron microscope JEOL 100 CX II (JEOL, Tokyo, Japan) with 80 kV.

Vascular Corrosion Casts

Animals were sacrificed by CO_2 inhalation. Vascular corrosion cast was performed as previously described by Houssier *et al.* [16]. Briefly, a perfusion was done with Mercox resin+catalyst (Ladd Research/Inland, Saint Loup sur Semouse, France) into the aorta through left heart ventricle. After removal, eye tissues were conserved overnight at 37°C in PBS to allow complete polymerisation and digested by 5% KOH during 2 weeks at 37°C until only the vascular corrosion casts remained. The specimens were prepared for electron microscopy, then scanned and analyzed using Image J Software (NIH). The avascular area was measured on frontal views and expressed as the percentage of intercapillary surface of the whole area. The thickness of choriocapillaries was measured on perpendicular views of the cast from the retinal to scleral side of the choriocapillary cast.

Reverse Transcription and Real Time Polymerase Chain Reaction

After tissues were separated (neural retina and choroid/RPE), total RNA was isolated with NucleoSpin RNA II Kit (Macherey-Nagel, Hoerdt, France). Single-stranded cDNA was synthesized from total RNA (pre-treated with DNaseI amplification grade) using oligodT as primer and superscript reverse transcriptase (Invitrogen, Cergy Pontoise, France). Subsequent real-time polymerase chain reaction (RT PCR) was performed using cDNA, qPCR SuperMix-UDG Platinum SYBR Green (Invitrogen), and the following primers (0.5 pmol/µl): mm actin sense: 5′-AAGGC-CAACCGTGAAAAGAT-3′; mm actin antisense : 5′-GTGGTACGACCAGAGGCATAC-3′; mm *Mfge8* sense : 5′-GGATAATCAGGGCAAGATCA-3′; mm *Mfge8* antisense : 5′-TAGGACGCCACATACTGGAT-3′

PCR reactions were performed in 40 cycles of 15 s at 95°C, 45 s at 60°C. Product was not generated in control reactions in which reverse transcriptase was omitted during cDNA synthesis.

Statistical Analysis

Graph Pad Prism 5 (GraphPad Software, San Diego, CA, USA) was used for the data analysis and graphic representations. All values are reported as means ± SEM. Statistical analysis was performed using the Mann-Whitney test for comparison among means between two groups or ANOVA test between more than two groups. Significance was set at $P<0.05$.

Results

MFGE8 single nucleotide polymorphism studies in two groups of wet AMD patients and their controls

Two common SNP were previously identified in the open reading frame of the *MFGE8* gene called *MFGE8* R3S (rs4945 for nucleotide C>A) and *MFGE8* M76L (rs1878326 for nucleotide 226 A>C), associated with an increased risk of systemic lupus erythematosus [7]. The fact that *Mfge8*$^{-/-}$ mice develop a spontaneous late onset lupus-like disease and glomerulonephritis [6] suggests that rs4945 and rs1878326 lead to a decrease of MFGE8 bioactivity, that would explain their association with the human disease.

We thus investigated the described *MFGE8* SNP in two DNA collections of "wet" AMD patients recruited in France (FAMD, 274 subjects) and in Germany (GAMD, 317 subjects) and their age matched controls (FCTL, 251 subjects; GCTL, 263 subjects). The mean age and gender distribution are summarized in Tables 1 and 2. All of the subjects were of caucasian origin or decent. Risk factors for "wet" AMD such as Factor H and smoking were more frequent among cases than among controls as previously described [31].

Genotype frequencies distribution of the rs4945 C>A (R3S) and rs1878326 A>C (M76L) are shown in Tables 3 and 4, respectively. All genotype distributions were compatible with Hardy-Weinberg equilibrium ($P>0.05$) in cases and in controls, from both French and German samples. In the French sample, the rs4945 -A allele was more frequent in cases than in controls (0.36 vs 0.29, $P=0.017$) but the inverse trend was observed in German (0.30 vs 0.33, $P=0.229$). Conversely, the pattern of association of the rs1878326 with AMD was homogeneous across populations. In both samples, the rs1878326-C allele tended to be more frequent in cases than in controls, 0.36 vs 0.32, $P=0.184$ and 0.41 vs 0.35, $P=0.053$, in French and German, respectively. The corresponding OR for AMD were then 1.19 [0.92–1.53] in French and 1.27 [1.00–1.61] in German. The two ORs were not significantly different ($P=0.92$). Even though statistical significance was not reached separately in each sample (likely due to small sample size), the resulting combined OR for AMD associated with the rs1878326-C allele was 1.23 [1.03–1.46] and achieved significance ($P=0.019$).

The pattern of linkage disequilibrium was homogeneous across populations and was characterized by a moderate linkage disequilibrium between the two studied SNP ($r^2=0.07$, $D'=-0.53$ in French and $r^2=0.10$, $D'=-0.60$) in German). As a consequence, the two SNP generated 4 common haplotypes (Table 5) among which the two haplotypes carrying the rs1878326-C allele were more frequent in cases than in controls in the German and the French study, confirming the association of the rs1878326-C allele with AMD observed in the univariate analysis.

MFGE8 expressing cells in the retina

In the litterature, immunohistochemistry using an anti-MFGE8 antibody localized MFGE8 protein mainly to the inner segments of photoreceptors and to a lesser extent to RPE cells in mice using

Table 3. Genotype distribution of MFGE8 rs4945 (R3S) polymorphism in AMD patients and controls.

MFGE8 rs4945	FCTL, n = 241	FAMD, n = 271	GCTL, n = 260	GAMD, n = 308
CC	122 (51%)	110 (41%)	118 (45%)	154 (50%)
CA	99 (41%)	128 (47%)	112 (43%)	125 (41%)
AA	20 (8%)	33 (12%)	30 (12%)	29 (9%)
MAF	0.29	0.36	0.33	0.30
OR [95%CI]	1.376 [1.056–1.791]		0.855 [0.665–1.100]	
P	0.017		0.229	

MAF: Minor Allele Frequency.
OR: Allelic Odds Ratio with its 95% Confidence Interval.
P: Cochran-Armitage trend test's p-value.

two different antibodies [14]. We identified MFGE8 expressing cells in *Mfge8*$^{+/-}$ mice thanks to the gene-trap insertion of ß-galactosidase in the *Mfge8* gene. The resulting fusion protein is retained in the cell and ß-galactosidase activity therefore allows to identify MFGE8 expressing cells [8]. ß-galactosidase, detected by a ß-galactosidase detection reagent, mainly localizes to the outer nuclear layer (ONL) containing photoreceptor cell bodies (Fig. 1A). Higher magnification reveals that staining is particularly strong in the outer part of the ONL and that the RPE does express little ß-galactosidase (Fig. 1B), confirming the previously published results using MFGE8 antibodies [14]. There was no endogenous ß-galactosidase detection in WT mice (data not shown). We confirmed this staining pattern using RT PCR in separated tissues (Fig. 1C). *Mfge8* mRNA was highly expressed in young and aged neural retina. In the RPE/choroid, basal mRNA expression was significantly lower than in the neural retina. A slight but significant increase in *Mfge8* mRNA expression at 18 month old compared to 3-month-old C57Bl6 mice was observed. Taken together, our results identify photoreceptors as the main source of MFGE8 in the eye and suggest that MFGE8 localization in the RPE cells [14] is due to uptake rather than RPE MFGE8 expression.

MFGE8 and retinal homeostasis

MFGE8 has been shown to be essential in diurnal OS phagocytosis [15] and disturbance of the phagocytosis of spent OS by the RPE, as observed in the RCS rat, leads to photoreceptor degeneration [10]. To evaluate if MFGE8 deficiency alters long-term retinal homeostasis, we first studied the fundoscopic appearance of 16–18 month old *Mfge8*$^{+/-}$ (Fig. 2A) and *Mfge8*$^{-/-}$ (Fig. 2B). Both fundi appeared smooth, devoid of any remarkable lesions, and similar to each other. Furthermore, histological sections of aged *Mfge8*$^{+/-}$ (Fig. 2C) and *Mfge8*$^{-/-}$ mice (Fig. 2D) showed a regular photoreceptor layer and quantification of the number of photoreceptor cell nuclei layers in the ONL revealed no signs of degeneration from the inferior to the superior pole in *Mfge8*$^{-/-}$ (Fig. 2E grey line) compared to *Mfge8*$^{+/-}$ mice (Fig. 2E black line). Labelling for RPE (phalloidine, red) and subretinal macrophages/microglial cells (IBA1, green) in aged *Mfge8*$^{+/-}$ (Fig. 2F) and *Mfge8*$^{-/-}$ mice (Fig. 2G) showed no morphological abnormalities of RPE cells and no pathological accumulation of phagocytes under the retina. Instead, we found a tendency of decreased subretinal phagocytes in 18-month-old *Mfge8*$^{-/-}$ compared to *Mfge8*$^{+/-}$ (Fig. 2H, quantification of subretinal IBA1 positive cells). Laminar deposits in the BM and Drusen in the RPE/BM complex are early signs of AMD that ultimately impact RPE and photoreceptor health [18,32]. To evaluate if MFGE8 is implicated in homeostasis of BM, we evaluated BM morphology of 16–18 month old *Mfge8*$^{+/-}$ (Fig. 2I and K) and *Mfge8*$^{-/-}$ (Fig. 2J and L) by electron microscopy. Although retina and RPE were ultrastructurally similar, we observed a very modest, but significant thickening of BM in *Mfge8*$^{-/-}$ mice by 22% (Fig. 2M). To evaluate possible differences in genes that are potentially involved in lipid clearance from the BM, we analyzed *Abca1*, *Abca4*, *Ldlr*, *cd36* and *Caveolin1* mRNA in aged *Mfge8*$^{+/-}$ and *Mfge8*$^{-/-}$. However, we were not able to detect an influence of MFGE8 on the expression of these genes (Figure S1). Since BM is rich in collagen, and MFGE8 has been shown to promote collagen phagocytosis to prevent reactive fibrosis [33], BM thickening observed in aged *Mfge8*$^{-/-}$ mice could be a result of a reactive fibrosis.

Table 4. Genotype distribution of MFGE8 rs1878326 (M76L) polymorphism in AMD patients and controls.

MFGE8 rs1878326	FCTL, n = 251	FAMD, n = 274	GCTL, n = 263	GAMD, n = 317
AA	108 (43%)	114 (42%)	112 (43%)	113 (35%)
AC	123 (49%)	121 (44%)	116 (44%)	148 (47%)
CC	20 (8%)	39 (14%)	35 (13%)	56 (18%)
MAF	0.32	0.36	0.35	0.41
OR [95%CI]	1.186 [0.919–1.531]		1.271 [1.001–1.613]	
P	0.184		0.053	

MAF: Minor Allele Frequency.
OR: Allelic Odds Ratio with its 95% Confidence Interval.
P: Cochran-Armitage trend test's p-value.

Table 5. Haplotype frequency distributions derived from MFGE8 rs1878326 (M76L) and rs4945 (R3S) polymorphisms in AMD patients and controls.

Polymorphisms		French		German	
rs1878326	**rs4945**	**FCTL (n = 238)**	**FAMD (n = 269)**	**GCTL (n = 253)**	**GAMD (n = 298)**
A	C	0.426	0.342	0.355	0.344
A	A	0.252	0.293	0.289	0.245
C	C	0.284	0.299	0.310	0.359
C	A	0.038	0.066	0.045	0.052

MFGE8 and choroidal homeostasis and neovascularization

Although MFGE8 deficiency did not lead to retinal degeneration, disturbances in RPE biology and diminished expression of trophic factors can lead to choroidal involution [16]. However, vascular corrosion casts of of 16–18 month old *Mfge8*$^{+/-}$ (Fig. 3 I and D) and *Mfge8*$^{-/-}$ (Fig. 3 B and E) showed no MFGE8-related vascular drop-out, measured as a percentage of intercapillary area of the total area, (Fig. 3C) or thinning, measured on pericentral, perpendicular sections through the vascular casts (Fig. 3F).

MFGE8 interacts with αvβ3 and αvβ5 on vascular endothelium and specifically promotes VEGF-driven ischemic neovascularization *in vivo*, but not bFGF induced neovascularization [8]. Since laser-induced CNV has been shown to be VEGF and integrin dependent [34,35], we quantified CNV in the MFGE8-deficient mice. Interestingly, FITC-dextran perfused choroidal flatmounts at 14 d after laser-induced neovascularization of *Mfge8*$^{+/-}$ (Fig. 3G) and *Mfge8*$^{-/-}$ (Fig. 3H), showed no difference of CNV in the two groups (Fig. 3I). These results are consistent with our recent observation that the promoting function of MFGE8 on development of bladder tumors is not linked with alterations in intratumor angiogenesis [36]. Thus, the interactions of MFGE8, integrin dimers and VEGF are possibly tissue dependent.

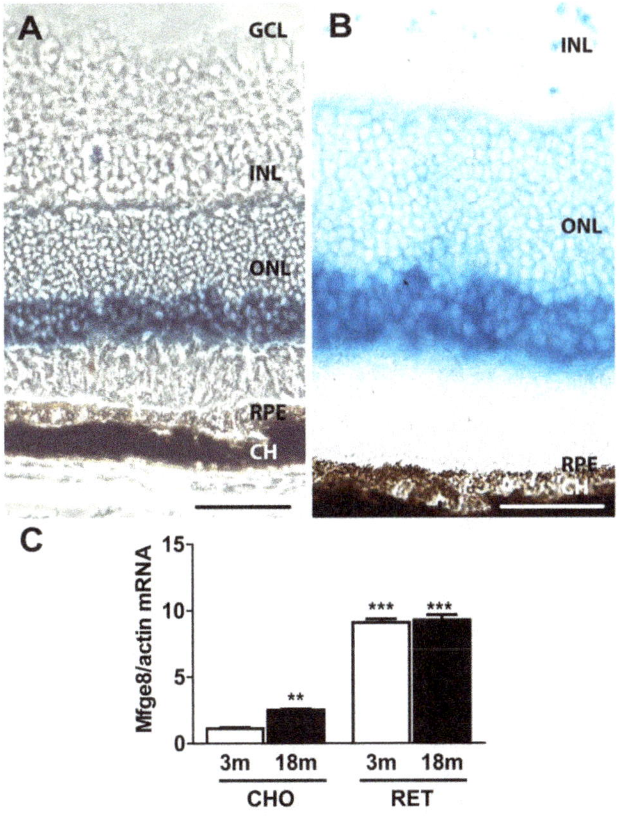

Figure 1. MFGE8 expressing cells in mouse retina. Representative micrographs of ß-galactosidase localization in MFGE8$^{+/GAL}$ mice detected by a ß-galactosidase detection reagent (blue staining). Phase contrast (A) image and light transmitted (B) image. CH: choroid; GCL: ganglion cell layer; INL: inner nuclear layer; ONL: outer nuclear layer; RPE: retinal pigment epithelium. Experiments were reproduced at least 3 times. Scale bars: 100 µm (A); 25 µm (B). *Mfge8* RT PCR in neural retina (RET) and choroid (CHO) at different time points in C57Bl6 mice (3 month old vs 18 month old, n = 6/group; Dunnett test with 3 m old CHO as control, **, $P \leq 0{,}01$ and ***, $P \leq 0{,}001$).

Discussion

MFGE8s essential role in diurnal OS phagocytosis [15] and critical involvement in VEGF-driven neovascularization [8] make it a candidate gene for an involvement in the pathogenesis of AMD, where photoreceptor degeneration, choroidal involution, or CNV can occur. We here show a suggestive statistical evidence for association of the rs1878326-C allele with increased risk of AMD in two European populations.

To evaluate the influence of MFGE8 dysfunction *in vivo* on retinal homeostasis and CNV we analyzed *Mfge8*$^{+/-}$ and *Mfge8*$^{-/-}$ mice with ageing and in a model of CNV. We first confirmed that MFGE8 is constitutively expressed by photoreceptors *in vivo*. Interestingly, the suppression of the diurnal peak of OS phagocytosis observed in *Mfge8*$^{-/-}$ mice [15] has very little negative effect on long term chorioretinal homeostasis in 18-month-old knockout mice, apart from a slight thickening of the BM. These findings confirm and extend the lack of retinal degeneration in 12-month-old *Mfge8*$^{-/-}$ mice [37]. Furthermore, even though MFGE8 interacts with αvβ3 and αvβ5 on the vascular endothelium and strongly promotes VEGF-driven neovascularization [8], it has no effect on laser-induced CNV which is VEGF and αvβ3 integrin dependent [34,35].

Taken together, our data shows that MFGE8 is expressed in the retina but not critically involved in retinal homeostasis or CNV. It seems unlikely that it is predominantly involved in the pathogenesis of AMD. Although we present mostly negative results, we feel that this extensive *in vivo* study is of interest to researchers in the field of AMD pathogenesis, due to its exclusion of a high potential candidate gene. We hope that the publication of these negative results are helpful to the community to exclude a valid hypothesis and avoid repetetion of expensive research in other laboratories.

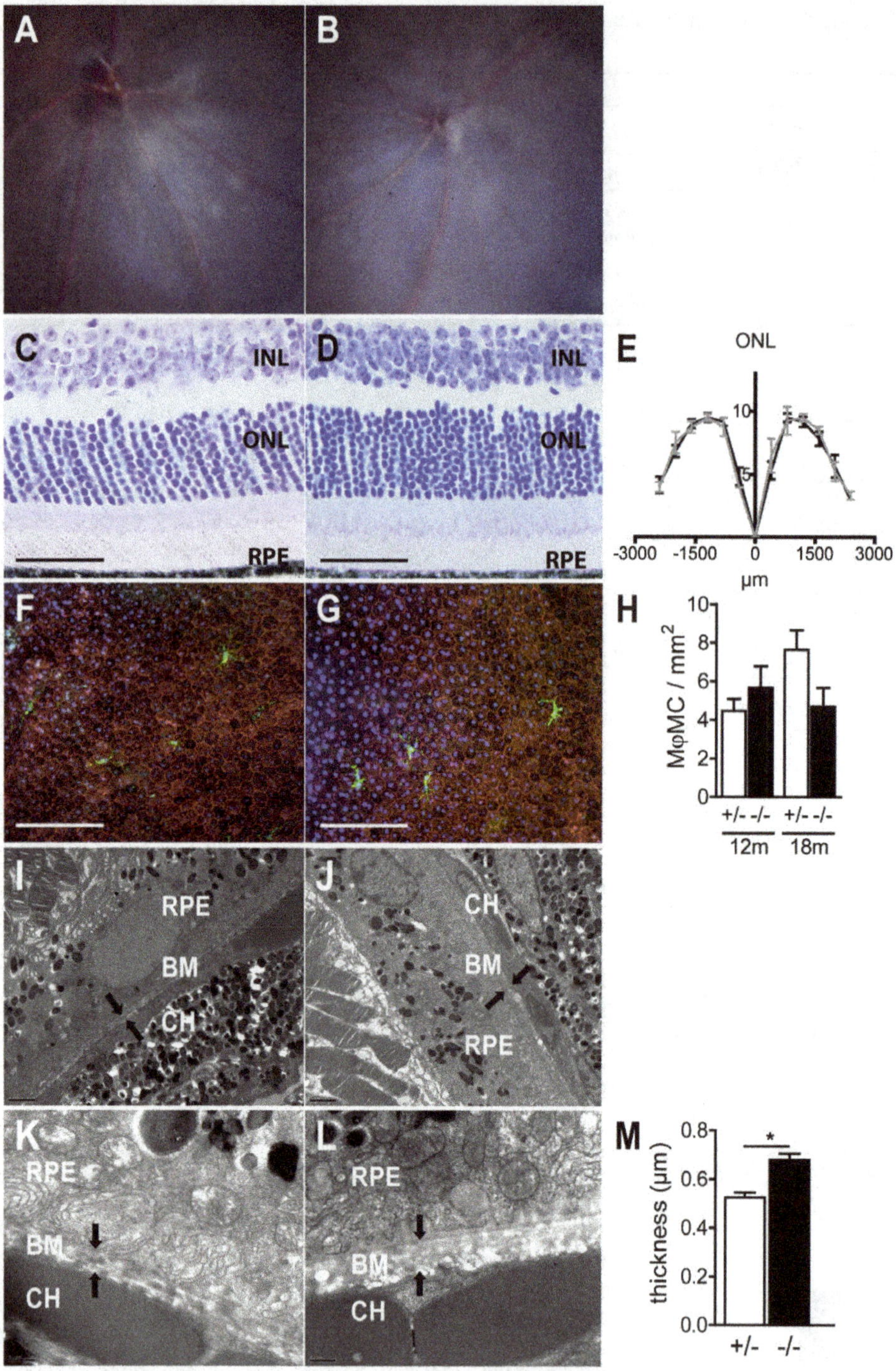

Figure 2. MFGE8 and retinal homeostasis. Fundus photographs of 18 month-old *Mfge8*$^{+/-}$ mice (A) and *Mfge8*$^{-/-}$ mice (B). Histological sections of historesin-embedded eyes from 18 months old *Mfge8*$^{+/-}$ mice (C) and *Mfge8*$^{-/-}$ mice (D). Quantification of the number of photoreceptor cell nuclei layers in the ONL from the inferior to the superior pole in 18 month old *Mfge8*$^{-/-}$ (E grey line) compared to *Mfge8*$^{+/-}$(E black line, n = 4 mice/group). Rhodamine phalloidine (red) IBA1 (green) stained RPE flatmounts of 18 month-old *Mfge8*$^{+/-}$ mice (F) and *Mfge8*$^{-/-}$ mice (G). Quantification of subretinal macrophages/microglia (Mφ/MC) IBA1 positive cells, (H, n = 6–8 mice/group). Representative transmission electron micrograph of Bruchs membrane (black arrows) of 18 month old *Mfge8*$^{+/-}$ (I and K) and *Mfge8*$^{-/-}$ (J and L) mice. Bruchs membrane thickness measurements in 18 month old *Mfge8*$^{+/-}$ and *Mfge8*$^{-/-}$ mice (M, $P \leq 0,05$, n = 4 mice/group) INL: inner nuclear layer; ONL: outer nuclear layer; RPE: retinal pigment epithelium; BM: Bruch membrane; CH: Choroid. Scale bars: 50 µm (C, D), 150 µm (F, G); 2 µm (I, J); 0,5 µm (K,L).

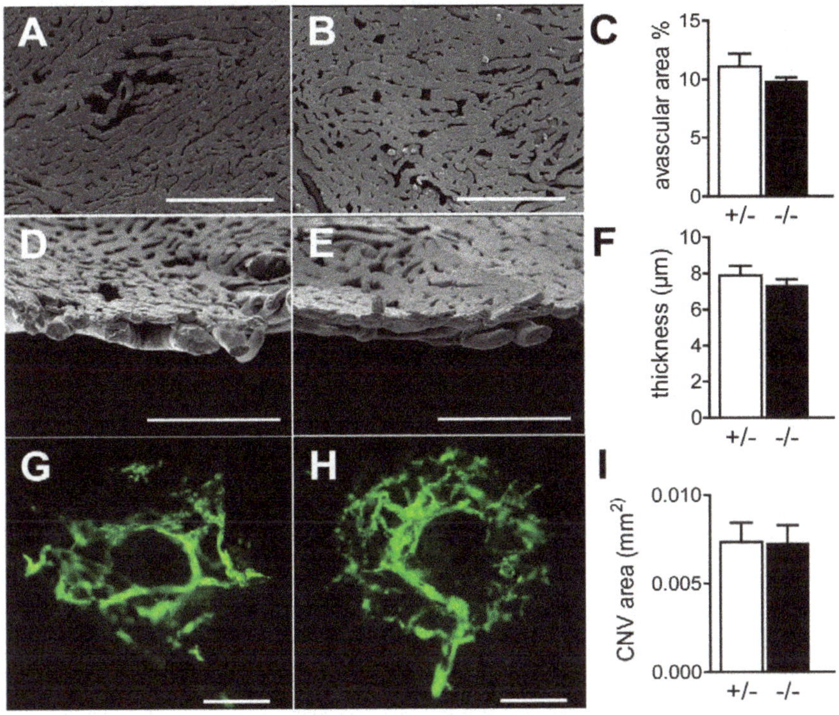

Figure 3. MFGE8 and choroidal homeostasis and neovascularization. Vascular corrosion casts of the retinal aspect of choriocapillaries of 16–18 month old *Mfge8*$^{+/-}$ (A) and *Mfge8*$^{-/-}$ mice (B). Quantification of the avascular intracapillary area in *Mfge8*$^{+/-}$ and *Mfge8*$^{-/-}$ mice (C, 5 mice/group). Vascular corrosion casts of perpendicularly cut choroid of 16–18 month old *Mfge8*$^{+/-}$ (D) and *Mfge8*$^{-/-}$ (E). Quantification of the thickness of the choriocapillaries in *Mfge8*$^{+/-}$ and *Mfge8*$^{-/-}$ mice (F, 3 mice/group). FITC-dextran perfused choroidal flatmounts at 14 d after laser-induced neovascularization of *Mfge8*$^{+/-}$ (G) and *Mfge8*$^{-/-}$ (H). Quantification of FITC positive choroidal neovascularizations in *Mfge8*$^{+/-}$ and *Mfge8*$^{-/-}$ mice (I, n = 8 mice/group). Scale bars: 200 µm (A, B); 100 µm (D, E); 50 µm (G, H).

Acknowledgments

The authors wish to thank Christopher Murray for critical review, Soazig Le Lay and Isabelle Dugail for data analysis and Isabel Le Disquet for scanning electron microscopy.

Author Contributions

Conceived and designed the experiments: WR FS. Performed the experiments: WR LP SL SC NK SK BC XG FS FBC SYC HB. Analyzed the data: WR DAT CC CT FS. Wrote the paper: WR FS.

References

1. Ceriani RL, Peterson JA, Lee JY, Moncada R, Blank EW (1983) Characterization of cell surface antigens of human mammary epithelial cells with monoclonal antibodies prepared against human milk fat globule. Somatic Cell Genet 9: 415–427.
2. Stubbs JD, Lekutis C, Singer KL, Bui A, Yuzuki D, et al. (1990) cDNA cloning of a mouse mammary epithelial cell surface protein reveals the existence of epidermal growth factor-like domains linked to factor VIII-like sequences. Proc Natl Acad Sci U S A 87: 8417–8421.
3. Oshima K, Aoki N, Kato T, Kitajima K, Matsuda T (2002) Secretion of a peripheral membrane protein, MFG-E8, as a complex with membrane vesicles. Eur J Biochem 269: 1209–1218.
4. Hanayama R, Tanaka M, Miwa K, Shinohara A, Iwamatsu A, et al. (2002) Identification of a factor that links apoptotic cells to phagocytes. Nature 417: 182–187.
5. Jinushi M, Nakazaki Y, Dougan M, Carrasco DR, Mihm M, et al. (2007) MFG-E8-mediated uptake of apoptotic cells by APCs links the pro- and antiinflammatory activities of GM-CSF. J Clin Invest 117: 1902–1913.
6. Hanayama R, Tanaka M, Miyasaka K, Aozasa K, Koike M, et al. (2004) Autoimmune disease and impaired uptake of apoptotic cells in MFG-E8-deficient mice. Science 304: 1147–1150.
7. Hu CY, Wu CS, Tsai HF, Chang SK, Tsai WI, et al. (2009) Genetic polymorphism in milk fat globule-EGF factor 8 (MFG-E8) is associated with systemic lupus erythematosus in human. Lupus 18: 676–681.
8. Silvestre JS, Thery C, Hamard G, Boddaert J, Aguilar B, et al. (2005) Lactadherin promotes VEGF-dependent neovascularization. Nat Med 11: 499–506.
9. Young RW, Bok D (1969) Participation of the retinal pigment epithelium in the rod outer segment renewal process. J Cell Biol 42: 392–403.
10. Edwards RB, Szamier RB (1977) Defective phagocytosis of isolated rod outer segments by RCS rat retinal pigment epithelium in culture. Science 197: 1001–1003.
11. Nandrot E, Dufour EM, Provost AC, Pequignot MO, Bonnel S, et al. (2000) Homozygous deletion in the coding sequence of the c-mer gene in RCS rats unravels general mechanisms of physiological cell adhesion and apoptosis. Neurobiol Dis 7: 586–599.
12. D'Cruz PM, Yasumura D, Weir J, Matthes MT, Abderrahim H, et al. (2000) Mutation of the receptor tyrosine kinase gene Mertk in the retinal dystrophic RCS rat. Hum Mol Genet 9: 645–651.
13. Finnemann SC, Bonilha VL, Marmorstein AD, Rodriguez-Boulan E (1997) Phagocytosis of rod outer segments by retinal pigment epithelial cells requires alpha(v)beta5 integrin for binding but not for internalization. Proc Natl Acad Sci U S A 94: 12932–12937.
14. Burgess BL, Abrams TA, Nagata S, Hall MO (2006) MFG-E8 in the retina and retinal pigment epithelium of rat and mouse. Mol Vis 12: 1437–1447.
15. Nandrot EF, Anand M, Almeida D, Atabai K, Sheppard D, et al. (2007) Essential role for MFG-E8 as ligand for alphavbeta5 integrin in diurnal retinal phagocytosis. Proc Natl Acad Sci U S A 104: 12005–12010.
16. Houssier M, Raoul W, Lavalette S, Keller N, Guillonneau X, et al. (2008) CD36 deficiency leads to choroidal involution via COX2 down-regulation in rodents. PLoS Med 5: e39.
17. Friedman DS, O'Colmain BJ, Munoz B, Tomany SC, McCarty C, et al. (2004) Prevalence of age-related macular degeneration in the United States. Arch Ophthalmol 122: 564–572.
18. Sarks SH (1976) Ageing and degeneration in the macular region: a clinico-pathological study. Br J Ophthalmol 60: 324–341.
19. Rosenfeld PJ, Brown DM, Heier JS, Boyer DS, Kaiser PK, et al. (2006) Ranibizumab for neovascular age-related macular degeneration. N Engl J Med 355: 1419–1431.
20. Klein R, Peto T, Bird A, Vannewkirk MR (2004) The epidemiology of age-related macular degeneration. Am J Ophthalmol 137: 486–495.

21. Ding X, Patel M, Chan CC (2009) Molecular pathology of age-related macular degeneration. Prog Retin Eye Res 28: 1–18.
22. Augood CA, Vingerling JR, de Jong PT, Chakravarthy U, Seland J, et al. (2006) Prevalence of age-related maculopathy in older Europeans: the European Eye Study (EUREYE). Arch Ophthalmol 124: 529–535.
23. Bird AC, Bressler NM, Bressler SB, Chisholm IH, Coscas G, et al. (1995) An international classification and grading system for age-related maculopathy and age-related macular degeneration. The International ARM Epidemiological Study Group. Surv Ophthalmol 39: 367–374.
24. Vinding T, Appleyard M, Nyboe J, Jensen G (1992) Risk factor analysis for atrophic and exudative age-related macular degeneration. An epidemiological study of 1000 aged individuals. Acta Ophthalmol (Copenh) 70: 66–72.
25. Klein R, Klein BE, Linton KL, DeMets DL (1993) The Beaver Dam Eye Study: the relation of age-related maculopathy to smoking. Am J Epidemiol 137: 190–200.
26. Combadiere C, Feumi C, Raoul W, Keller N, Rodero M, et al. (2007) CX3CR1-dependent subretinal microglia cell accumulation is associated with cardinal features of age-related macular degeneration. J Clin Invest 117: 2920–2928.
27. Baatz H, Poupel L, Coudert M, Sennlaub F, Combadiere C (2009) [Polymorphisms of complement factor genes and age-related macular degeneration in a German population]. Klin Monbl Augenheilkd 226: 654–658.
28. Sasieni PD (1997) From genotypes to genes: doubling the sample size. Biometrics 53: 1253–1261.
29. Tregouet DA, Garelle V (2007) A new JAVA interface implementation of THESIAS: testing haplotype effects in association studies. Bioinformatics 23: 1038–1039.
30. Paques M, Guyomard JL, Simonutti M, Roux MJ, Picaud S, et al. (2007) Panretinal, high-resolution color photography of the mouse fundus. Invest Ophthalmol Vis Sci 48: 2769–2774.
31. Swaroop A, Branham KE, Chen W, Abecasis G (2007) Genetic susceptibility to age-related macular degeneration: a paradigm for dissecting complex disease traits. Hum Mol Genet 16 Spec No. 2: R174–182.
32. Green WR, Enger C (1993) Age-related macular degeneration histopathologic studies. The 1992 Lorenz E. Zimmerman Lecture. Ophthalmology 100: 1519–1535.
33. Atabai K, Jame S, Azhar N, Kuo A, Lam M, et al. (2009) Mfge8 diminishes the severity of tissue fibrosis in mice by binding and targeting collagen for uptake by macrophages. J Clin Invest 119: 3713–3722.
34. Kwak N, Okamoto N, Wood JM, Campochiaro PA (2000) VEGF is major stimulator in model of choroidal neovascularization. Invest Ophthalmol Vis Sci 41: 3158–3164.
35. Kamizuru H, Kimura H, Yasukawa T, Tabata Y, Honda Y, et al. (2001) Monoclonal antibody-mediated drug targeting to choroidal neovascularization in the rat. Invest Ophthalmol Vis Sci 42: 2664–2672.
36. Sugano G, Bernard-Pierrot I, Lae M, Battail C, Allory Y, et al. (2010) Milk fat globule–epidermal growth factor–factor VIII (MFGE8)/lactadherin promotes bladder tumor development. Oncogene 30: 642–653.
37. Nandrot EF, Finnemann SC (2008) Lack of alphavbeta5 integrin receptor or its ligand MFG-E8: distinct effects on retinal function. Ophthalmic Res 40: 120–123.

14

Decreased Fixation Stability of the Preferred Retinal Location in Juvenile Macular Degeneration

Richard A. I. Bethlehem[1,4]*, Serge O. Dumoulin[1], Edwin S. Dalmaijer[1], Miranda Smit[1,2], Tos T. J. M. Berendschot[3], Tanja C. W. Nijboer[1,2], Stefan Van der Stigchel[1]

1 Experimental Psychology, Helmholtz Institute, Utrecht University, Utrecht, The Netherlands, **2** Rudolf Magnus Institute of Neuroscience and Centre of Excellence for Rehabilitation Medicine, University Medical Centre Utrecht and Rehabilitation Centre De Hoogstraat, Utrecht, The Netherlands, **3** University Eye Clinic Maastricht, Maastricht, The Netherlands, **4** Autism Research Centre, Department of Psychiatry, University of Cambridge, Cambridge, United Kingdom

Abstract

Macular degeneration is the main cause for diminished visual acuity in the elderly. The juvenile form of macular degeneration has equally detrimental consequences on foveal vision. To compensate for loss of foveal vision most patients with macular degeneration adopt an eccentric preferred retinal location that takes over tasks normally performed by the healthy fovea. It is unclear however, whether the preferred retinal locus also develops properties typical for foveal vision. Here, we investigated whether the fixation characteristics of the preferred retinal locus resemble those of the healthy fovea. For this purpose, we used the fixation-offset paradigm and tracked eye-position using a high spatial and temporal resolution infrared eye-tracker. The fixation-offset paradigm measures release from fixation under different fixation conditions and has been shown useful to distinguish between foveal and non-foveal fixation. We measured eye-movements in nine healthy age-matched controls and five patients with juvenile macular degeneration. In addition, we performed a simulation with the same task in a group of five healthy controls. Our results show that the preferred retinal locus does not adopt a foveal type of fixation but instead drifts further away from its original fixation and has overall increased fixation instability. Furthermore, the fixation instability is most pronounced in low frequency eye-movements representing a slow drift from fixation. We argue that the increased fixation instability cannot be attributed to fixation under an unnatural angle. Instead, diminished visual acuity in the periphery causes reduced oculomotor control and results in increased fixation instability.

Editor: Chris I. Baker, National Institute of Mental Health, United States of America

Funding: This research was funded by a grant from the Dutch MD-foundation to authors SD, TN, and SvS. The funders had no role in study design, data collection and analysis, decision to publish, or preparation of the manuscript.

Competing Interests: The authors have declared that no competing interests exist.

* E-mail: rb643@cam.ac.uk

Introduction

Juvenile macular degeneration (JMD) affects approximately 1 in 10.000 individuals [1]. Most often it is caused by mutations in the ABCA4 gene, which transcribes a large retina-specific protein, leading to Stargardt disease [2,3,4]. As a result patients commonly develop a central scotoma that involves the fovea. The resulting loss of foveal vision has a severe impact on patients visual acuity. Early research has shown that this can be accompanied by a shift in the oculomotor reference from the fovea to a nonfoveal locus [5]. Subsequently patients suffering from macular degeneration often adopt one or multiple preferred retinal loci (PRL) that can serve as a 'pseudo-fovea' [6,7]. This PRL is an eccentric location on the retina that is used for fixation in favor of the fovea. Crossland et al. [8] have shown that this PRL can develop within six months of visual loss onset and further research shows that the PRL location can remain relatively stable in people with age-related macular degeneration [9]. Additionally, strategies for developing a PRL appear to be slightly different for different causes of macular degeneration [10], with Stargardts disease being the more variable one. Apart from the obvious poorer resolution of the visual retina in the periphery, fixation with the PRL in patients with MD (Throughout this manuscript we use JMD to refer to juvenile macular degeneration, MD to refer to non-specific macular degeneration and AMD to refer to age-related macular degeneration) also tends to be unstable [11,12]. In healthy individuals fixation instability can be beneficial in the central retina because of a low tolerance for image motion [13,14]. As resolution decreases with higher velocity eye movements [14] fixation instability recovers some of this loss [13]. During stable fixation peripheral vision also tends to decrease (Troxler fading) and unstable fixation partially recovers this fading. As Deruaz et al point out this has led to the suggestion that increased fixation instability for people that use peripheral fixation (such as people with MD) might be equally beneficial [15]. However, Macedo et al. have showed that this is not necessarily the case for patients with MD using peripheral vision [16]. Specifically, Macedo and colleagues [16] showed that fixation instability does not reduce crowded or non-crowded visual acuity. Thus, in standard reading or acuity test this instability does not produce any net benefit for people with MD. At the same time, paradigms utilizing visual acuity types of tests might not be the best predictors in determining fixation patterns and rehabilitation outcomes in patients with macular degeneration [17].

Most studies to date have not explicitly focused on the juvenile form of macular degeneration but on age-related macular degeneration (AMD) [10,17,18,19,20,21,22,23,24]. AMD is the most common form and is considered to be the main cause of diminished visual acuity in the elderly [25]. One study has shown that in AMD training can significantly improve fixation stability [24]. It has also been shown that fixation stability can be strongly correlated with PRL eccentricity [23]. In addition, Tarita-Nistor et al. [21] have shown that patients with AMD generally have good ocular motor coordination and fixation control, but that this disappears when one eye is covered. In addition, it has been shown that fixation characteristics may differ between monocular and binocular viewing in patients with AMD when asked to fixate for relatively long time periods [26]. It is possible that the relative late onset of AMD compared to JMD allows for some sustaining of oculomotor control and that this is better during binocular viewing [21]. In the present study we will focus specifically on the ability to keep fixation steady for short periods during binocular viewing by individuals with JMD.

Most studies which have investigated fixation characteristics of patients with macular degeneration have used a microperimeter [18,19,23,24,27] to assess fixation stability of the PRL. This measure generally has a low temporal resolution (<25 Hz) and as a result partial saccades (start or end points) are often difficult to take into account, let alone remove from the data. Additionally, long fixation periods are often used (exceeding 10s) which might make it harder for participants to stay focused. In contrast, short fixation phases might give a more accurate account of fixation characteristics under ecologically important and valid conditions such as during reading, visual search, visual scene processing or even typing. These types of fixation phases generally fall well within a 150 to 450 ms. time-scale [28]. In addition, precisely these types of viewing conditions have been shown to be impaired in MD [11,29]. Infrared eye-trackers allow short but detailed recording at this high temporal resolution as well as detection of trials containing saccades that can subsequently be removed. Infrared eye-trackers have already shown high test-retest reliability and have been proven useful in the assessment of fixation characteristics when compared to standard Scanning Laser Ophthalmoscope (SLO) measurements [30]. Although Crossland and Rubin [30] show that the eye-tracker methodology tends to overestimate the fixation instability, they also argue that this overestimation might be caused by small compensatory eye-movements. These are a result of the fact that participants' heads were completely unrestrained during testing. In addition, because infrared eye-trackers can record at high temporal resolutions, the need for long fixation periods becomes unnecessary and paves the way for more ecologically valid ways of assessing fixation in patients with MD. Furthermore, they allow for more fine-grained analyses of eye-tracking data such as power spectral densities with high temporal resolution that can further elucidate underlying fixation characteristics [31].

In the present study we aim to investigate the fixation characteristics in a group of patients with JMD that have stable PRL's during a paradigm that can potentially distinguish between foveal and peripheral types of fixation using an infrared eye-tracker. To this end we adopted a fixation offset paradigm [32]. This paradigm includes a short fixation phase that covers the range of fixation times reported during various different types of viewing [28] without explicitly restraining the fixation characteristics by a specific cue. In this paradigm participants do not focus explicitly on a fixation cross but instead are shown fixation anchors at a distance of either 1° degree or 3°. Machado and Rafal [32] have shown that in healthy controls the 1° condition represents a foveal specific type of fixation whereas the 3° does not. In the 1° condition, introducing a gap between target onset and fixation offset results in a decrease in saccade latencies which does not occur in the 3° condition [33]. Fendrich et al. [33] argue that the 1° anchor falls within foveal fixation and the gap-effect thus only occurs for foveal fixation. In a previous study we have shown that a central scotoma combined with peripheral viewing impairs search efficiency and that these results can be explained without the necessity of reorganisation in the visual system [29]. Since the JMD group will use their periphery for both the foveal as well as the peripheral fixation anchor conditions the difference in fixation stability should be minimal. For the control group we would expect a difference for foveal (1 degree condition) versus non-foveal (3 degree condition) fixation, whereby the non-foveal fixation may resemble the general fixation of the patient group more closely.

We hypothesize that patients with JMD will have greater overall fixation instability due the use of peripheral viewing when compared to controls. Based on our previous study [29] using a visual search paradigm we do not expect that the PRL will have adopted foveal fixation properties and thus we do not expect an effect of fixation anchor-size. In contrast, we expect healthy controls to have an overall more stable fixation pattern that is strongest in the foveal (1 degree) fixation condition. To assess this instability, we will first look at the number of intrusive saccades, defined as a saccade during a moment in the task where stable fixation is required. Second, as a measure of fixation instability we use a bivariate contour ellipse area (BCEA) [23,30,34,35] and the overall displacement during the course of the fixation period. Finally, to further investigate the nature of fixation in JMD we will analyze the power spectral densities [31]. To ensure that any fixation instability is not explained by an 'unnatural' position of the eye during eccentric viewing we also tested a simulated PRL version of this paradigm in healthy controls.

Methods

Ethics Statement

The ethical institutional review board of the University Medical Centre Utrecht approved this study, and all subjects gave written informed consent prior to participation. All study procedures have been conducted according to the principles expressed in the Declaration of Helsinki.

Participants

For this study, we recruited 10 patients with juvenile MD. Additionally, 10 healthy age-matched controls participated in the same paradigm and another 6 healthy controls were recruited for participation in a simulation version of this paradigm. The JMD participants had an official diagnosis of JMD (assessed by their own physician and confirmed by means of a questionnaire) and had no history of neurological and/or psychiatrical disorders or substance abuse. Controls had normal or corrected to normal acuity and had no history of neurological and/or psychiatrical disorders or substance abuse either. All participants received 20 euro and travel expenses for their participation.

Procedure, Stimuli and Design

Clinical characteristics of the JMD patients were verbally interrogated by means of a questionnaire, see Table 1. After filling out the questionnaire, the experimental procedure started. All measurements were conducted in a sound-attenuated, dimly lit room. Eye movements were recorded by an Eyelink1000 system (SR Research Ltd, Canada), an infrared video-based eye-tracker.

The dominant eye, which was verified with a visual alignment task [36], was monitored and analysed in all participants. The non-dominant eye was not occluded during the course of the experiment to allow for naturalistic viewing. Although no research to date has established a clear link between eye dominance as measured by an alignment task and the dominant eye for fixation, this was the least arbitrary way to determine which eye to track. The participants' heads were stabilized using a chin rest to control for compensatory head movements. We acknowledge that head stabilization may somewhat limit the ecological validity, but it was necessary to make full use of the eye trackers temporal and spatial specificity. The distance between monitor and chin rest was 57 cm. A nine-point grid calibration and subsequent validation procedure was utilized before the start of the experiment.

Scanning Laser Opthalmology

In order to gain information about fixation stability and absolute locus of the PRL, patients were invited for a separate Scanning Laser Ophthalmoscope measurement (SLO) at the University Eye Clinic Maastricht [37]. We used a custom build Scanning Laser Ophthalmoscope [37,38] to image the fundus and to present the stimulus. The subjects fixated on a red cross that was presented in the SLO. To determine the absolute location of the PRL at the retina and its stability, we acquired 60 SLO images per participant with the use of a frame grabber, having a 1 sec interval in between. Similarly as described in Reinhard et al. [39] we used an SLO that shows the fundus and the fixation cross simultaneously on a video monitor. Further analysis was done also similar as described in the Reinhard et al. paper [39]. We aligned the subsequent images and calculated the PRL and its movement. Images are shown in Figure 1. The fundus photographs show the location of this PRL over time.

Visual Field Test

In addition, we used a visual field test to confirm the absolute visual field defect. In the visual field test, one target at a time was shown and a fixation cross was used which remained on screen during presentation of the target. The target was a black 1.5° dot and could appear at 33 possible stimulus locations with a background luminance of 52.95 cd/m2. The target was presented for 1500 ms. The 33 locations were organised in five rows; three rows consisted of seven locations and two rows of six locations. The centre-to-centre distance, both within and between rows of each location had a visual angle of 5°. Participants were instructed to remain fixated on the fixation cross and report, using the 'z' and '/' keys, whether they had seen a target or not. After their response a confirmation of their choice was presented on screen. Target present trials were mixed with 'catch' trials in which no target was presented. All target locations were presented four times along with 16 catch trials, making for 148 trials in total [29]. The visual field defect has been incorporated in Figure 1. MD case number 6 was excluded based on converging evidence from both the SLO and visual field test that the fixation overlapped with the fovea. For MD 3 there was a technical issue with the visual field data, but the SLO showed clear use of a PRL.

Fixation Offset Paradigm

To test fixation characteristics we used a fixation-offset paradigm [32]. All trials started with a drift check to ensure the calibration was still accurate. Participants were instructed to fixate on an unmarked centre containing four eccentric anchors surrounding the *unmarked* centre (background luminance of 32.07 cd/m2). The unmarked centre served as the fixation point and was located at the centre of the display. The eccentric fixation anchors consisted of four black crosses (0.64°×0.64°) and were presented on the corners of an unmarked square. The distance from the crosses to the centre of the screen was either 3° or 1°. After a pseudo-random interval (between 550 and 950 ms.), a black target circle appeared (diameter of 1.43°). See figure 2A for an overview. In the patient group the location of target dots was dependent of the scotomatous area (either left, right, above or below the eccentric fixation anchor) as target locations that fell within the scotoma, as assessed with a visual field test, were removed from the location possibilities. The eccentric anchors were the same as in the control group to minimize potentially biasing the fixation stability by using different fixation anchors. In the control group targets were presented in all four (left, right, above and below the fixation anchor) possible locations. Participants were instructed to fixate at the *unmarked* centre until the target dot appeared, and subsequently were to move their eyes as fast as possible to the target circle. The target display was presented for 1500 ms. Afterwards all objects were removed from the display. The experiment consisted of 240 experimental trials and 24 practice trials.

Fixation Offset Simulation Paradigm

To investigate whether any difference in fixation might be caused by an unnatural eye-position in the patient group we also conducted a separate simulation in healthy controls. In this adaptation a para-foveal fixation cross at 8° eccentricity is presented at the right side of the true fixation. This eccentric fixation is an offset of the eye-position as measured with the eye-tracker and is thus controlled by participants' eye-movement. Participants are instructed to move this alternative fixation point over a centrally located fixation cross, hold their fixation steady and press the spacebar. When this alternative fixation was stable

Table 1. Clinical characteristics of individual patients.

Patient	Gender	Official Diagnosis	Age (y)	Age onset (y)
MD1	F	Stargardt	33	23
MD2	F	Stargardt	29	12
MD3	M	X-Chromosal schisis*	48	congenital
MD4	M	Stargardt	47	gradual
MD5	M	Stargardt	23	6
MD6	F	Best's Disease	38	20

*X-chromosome-linked juvenile retino- schisis.

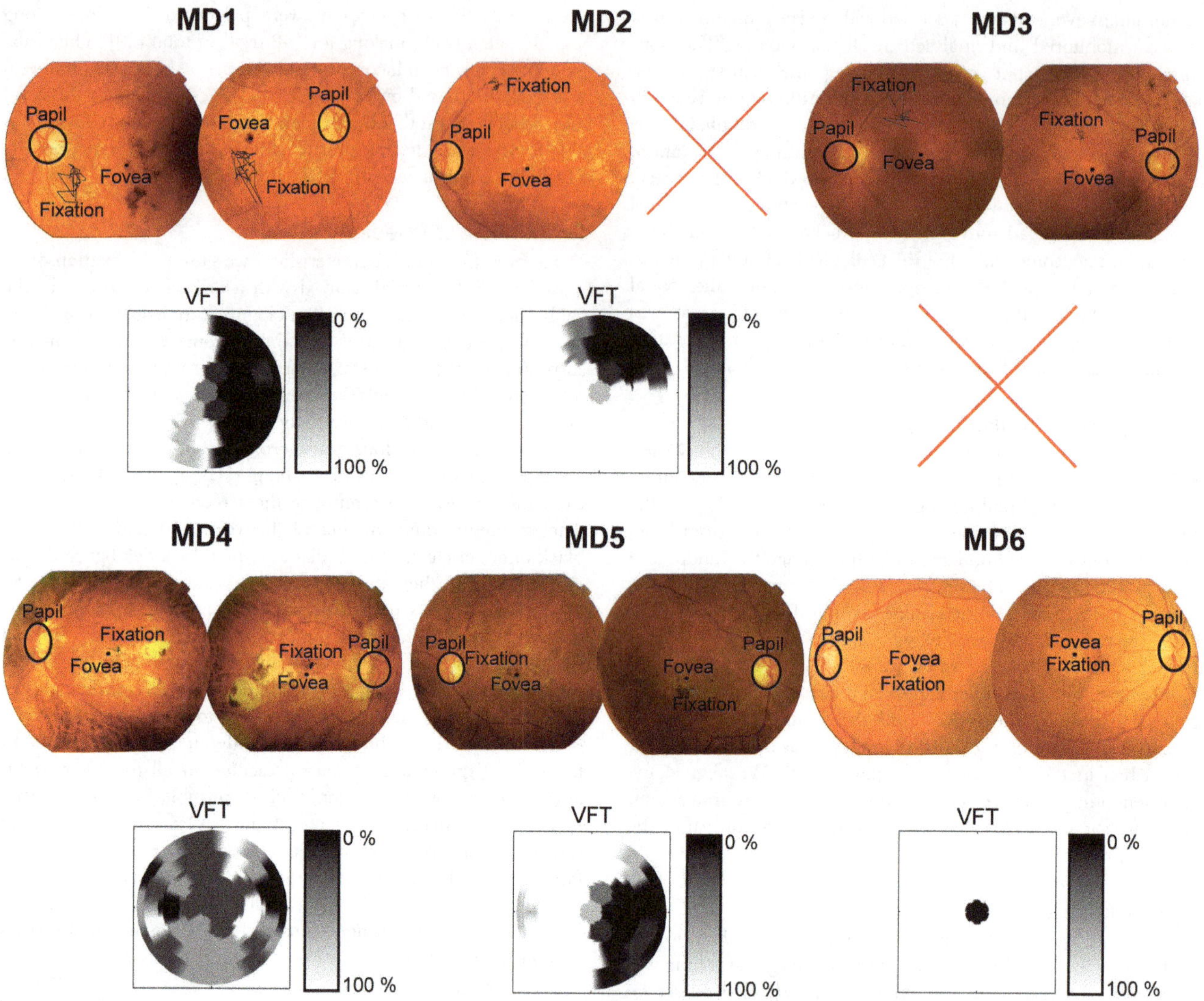

Figure 1. Scanning Laser Opthalmoscope photo's. SLO photographs of all JMD participants. Participant 6 (lower right) was excluded due to the evident overlap of fixation and fovea. Interpolated visual field task images are shown below each respective SLO image. These show the visual field defect (VFT) for an 18° by 18° degrees visual field. Dark areas represent the point in the visual field where there was a defect, white represent no defect (ranging from 0–100%). Because the VFT measurements are based on binocular viewing and the SLO images are from each eye separately they not always clearly translate to one another [21,26].

within 2° degrees of the central fixation cross the trial started by removal of the central fixation point. See figure 2B for a graphical overview. At the same time as the central fixation cross disappeared, fixation anchors were presented at either 1° or 3° degrees eccentricity from fixation. These were exactly the same as in the original paradigm and were presented for the same pseudorandom interval (550 ms-950 ms). After this a target was presented above, below or to the left of the true fixation and participants were instructed to move the eyes there as fast as possible and press the spacebar once they had done so. Size of the target dots, fixation crosses and fixation anchors as well as all luminance ratios was kept the same as in the original paradigm. This task was programmed using PyGaze [40]. We acknowledge that the simulation group cannot be considered the ideal comparison to the behaviour observed in the MD group. A gaze-contingent eccentric fixation anchor might not be the best reflection of the deficit that people with MD experience and an alternative might have been the use of a gaze-contingent artificial scotoma. However, we chose not to use a gaze-contingent artificial scotoma because this would have provided the healthy participants of the simulation study with a strong cue (namely the border of the artificial scotoma) to be aligned with the eccentric fixation anchors. Furthermore, an artificial gaze-contingent scotoma is still always visible to a healthy control subject and is thus likely to affect the oculomotor programming. Also, healthy subjects might not necessarily deviate attention to a peripheral location when the artificial scotoma is visible. Instead they might simply attend to the borders of the artificial scotoma. We aimed to minimize these effects by using a gaze-contingent eccentric anchor instead.

Data Analysis

Our main question concerned the fixation behaviour with patients with JMD and a stable PRL in the absence of a clear fixation point. Therefore we focussed our analysis on the pseudo-random fixation phase at the start of each trial during which participants have to keep their fixation steady and within which the anchor points are presented on screen (Figure 2A).

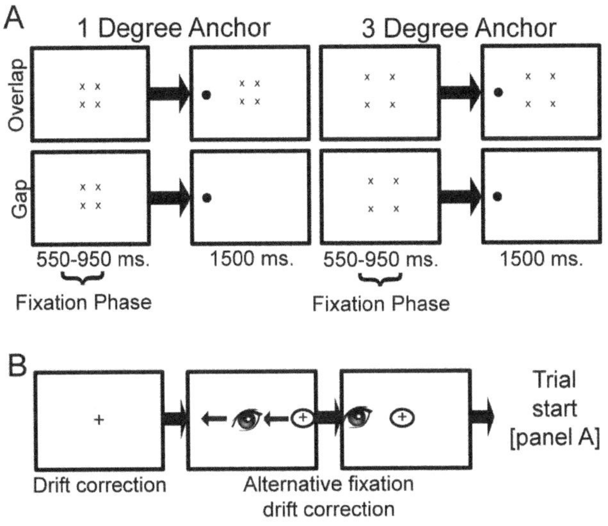

Figure 2. Paradigm overview. Panel A shows a schematic overview of the fixation-offset paradigm as used by Machado & Rafal [32]. After drift correction participants are instructed to keep a steady fixation within the four anchors. As soon as a target appears they are instructed to make an eye-movement to that target as fast as possible. Presently, we focussed on the fixation phase (before target presentation) of this paradigm. Panel B shows the adaptation used in the PRL simulation version of this paradigm. Prior to the normal trial procedure (but after drift correction), participants had to align a gaze-controlled alternate eccentric fixation point over a central fixation cross. This led them to use their peripheral vision to fixate on the central fixation cross before the start of the trial. In panel B the "eyeball" symbol represent the true fixation, the '+' sign represents the central fixation and the circled '+' sign represents the eccentric fixation point that was controlled by the participants eye movement. There was no minimum fixation time during alignment of the eccentric fixation point that participants had to maintain for the trial to start. However, should participants make a saccade directing the eccentric fixation to the central fixation cross and then press the spacebar, the subsequent saccade parser would have detected a saccade at trial start and the trial would have been removed from subsequent analysis.

Three main measures were taken during this period. First, we determined the number of saccades during the fixation phase (figure 2A). Thresholds for detecting the onset of a saccadic movement were an acceleration of 8000°/s2 and a velocity of 30°/s. These are the standard criteria used by SR Research's Eyelink systems to detect saccades. During this part of the task people are explicitly instructed to keep a steady fixation, thus we termed saccades during this period 'intrusive saccades' as opposed to the subsequent saccade made to the target after the fixation phase. Trials containing such 'intrusive saccades' were subsequently removed from further analysis and these trials are thus not included in any of the other reported measures. Second, we determined the total displacement of the fixation position at a single point in time as the distance between the original fixation and the position of the eye at target onset in degrees. The total displacement measure is potentially more sensitive to slow one-directional drift as opposed to fixation area. The rationale behind this measure was that if an eye movement (below saccade thresholds described above) would go in a single direction then the overall fixation instability, as determined by the BCEA, would be relatively small since this measure is largely determined by the standard deviation of eye-movement in x and y directions. Thus the total displacement might reflect a different type of fixation instability. Third, fixation stability was calculated using the method of determining a bivariate contour ellipse area the methodology of which is extensive described elsewhere [23,30,34,35].

To investigate the nature of the instability we analysed the power spectral density (using a fast fourier transformation) of the time-courses of the displacement [31,41] of trials without saccades and blinks. The rationale behind this approach is that it might be more sensitive to detect a slow displacement drift as opposed to faster 'jerky' eye-movement instability that might be the result of reduced oculomotor control.

All measures were analysed using 2x3 mixed ANOVA with condition (1degree anchor vs. 3degree anchor) as within subjects factor and group (Control vs. MD vs. Simulation) as between subjects factor. Post-hoc t-tests (two-sided) were conducted using Bonferroni correction for multiple comparisons.

Apart from a diagnosis of JMD, inclusion criteria for the JMD group included a clear usage of a stable PRL as measured with the SLO and the ability to perform both a nine-grid calibration and validation on the Eyelink system prior to the start of the experiment. Four participants from the JMD group were unable to attend an SLO measurement and were thus excluded from the final analysed sample. In one case the PRL overlapped almost perfectly and was thus also excluded (MD6 in figure 1). If the number of valid trials, after removal of trials including an intrusive saccade, was more than 3 standard deviations away from the group mean, that subject was considered an extreme outlier. In the control and simulation group one extreme outlier on the intrusive saccade measure was excluded. In total our exclusion criteria thus led to a loss of 5 JMD participants, 1 control participant and 1 control participant performing the simulation experiment. The final analysed sample thus included 5 JMD participants (see Table 1 for clinical characteristics of the JMD group) and 9 controls matched for age and 5 controls participating in the simulation experiment. This relatively small number of JMD participants is not uncommon in the literature [16,24,29,42,43,44]. In addition all our results figures include individual data points showing that our results are consistent across patients and that the behaviour of nearly each patient deviates from the control group.

Results

Example eye-movement recordings and BCEA computation are shown in Figure 3. Figure 3 depicts three types of trials. The top trial (3A and 3B) is an example of a trial with an intrusive saccade. The scatterplot (3B) shows how an intrusive saccade influences the spread of the displacement and thus the BCEA and overall displacement. Intrusive saccades can greatly bias the displacement and fixation stability measures and therefore all trials that included intrusive saccades were removed from the remaining analysis. The two other trials show a 'normal' time-course (3C) and scatterplot (3D) of a healthy control and a time-course (3E) and scatterplot (3F) of a patient with JMD. In the scatterplots of the included trial types (3D and 3F) examples of a BCEA are shown.

Intrusive Saccades

We measured the amount of intrusive saccades, as defined above, during the fixation phase (figure 2A) of the fixation-offset paradigm. JMD patients made more intrusive saccades than both the control and simulation groups as is evident from a main effect of Group $F(2,16) = 46.243$, $p<0.001$ and Post-hoc tests: JMD> Control ($p<0.001$) and JMD>Simulation ($p<0.001$), see figure 4. There was no apparent Post-hoc difference between the control group and the simulation group. These results clearly show that

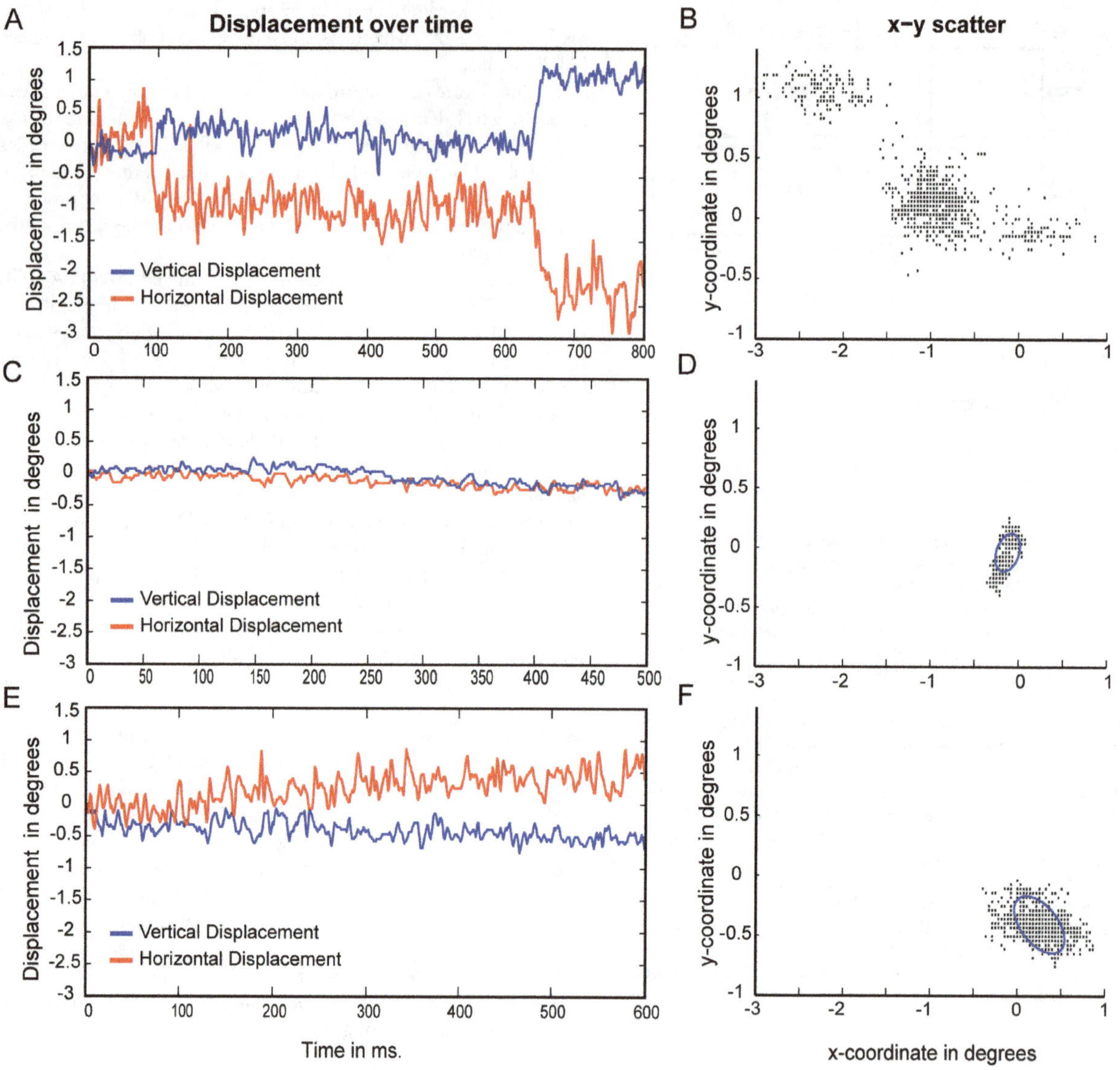

Figure 3. Time-course and scatterplot examples for different types of trials. Panels A, C and E show example time-courses of eye-position over time, lines indicate horizontal (red) and vertical (blue) displacement over time. The example time-courses illustrate measurement with (A) and without (C) an intrusive saccade in control subjects and a typical trial without saccades or blinks of a JMD patient (E). Panels B, D and F show the corresponding eye-positions across the entire measurement duration, indicating the effect of saccade and blinks on the displacement spread (Panel B). Displacement was summarized by the BCEA and examples are shown in blue circles in panels D and E. Only trials that did not include these intrusive saccades or blinks were included in the analysis of the BCEA, displacement and power spectral densities.

patients with JMD have difficulty in maintaining fixation even for a very short duration.

Our within subjects factor of fixation anchor-size also showed a main effect: $F(2,16) = 8.746$, $p = 0.009$. The interaction between the size of the fixation anchor and Group was not significant $F(2,16) = 3.373$, $p = 0.060$.

Displacement

Second, we measured the displacement between the start- and end-point of the eye at the onset of the fixation phase. Here, results show a main effect of Group $F(2,16) = 16.904$, $p < 0.001$. This effect also seems to be mainly driven by the JMD group as Post-Hoc tests show: JMD>Control ($p < 0.001$) and JMD>Simulation ($p < 0.001$), see figure 5. There was no main effect of Anchorsize, nor an interaction effect on the total displacement. These results confirm that patients with JMD have an unstable fixation pattern even when trials that contained saccades were removed from the analysis.

Fixation Stability

Third, we determined the total fixation area using a BCEA for all time-points during the fixation-phase of the fixation-offset paradigm (Figure 3D & F). The results show that fixation stability as measured with a bivariate contour ellipse during a short fixation phase was significantly different across the three groups $F(2,16) = 4.476$, $p = 0.029$, see figure 6. Post-hoc tests show that this effect is mainly caused by the JMD group: JMD>Control ($p = 0.047$) and that there was no significant effect for the JMD group compared to the simulation JMD>Simulation ($p = 0.059$). There was no main effect of Anchorsize, nor an interaction effect

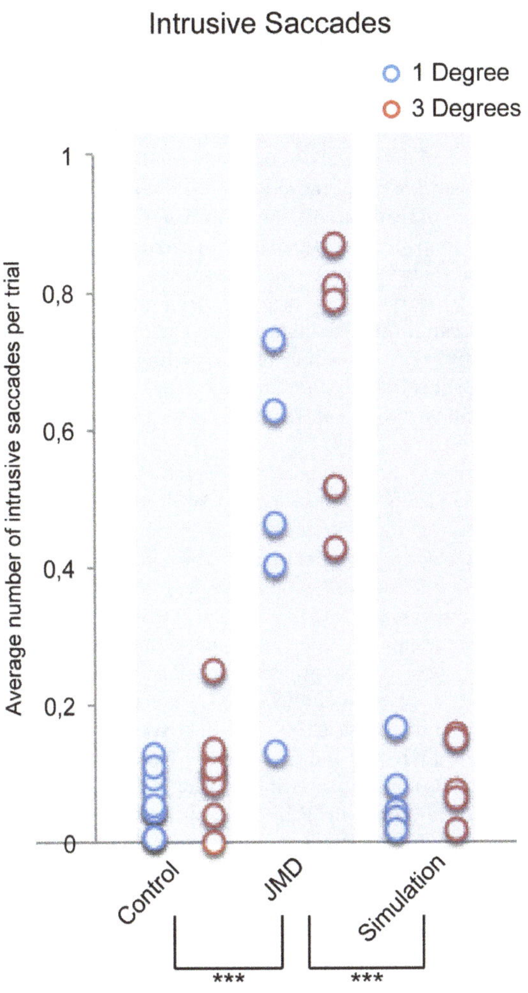

Figure 4. Number of intrusive saccades during fixation. The average number of intrusive saccades per trial are shown. Significant differences are marked: p<0.001 = ***, p<0.01 = ** & p<0.05 = *. This figure shows that the JMD group (1 degree [M: 0.47 SD: 0.23], 3 degrees [M: 0.68 SD: 0.20]) made significantly more intrusive saccades compared to healthy controls (1 degree [M: 0.06 SD: 0.04], 3 degrees [M: 0.11 SD: 0.07]) and controls performing the simulation (1 degree [M: 0.07 SD: 0.06], 3 degrees [M: 0.09 SD: 0.06]). It also shows that in the control group people made less intrusive saccade in the 1-degree condition.

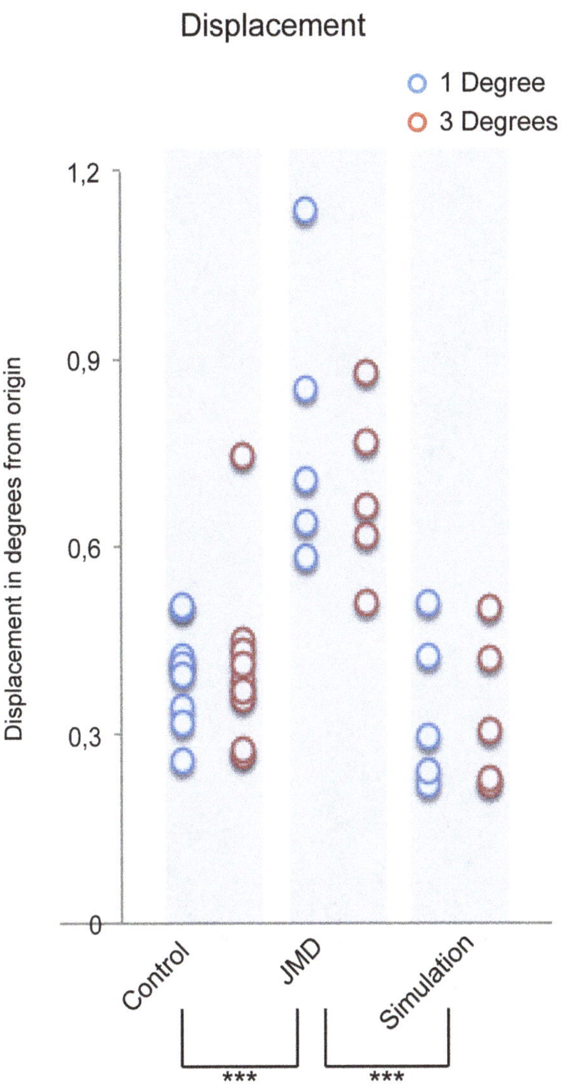

Figure 5. Displacement during fixation. The start-to-end displacement in degrees of visual angle is shown. Significant differences are marked: p<0.001 = ***, p<0.01 = ** & p<0.05 = *. This figure shows that patients with JMD (1 degree [M: 0.78 SD: 0.22], 3 degrees [M: 0.69 SD: 0.14]) deviated more from their original fixation at the end of the fixation phase compared to controls in both the normal (1 degree [M: 0.40 SD: 0.08], 3 degrees [M: 0.41 SD: 0.14]) and simulation (1 degree [M: 0.34 SD: 0.12], 3 degrees [M: 0.34 SD: 0.12]) paradigm.

on the fixation stability. The results remained statistically significant even with the JMD outlier removed (main effect of Group *(F2,15) = 11.537, p = 0.001* and Post-Hoc differences: JMD>Control, *p = 0.003* and JMD>Simulation, *p = 0.001*). Again, these results show that patients with JMD have an unstable fixation that cannot directly be related to an unnatural eye-position.

Power Spectral Density

In order to measure the nature of the fixation instability we measured the power spectral density of the first 500 ms. of the fixation time-courses [31,41]. The results from our power spectral density analyses are plotted in figure 7. This analysis suggests that the difference in fixation stability reported above is primarily driven by low frequency eye-movements. Figure 7 shows that below 10 Hz all patients from the JMD group fall well outside the 95% confidence interval of the healthy control group. Although the saccade parser used in the present study did not explicitly detect micro-saccades, low-frequency eye movements are often interpreted as slow variations in eye position such as drift [31,45]. These low frequency differences can thus not be attributed to potential contamination with high-frequency eye movements such as micro-saccades or tremors [46].

Discussion

The PRL in individuals with JMD exhibits unstable fixation patterns compared to fixation patterns of the healthy fovea. This instability is reflected in more intrusive saccades and decreased fixation stability. The decreased fixation stability is driven by slow variations in eye-position. The intrusive saccades measure we used in the present study might also reflect the fact that a decrease in visual acuity causes a deficit in terms of maintaining attention on

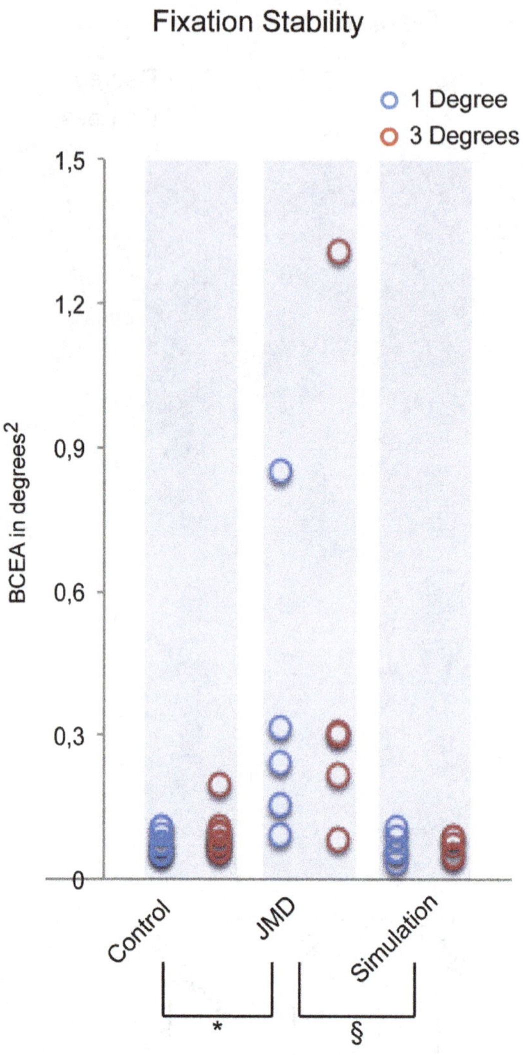

Figure 6. Fixation stability during fixation. The fixation stability in squared degrees as measured with a bivariate contour ellipse area (see figures 3B and 3D for an example). Significant differences are marked: $p<0.001$ = ***, $p<0.01$ = ** & $p<0.05$ = *. The "§" marks a trend. This figure shows that fixation was more unstable in the JMD group (1 degree [M: 0.33 SD: 0.20], 3 degrees [M: 0.44 SD: 0.49]) compared to the healthy control group (1 degree [M: 0.08 SD: 0.02], 3 degrees [M: 0.09 SD: 0.04]). The difference between the JMD group and the simulation group (1 degree [M: 0.07 SD: 0.03], 3 degrees [M: 0.07 SD: 0.02]) was not significant but a Bonferroni corrected p-value of 0.067 might be considered a trend.

the fixation stimulus. The decreased visual acuity might lead to uncertainty concerning the possible offset of the fixation cross, resulting in an increase in preliminary saccades away from the fixation stimulus, even though it is still physically present on the screen. Since all trials that contained such saccades were subsequently removed from further analysis this would not directly explain differences in fixation stability. Another potential cause for the detection of these saccades might have been a switch to a different PRL. Such a switch might be detected by the eye tracker as a rapid saccade, although it is unlikely that PRL switch will occur in such a short time-frame. If participants indeed switched to a different PRL the eye-tracker would have to be re-calibrated. Because it was calibrated for another PRL the drift check preceding each trial would fail after a PRL switch and would only continue after re-calibrating for the new PRL. Since no re-calibration was needed we assume that the final analysed trials were all from the same PRL.

The simulation suggest that it is unlikely that the present results can be explained by the notion that during peripheral viewing the eye-muscles are in an unnatural position and are thus more prone to saccadic behavior back to a more natural position. The control group performing the simulation shows similar fixation characteristics as the group performing the normal paradigm. Consequently, they also show the same differences when compared with the JMD group performing the normal paradigm. This is in line with previous research using simulated scotomas that show intact oculomotor control during reading [47] as well as during visual search [48]. Thus it is unlikely that any differences in oculomotor control in the patient group can be ascribed to peripheral vision alone.

Recently, there is a debate about the degree of plasticity and stability in the human brain following retinal degeneration. This debate is centred on the observation that regions deprived of retinal input, such as the foveal projection zone, can still respond to visual stimulation. Some authors have argued that these signals reflect cortical reorganization [42,43,49] whereas others don't [29,44,50]. In the present study we found that in the control group fixation is more stable during presentation of foveal anchors (1 degree) compared to parafoveal anchors (3 degrees) as measured by the number of intrusive saccades. This increased stability was absent in both the JMD and the simulation group. Furthermore, the present results also show that peripheral fixation using a PRL is significantly more unstable in JMD patients compared to the simulation group. This indicates that the instability cannot be attributed to peripheral fixation alone. Thus even in the periphery where the PRL is located patients with JMD suffer from reduced fixation stability. This is in contrast to a previous study by White and Bedell [5] showing relatively stable fixation patterns in patients with bilateral macular disease. This study however used a much lower temporal resolution and might have been unable to accurately filter out intrusive saccades nor detect slow drift. Our results align with a more recent study that also showed decreased fixation stability in patients with JMD [51]. Given results from our previous study [29] it is likely that diminished visual acuity in the periphery contributes to this decreased fixational control. Although acuity was not measured in the present study, we assume that acuity diminishes at increased eccentricity for both controls and patients. With regards to plasticity, the behavioural eye-movement characteristics in the present study do not mimic the characteristics of the fovea when compared in a fixation-offset paradigm with foveal and parafoveal anchors. Therefore, the present results can be explained without the need for plasticity and instead be attributed to eccentric viewing with possible additional reduced visual acuity. We note, however, that current results might not extent to the non-dominant eye, as we only measured the oculomotor characteristics of the dominant eye Previous studies that focussed on AMD have shown that oculomotor control can differ between monocular and binocular viewing [21,26]. Interestingly and in contrast to the present study, in AMD oculomotor control seems to be relatively good during binocular viewing [21]. As stated before it is possible that the relative late onset of AMD might allow for some sustaining of oculomotor control. In the present study we did however not test the effects of monocular versus binocular viewing. Future studies investigating oculomotor control of the PRL in individuals with macular degeneration should therefore carefully control for acuity and test both eyes separately to make such a direct comparison possible.

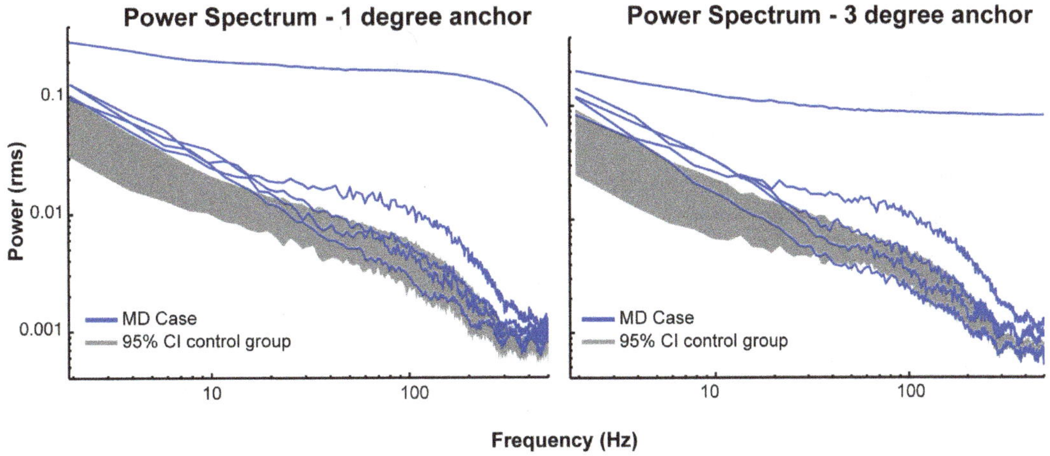

Figure 7. Power spectral density plots. Power spectral densities for the one and three degrees condition. The grey bars represent the 95% confidence interval (CI) of the control group mean. Each blue line represents one JMD patient. This figure shows that JMD patients had significant more power in the lower frequencies, indicating that low frequency eye-movements dominate the differences in displacement and fixation stability.

The differences in low-frequency eye-movements, interpreted as drift, provide another clue about the effect of macular degeneration on fixation characteristics. Under normal conditions drift is sometimes termed 'slow control' [52]. This refers to the balance between maintaining fixation on a certain object while allowing some eye-movements oscillation to prevent perceptual fading [13,45]. As such, it is possible that the increased power of these types of eye-oscillations in JMD reflects a compensatory mechanism for loss of visual acuity due to peripheral viewing. It is also possible that this increased drift is simply a result of decreased oculomotor control as drift can sometimes also be triggered by spontaneous activation of peripheral oculomotor mechanisms [45]. Because we also observed an increased number of intrusive saccades in the JMD group the latter explanation seems the most likely. This finding is further supported by early findings showing that especially slow eye-movements are normally controlled by the fovea [53], although this study investigated fixation during a fairly long interval of 12 seconds and with considerably lower temporal resolution (<100 Hz).

In sum, our findings show a clear deficit in oculomotor control in patients with JMD during fixation. Given that we ruled out an unnatural eye-position as the cause for this instability we suggest that diminished peripheral acuity may be the most likely explanation. This may also be the factor underlying increased low-frequency drift. Perhaps, the adoption of a fixation stimulus that is scaled, such that is easier to see for the patients with JMD, might restore normal fixation behaviour.

Author Contributions

Conceived and designed the experiments: RB SD ED MS TB TN SvS. Performed the experiments: RB MS TB TN. Analyzed the data: RB SD MS TB SvS. Contributed reagents/materials/analysis tools: RB SD ED MS TB TN SvS. Wrote the paper: RB SD ED MS TB TN SvS.

References

1. Bither PP, Berns LA (1985) Stargardt's disease: A review of the literature. Journal of the American Optomology Association 59: 106–111.
2. Allikmets R (1997) A photoreceptor cell-specific ATP-binding transporter gene (ABCR) is mutated in recessive Stargardt macular dystrophy. Nature genetics 17: 122.
3. Allikmets R, Shroyer NF, Singh N, Seddon JM, Lewis RA, et al. (1997) Mutation of the Stargardt disease gene (ABCR) in age-related macular degeneration. Science 277: 1805–1807.
4. Koenekoop RK (2003) The gene for Stargardt disease, ABCA4, is a major retinal gene: a mini-review. Ophthalmic genetics 24: 75–80.
5. White JM, Bedell HE (1990) The oculomotor reference in humans with bilateral macular disease. Investigative ophthalmology & visual science 31: 1149–1161.
6. Crossland MD, Engel SA, Legge GE (2011) The preferred retinal locus in macular disease: toward a consensus definition. Retina 31: 2109–2114.
7. Greenstein VC, Santos RA, Tsang SH, Smith RT, Barile GR, et al. (2008) Preferred retinal locus in macular disease: characteristics and clinical implications. Retina 28: 1234–1240.
8. Crossland MD, Culham LE, Kabanarou SA, Rubin GS (2005) Preferred retinal locus development in patients with macular disease. Ophthalmology 112: 1579–1585.
9. Sunness JS, Applegate CA (2005) Long-term follow-up of fixation patterns in eyes with central scotomas from geographic atrophy that is associated with age-related macular degeneration. American journal of ophthalmology 140: 1085–1093.
10. Sunness JS, Applegate CA, Haselwood D, Rubin GS (1996) Fixation patterns and reading rates in eyes with central scotomas from advanced atrophic age-related macular degeneration and Stargardt disease. Ophthalmology 103: 1458–1466.
11. Crossland MD, Culham LE, Rubin GS (2004) Fixation stability and reading speed in patients with newly developed macular disease. Ophthalmic & physiological optics : the journal of the British College of Ophthalmic Opticians 24: 327–333.
12. Timberlake GT, Mainster MA, Peli E, Augliere RA, Essock EA, et al. (1986) Reading with a macular scotoma. I. Retinal location of scotoma and fixation area. Investigative ophthalmology & visual science 27: 1137–1147.
13. Martinez-Conde S, Macknik SL, Hubel DH (2004) The role of fixational eye movements in visual perception. Nature reviews Neuroscience 5: 229–240.
14. Morgan MJ, Benton S (1989) Motion-deblurring in human vision. Nature 340: 385–386.
15. Deruaz A, Matter M, Whatham AR, Goldschmidt M, Duret F, et al. (2004) Can fixation instability improve text perception during eccentric fixation in patients with central scotomas? The British journal of ophthalmology 88: 461–463.
16. Macedo AF, Crossland MD, Rubin GS (2011) Investigating unstable fixation in patients with macular disease. Investigative ophthalmology & visual science 52: 1275–1280.
17. Cacho I, Dickinson CM, Reeves BC, Harper RA (2007) Visual acuity and fixation characteristics in age-related macular degeneration. Optometry and vision science 84: 487–495.
18. Gonzalez EG, Tarita-Nistor L, Mandelcorn ED, Mandelcorn M, Steinbach MJ (2011) Fixation control before and after treatment for neovascular age-related macular degeneration. Investigative ophthalmology & visual science 52: 4208–4213.
19. Sivaprasad S, Pearce E, Chong V (2011) Quality of fixation in eyes with neovascular age-related macular degeneration treated with ranibizumab. Eye 25: 1612–1616.

20. Tarita-Nistor L, Brent MH, Steinbach MJ, Gonzalez EG (2011) Fixation stability during binocular viewing in patients with age-related macular degeneration. Investigative ophthalmology & visual science 52: 1887–1893.
21. Tarita-Nistor L, Brent MH, Steinbach MJ, Gonzalez EG (2012) Fixation patterns in maculopathy: from binocular to monocular viewing. Optometry and vision science 89: 277–287.
22. Tarita-Nistor L, Gonzalez EG, Markowitz SN, Steinbach MJ (2006) Binocular function in patients with age-related macular degeneration: a review. Canadian journal of ophthalmology Journal canadien d'ophtalmologie 41: 327–332.
23. Tarita-Nistor L, Gonzalez EG, Markowitz SN, Steinbach MJ (2008) Fixation characteristics of patients with macular degeneration recorded with the mp-1 microperimeter. Retina 28: 125–133.
24. Tarita-Nistor L, Gonzalez EG, Markowitz SN, Steinbach MJ (2009) Plasticity of fixation in patients with central vision loss. Visual neuroscience 26: 487–494.
25. Leibowitz HM, Krueger DE, Maunder LR, Milton RC, Kini MM, et al. (1980) The Framingham Eye Study monograph: An ophthalmological and epidemiological study of cataract, glaucoma, diabetic retinopathy, macular degeneration, and visual acuity in a general population of 2631 adults, 1973–1975. Survey of ophthalmology 24: 335–610.
26. Kabanarou SA, Crossland MD, Bellmann C, Rees A, Culham LE, et al. (2006) Gaze changes with binocular versus monocular viewing in age-related macular degeneration. Ophthalmology 113: 2251–2258.
27. Crossland MD, Crabb DP, Rubin GS (2011) Task-specific fixation behavior in macular disease. Investigative ophthalmology & visual science 52: 411–416.
28. Rayner K (1998) Eye movements in reading and information processing: 20 years of research. Psychological bulletin 124: 372–422.
29. Van der Stigchel S, Bethlehem RA, Klein BP, Berendschot TT, Nijboer TC, et al. (2013) Macular degeneration affects eye movement behavior during visual search. Frontiers in psychology 4: 579.
30. Crossland MD, Rubin GS (2002) The use of an infrared eyetracker to measure fixation stability. Optometry and vision science 79: 735–739.
31. Eizenman M, Hallett PE, Frecker RC (1985) Power spectra for ocular drift and tremor. Vision research 25: 1635–1640.
32. Machado L, Rafal RD (2000) Strategic control over saccadic eye movements: studies of the fixation offset effect. Perception & psychophysics 62: 1236–1242.
33. Fendrich R, Demirel S, Danziger S (1999) The oculomotor gap effect without a foveal fixation point. Vision research 39: 833–841.
34. Steinman RM (1965) Effect of Target Size, Luminance, and Color on Monocular Fixation. J Opt Soc Am 55: 1158–1164.
35. Timberlake GT, Sharma MK, Grose SA, Gobert DV, Gauch JM, et al. (2005) Retinal location of the preferred retinal locus relative to the fovea in scanning laser ophthalmoscope images. Optometry and vision science 82: 177–185.
36. Porac C, Coren S (1976) The dominant eye. Psychological bulletin 83: 880–897.
37. Ossewaarde-Van Norel J, van Den Biesen PR, van De Kraats J, Berendschot TT, van Norren D (2002) Comparison of fluorescence of sodium fluorescein in retinal angiography with measurements in vitro. J Biomed Opt 7: 190–198.
38. van Norren D, van de Kraats J (1989) Imaging retinal densitometry with a confocal Scanning Laser Ophthalmoscope. Vision research 29: 1825–1830.
39. Reinhard J, Messias A, Dietz K, Mackeben M, Lakmann R, et al. (2007) Quantifying fixation in patients with Stargardt disease. Vision research 47: 2076–2085.
40. Dalmaijer ES, Mathot S, Van der Stigchel S (2013) PyGaze: An open-source, cross-platform toolbox for minimal-effort programming of eyetracking experiments. Behavior research methods.
41. Findlay JM (1971) Frequency analysis of human involuntary eye movement. Kybernetik 8: 207–214.
42. Baker CI, Peli E, Knouf N, Kanwisher NG (2005) Reorganization of visual processing in macular degeneration. The Journal of neuroscience 25: 614–618.
43. Dilks DD, Baker CI, Peli E, Kanwisher N (2009) Reorganization of visual processing in macular degeneration is not specific to the "preferred retinal locus". The Journal of neuroscience 29: 2768–2773.
44. Masuda Y, Dumoulin SO, Nakadomari S, Wandell BA (2008) V1 projection zone signals in human macular degeneration depend on task, not stimulus. Cerebral cortex 18: 2483–2493.
45. Murakami I (2010) Eye movements during fixation as velocity noise in minimum motion detection. Japanese Psychological Research 52: 54–66.
46. Steinman RM, Cunitz RJ, Timberlake GT, Herman M (1967) Voluntary control of microsaccades during maintained monocular fixation. Science 155: 1577–1579.
47. Lingnau A, Schwarzbach J, Vorberg D (2008) Adaptive strategies for reading with a forced retinal location. Journal of vision 8: 6 1–18.
48. Lingnau A, Schwarzbach J, Vorberg D (2010) (Un-) coupling gaze and attention outside central vision. Journal of vision 10: 13.
49. Baker CI, Dilks DD, Peli E, Kanwisher N (2008) Reorganization of visual processing in macular degeneration: replication and clues about the role of foveal loss. Vision research 48: 1910–1919.
50. Baseler HA, Gouws A, Haak KV, Racey C, Crossland MD, et al. (2011) Large-scale remapping of visual cortex is absent in adult humans with macular degeneration. Nature neuroscience 14: 649–655.
51. Macedo AF, Nascimento SM, Gomes AO, Puga AT (2007) Fixation in patients with juvenile macular disease. Optometry and vision science : official publication of the American Academy of Optometry 84: 852–858.
52. Steinman RM, Haddad GM, Skavenski AA, Wyman D (1973) Miniature eye movement. Science 181: 810–819.
53. Whittaker SG, Budd J, Cummings RW (1988) Eccentric fixation with macular scotoma. Investigative ophthalmology & visual science 29: 268–278.

15

Effect of Intravitreal Anti-Vascular Endothelial Growth Factor Therapy on the Risk of Arterial Thromboembolic Events

Jin-Wei Cheng[1,⁹], Shi-Wei Cheng[2,⁹], Guo-Cai Lu[3]*, Rui-Li Wei[1]*

1 Department of Ophthalmology, Shanghai Changzheng Hospital, Second Military Medical University, Shanghai, China, 2 School of Life Sciences, Ludong University, Yantai, China, 3 Center for New Drug Evaluation, Institute of Basic Medical Science, Second Military Medical University, Shanghai, China

Abstract

Background: Intravitreal anti-vascular endothelial growth factor (VEGF) monoclonal antibodies are used in ocular neovascular diseases. A consensus has emerged that intravenous anti-VEGF can increase the risk of arterial thromboembolic events. However, the role of intravitreal anti-VEGF in arterial thromboembolism is controversial. Therefore, we did a systematic review and meta-analysis to investigate the effects of intravitreal anti-VEGF on the risk of arterial thromboembolic events.

Methods: Electronic databases were searched to identify relevant randomized clinical trials comparing intravitreal anti-VEGF with controls. Criteria for inclusion in our meta-analysis included a study duration of no less than 12 months, the use of a randomized control group not receiving any intravitreal active agent, and the availability of outcome data for arterial thromboembolic events, myocardial infarction, cerebrovascular accidents, and vascular death. The risk ratios and 95% CIs were calculated using a fixed-effects or random-effects model, depending on the heterogeneity of the included studies.

Results: A total of 4942 patients with a variety of ocular neovascular diseases from 13 randomized controlled trials were identified and included for analysis. There was no significant difference between intravitreal anti-VEGF and control in the risk of all events, with risk ratios of 0.87 (95% CI, 0.64 to 1.19) for arterial thromboembolic events, 0.96 (95% CI, 0.55–1.68) for cerebrovascular accidents, 0.69 (95% CI 0.40–1.21) for myocardial infarctions, and 0.68 (95% CI, 0.37–1.27) for vascular death.

Conclusions: The strength evidence suggests that the intravitreal use of anti-VEGF antibodies is not associated with an increased risk of arterial thromboembolic events.

Editor: Bang V. Bui, Univeristy of Melbourne, Australia

Funding: This study is supported by Shanghai Municipal Natural Science Foundation (Grant No. 10ZR1439300), and National Natural Science Foundation of China (Grant No. 81000374 and 81170874). The funders had no role in study design, data collection and analysis, decision to publish, or preparation of the manuscript.

Competing Interests: The authors have declared that no competing interests exist.

* E-mail: ruiliwei@gmail.com (RLW); newdrug@smmu.edu.cn (GCL)

⁹ These authors contributed equally to this work.

Introduction

Angiogenesis, a process involving the proliferation of new blood vessels, plays a crucial role in many pathologic states [1]. This process is mainly driven by vascular endothelial growth factor (VEGF), whose signaling pathway has been a target of many new antiangiogenic agents [2]. Currently used monoclonal antibodies against VEGF included pegaptanib, ranibizumab, and bevacizumab. Bevacizumab (Avastin®) is a recombinant full length humanized antibody that binds to all types of VEGF and is used successfully in the treatment of many types of malignancy as a systemic drug [3,4]. Pegaptanib (Macugen®), a 28-base ribonucleic acid aptamer covalently linked to two branched 20-kD polyethylene glycol moieties, binds to extracellular VEGF, specifically the 165-amino-acid isoform (VEGF-165), and antagonizes its biological effects [5]. Ranibizumab (Lucentis®) is a recombinant humanized monoclonal antibody Fab that neutralizes all active forms of VEGF-A [6]. All three anti-VEGF agents have been proven promise in the treatment of various ocular neovascular diseases, such as age-related macular degeneration, diabetic retinopathy, and retinal vein occlusion [7,8].

Because VEGF plays many roles in physiologic processes, its inhibition could have potentially serious systemic consequences. While the use of intravenous bevacizumab is recognized to be associated with an increased risk of arterial and venous thromboembolic events [9,10], it is controversial whether intravitreal anti-VEGF agents contribute to the development of arterial thromboembolic events, such as myocardial infarction and cerebrovascular accidents, common comorbidities leading to mortality in patients with ocular neovascular diseases [11,12]. A pooled analysis from three randomized clinical trials (RCTs) that included 859 patients with age-related macular degeneration showed that intravitreal ranibizumab was associated with an increased risk of cerebrovascular accidents (odds ratios [OR],

3.24; 95% confidence interval [CI], 0.96–10.95; P = 0.045), when compared with sham treatment, whereas there was no apparent association between intravitreal ranibizumab and myocardial infarction (OR, 0.61 [95%CI, 0.29–1.29]; P = 0.193) [13]. Because the number of patients included in this analysis is limited, the contribution of intravitreal anti-VEGF therapy to arterial thromboembolic events remains poorly defined.

Recently, many more RCTs of intravitreal anti-VEGF therapy in ocular neovascular diseases have been performed. However, no significant association between intravitreal anti-VEGF therapy and arterial thromboembolic events has been shown in any RCTs. We hypothesized that these studies were not powered sufficiently to reveal a significantly increased risk due to the low incidences of arterial thromboembolic events. Therefore, we performed a systematic review of the published RCTs for a meta-analysis to determine the risk of arterial thromboembolic events associated with intravitreal anti-VEGF treatment.

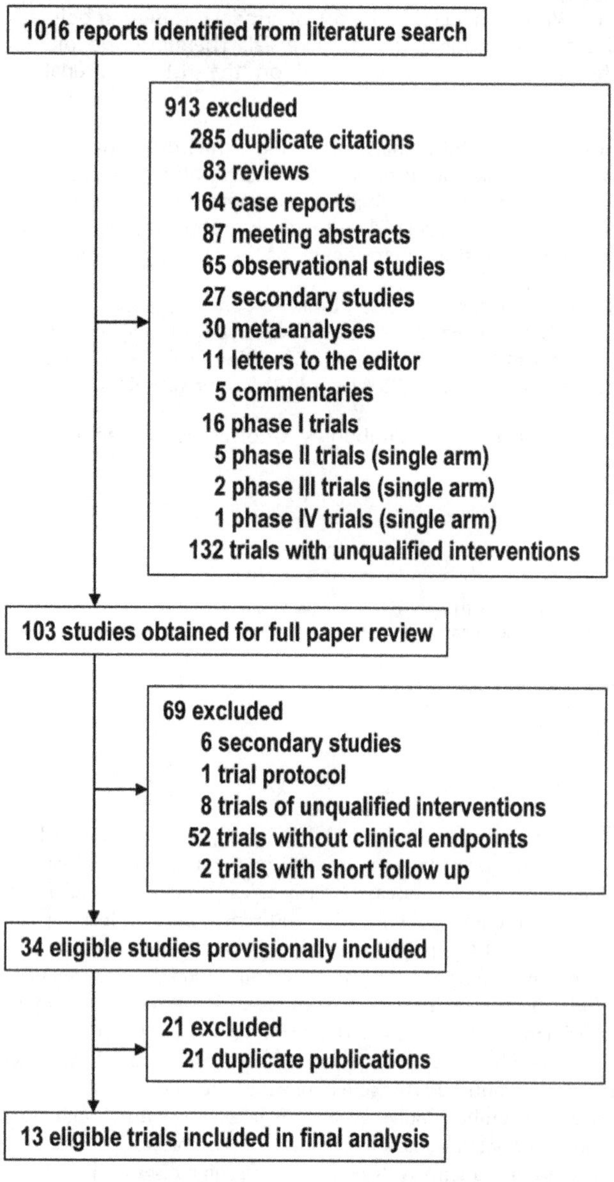

Figure 1. Flow diagram showing citations retrieved from literature searches and number of trials included in the meta-analysis.

Methods

Data Source

Published RCTs were identified through a comprehensive search of PubMed, EMBASE, and the Cochrane central register of controlled trials, each from inception to October 31, 2011. The search combined terms related to drugs (bevacizumab, pegaptanib, and ranibizumab), and terms related to diseases (macular degeneration, diabetic retinopathy, macular edema, retinal vein occlusion, retinal neovascularization, and choroidal neovascularization), with a filter to restrict results to clinical trial. The reference lists of identified articles were examined for additional publications.

We reviewed each publication and only the most recent or complete report of clinical trials was included when duplicate publications were identified. Efforts also were made to contact the investigators when relevant data were not clear.

Study Selection

The goal of this study was to determine whether intravitreal anti-VEGF therapy contributes to the development of arterial thromboembolic events. Therefore, only RCTs with a direct comparison between patients treated with and without intravitreal injection of anti-VEGF agents were included for analysis. Specifically, clinical trials fulfilling the following criteria were included in the meta-analysis: (i) study design – randomized clinical trials, which all should have adequate IRB review and consent processes; (ii) population – patients with ocular neovascular diseases, such as age-related macular degeneration, diabetic retinopathy, and retinal vein occlusion; (iii) intervention – intravitreal anti-VEGF agents versus control, and the use of a randomized control group not receiving any intravitreal active agent; (iv) outcome measurement – the incidence of arterial thromboembolic events, myocardial infarction, cerebrovascular accidents, and vascular death; (v) duration – the minimum length of follow up was 12 months.

After completion of the searches, two review authors (JWC and SWC) working independently assessed the titles and abstracts of all obtained reports for a rough judgment of an article's eligibility. The full text copies of possibly and definitely relevant trials were obtained and assessed by the three authors independently according to the definitions in the criteria. Only trials meeting these criteria were assessed for methodological quality.

Data Extraction and Clinical Endpoints

Data extraction was performed by two reviewers (JWC and SWC) independently. Any disagreement was resolved by discussion. For each study and each type of treatment, the following data were extracted: information on study design (whether randomization, allocation concealment, intention to treat analysis, double blind or single blind, parallel or crossover), location of trial, length of study, sample size, patient age, sex, race, type of diagnosis, and events of arterial thromboembolic events, myocardial infarction, cerebrovascular accidents, and vascular death.

The clinical endpoints included arterial thromboembolic events, non-fatal cerebrovascular accidents, non-fatal myocardial infarction, and vascular death. Arterial thromboembolic events included nonfatal myocardial infarction, nonfatal stroke, and death from a vascular or unknown cause, on the basis of the classification system of the Antiplatelet Trialists' Collaboration (APTC) [14]. All

Table 1. Characteristics of randomized controlled clinical trials in the meta-analysis.

Acronym	Design	Treatment arm	Control arm	Concurrent treatment	Number of patients	Disease	Mean age (range, years)	Women (%)	Follow up (months)	Lost to follow-up (%)	Quality score
VISION[22]	DB-P	Pegaptanib	Placebo	Verteporfin	1190	Neovascular AMD	NA	696 (58.5)	12	11.5	5
MARINA[23]	DB-P	Ranibizumab	Placebo	Verteporfin	716	Neovascular AMD	77 (52–95)	464 (64.8)	24	14.1	5
FOCUS[24]	SB-P	Ranibizumab	Placebo	Verteporfin	162	Neovascular AMD	74 (50–93)	86 (53.1)	24	14.8	4
ANCHOR[25]	DB-P	Ranibizumab	Verteporfin	Laser	423	Neovascular AMD	77 (53–97)	211 (49.9)	24	22.2	5
BOLT[26]	SB-P	Bevacizumab	Laser	None	80	DME	64 (40–86)	25 (31.3)	12	2.5	4
ABC Trial[27]	DB-P	Bevacizumab	Placebo, verteporfin, pegaptanib	None	131	Neovascular AMD	81 (NA)	80 (61.1)	12	4.8	5
PIER[28]	DB-P	Ranibizumab	Placebo	Verteporfin	184	Neovascular AMD	78 (54–94)	110 (59.8)	24	16.8	5
RESOLVE[29]	DB-P	Ranibizumab	Placebo	None	151	DME	64 (32–85)	70 (46.4)	12	12.6	5
BRAVO[30]	DB-P	Ranibizumab	Placebo	Laser	397	BRVO	66 (26–91)	185 (46.6)	12	10.3	5
CRUISE[31]	DB-P	Ranibizumab	Placebo	None	392	CRVO	68 (20–91)	169 (43.1)	12	11.0	5
DRCR[32]	DB-P	Ranibizumab	Placebo, triamcinolone	Laser	691	DME	63 (NA)	304 (44.0)	24	6.4	5
RESTORE[33]	DB-P	Ranibizumab	Placebo	Laser	345	DME	63 (NA)	144 (41.7)	12	12.2	5
Macugen 1013[34]	DB-P	Pegaptanib	Placebo	Laser	260	DME	62 (20–83)	111 (42.7)	24	32.5	5

NA = data not available. DB-P = double blind parallel; SB-P = single blind parallel. AMD = age-related macular degeneration; DME = diabetic macular edema; CRVO = central retinal vein occlusion; BRVO = branch retinal vein occlusion.

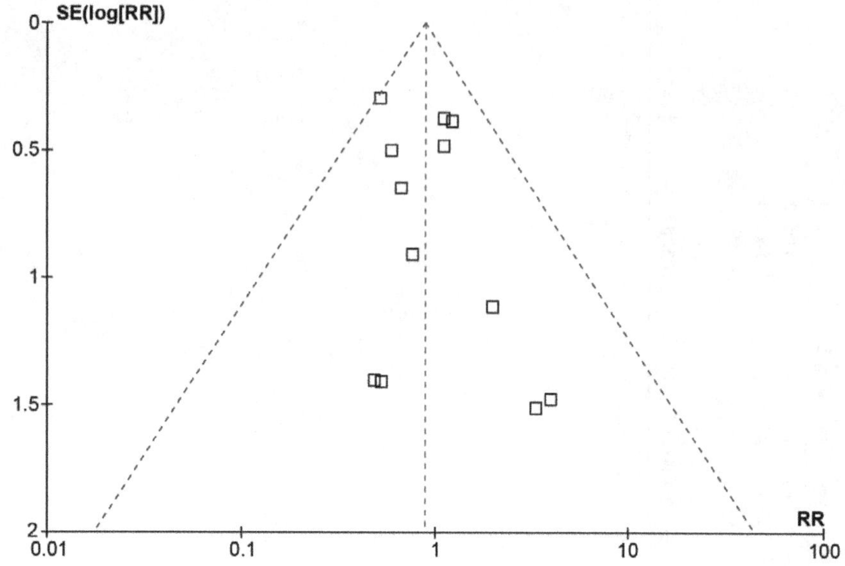

Figure 2. Funnel plot of studies on arterial thromboembolic events.

reported strokes, transient ischemic attacks, or cerebral ischemic incidents were regarded as cerebrovascular accidents.

Qualitative Assessment

Two authors (in duplicate by JWC and SWC) used standard criteria (allocation concealment, blinding, intention to treat analysis, loss to follow-up) to appraise study quality, in addition to quantitative quality assessment by using the scoring system developed by Jadad [15]. The quality scoring system was followed as: (i) allocation concealment, coded as adequate (1 score), inadequate or unclear (0 score); (ii) blinding, coded as double-blind (2 scores), single-blind (1 score), and open label (0 score); (iii) intention to treat analysis, coded as used (1 score), not used or unable to assess (0 score); and (iv) lost to follow-up, coded as given (1 score), and not given (0 score). "Poor quality" refers to a Jadad score less than 3, and the impact of excluding low quality studies was assessed by a sensitivity analysis.

Statistical Analysis

Outcome measure was assessed on an intent-to-treat (ITT) basis, the ITT population comprising all randomized patients who received a minimum of one dose of active treatment and provided a valid baseline measurement.

All statistical analyses were performed using version 2 of the Comprehensive Meta-analysis program (Biostat, Englewood Cliffs, New Jersey). For each study, risk ratio (RR) of arterial thromboembolic events, non-fatal cerebrovascular accidents, non-fatal myocardial infarction, and vascular death with exact 95% CI were calculated. The heterogeneity across all eligible comparisons was estimated using the X^2-based Q statistic. Heterogeneity was checked by *P*-value [16]. I^2 metrics, which quantify heterogeneity irrespective of the number of studies, were also reported [17]. If no heterogeneity detected ($P>0.1$), we combined the results in a meta-analysis using the Mantel-Haenszel fixed effects model [18], otherwise, the DerSimonian-Laird random effects model were used to pool the data after exploring the causes of heterogeneity [19,20].

Source	Arterial thromboembolic events Anti-VEGF	Control	Weight (%)	Risk ratio (95% CI)	*P* value
VISION[22]	30 / 892	9 / 298	16.44	1.11 (0.54, 2.32)	0.774
MARINA[23]	22 / 478	9 / 238	14.65	1.22 (0.57, 2.60)	0.612
FOCUS[24]	5 / 106	4 / 56	6.38	0.66 (0.18, 2.36)	0.523
ANCHOR[25]	13 / 280	6 / 143	9.68	1.11 (0.43, 2.85)	0.834
ABC Trial[27]	4 / 65	0 / 28	0.85	3.95 (0.22, 71.08)	0.351
PIER[28]	1 / 121	1 / 63	1.60	0.52 (0.03, 8.19)	0.642
RESOLVE[29]	1 / 102	1 / 49	1.65	0.48 (0.03, 7.52)	0.601
BRAVO[30]	3 / 265	2 / 132	3.25	0.75 (0.13, 4.42)	0.748
CRUISE[31]	4 / 262	1 / 130	1.63	1.98 (0.22, 17.58)	0.538
DRCR[32]	25 / 375	17 / 130	30.77	0.51 (0.28, 0.91)	0.024
RESTORE[33]	3 / 234	0 / 111	0.83	3.34 (0.17, 64.04)	0.424
Macugen 1013[34]	6 / 144	10 / 142	12.27	0.59 (0.22, 1.58)	0.296
Overall (fixed)	**117 / 3324**	**60 / 1520**		**0.87 (0.64, 1.19)**	**0.387**

Test for heterogeneity: I^2=0.00%, *P*=0.696, Q=8.190

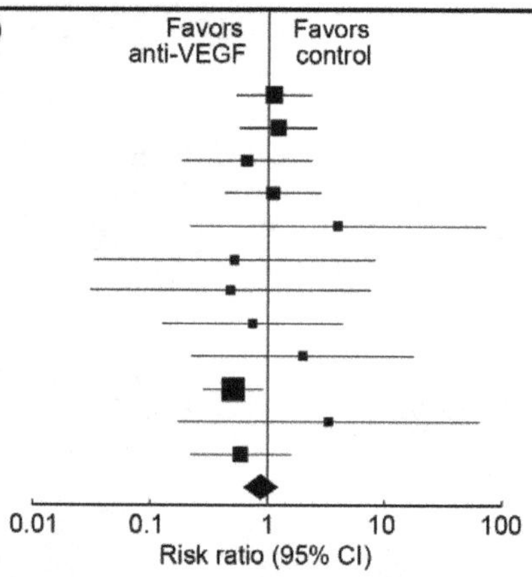

Figure 3. Risk ratio of arterial thromboembolic events associated with intravitreal anti-VEGF treatment compared with control treatment.

Table 2. Risk ratio of arterial thromboembolic events.

		Number of events/total number (%)			
	No of Trials	**Anti-VEGF**	**Control**	**Risk ratio (95% CI)**	**P value**
Arterial thromboembolic events					
Overall	12	117/3324 (3.5)	60/1520 (3.9)	0.87 (0.64, 1.19)	0.387
Neovascular AMD	6	75/1942 (3.9)	29/826 (3.5)	1.14 (0.73, 1.70)	0.615
DME	4	35/885 (4.1)	28/432 (6.5)	0.58 (0.36, 0.94)	0.028
RVO	2	7/527 (1.3)	3/262 (1.2)	1.16 (0.30, 4.45)	0.829
Ranibizumab	9	77/2223 (3.5)	41/1052 (3.9)	0.83 (0.58, 1.19)	0.315
Pegaptanib	2	36/1036 (3.5)	19/440 (4.3)	0.89 (0.50, 1.59)	0.696
Bevacizumab	1	4/65 (6.2)	0/28 (0.0)	3.96 (0.22, 71.08)	0.351
Cerebrovascular accidents					
Overall	10	32/2288 (1.4)	15/1169 (1.3)	0.96 (0.55, 1.68)	0.891
Neovascular AMD	3	18/864 (2.1)	4/437 (0.9)	2.10 (0.76, 5.83)	0.155
DME	5	11/897 (1.2)	10/470 (2.1)	0.51 (0.24, 1.09)	0.083
RVO	2	3/527 (0.6)	1/262 (0.4)	1.16 (0.17, 7.82)	0.877
Ranibizumab	8	30/2102 (1.2)	17/1052 (1.6)	0.96 (0.53, 1.74)	0.899
Pegaptanib	1	2/144 (1.4)	1/142 (0.7)	1.97 (0.18, 21.51)	0.577
Bevacizumab	1	0/42 (0.0)	1/38 (2.6)	0.30 (0.01, 7.21)	0.460
Myocardial infarction					
Overall	11	29/2432 (1.2)	20/1222 (1.6)	0.69 (0.40, 1.21)	0.195
Neovascular AMD	5	18/1050 (1.7)	10/528 (1.9)	0.86 (0.41, 1.81)	0.700
DME	4	8/855 (0.9)	8/432 (1.9)	0.46 (0.18, 1.23)	0.121
RVO	2	3/527 (0.6)	2/262 (0.8)	0.75 (0.13, 4.43)	0.747
Ranibizumab	9	27/2223 (1.2)	17/1052 (1.6)	0.73 (0.41, 1.31)	0.292
Pegaptanib	1	0/144 (0.0)	3/142 (2.1)	0.14 (0.01, 2.70)	0.194
Bevacizumab	1	2/65 (3.1)	0/28 (0.0)	2.20 (0.11, 44.34)	0.608
Vascular death					
Overall	4	25/1198 (2.1)	15/539 (2.8)	0.68 (0.37, 1.27)	0.225
Neovascular AMD	3	12/823 (1.4)	7/409 (1.7)	0.79 (0.31, 2.01)	0.626
DME	1	13/375 (3.5)	8/130 (6.2)	0.55 (0.22, 1.35)	0.192
Ranibizumab	3	23/1133 (2.0)	15/511 (2.9)	0.63 (0.33, 1.20)	0.159
Bevacizumab	1	2/65 (3.1)	0/28 (0.0)	2.20 (0.11, 44.34)	0.608

AMD = age-related macular degeneration; DME = diabetic macular edema; RVO = retinal vein occlusion.

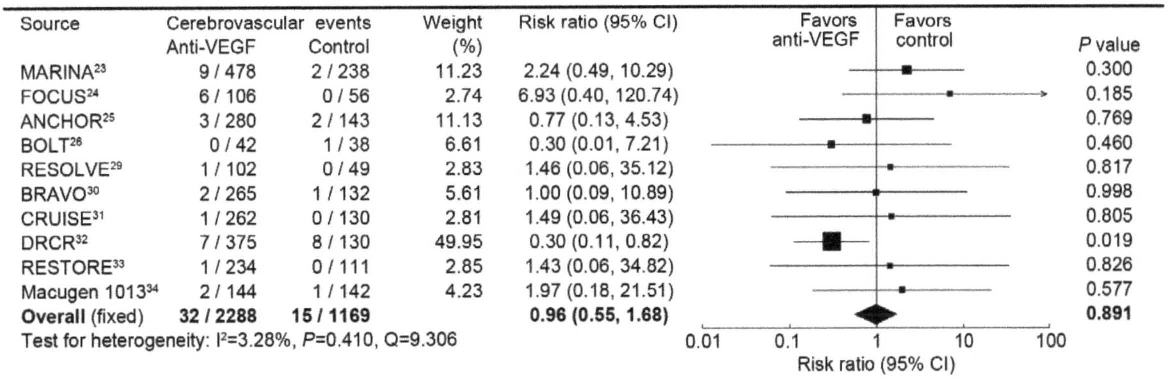

Figure 4. Risk ratio of cerebrovascular accidents associated with intravitreal anti-VEGF treatment compared with control treatment.

Source	Myocardial infarction Anti-VEGF	Control	Weight (%)	Risk ratio (95% CI)	P value
MARINA[23]	9 / 478	4 / 238	18.58	1.12 (0.35, 3.60)	0.849
FOCUS[24]	1 / 106	3 / 56	13.66	0.18 (0.02, 1.65)	0.129
ANCHOR[25]	6 / 280	2 / 143	9.21	1.53 (0.31, 7.50)	0.598
ABC Trial[27]	2 / 65	0 / 28	2.42	2.20 (0.11, 44.34)	0.608
PIER[28]	0 / 121	1 / 63	6.85	0.17 (0.01, 4.23)	0.283
RESOLVE[29]	1 / 102	1 / 49	4.70	0.48 (0.03, 7.52)	0.601
BRAVO[30]	1 / 265	1 / 132	4.64	0.50 (0.03, 7.90)	0.621
CRUISE[31]	2 / 262	1 / 130	4.65	0.99 (0.09, 10.84)	0.995
DRCR[32]	5 / 375	4 / 130	20.67	0.43 (0.12, 1.59)	0.207
RESTORE[33]	2 / 234	0 / 111	2.36	2.38 (0.12, 49.22)	0.574
Macugen 1013[34]	0 / 144	3 / 142	12.26	0.14 (0.01, 2.70)	0.194
Overall (fixed)	**29 / 2432**	**20 / 1222**		**0.69 (0.40, 1.21)**	**0.195**

Test for heterogeneity: I^2=0.00%, P=0.744, Q=6.798

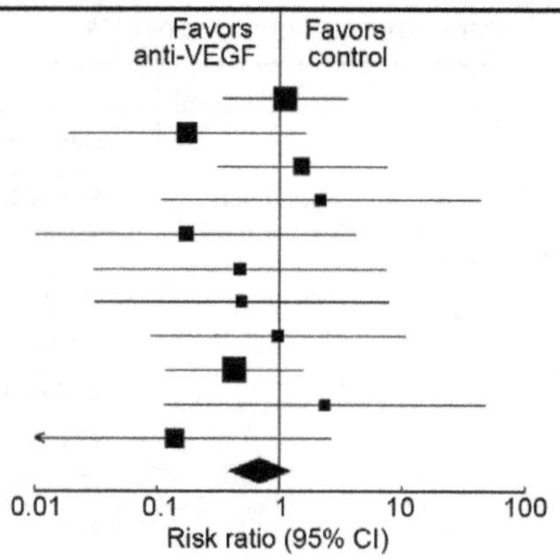

Figure 5. Risk ratio of myocardial infarctions associated with intravitreal anti-VEGF treatment compared with control treatment.

We constructed standard funnel plots to investigate the potential for publication bias, by examining visually the asymmetry. Furthermore, Egger's linear regression method was used to detect the presence of publication bias regarding primary endpoint (arterial thromboembolic events) [21].

Results

The flow of the randomized controlled trials included in our analysis is shown in the **Figure 1**. We reviewed the full text of 103 articles from 1016 studies identified from our initial literature search. After excluding secondary studies, trial protocols, trials of unqualified interventions, trials without clinical endpoints, and duplicate publications, totally 13 randomized controlled trials were included in the final meta-analysis (**Table 1**) [22–34].

All trials had a prospective, parallel design. Randomized treatment allocation sequences were generated in all trials. Eleven trials were double-blinded, and two other trials were single-blinded. Nine trials had placebo as controls; two other trials had active controls; the rest of the trials were placebo and active controls. Patients were analyzed by the intention to treat principle in all trials. The quality of all the trials was acceptable: eleven trials scored 5, two trials scored 4.

Funnel plot for the studies on arterial thromboembolic events was qualitatively symmetrical (**Figure 2**), and no publication bias was detected for the primary endpoint by Egger's test (one-tailed, P = 0.13; two-tailed, P = 0.27).

There were 38 patients treated with pegaptanib in ABC Trial [27], and 142 patients treated with triamcinolone in DRCR study [32]; we excluded the two arms from the final analysis. Therefore, a total of 4942 patients from 13 randomized clinical trials were included for analysis. The baseline characteristics of patients in the 13 studies are summarized in **Table 1**. Six studies included neovascular age-related macular degeneration, five included diabetic macular edema, and each one included central retinal vein occlusion and branch retinal vein occlusion.

Our meta-analysis calculated the overall risk ratio for arterial thromboembolic events associated with intravitreal anti-VEGF treatment compared with control treatment, and twelve trials were included in this analysis (**Figure 3**). There were 117 (3.5%) arterial thromboembolic events of 3324 patients in the intravitreal anti-VEGF group, and 60 (3.9%) of 1520 patients in the control group. No significant heterogeneity was found in this analysis. Intravitreal anti-VEGF therapy was not associated with the risk of arterial thromboembolic events, with a pooled risk ratio of 0.87 (95% CI, 0.64 to 1.19) using a fixed-effects model. Analysis using the random effects model similarly showed no association between intravitreal anti-VEGF therapy and the risk of arterial thromboembolic events (pooled risk ratio 0.83, 0.61 to 1.13). **Table 2** lists the risk ratios and 95% confidence intervals for arterial thromboembolic events from all the trials; results from the pooled group according to the type of diseases and the type of interventions are shown separately.

The results of the meta-analysis for cerebrovascular accidents are shown in **Figure 4**, and ten trials were included in this analysis, involving a total of 3457 patients. 32 (1.4%) of 2288 patients in receiving intravitreal anti-VEGF experienced cerebrovascular accidents, compared with 15 (1.3%) of 1169 patients receiving control. There was not a significant heterogeneity in this analysis. Intravitreal anti-VEGF was not associated with the risk of cerebrovascular accidents, with a pooled RR of 0.96 (0.55 to 1.68) by fixed effects analysis and 0.83 (0.44 to 1.57) by random effects analysis. **Table 2** shows the sub-pooled risk ratio, which also suggested that intravitreal anti-VEGF was not associated with the risk of cerebrovascular accidents.

Source	Vascular death Anti-VEGF	Control	Weight (%)	Risk ratio (95% CI)	P value
MARINA[23]	6 / 478	4 / 238	24.40	0.75 (0.21, 2.62)	0.649
ANCHOR[25]	4 / 280	3 / 143	18.14	0.68 (0.15, 3.00)	0.612
ABC Trial[27]	2 / 65	0 / 28	3.17	2.20 (0.11, 44.34)	0.608
DRCR[32]	13 / 375	8 / 130	54.28	0.56 (0.24, 1.33)	0.190
Overall (fixed)	**25 / 1198**	**15 / 539**		**0.68 (0.37, 1.27)**	**0.225**

Test for heterogeneity: I^2=0.00%, P=0.851, Q=0.793

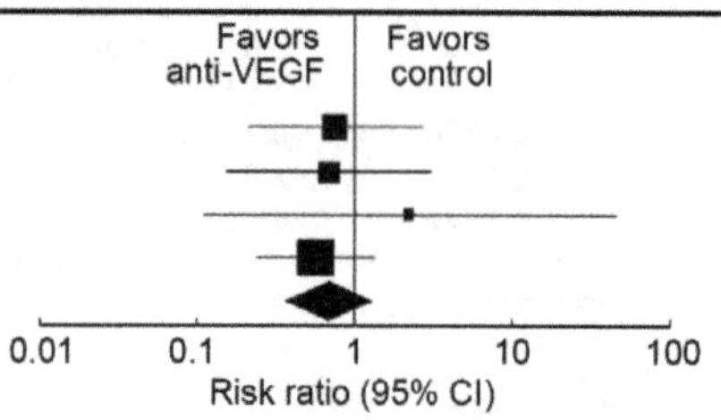

Figure 6. Risk ratio of vascular death associated with intravitreal anti-VEGF treatment compared with control treatment.

Eleven trials comparing intravitreal anti-VEGF with control reported the rate of myocardial infarction, with a total of 3654 patients included in this analysis. Myocardial infarctions occurred in 29 (1.2%) of 2432 patients receiving intravitreal anti-VEGF, and 20 (1.6%) of 1222 patients receiving control. There was no significant difference between anti-VEGF and control in the risk of myocardial infarctions, with a risk ratio being 0.69 (0.40–1.21) by fixed-effects analysis and 0.70 (0.39 to 1.28) by random effects analysis (**Figure 5**). Intravitreal anti-VEGF was also not associated with the risk of myocardial infarctions for neovascular age-related macular degeneration, diabetic macular edema, and retinal vein occlusion (**Table 2**).

Figure 6 shows the results of the meta-analysis for vascular death comparing anti-VEGF with control. There were 25 (2.1%) of 1198 patients allocated to treatment with intravitreal anti-VEGF, and 15 (2.8%) of 539 patients allocated to control, who experienced vascular death. No significant heterogeneity was found in this analysis. Intravitreal anti-VEGF was not associated with the risk of vascular death, with a risk ratio of 0.68 (0.37–1.27) from the fixed-effects model, and 0.66 (0.35 to 1.24) from the random-effects model. Sub-group analyses using the fixed-effects model also suggested that intravitreal anti-VEGF was not associated with the risk of vascular death (**Table 2**).

Discussion

The results of this programme of prospectively designed overviews of data from 13 randomized clinical trials revealed that, as compared with control, intravitreal anti-VEGF therapy was not associated with the risk of arterial thromboembolic events, non-fatal cerebrovascular accidents, non-fatal myocardial infarction, and vascular death.

The previous meta-analyses suggested the use of intravenous bevacizumab was recognized to be associated with an increased risk of arterial and venous thromboembolic events [9,10]. Because of the high association of the risk of cardiovascular events with age-related macular degeneration, diabetes, and retinal vein occlusion [35–37], the results of a previous meta-analysis [13], which revealed intravitreal anti-VEGF was also associated with an increased risk of cerebrovascular accidents, was worrisome. However, another previous systematic review [38], as well as two non-randomized studies [39,40], suggested that intravitreal anti-VEGF use was not associated with increased risks of mortality, myocardial infarction, or stroke. Therefore, the success to detect such an increase in cerebrovascular accidents risk is likely due to the limited number of trials included for the analysis. Furthermore, risk ratios might be affected by small changes in the classification of events, due to the results based on a relatively small number of events.

In the overview for arterial thromboembolic events, no difference in this risk between the arms receiving intravitreal anti-VEGF and control, with the 95% confidence interval included an up to 19% increased risk of arterial thromboembolic events down to a 36% reduction with intravitreal anti-VEGF. In the overviews for non-fatal cerebrovascular accidents, non-fatal myocardial infarction, and vascular death, there was also no clear difference between intravitreal anti-VEGF and control.

In the present meta-analysis, several ocular neovascular diseases, such as age-related macular degeneration, diabetic retinopathy, and retinal vein occlusion, were included. Sensitivity analysis was undertaken to evaluate the variation of the risk of arterial thromboembolic events with anti-VEGF among different diseases. Intravitreal anti-VEGF significantly decreased the risk of arterial thromboembolic events by 32% in patients with diabetic macular edema, with the 95% confidence intervals of 6% to 64%; no difference in this risk was detected in patients with neovascular age-related macular degeneration and retinal vein occlusion. In patients with diabetes mellitus, increased VEGF-mediated angiogenesis has been implicated in retinopathy and nephropathy, whereas a defective angiogenic response to ischemia, which might be attributable to a VEGF signaling defect in which there is reduced receptor signaling despite higher ligand expression, could lead to poor clinical outcomes [41]. Therefore, the targets within the system that lead to altered VEGF signaling, such as low dose systemic anti-VEGF, may be beneficial in diabetic patients.

The sensitivity analysis according to the type of diseases showed that intravitreal anti-VEGF increased the risks of cerebrovascular accidents by 52% in neovascular age-related macular degeneration, with the 95% confidence intervals of -32% to 83%. However, the point estimates of all three trials were distributed across the 1.0 risk ratio [23–25]. Two estimates have shown a possible risk of cerebrovascular accidents of intravitreal anti-VEGF [23,24]. However, a larger epidemiological study found that no statistically significant relationship between intravitreal anti-VEGF use and stroke [39]. Therefore, the small differences of cerebrovascular accidents between intravitreal anti-VEGF and placebo in the two trials might be due to chance finding, but not drug-related [38].

Although we tried to conduct a thorough review of the existing literature, this present analysis has limitations inherent to any systematic review. First, the incidences of arterial thromboembolic events showed significant heterogeneity among the included studies. This may reflect differences in sample sizes, disease types, interventions, concomitant treatment, study durations, and many other factors among these studies. Despite these differences, the risk ratios reported by all of these studies showed remarkable homogeneity. In addition, combination data by using a random-effects model may be able to achieve more conservative estimates. Second, the included trials were done at various clinical centers, and the ability to detect arterial thromboembolic events and the classification of events might vary among these institutions, which could result in a bias of reported incidence rates. Third, only published studies were included in the present meta-analysis. To avoid the publication bias, we searched in multiple databases. In addition, to find potential publication biases, we explored asymmetry in funnel plots and detect heterogeneity using Egger's linear regression, and no publication bias was found. Finally, the findings of this meta-analysis are based on the study level, not on patient-level source data, and some confounding factors cannot be properly assessed and incorporated into the results.

Despite these limitations, the strength evidence from the present meta-analysis data suggests that the intravitreal use of anti-VEGF agents is not associated with an increased risk of arterial thromboembolic events.

Author Contributions

Conceived and designed the experiments: JWC SWC GCL RLW. Performed the experiments: JWC SWC. Analyzed the data: JWC SWC GCL. Contributed reagents/materials/analysis tools: JWC. Wrote the paper: JWC SWC GCL RLW.

References

1. Folkman J (1995) Angiogenesis in cancer, vascular, rheumatoid and other disease. Nat Med 1:27–31.
2. Hicklin DJ, Ellis LM (2005) Role of the vascular endothelial growth factor pathway in tumor growth and angiogenesis. J Clin Oncol 23:1011–27.

3. Hurwitz H, Fehrenbacher L, Novotny W, Cartwright T, Hainsworth J, et al. (2004) Bevacizumab plus irinotecan, fluorouracil, and leucovorin for metastatic colorectal cancer. N Engl J Med 350:2335–42.
4. Sandler A, Gray R, Perry MC, Brahmer J, Schiller JH, et al. (2006) Paclitaxel-carboplatin alone or with bevacizumab for non-small-cell lung cancer. N Engl J Med 355:2542–50.
5. Moshfeghi AA, Puliafito CA (2005) Pegaptanib sodium for the treatment of neovascular age-related macular degeneration. Expert Opin Investig Drugs 14:671–82.
6. Pieramici DJ, Avery RL (2006) Ranibizumab: treatment in patients with neovascular age-related macular degeneration. Expert Opin Biol Ther 6:1237–45.
7. Andreoli CM, Miller JW (2007) Anti-vascular endothelial growth factor therapy for ocular neovascular disease. Curr Opin Ophthalmol. 18:502–8.
8. Ciulla TA, Rosenfeld PJ (2009) Anti-vascular endothelial growth factor therapy for neovascular ocular diseases other than age-related macular degeneration. Curr Opin Ophthalmol 20:166–74.
9. Scappaticci FA, Skillings JR, Holden SN, Gerber HP, Miller K, et al. (2007) Arterial thromboembolic events in patients with metastatic carcinoma treated with chemotherapy and bevacizumab. J Natl Cancer Inst 99:1232–9.
10. Nalluri SR, Chu D, Keresztes R, Zhu X, Wu S (2008) Risk of venous thromboembolism with the angiogenesis inhibitor bevacizumab in cancer patients: a meta-analysis. JAMA 300:2277–85.
11. Hyman L, Schachat AP, He Q, Leske MC (2000) Hypertension, cardiovascular disease, and age-related macular degeneration. Arch Ophthalmol 118:351–8.
12. Hogg RE, Woodside JV, Gilchrist SE, Graydon R, Fletcher AE, et al. (2008) Cardiovascular disease and hypertension are strong risk factors for choroidal neovascularization. Ophthalmology 115:1046–1052.e2.
13. Ueta T, Yanagi Y, Tamaki Y, Yamaguchi T (2009) Cerebrovascular accidents in ranibizumab. Ophthalmology 116:362.
14. Antiplatelet Trialists' Collaboration (1994) Collaborative overview of randomised trials of antiplatelet therapy–I: Prevention of death, myocardial infarction, and stroke by prolonged antiplatelet therapy in various categories of patients. BMJ 308:81–106.
15. Jadad AR, Moore RA, Carroll D, Jenkinson C, Reynolds DJ, et al. (1996) Assessing the quality of reports of randomized clinical trials: is blinding necessary? Control Clin Trials 17:1–12.
16. Higgins JP, Thompson SG, Deeks JJ, Altman DG (2003) Measuring inconsistency in meta-analyses. BMJ 327:557–560.
17. Higgins JP, Thompson SG (2002) Quantifying heterogeneity in a meta-analysis. Stat Med 21:1539–58.
18. Mantel N, Haenszel W (1959) Statistical aspects of the analysis of data from retrospective studies of disease. J Natl Cancer Inst 22:719–48.
19. DerSimonian R, Laird N (1986) Meta-analysis in clinical trials. Control Clin Trials 7:177–88.
20. Lau J, Ioannidis JP, Schmid CH (1997) Quantitative synthesis in systematic reviews. Ann Intern Med 127:820–6.
21. Egger M, Davey Smith G, Schneider M, Minder C (1997) Bias in meta-analysis detected by a simple, graphical test. BMJ 315:629–34.
22. VEGF Inhibition Study in Ocular Neovascularization (V.I.S.I.O.N.) Clinical Trial Group, D'Amico DJ, Masonson HN, Patel M, Adamis AP, et al. (2006) Pegaptanib sodium for neovascular age-related macular degeneration: two-year safety results of the two prospective, multicenter, controlled clinical trials. Ophthalmology 113:992–1001.e6.
23. Rosenfeld PJ, Brown DM, Heier JS, Boyer DS, Kaiser PK, et al. (2006) Ranibizumab for neovascular age-related macular degeneration. N Engl J Med 355:1419–31.
24. Antoszyk AN, Tuomi L, Chung CY, Singh A; FOCUS Study Group (2008) Ranibizumab combined with verteporfin photodynamic therapy in neovascular age-related macular degeneration (FOCUS): year 2 results. Am J Ophthalmol 145:862–74.
25. Brown DM, Michels M, Kaiser PK, Heier JS, Sy JP, et al. (2009) Ranibizumab versus verteporfin photodynamic therapy for neovascular age-related macular degeneration: Two-year results of the ANCHOR study. Ophthalmology 116:57–65.e5.
26. Michaelides M, Kaines A, Hamilton RD, Fraser-Bell S, Rajendram R, et al. (2010) A prospective randomized trial of intravitreal bevacizumab or laser therapy in the management of diabetic macular edema (BOLT study) 12-month data: report 2. Ophthalmology. 117:1078–1086.e2.
27. Tufail A, Patel PJ, Egan C, Hykin P, da Cruz L, et al. (2010) Bevacizumab for neovascular age related macular degeneration (ABC Trial): multicentre randomised double masked study. BMJ 340:c2459.
28. Abraham P, Yue H, Wilson L (2010) Randomized, double-masked, sham-controlled trial of ranibizumab for neovascular age-related macular degeneration: PIER study year 2. Am J Ophthalmol. 150:315–324.e1.
29. Massin P, Bandello F, Garweg JG, Hansen LL, Harding SP, et al. (2010) Safety and efficacy of ranibizumab in diabetic macular edema (RESOLVE Study): a 12-month, randomized, controlled, double-masked, multicenter phase II study. Diabetes Care 33:2399–405.
30. Brown DM, Campochiaro PA, Bhisitkul RB, Ho AC, Gray S, et al. (2011) Sustained benefits from ranibizumab for macular edema following branch retinal vein occlusion: 12-month outcomes of a phase III study. Ophthalmology 118:1594–602.
31. Campochiaro PA, Brown DM, Awh CC, Lee SY, Gray S, et al. (2011) Sustained benefits from ranibizumab for macular edema following central retinal vein occlusion: twelve-month outcomes of a phase III study. Ophthalmology 118:2041–9.
32. Elman MJ, Bressler NM, Qin H, Beck RW, Ferris FL 3rd, et al. (2011) Expanded 2-year follow-up of ranibizumab plus prompt or deferred laser or triamcinolone plus prompt laser for diabetic macular edema. Ophthalmology 118:609–14.
33. Mitchell P, Bandello F, Schmidt-Erfurth U, Lang GE, Massin P, et al. (2011) The RESTORE study: ranibizumab monotherapy or combined with laser versus laser monotherapy for diabetic macular edema. Ophthalmology 118:615–25.
34. Sultan MB, Zhou D, Loftus J, Dombi T, Ice KS; Macugen 1013 Study Group (2011) A phase 2/3, multicenter, randomized, double-masked, 2-year trial of pegaptanib sodium for the treatment of diabetic macular edema. Ophthalmology 118:1107–18.
35. Trempe C (2011) Ranibizumab for age-related macular degeneration. N Engl J Med 364:581–2.
36. Nissen SE, Wolski K (2007) Effect of rosiglitazone on the risk of myocardial infarction and death from cardiovascular causes. N Engl J Med 356:2457–71.
37. Wong TY, Larsen EK, Klein R, Mitchell P, Couper DJ, et al. (2005) Cardiovascular risk factors for retinal vein occlusion and arteriolar emboli: the Atherosclerosis Risk in Communities & Cardiovascular Health studies. Ophthalmology 112:540–7.
38. Schmucker C, Loke YK, Ehlken C, Agostini HT, Hansen LL, et al. (2011) Intravitreal bevacizumab (Avastin) versus ranibizumab (Lucentis) for the treatment of age-related macular degeneration: a safety review. Br J Ophthalmol 95:308–17.
39. Curtis LH, Hammill BG, Schulman KA, Cousins SW (2010) Risks of mortality, myocardial infarction, bleeding, and stroke associated with therapies for age-related macular degeneration. Arch Ophthalmol128:1273–9.
40. French DD, Margo CE (2011) Age-related macular degeneration, anti-vascular endothelial growth factor agents, and short-term mortality: a postmarketing medication safety and surveillance study. Retina 31:1036–42.
41. Hazarika S, Dokun AO, Li Y, Popel AS, Kontos CD, et al. (2007) Impaired angiogenesis after hindlimb ischemia in type 2 diabetes mellitus: differential regulation of vascular endothelial growth factor receptor 1 and soluble vascular endothelial growth factor receptor 1. Circ Res 101:948–56.

16

A Genome-Wide Association Study for Primary Open Angle Glaucoma and Macular Degeneration Reveals Novel Loci

Todd E. Scheetz[1,2,3], John H. Fingert[1], Kai Wang[4], Markus H. Kuehn[1], Kevin L. Knudtson[5], Wallace L. M. Alward[1], H. Culver Boldt[1], Stephen R. Russell[1], James C. Folk[1], Thomas L. Casavant[1,2,3,6], Terry A. Braun[1,2,3], Abbot F. Clark[7,8], Edwin M. Stone[1,10], Val C. Sheffield[1,9,10]*

1 Department of Ophthalmology and Visual Sciences, The University of Iowa, Iowa City, Iowa, United States of America, **2** Department of Biomedical Engineering, The University of Iowa, Iowa City, Iowa, United States of America, **3** Center for Bioinformatics and Computational Biology, The University of Iowa, Iowa City, Iowa, United States of America, **4** Department of Biostatistics, The University of Iowa, Iowa City, Iowa, United States of America, **5** DNA Core Facility, The University of Iowa, Iowa City, Iowa, United States of America, **6** Department of Electrical and Computer Engineering, The University of Iowa, Iowa City, Iowa, United States of America, **7** Department of Cell Biology and Anatomy, The University of Iowa, Iowa City, Iowa, United States of America, **8** North Texas Eye Research Institute, University of North Texas Health Sciences Center, Fort Worth, Texas, United States of America, **9** Department of Pediatrics, Howard Hughes Medical Institute, Iowa City, Iowa, United States of America, **10** Howard Hughes Medical Institute, Iowa City, Iowa, United States of America

Abstract

Glaucoma and age-related macular degeneration (AMD) are the two leading causes of visual loss in the United States. We utilized a novel study design to perform a genome-wide association for both primary open angle glaucoma (POAG) and AMD. This study design utilized a two-stage process for hypothesis generation and validation, in which each disease cohort was utilized as a control for the other. A total of 400 POAG patients and 400 AMD patients were ascertained and genotyped at 500,000 loci. This study identified a novel association of complement component 7 (C7) to POAG. Additionally, an association of central corneal thickness, a known risk factor for POAG, was found to be associated with ribophorin II (RPN2). Linked monogenic loci for POAG and AMD were also evaluated for evidence of association, none of which were found to be significantly associated. However, several yielded putative associations requiring validation. Our data suggest that POAG is more genetically complex than AMD, with no common risk alleles of large effect.

Editor: Pedro Gonzalez, Duke University, United States of America

Funding: This work was supported by the National Institutes of Health [R01-EY-010564 to VCS, R01-EY-016822 to EMS, R01-EY-018825 to JHF]; the Carver Endowment for Molecular Ophthalmology to EMS and VCS; Research to Prevent Blindness (Department of Ophthalmology, University of Iowa, Career Development Awards to TES and JHF, and the Lew Wasserman Award to WLMA); and Foundation Fighting Blindness. VCS and EMS are investigators of the Howard Hughes Medical Institute. Alcon Research, Ltd. (Ft. Worth, Texas) provided funds for the purchase of the SNP genotyping chips used in this study. The funders had no role in study design, data collection and analysis, decision to publish, or preparation of the manuscript.

Competing Interests: This research was supported in part by Alcon Research Ltd, specifically in acquisition of the genotyping arrays.

* E-mail: val-sheffield@uiowa.edu

Introduction

Age-related macular degeneration (AMD) and glaucoma are leading causes of blindness and visual disability in aging populations. Although these conditions are unrelated, each has a strong genetic component. The glaucomas are a group of diseases that are characterized by injury to the optic nerve and a corresponding pattern of visual loss. These disorders are the second most common cause of irreversible blindness and visual impairment in the United States.[1] The most common form of glaucoma in the United States is primary open angle glaucoma (POAG). Epidemiological studies have shown that POAG is caused, at least in part, by heritable factors. Classic risk factors for glaucoma include advanced age, ethnicity, elevated intraocular pressure, and family history. More recently individuals with relatively thin corneas have been shown to have a three-fold greater risk of developing glaucoma than individuals with normal corneal thickness[2]. Most cases of POAG, and indeed the risk factors of elevated IOP and thin central corneal thickness, are thought to be inherited in a complex fashion[3,4].

While the genetics of glaucoma are overall complex, a fraction of glaucoma is caused primarily by defects or mutations in single genes. Linkage studies of large families exhibiting autosomal dominant inheritance of glaucoma have mapped the chromosomal locations of multiple different genes capable of causing glaucoma (GLC1A-P; [5–17]). The causative genes at six loci have been reported: myocilin (*MYOC*) [18], optineurin (*OPTN*) [19], WD repeat domain 36 (*WDR36*) [14], neurotrophin 4 (*NTF4*) [20], TANK binding kinase 1 (*TBK1*) [17], and ankyrin repeat and SOCS-box containing 10 (*ASB10*) [21]. Mutations in *MYOC* are responsible for ~4% of cases of POAG. MYOC-associated POAG cases are usually characterized by markedly elevated IOP.[22] Mutations in *OPTN* have been associated with 1–2% of cases of normotensive glaucoma (NTG).[19,23,24] The extent to which *WDR36*, *NTF4*, *ASB10* and *TBK1* play a role in the high incidence of POAG is unclear.[14,20,21,25–30] Loci and genes have also been reported for primary congenital glaucoma[31–36]. In addition, several genetic syndromes are associated with glaucoma.[37,38]

Genome-wide association studies (GWAS) have begun to identify genes that confer some risk for complex forms of glaucoma (*i.e. caused by the combined actions of multiple genes*). Genes that have been reported to confer an increased risk for POAG or NTG include: *CAV1/2*,[39] *CDKN2B-AS1*,[40–43] *ATOH7*,[41,42], *SIX1*,[41] *TMCO1*,[40] *TLR4*,[44] *SRBD1* and *ELOVL5*[45].

Genetic studies of AMD have also identified many important disease-causing genes and risk factors. Linkage analysis and positional cloning studies of pedigrees with Mendelian forms of macular degeneration have identified genes that are likely the primary cause of disease in some patients. For example, a family-based study identified fibulin 5 mutations in members of a large AMD pedigree.[46] GWAS studies have also been highly successful in identifying risk factors of major effect for AMD. The first AMD risk factor to be discovered was a coding sequence variant (Tyr402His) in the complement factor H (CFH) gene.[47–50]. Another major AMD risk factor was subsequently identified on chromosome 10. Two genes at this locus (*ARMS2* and *HTRA1*) have been investigated as the source of the AMD risk.[51,52] Additional AMD risks have been reported for other genes involved in the complement pathway including C2/CFB; C3; C5; C7; SERPING1; CFHR1 +3; CFHR2,4,5; CFI [53–60].

The goal of the current study was to use a novel GWAS design to identify additional loci involved in glaucoma and age-related macular degeneration. Importantly, there is no known comorbidity between AMD and glaucoma. We compared the SNP allele and genotype frequencies between two independent cohorts, each with 200 glaucoma patients and 200 AMD patients - a total of 800 patients. Both disease populations were selected to be without a history, clinical signs or symptoms of the other disease. Specifically, the glaucoma patients had no evidence of AMD, and the AMD patients had no evidence of glaucoma. AMD patients were then able to serve as the control (normal) population for the glaucoma cohort and vice versa. This design also incorporated a replication phase. This second 200 versus 200 comparison allowed the validation of the statistically-supported hypotheses generated by the first 200 versus 200 comparison. As all 800 patient samples were evaluated on a genome-wide collection of SNPs (Affymetrix 500k and Mapping 5.0 arrays), a comprehensive comparison of all 400 glaucoma versus 400 AMD patients was also performed in order to maximize our ability to detect associations found through this experiment.

This methodology allowed two simultaneous analyses to be performed, with both cost and time benefits. The disadvantages of this design are that it may be difficult to distinguish the 'disease phase' of a given association (i.e., if a given genotypic difference is associated with AMD or glaucoma risk), and that the identification of associations may be confounded by similar disease pathophysiology. Much of the challenge in determining the disease corresponding to a given association was alleviated through the use of expected normal genotypes – for example, the allele and genotype frequencies available as part of HapMap[61] and the Exome Sequencing Project[62]. The design also requires that both cohorts be rigorously assessed to ensure that the AMD patients are free of glaucoma, and vice versa. The number of patients assessed for each phenotype is then equivalent to that of two independent case-control designs.

Materials and Methods

Patient Samples

The University of Iowa's Institutional Review Board approved the research study and written informed consent was obtained from study participants. All patients were ascertained in the Department of Ophthalmology and Visual Sciences at the University of Iowa Carver College of Medicine. Blood samples were obtained from study participants and DNA was prepared using a non-organic method as previously described[63].

The primary and validation cohorts within each phenotype category (AMD, glaucoma) were matched for age, disease, gender and sub-phenotypes (dry, unilateral choroidal neovascularization (UCNV), bilateral choroidal neovascularization (BCNV) for AMD; normal tension glaucoma (NTG), high tension glaucoma (HTG) for glaucoma). These cohorts were designed such that the prevalence of disease, sub-phenotype, age and gender were equally represented as shown in Table 1.

Selection of normative data sets

Two normative data sets were utilized in assessing the results of the study. The first was the HapMap[61] CEU population which is comprised of Centre d' Etude du Polymorphisme Humain (CEPH) individuals of Caucasian ethnicity. Population-based allele frequencies for each SNP were provided as part of the annotations available for the Affymetrix genotyping platforms. This population is a representative sample of the general population, and is therefore expected to have the population prevalence of AMD and glaucoma within that population. The second normative population used was a disease-free set of 100 patients drawn from the University of Iowa Ophthalmology clinic. These patients were all over the age of 59 at the time of ascertainment, and had no signs or history of either glaucoma or AMD, as defined below.

Clinical Criteria – Primary Open Angle Glaucoma

The cohort of glaucoma subjects underwent complete ophthalmologic evaluation including a dilated stereoscopic examination of the optic nerve heads, Goldmann applanation tonometry, gonioscopy, optic nerve head photography, perimetry and slit lamp examination. Visual fields were assessed in using the SITA 24-2 program on the Humphrey Field Analyzer (Humphrey-Zeiss, Dublin, Ca.). Patients that were unable to perform automated perimetry were tested with Goldmann manual kinetic perimetry (Haag-Streit Instruments, Koeniz, Switzerland).

Patients exhibiting excavation of their optic nerve head and associated glaucomatous visual field loss in at least one eye were considered to have glaucoma. Glaucomatous optic nerves were

Table 1. Distribution of patient phenotypes among the primary and validation cohorts.

		AMD			POAG
Phase	**Gender**	**Dry[a]**	**UCNV[b]**	**BCNV[c]**	
Primary	Female	29	49	48	114
	Male	19	28	27	83
Validation	Female	35	48	45	111
	Male	20	27	25	89

[a]No evidence for choroidal neovascularization found in either eye.
[b]Evidence for choroidal neovascularization found in one eye.
[c]Evidence for choroidal neovascularization found in both eyes.

defined as nerves with cup-to-disc ratios of greater than 0.7, thinning of the neural rim, asymmetry of the optic nerve cup-to-disc ratio of >0.2, or photographic documentation of progressive loss of the neural rim. Patients were required to have visual fields of adequate quality for interpretation. For Humphrey visual fields this required a false positive rate, false negative rate and fixation loss rate of less than 33% [64]. Humphrey visual field evidence of glaucoma was based on the Collaborative Normal Tension Glaucoma Treatment Trial criteria[65]. Patients screened using manual kinetic perimetry were required to exhibit depression of the visual field in an arcuate pattern respecting the nasal horizontal meridian. Central corneal thickness was measured using a Pachette 3 ultrasound pachymeter (DGH technology, Inc., Exton, PA). Topical proparicaine was used for anesthesia, the ultrasound probe was placed in apposition to patient corneas and 25 measurements of the corneal thickness were automatically obtained from each eye. The mean of thickness measurements obtained from both eyes was used as the central corneal thickness for each subject.

The medical records of glaucoma patients were reviewed for evidence of macular degeneration. Subjects were excluded from the glaucoma cohort if: 1) they had a prior diagnosis of macular degeneration; 2) they take oral medications for macular degeneration (i.e. AREDS vitamins); or 3) they have a history of treatment with anti-VEGF therapies.

Clinical Criteria - AMD

Candidates for this project were selected from a pool of patients diagnosed with age-related macular degeneration (AMD) by a faculty ophthalmologist at the University of Iowa. Their charts and photofiles were reviewed by a retinal expert with extensive experience in AMD and AMD trials. For inclusion in this study, a patient had to have either Category 3 or 4 AMD as defined by the Age-Related Treatment Trial in both eyes[66,67]. For an eye to be classified as Category 3 it must have at least one large (≥125μ) druse, or enough intermediate size (63–125μ) drusen that when the area occupied would be at least 0.5 disc area. A Category 4 eye has advanced AMD defined as geographic atrophy of the retinal pigment epithelium (RPE) in the center of the fovea or choroidal neovascularization. Geographic atrophy of the RPE is defined in the AREDS as the presence of at least two of the three following characteristics: a circular area, sharply defined margins, and visible choroidal vessels. Signs of choroidal neovascularization include elevation of the retinal pigment epithelium, subretinal hemorrhage or fibrosis, serous retinal detachment, hard exudation and leakage of new vessels on fluorescein angiography. If a patient had Category 4 AMD in both eyes, at least one eye had to have at least one large drusen or a 0.5 disc area of intermediate drusen when added together.

Patients with evidence of myopic degeneration, chorioretinal scars in the macula, angioid streaks, or diabetic retinopathy consisting of more than five microaneursyms or hemorrhages were excluded from the study. The few patients who had equivocal findings, no photos, or poor quality photos that could not be evaluated were excluded from the study.

Patients were subdivided into groups based on past or present evidence of CNV up to and including their last follow-up examination. Patients with CNV in both eyes were placed in group one. Patients with CNV in only one eye were placed into group two. Patients with no CNV and were age 70 or older were placed into group three.

The AMD patients were rigorously evaluated for glaucoma to ensure that they could serve as a glaucoma depleted control group. AMD patients were examined and medical records were reviewed by an ophthalmologist that judged them to be free of glaucoma based on the following criteria: 1) history of medication to lower their intraocular pressure; 2) history of any type of glaucoma or status as a glaucoma suspect; 3) cup to disc ratio in either eye of 0.5 or greater unless they had been evaluated by the glaucoma service at UIHC and deemed not to have glaucoma; and 4) intraocular pressure of 25 mm Hg or higher. Patients with an intraocular pressure of 22–24 mm Hg in either eye were included only if there were at least three other measurements that were below this mark.

SNP Array Genotyping

Genome-wide SNP genotypes were obtained for all samples with the Affymetrix 500 K set and Mapping 5.0 arrays (Affymetrix Inc., Santa Clara, CA) using the manufacturer's recommended protocols. The BRLMM[68] and BRLMM-P[69] algorithms within the Affymetrix Power Tools suite[70] were used to calculate the individual genotypes. Genotypes were called on the 500 K SNP array hybridizations with the BRLMM algorithm as a single group using default parameters. Genotypes were called on the Mapping 5.0 array hybridizations with the BRLMM-P algorithm using default parameters.

Data management and quality control

SNPs with a call rate less than 85% were eliminated from the analysis. All SNP genotypes were analyzed for Hardy-Weinberg Equilibrium (HWE). A p-value threshold of 0.001 was used to identify SNPs not in HWE. Deviations from HWE may be caused by genuine associations or genotyping errors. Thus all SNPs determined not to be in HWE were manually inspected for evidence of genotyping errors.

Genetic Analysis

Gender is a known confounder for both glaucoma and AMD. The balanced construction of our populations, however, was designed to minimize gender as a covariate. The Cochran-Armitage test for trend was used to evaluate the genetic variations between the groups of discrete traits (e.g., glaucoma, ocular hypertension) with a correction for population stratification [71] (the 0.1-trimmed variance estimate was used). For continuous traits, genetic association was evaluated through a linear regression in which the dependent variable was the quantitative trait and the predictor variable was the SNP genotype. The possibility of population stratification was corrected for in a similar manner[71]. An uncorrected p-value of 5×10^{-7} was used as the threshold for statistical significance of the associations[72]. P-values less than 1×10^{-5} were classified as suggestive of an association. Only SNPs that were reproducibly associated in both cohorts were considered significant. A cluster of at least three statistically significant (or suggestive) SNPs was required to define an associated (or suggestive) locus, with an inter-SNP distance of at most 200 kb. Associated loci were classified as AMD or POAG using a Fisher's Exact test versus the control populations. To classify the locus, a p-value <0.05 was required for a disease population in both the primary and validation cohorts, with the other disease yielding non-significant p-values (p>0.05).

Results

Patient Demographics

Age, gender, and sub-phenotype(s) were evenly distributed within each 200×200 comparison (see Table 1). The absence of inadvertent bias was validated by comparing the distribution of genotypes among the populations using several hundred of the most informative SNPs. These SNPs showed no significant associations, indicating that the hypothesis generating and validating populations had similar ethnic compositions. This was confirmed using the protocol described in by Stokowski et al.[73] using STRUCTURE with a set of genome-wide genomic control SNPs.

Associated Loci

Eight hundred patients were genotyped and analyzed in a genome-wide association study design. The resulting associations are summarized in Table 2, ranked by significance. This table lists the associated loci, the p-values from the hypothesis-generating (primary) cohorts, the p-values from the validation cohorts, and the p-values from the combined cohorts. A list of genes within each associated locus is also provided. A graphic depiction of the genome-wide associations is provided in Figure 1. The significance of the associations is represented by red lines to the right of the chromosomes, with stronger associations resulting in longer lines. The associated regions from Table 2 are annotated on this figure in green to the left of the chromosome lines. The associations in Table 2 are classified as either AMD or glaucoma. This assessment was based upon comparison with the expected allele frequencies in Caucasian populations as determined by the two control datasets described previously.

As Figure 1 and Table 2 show, the strongest associations are between the two previously reported AMD risk loci on chromosome 1 (complement factor H;[47,49,50,74]) and chromosome 10 (ARMS2; [75,76]). The strongest association found was that of the Y402H AMD risk-allele in CFH. The reproduction of the two major AMD loci within this analysis served as additional verification of the validity of our study design. Both the CFH and ARMS2 loci are clearly visible with peak associations of $p<10^{-16}$. Also of note based upon previously published results, we carefully evaluated several recently published glaucoma associations [39,40,77–80]. None of the published associations reached genome-wide significance in our study, however associations to CDKN2B-AS1 and SRBD1 satisfied a gene-level Bonferroni correction with p-values of 0.0002 and 0.0001 respectively. Of the 47 SNPs at the SRBD1 locus only one SNP, rs3213787, produced a significant p-value. This association data provides some support for the previously reported POAG association at the SRBD1 locus. However, the absence of a significant association with other neighboring SNPs suggests our finding at the SRBD1 may be a false positive signal. In contrast, of the 35 SNPs at the CDKN2B-AS1 locus, four produced significant p-values (0.0004, 0.0002, 0.001, 0.0049). This lends additional confidence to the bona fide association of this locus to POAG in our cohort.

Because both populations were selected from the extant clinical population, the relative gender distribution differs slightly between the two disease populations. While the difference is small, we performed a logistic regression as part of the association analysis to address this issue. The resulting p-values were virtually identical to the original analysis, with the expected decrease in significance due to the additional degree of freedom.

Novel Glaucoma Loci

The genome-wide association analysis identified one glaucoma-associated loci, as shown in Table 2. The peak of the glaucoma association on chromosome 5 occurs within the C7 gene – one of the components of the complement system. This finding is of interest because several complement components have previously been reported as risk-associated factors for AMD. However, based upon the expected allele frequency from HapMap and based upon additional genotyping in a population of normal control individuals, our data strongly suggest that the observed locus is not

Table 2. Summary of associated loci.

Position	Class[a]	SNPs[b]	Best SNP & MAF[c] (AMD/NL/POAG)	Odds ratio (95% CI)	Joint p-value	p-value (primary)	p-value (replicate)	Genes
chr1 194664398-195393272	AMD	31	SNP_A-2171106 (0.16/0.39/0.39)	3.75 (2.91,4.82)	$<10^{-16}$	6.7×10^{-13}	1.2×10^{-8}	KCNT2, **CFH**, CFHR3, CFHR1P, CFHR4, CFHR2, CFHR5, F13B, ASPM, ZBTB41
chr10 124139342-124225345	AMD	7	SNP_A-1841655 (0.45/0.18/0.20)	3.14 (2.49,3.97)	$<10^{-16}$	1.1×10^{-7}	3.1×10^{-11}	PLEKHA1, **ARMS2**, HTRA1
chr5 40965351-40991318	POAG	6	SNP_A-1838573 (0.36/0.36/0.48)	1.65 (1.34,2.03)	5.6×10^{-5}	2.2×10^{-3}	9.8×10^{-3}	**C7**

[a]Disease classification (AMD or POAG)
[b]Number of associated SNPs.
[c]Minor Allele Frequencies (MAFs) presented for AMD, normal controls, and POAG respectively.

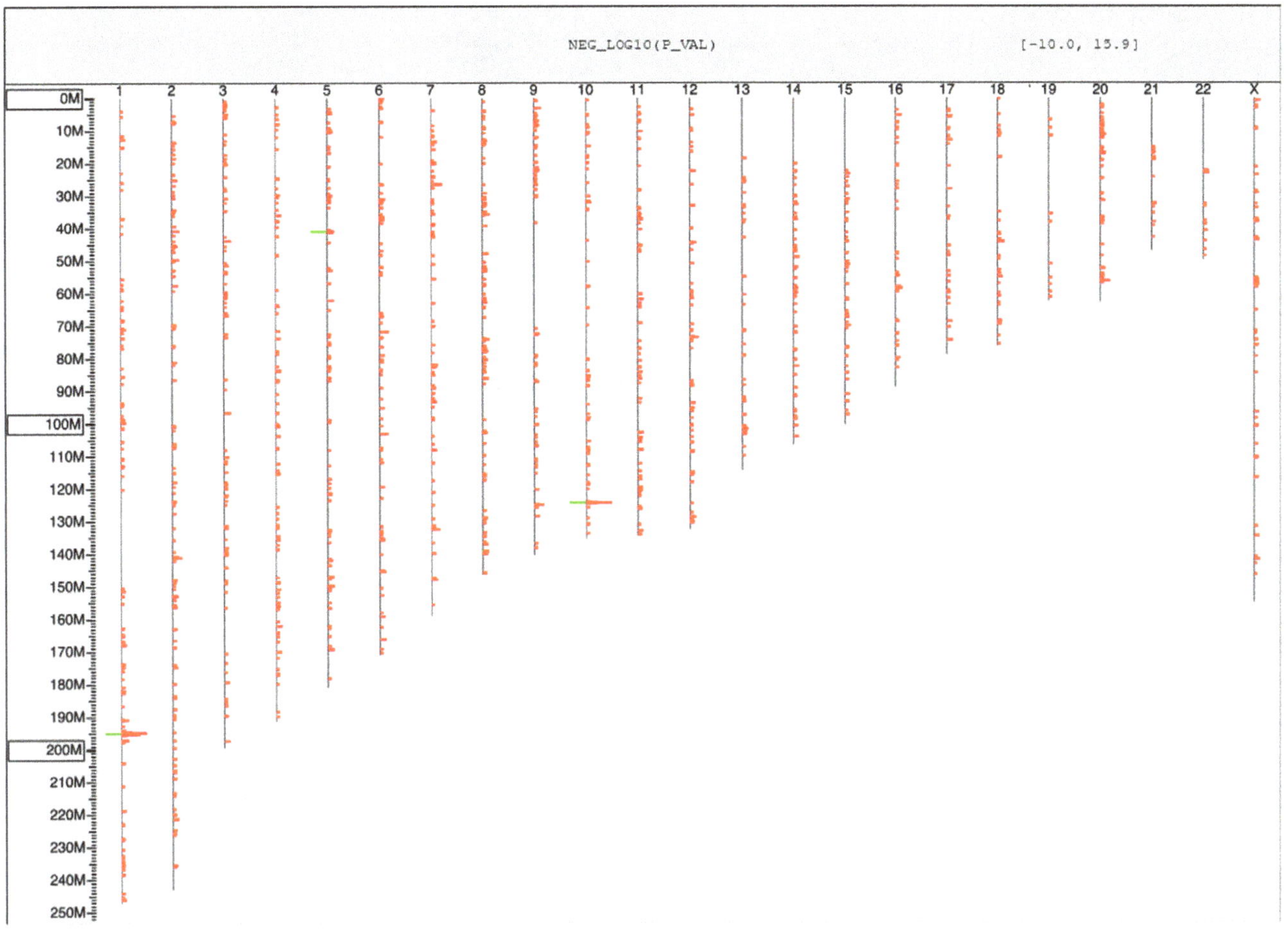

Figure 1. Genome-wide summary of associations. This figure presents the associations identified across all 22 autosomes and the X chromosome. Each vertical line represents a chromosome and the position within that chromosome is given based upon the position along the vertical axis. The length of the red bars represents the strength of the association for individual SNPs, calculated as the negative $\log_{10}$ of the association p-value. Only SNPs with $p < 10^{-3}$ are shown. The green bars denote the position of the associated SNP clusters, as summarized in Table 2.

associated with AMD but represents a novel glaucoma locus. Of the SNPs at the C7 locus showing association with glaucoma, four are found in introns of the gene, and one results in a highly conserved amino acid change (Ser389Thr). While little is known regarding the function of individual protein domains of C7, Ser389 exhibits remarkable conservation in orthologous genes from vertebrate species, suggesting that this region may be functionally important (Figure 2).

```
                            *
KAASGTQNNVLRGEPFIRGGGAGFISGLSYLELDNPAGNKRRYSAWAESV   Human
KSASGTQSNVLRGVPFVRGGRPGFVSGLSYLELDNPDGNKQRYSSWAGSV   Pig
KSDSGTQGNMVRGDPYVRGGSLDFVAGLSKLQLDNPAGNKGRYASWAESV   Dog
KSNSGNQGRVLRGEPSVIGGGPGFVADLSFLDLDNPAGNRQRYSSWASSV   Rat
KSTSGNKGRLLRGKPLVRGGDSGFVADLSFLDLDNPAGNKQRYSSWAGSV   Mouse
-APPGSSGNELRGDPYIEGGNPAGVAGLSYLDLNNPAGNSARYSSWAGSN   Platypus
QTSSGSSGSKIRGDPYIEGGSPSAVAGLSYLDLDDPAGNNQRYSTWARSV   Chicken
RQSSGSTDREVRGDVFVQGGEAKFVAGLSYFSLDNPLSNENRYAAWAGSV   Xenopus
----------------IIGGNSAYIAGLSLLDLENPDNNKQMYTKWAGSV   Danio
KTSKEYNNNKLPIKTNVIGGDPSFIAGLSVLDLENPEANGQMYDKWARSV   Salmon
```

Figure 2. Conservation of the complement component 7 protein. Multiple sequence alignment highlighting the amino acid conservation of the complement component 7 protein (C7) across a broad spectrum of animal species, including mammal, bird, amphibian and fish. The SNP rs1063499 (asterisk) is conserved across these species, suggesting functional conservation of this amino acid.

Evaluation of Mendelian POAG intervals

All previously reported loci for monogenic forms of POAG (GLC1A – GLC1P [5–16]) were considered *a priori* candidates for association with POAG. Of note, the novel glaucoma-associated regions described above do not overlap this set of published monogenic glaucoma intervals. In this association study, only one of the previously linked loci, GLC1N, exhibited an association ($p = 0.00013$) to the SNP rs872476. This SNP lies within the THSD4 gene, which is expressed in several ocular tissues including the trabecular meshwork and optic nerve (data not shown).

Evaluation of Candidate Glaucoma Genes

A set of candidate glaucoma genes was assessed for association in this study. This set of candidate genes consisted of 73 genes localized to the peroxisome, or involved in peroxisome biology as annotated in the Gene Ontology[81], and were selected based upon a recently proposed mechanism for MYOC glaucoma[82]. No associations were found to be both significant and reproducible for these candidates in both cohorts. The best association was found to a SNP (rs2142697) in the hydroxyacid oxidase 1 (HAO1) gene ($p = 0.0022$). HAO1 was not expressed in any ocular tissues in a high-density gene expression survey of ten ocular tissues (data not shown).

Central Cornea Thickness

Central cornea thickness (CCT) is one of several quantitative traits reported to be a risk factor for glaucoma. Patients with thin corneas were shown to have a higher prevalence of glaucoma[2]. In this study, CCT data were available for 280 of the 800 patients genotyped. A genome-wide scan was performed to search for genetic variations that modulate corneal thickness. We identified one major QTL on chromosome 20, centered at 35.2 Mb consisting of nine associated SNPs. The distribution of CCT values in the three genotype classes of rs6124577 is shown in Figure 3. This figure shows that AA homozygotes and AB heterozygotes have significantly thinner corneas compared to BB homozygotes. This locus contains the RBL1, C20ORF132 and RPN2 genes, with the strongest association within the RPN2 gene. Although the p-values are not significant at the genome-wide level, this cluster is reproducibly observed in the primary and validation cohorts.

AMD Loci

This study identified the two previously reported AMD loci CFH[47,49,50,74] and chromosome 10[75] (Table 2). The chromosome 10 locus contains the PLEKHA1, ARMS2 (LOC387715) and HTRA1 genes. There is evidence for each of these genes to be the risk-associated gene[51,75,83]. Our analysis found the strongest association to the Arg69Ser variation in ARMS2 reported by Swaroop et al. [76].

A set of previously reported AMD causing or AMD risk associated loci (RetNet.org; [84]) were also evaluated. The analysis of these loci is presented in Table 3. Three of the loci (BSMD, MCDR3 and MCDR4) were associated with AMD in the primary and validation cohorts. The BSMD locus contains a cluster of associated SNPs with a peak p-value of 6.2×10^{-5}. The associated SNPs localize within the first intron of the CAMK2A gene, a calcium-dependent serine/threonine kinase. The MCDR3 locus contains a cluster of eight associated SNPs with a peak p-value of 2×10^{-4}. This associated locus contains the CCT5 gene, part of the chaperonin containing TCP1 complex, and the first exon of the FAM173B gene. The MCDR4 locus contains three associated SNPs with a peak p-value of 0.002. There are no annotated genes within the MCDR4 associated SNP cluster.

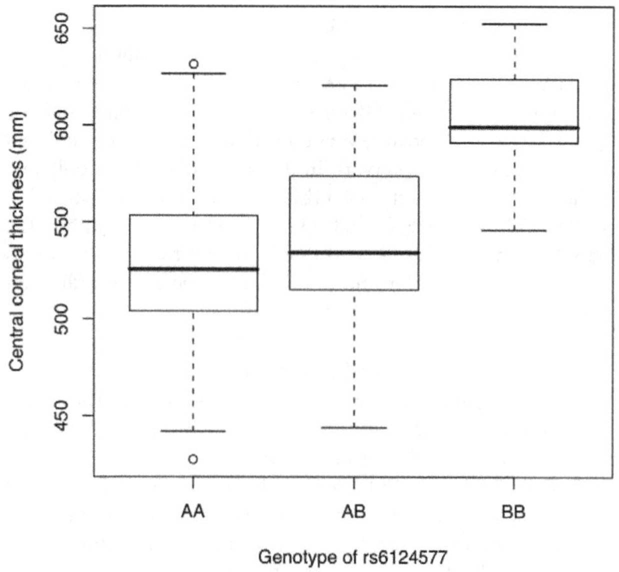

Figure 3. Distribution of central corneal thickness. A boxplot of CCT measurements is presented, demonstrating the differential thickness based upon the observed genotype at rs6124577.

AMD associated genes

We also assessed the set of published AMD-causing or risk-associated genes, as well as complement-related genes for evidence of an AMD association. These results are summarized in Table 3. As described above, both CFH and ARMS2 are significantly associated in the genome-wide screen. From the set of AMD causing and risk-associated genes, suggestive and reproducible associations were detected for C2/CFB, C3, HTRA1 and PROM1. The association to C2 and CFB comes from a SNP (rs522162) that is immediately 3′ of CFB. However, given the proximity of C2 and CFB this SNP may be in linkage disequilibrium with a causative variation in either or both genes. Eight additional complement associated genes were identified with suggestive, reproducible AMD associations, specifically ADCY3, CFHR2, CFHR3, CFHR4, CFHR5, F13B, ASPH and CSMD1. It should be noted that the apparent association for CFHR2-5 and F13B may be due to their proximity to CFH.

Discussion

The design of this study utilized two separate affected populations, glaucoma patients and macular degeneration patients. Each patient population served as the normal control for the other. This study design allowed maximum efficiency in utilization of the genetic data in the assessment of genetic associations. A limitation of this study design is that the diseases to be studied should not share genetic risk factors with each other. Without this constraint, loci contributing to both disorders would likely go undetected. For example, if the Y402H variation in complement factor H was a risk allele for both glaucoma and AMD, the likelihood for identification of this variation as a risk allele for either disorder would be diminished compared to studies using normal controls (patients with neither glaucoma or AMD).

Provided that two diseases do not share risk associations, the study design used here allows the identification of SNPs that are statistically associated to one of the diseases or the other. However, the *disease classification* of each individual association (i.e., in which disease the genetic variant is acting) is not immediately apparent. In such instances, it is possible to utilize the expected allele and genotype frequencies based upon other studies such as the HapMap project[61]. The disease population differing from the 'normal' frequency determines the disease classification of the association. It is possible that, in rare instances, a given allele could be a risk factor for one disorder and a protective allele for the second disorder. In such an instance the risk allele would be enriched in one population and depleted in the other (compared to normal controls), providing an increase in statistical power to detect the association. In the current study, the previously reported AMD associations, CFH and ARMS2, were readily detected as AMD associated loci using the glaucoma cohort as the control, with allele frequencies similar to those reported in other studies. These findings validate the use of glaucoma controls for AMD studies, and indicate that CFH and ARMS2 are not involved in glaucoma.

The primary advantage of the two-disease study design is that genotyping costs can be conserved in the initial phase of the study (genotyping of the primary cohorts). This allows hypotheses to be developed for both diseases for a specific population without genotyping an additional normal control cohort. The power to detect association is based upon the size of the two disease cohorts.

Table 3. Evidence for association to linked AMD loci.

Linked Locus	Genomic Position	Peak p-value	Primary p-value	Validation p-value
BCMAD	chr6:45098201-104690621	1.1×10^{-6}	8.0×10^{-1}	1.1×10^{-10}
BSMD	chr5:121308199-155661743	6.2×10^{-5}	4.9×10^{-3}	5.1×10^{-3}
MCDR1	chr6:75845485-99792538	3.4×10^{-4}	1.0×10^{-4}	8.2×10^{-1}
MCDR3	chr5:988510-21094862	2.5×10^{-4}	2.4×10^{-2}	4.0×10^{-3}
MCDR4	chr14:20983113-21023115	2.9×10^{-3}	4.1×10^{-2}	3.4×10^{-2}
MCDR5	chr19:44719578-46244168	3.3×10^{-3}	2.2×10^{-4}	N/A
MDDC	chr7:22317857-26483126	5.4×10^{-8}	6.6×10^{-1}	1.2×10^{-11}
TEAD1	chr11:12703561-12963122	1.2×10^{-2}	4.9×10^{-2}	1.2×10^{-1}

Hypotheses developed in the initial phase, can then be pursued using a validation cohort. A control cohort can be included for limited genotyping at loci of interest and to clarify the specific disease associations. In this study two control cohorts were utilized – the CEU population from HapMap and a set of normal patients from the same clinic population as the POAG and AMD cohorts. The allele and genotype frequencies from the normal cohorts were in close agreement with each other.

In this study, no single, large risk allele for glaucoma on the order of the CFH AMD risk allele was detected. Therefore it is likely that this disorder is very genetically heterogeneous and that no single locus with a high genotype relative risk (GRR) exists for POAG in the population studied. A key factor in the power to detect associated loci in a GWAS analysis is the genotype relative risk. The GRR reported for CFH and ARMS2 (2.44–5.93 and 3.2–7.9, respectively) contribute substantially to the ability to detect those associations[74,75]. In contrast to POAG, a single locus on the LOXL1 gene significantly contributes to elevated risk for developing exfoliation syndrome[85], a condition that is highly prevalent in some populations and may lead to secondary glaucoma.

The findings highlight the genetic complexity of glaucoma. Known Mendelian genes account for between three to five percent of glaucoma, with the remainder of disease most likely resulting from a combination of many risk factors, each with a small effect. Previous GWAS reports have identified several glaucoma risk associated genes (*CAV1/2*,[39] *CDKN2B-AS1*,[40–43] *ATOH7*,[41,42], *SIX1*,[41] *TMCO1*,[40] *TLR4*,[44] *SRBD1* and *ELOVL5* [45]). However, none of these risk factors were associated with glaucoma in our study at genome-wide significance. A single gene, SRBD1, was found to be significant under a more permissive multiple hypothesis correction strategy, in which only the eight risk-associated genes were evaluated ($p<0.00625$). These data underscore key features of the genetic complexity of glaucoma. No genetic risk factors of major effect have been discovered for POAG, and the identified risk factors of smaller effect are more important in some populations than others.

This study is adequately powered to detect genetic effects where additional copies of the disease allele increase the odds of disease by a factor of 2 or larger unless the disease-associated allele is rare. For instance, OR> = 2 and MAF>0.1 (Table 4). For smaller odds ratios, the power is lower unless the disease-associated allele is common, for instance, OR = 1.75 and MAF = 0.4 (Table 4).

Complement factor 7 (C7)

Despite the lack of strongly associated loci for POAG or strongly associated novel loci for AMD, several loci and genes of interest were identified. Of particular interest to the study of glaucoma is the association of C7. C7 has several features that make it an interesting glaucoma candidate. Although C7 is widely expressed, it is highly expressed in optic nerve (data not shown), a tissue of critical relevance to glaucoma. Our data indicate that there are several SNPs within the C7 gene that are significantly associated with glaucoma. Four associated SNPs are located in an intron. An additional SNP encodes an amino acid change (Ser389Thr), which is phylogenetically highly conserved in many vertebrates, including mammals, fish, amphibians, and birds. Chou-Fasman modeling predicts that this mutation results in a change in the secondary structure of C7 and may affect the activity of the protein. C7 is required for assembly of C5b-9.

We and others have demonstrated that complement components, including the C1q, C3, and the C5b-9 complex, are deposited in the glaucomatous retina and optic nerve head[86,87]. C1q and C3 are involved in the 'pruning' of retinal ganglion cells dendrites during development and have been implicated in glaucomatous damage to the retina and optic nerve[88]. Although the physiological role of complement activation in glaucoma is not entirely understood, studies in a mouse model of ischemic neuropathy indicate that complement inhibition delays retinal ganglion cell degeneration[89]. These findings suggest that complement may specifically target damaged retinal ganglion cells for rapid disruption and removal, possibly to avoid the initiation of an adaptive auto-immune response to retinal antigens as has been described in other diseases[90]. On the other hand, sublytic complement activation may be beneficial for cell survival[91] and it is conceivable that the C5b-9 deposition observed in glaucoma is part of a neuroprotective response of stressed retinal ganglion cells.

In addition to evaluating SNP associations for the primary phenotypes, it is also of interest to identify associations with known disease risk factors, subclasses of disease, and disease complications. For example, central corneal thickness (CCT) has been shown to be a risk factor for glaucoma[2]. In one study eyes with thin corneas (less than 556 microns) have a three-fold greater risk of developing glaucoma than eyes with thick corneas (more than 588 microns). Thus the presence of thin corneas is considered a glaucoma risk factor. In our study, CCT data was available for a subset of patients. Despite the relatively small size of the data set, we observed significant association with CCT at a locus on chromosome 20. Our data indicate that there may be at least one strong genetic locus involved in CCT. It is known that corneal thickness influences intraocular pressure, another risk factor for glaucoma. Thus further study will be required to determine if the chromosome 20 locus is an independent risk locus for glaucoma.

Table 4. Power to detect genetic effect.

OR	Minor Allele Frequency	Power ($\alpha=5\times10^{-7}$)	Power ($\alpha=1\times10^{-5}$)	Power ($\alpha=5\times10^{-5}$)
1.75	0.10	0.011	0.044	0.104
	0.20	0.149	0.367	0.509
	0.30	0.343	0.625	0.773
	0.40	0.535	0.792	0.865
2.00	0.10	0.042	0.164	0.277
	0.20	0.417	0.665	0.798
	0.30	0.758	0.912	0.960
	0.40	0.892	0.971	0.990
2.50	0.10	0.221	0.480	0.636
	0.20	0.866	0.961	0.986
	0.30	0.984	0.995	0.999
	0.40	0.998	0.999	1.000

OR is the odds ratio of disease risk for genotype Dd versus genotype dd (assumed to be equal to the odds ratio for genotype DD versus Dd). The disease risk for genotype dd is assumed to be 0.001. Power is simulated over 1000 replications.

An important subclass of glaucoma is normal tension glaucoma. The current study had limited power to detect association for normal tension glaucoma, due to a limited number of patients with this subclass of disease. A major complication of AMD is the presence of CNV. This study identified a suggestive risk locus for CNV. Although there are no reported genes at the associated locus, multiple ESTs map to this region.

Conclusions

This study reports a genome-wide association study in primary open angle glaucoma. A novel association of POAG to a variation in complement component 7 was identified. In addition, an association of central corneal thickness, a quantitative risk factor for glaucoma, to a SNP in the ribophorin II gene was identified. This study utilized a novel design to maximize the utility of the available genotyping resources and patient cohorts. This design was validated through the observation of AMD associations to the most significant AMD-risk associated alleles – Tyr402His in CFH and Arg69Ser in ARMS2. However, further investigation of this study design is needed to better characterize the power to detect bona fide associations and to correctly reject false associations in comparison to a traditional case-control design. Future work includes focused genotyping in additional large cohorts to further validate the genetic associations.

Acknowledgments

The authors are grateful to the patients and their families for participating in this study. The authors thank J. Beck and A.J. Grundstad for technical assistance, and Drs. D. Nishimura and R. Swiderski for helpful discussions.

Author Contributions

Conceived and designed the experiments: VCS EMS AFC TES TAB JHF TLC. Performed the experiments: TES JHF KW KLK TAB. Analyzed the data: TES KW TAB. Contributed reagents/materials/analysis tools: JHF EMS JCF SRR HCB WLMA TES TAB TLC. Wrote the paper: TES JHF VCS EMS KW MHK AFC TLC.

References

1. Leske MC (1983) The epidemiology of open-angle glaucoma: a review. Am J Epidemiol 118: 166–191.
2. Gordon MO, Beiser JA, Brandt JD, Heuer DK, Higginbotham EJ, et al. (2002) The Ocular Hypertension Treatment Study: baseline factors that predict the onset of primary open-angle glaucoma. Arch Ophthalmol 120: 714–720; discussion 829–730.
3. Libby RT, Gould DB, Anderson MG, John SW (2005) Complex genetics of glaucoma susceptibility. Annu Rev Genomics Hum Genet 6: 15–44.
4. Hewitt AW, Craig JE, Mackey DA (2006) Complex genetics of complex traits: the case of primary open-angle glaucoma. Clin Experiment Ophthalmol 34: 472–484.
5. Sheffield VC, Stone EM, Alward WL, Drack AV, Johnson AT, et al. (1993) Genetic linkage of familial open angle glaucoma to chromosome 1q21–q31. Nat Genet 4: 47–50.
6. Stoilova D, Child A, Trifan OC, Crick RP, Coakes RL, et al. (1996) Localization of a locus (GLC1B) for adult-onset primary open angle glaucoma to the 2cen-q13 region. Genomics 36: 142–150.
7. Wirtz MK, Samples JR, Kramer PL, Rust K, Topinka JR, et al. (1997) Mapping a gene for adult-onset primary open-angle glaucoma to chromosome 3q. American Journal of Human Genetics 60: 296–304.
8. Sarfarazi M, Child A, Stoilova D, Brice G, Desai T, et al. (1998) Localization of the fourth locus (GLC1E) for adult-onset primary open-angle glaucoma to the 10p15-p14 region. American Journal of Human Genetics 62: 641–652.
9. Trifan OC, Traboulsi EI, Stoilova D, Alozie I, Nguyen R, et al. (1998) A third locus (GLC1D) for adult-onset primary open-angle glaucoma maps to the 8q23 region. Am J Ophthalmol 126: 17–28.
10. Wirtz MK, Samples JR, Rust K, Lie J, Nordling L, et al. (1999) GLC1F, a new primary open-angle glaucoma locus, maps to 7q35–q36. Arch Ophthalmol 117: 237–241.
11. Wiggs JL, Lynch S, Ynagi G, Maselli M, Auguste J, et al. (2004) A genomewide scan identifies novel early-onset primary open-angle glaucoma loci on 9q22 and 20p12. American Journal of Human Genetics 74: 1314–1320.
12. Allingham RR, Wiggs JL, Hauser ER, Larocque-Abramson KR, Santiago-Turla C, et al. (2005) Early adult-onset POAG linked to 15q11–13 using ordered subset analysis. Invest Ophthalmol Vis Sci 46: 2002–2005.
13. Baird PN, Foote SJ, Mackey DA, Craig J, Speed TP, et al. (2005) Evidence for a novel glaucoma locus at chromosome 3p21–22. Hum Genet 117: 249–257.
14. Monemi S, Spaeth G, DaSilva A, Popinchalk S, Ilitchev E, et al. (2005) Identification of a novel adult-onset primary open-angle glaucoma (POAG) gene on 5q22.1. Hum Mol Genet 14: 725–733.
15. Wang DY, Fan BJ, Chua JK, Tam PO, Leung CK, et al. (2006) A genome-wide scan maps a novel juvenile-onset primary open-angle glaucoma locus to 15q. Invest Ophthalmol Vis Sci 47: 5315–5321.
16. Fan BJ, Ko WC, Wang DY, Canlas O, Ritch R, et al. (2007) Fine mapping of new glaucoma locus GLC1M and exclusion of neuregulin 2 as the causative gene. Mol Vis 13: 779–784.

17. Fingert JH, Robin AL, Stone JL, Roos BR, Davis LK, et al. (2011) Copy number variations on chromosome 12q14 in patients with normal tension glaucoma. Hum Mol Genet 20: 2482–2494.
18. Stone EM, Fingert JH, Alward WL, Nguyen TD, Polansky JR, et al. (1997) Identification of a gene that causes primary open angle glaucoma. Science 275: 668–670.
19. Rezaie T, Child A, Hitchings R, Brice G, Miller L, et al. (2002) Adult-onset primary open-angle glaucoma caused by mutations in optineurin. Science 295: 1077–1079.
20. Pasutto F, Matsumoto T, Mardin CY, Sticht H, Brandstatter JH, et al. (2009) Heterozygous NTF4 mutations impairing neurotrophin-4 signaling in patients with primary open-angle glaucoma. American Journal of Human Genetics 85: 447–456.
21. Pasutto F, Keller KE, Weisschuh N, Sticht H, Samples JR, et al. (2012) Variants in ASB10 are associated with open-angle glaucoma. Hum Mol Genet 21: 1336–1349.
22. Fingert JH, Heon E, Liebmann JM, Yamamoto T, Craig JE, et al. (1999) Analysis of myocilin mutations in 1703 glaucoma patients from five different populations. Hum Mol Genet 8: 899–905.
23. Alward WL, Kwon YH, Kawase K, Craig JE, Hayreh SS, et al. (2003) Evaluation of optineurin sequence variations in 1,048 patients with open-angle glaucoma. Am J Ophthalmol 136: 904–910.
24. Fingert JH (2011) Primary open-angle glaucoma genes. Eye (Lond) 25: 587–595.
25. Hewitt AW, Dimasi DP, Mackey DA, Craig JE (2006) A Glaucoma Case-control Study of the WDR36 Gene D658G sequence variant. Am J Ophthalmol. pp. 324–325.
26. Fingert JH, Alward WL, Kwon YH, Shankar SP, Andorf JL, et al. (2007) No association between variations in the WDR36 gene and primary open-angle glaucoma. Arch Ophthalmol 125: 434–436.
27. Hauser MA, Allingham RR, Linkroum K, Wang J, LaRocque-Abramson K, et al. (2006) Distribution of WDR36 DNA sequence variants in patients with primary open-angle glaucoma. Invest Ophthalmol Vis Sci. pp. 2542–2546.
28. Liu Y, Liu W, Crooks K, Schmidt S, Allingham RR, et al. No evidence of association of heterozygous NTF4 mutations in patients with primary open-angle glaucoma. Am J Hum Genet 86: 498–499; author reply 500.
29. Fingert JH, Roos BR, Solivan-Timpe F, Miller KA, Oetting TA, et al. (2012) Analysis of ASB10 variants in open angle glaucoma. Hum Mol Genet.
30. Kawase K, Allingham RR, Meguro A, Mizuki N, Roos B, et al. (2012) Confirmation of TBK1 duplication in normal tension glaucoma. Exp Eye Res 96: 178–180.
31. Sarfarazi M, Akarsu AN, Hossain A, Turacli ME, Aktan SG, et al. (1995) Assignment of a locus (GLC3A) for primary congenital glaucoma (Buphthalmos) to 2p21 and evidence for genetic heterogeneity. Genomics 30: 171–177.
32. Akarsu AN, Turacli ME, Aktan SG, Barsoum-Homsy M, Chevrette L, et al. (1996) A second locus (GLC3B) for primary congenital glaucoma (Buphthalmos) maps to the 1p36 region. Hum Mol Genet 5: 1199–1203.
33. Stoilov I, Sarfarazi M (2002) The third genetic locus (GLC3C) for primary congenital glaucoma (PCG) maps to chromosome 14q24.3. Association for Vision Research and Ophthalmology. pp. 43.
34. Stoilov I, Akarsu AN, Sarfarazi M (1997) Identification of three different truncating mutations in cytochrome P4501B1 (CYP1B1) as the principal cause of primary congenital glaucoma (Buphthalmos) in families linked to the GLC3A locus on chromosome 2p21. Hum Mol Genet 6: 641–647.
35. Firasat S, Riazuddin SA, Hejtmancik JF, Riazuddin S (2008) Primary congenital glaucoma localizes to chromosome 14q24.2–24.3 in two consanguineous Pakistani families. Mol Vis 14: 1659–1665.
36. Ali M, McKibbin M, Booth A, Parry DA, Jain P, et al. (2009) Null mutations in LTBP2 cause primary congenital glaucoma. Am J Hum Genet 84: 664–671.
37. Nishimura DY, Swiderski RE, Alward WL, Searby CC, Patil SR, et al. (1998) The forkhead transcription factor gene FKHL7 is responsible for glaucoma phenotypes which map to 6p25. Nat Genet 19: 140–147.
38. Semina EV, Reiter R, Leysens NJ, Alward WL, Small KW, et al. (1996) Cloning and characterization of a novel bicoid-related homeobox transcription factor gene, RIEG, involved in Rieger syndrome. Nat Genet 14: 392–399.
39. Thorleifsson G, Walters GB, Hewitt AW, Masson G, Helgason A, et al. (2010) Common variants near CAV1 and CAV2 are associated with primary open-angle glaucoma. Nat Genet 42: 906–909.
40. Burdon KP, Macgregor S, Hewitt AW, Sharma S, Chidlow G, et al. (2011) Genome-wide association study identifies susceptibility loci for open angle glaucoma at TMCO1 and CDKN2B-AS1. Nat Genet 43: 574–578.
41. Ramdas WD, van Koolwijk LM, Lemij HG, Pasutto F, Cree AJ, et al. (2011) Common genetic variants associated with open-angle glaucoma. Hum Mol Genet 20: 2464–2471.
42. Fan BJ, Wang DY, Pasquale LR, Haines JL, Wiggs JL (2011) Genetic variants associated with optic nerve vertical cup-to-disc ratio are risk factors for primary open angle glaucoma in a US Caucasian population. Invest Ophthalmol Vis Sci 52: 1788–1792.
43. Wiggs JL, Yaspan BL, Hauser MA, Kang JH, Allingham RR, et al. (2012) Common variants at 9p21 and 8q22 are associated with increased susceptibility to optic nerve degeneration in glaucoma. PLoS Genet 8: e1002654.
44. Shibuya E, Meguro A, Ota M, Kashiwagi K, Mabuchi F, et al. (2008) Association of Toll-like receptor 4 gene polymorphisms with normal tension glaucoma. Invest Ophthalmol Vis Sci 49: 4453–4457.
45. Meguro A, Inoko H, Ota M, Mizuki N, Bahram S (2010) Genome-wide association study of normal tension glaucoma: common variants in SRBD1 and ELOVL5 contribute to disease susceptibility. Ophthalmology 117: 1331–1338 e1335.
46. Stone EM, Braun TA, Russell SR, Kuehn MH, Lotery AJ, et al. (2004) Missense variations in the fibulin 5 gene and age-related macular degeneration. N Engl J Med 351: 346–353.
47. Klein RJ, Zeiss C, Chew EY, Tsai JY, Sackler RS, et al. (2005) Complement factor H polymorphism in age-related macular degeneration. Science 308: 385–389.
48. Haines JL, Hauser MA, Schmidt S, Scott WK, Olson LM, et al. (2005) Complement factor H variant increases the risk of age-related macular degeneration. Science 308: 419–421.
49. Edwards AO, Ritter R, 3rd, Abel KJ, Manning A, Panhuysen C, et al. (2005) Complement factor H polymorphism and age-related macular degeneration. Science 308: 421–424.
50. Hageman GS, Anderson DH, Johnson LV, Hancox LS, Taiber AJ, et al. (2005) A common haplotype in the complement regulatory gene factor H (HF1/CFH) predisposes individuals to age-related macular degeneration. Proc Natl Acad Sci U S A 102: 7227–7232.
51. Rivera A, Fisher SA, Fritsche LG, Keilhauer CN, Lichtner P, et al. (2005) Hypothetical LOC387715 is a second major susceptibility gene for age-related macular degeneration, contributing independently of complement factor H to disease risk. Hum Mol Genet 14: 3227–3236.
52. Dewan A, Liu M, Hartman S, Zhang SS, Liu DT, et al. (2006) HTRA1 promoter polymorphism in wet age-related macular degeneration. Science 314: 989–992.
53. Gold B, Merriam JE, Zernant J, Hancox LS, Taiber AJ, et al. (2006) Variation in factor B (BF) and complement component 2 (C2) genes is associated with age-related macular degeneration. Nat Genet 38: 458–462.
54. Yates JR, Sepp T, Matharu BK, Khan JC, Thurlby DA, et al. (2007) Complement C3 variant and the risk of age-related macular degeneration. N Engl J Med 357: 553–561.
55. Baas DC, Ho L, Ennis S, Merriam JE, Tanck MW, et al. (2010) The complement component 5 gene and age-related macular degeneration. Ophthalmology 117: 500–511.
56. Gibson J, Cree A, Collins A, Lotery A, Ennis S (2010) Determination of a gene and environment risk model for age-related macular degeneration. Br J Ophthalmol 94: 1382–1387.
57. Ennis S, Jomary C, Mullins R, Cree A, Chen X, et al. (2008) Association between the SERPING1 gene and age-related macular degeneration: a two-stage case-control study. Lancet 372: 1828–1834.
58. Hughes AE, Orr N, Esfandiary H, Diaz-Torres M, Goodship T, et al. (2006) A common CFH haplotype, with deletion of CFHR1 and CFHR3, is associated with lower risk of age-related macular degeneration. Nat Genet 38: 1173–1177.
59. Zhang H, Morrison MA, Dewan A, Adams S, Andreoli M, et al. (2008) The NEI/NCBI dbGAP database: genotypes and haplotypes that may specifically predispose to risk of neovascular age-related macular degeneration. BMC Med Genet 9: 51.
60. Fagerness JA, Maller JB, Neale BM, Reynolds RC, Daly MJ, et al. (2009) Variation near complement factor I is associated with risk of advanced AMD. Eur J Hum Genet 17: 100–104.
61. The International HapMap Consortium. (2003) The International HapMap Project. Nature 426: 789–796.
62. NHLBI GO Exome Sequencing Project. (2012) Exome Variant Server, Seattle, WA (URL: http://evs.gs.washington.edu/EVS/).
63. Grimberg J, Nawoschik S, Belluscio L, Mckee R, Turck A, et al. (1989) A Simple and Efficient Non-Organic Procedure for the Isolation of Genomic DNA from Blood. Nucleic Acids Res 17: 8390–8390.
64. Gordon MO, Kass MA (1999) The Ocular Hypertension Treatment Study: design and baseline description of the participants. Arch Ophthalmol 117: 573–583.
65. Collaborative Normal-Tension Glaucoma Study Group. (1998) Comparison of glaucomatous progression between untreated patients with normal-tension glaucoma and patients with therapeutically reduced intraocular pressures. Collaborative Normal-Tension Glaucoma Study Group. Am J Ophthalmol 126: 487–497.
66. Age-related Eye Disease Study Research Group. (2000) Risk factors associated with age-related macular degeneration. A case-control study in the age-related eye disease study: Age-Related Eye Disease Study Report Number 3. Ophthalmology 107: 2224–2232.
67. Age-related Eye Disease Study Research Group. (2001) A randomized, placebo-controlled, clinical trial of high-dose supplementation with vitamins C and E, beta carotene, and zinc for age-related macular degeneration and vision loss: AREDS report no. 8. Arch Ophthalmol 119: 1417–1436.
68. Rabbee N, Speed TP (2006) A genotype calling algorithm for affymetrix SNP arrays. Bioinformatics 22: 7–12.
69. Affymetrix (2007) BRLMM-P: a Genotype Calling Method for the SNP 5.0 Array.
70. Affymetrix (2009) Affymetrix Power Tools.
71. Wang K (2009) Testing for genetic association in the presence of population stratification in genome-wide association studies. Genet Epidemiol 33: 637–645.

72. Wellcome Trust Case Control Consortium. (2007) Genome-wide association study of 14,000 cases of seven common diseases and 3,000 shared controls. Nature 447: 661–678.
73. Stokowski RP, Pant PV, Dadd T, Fereday A, Hinds DA, et al. (2007) A genomewide association study of skin pigmentation in a South Asian population. American Journal of Human Genetics 81: 1119–1132.
74. Zareparsi S, Branham KE, Li M, Shah S, Klein RJ, et al. (2005) Strong association of the Y402H variant in complement factor H at 1q32 with susceptibility to age-related macular degeneration. American Journal of Human Genetics 77: 149–153.
75. Jakobsdottir J, Conley YP, Weeks DE, Mah TS, Ferrell RE, et al. (2005) Susceptibility genes for age-related maculopathy on chromosome 10q26. American Journal of Human Genetics 77: 389–407.
76. Kanda A, Chen W, Othman M, Branham KE, Brooks M, et al. (2007) A variant of mitochondrial protein LOC387715/ARMS2, not HTRA1, is strongly associated with age-related macular degeneration. Proc Natl Acad Sci U S A 104: 16227–16232.
77. Nakano M, Ikeda Y, Taniguchi T, Yagi T, Fuwa M, et al. (2009) Three susceptible loci associated with primary open-angle glaucoma identified by genome-wide association study in a Japanese population. Proc Natl Acad Sci U S A 106: 12838–12842.
78. Wiggs JL, Kang JH, Yaspan BL, Mirel DB, Laurie C, et al. (2011) Common variants near CAV1 and CAV2 are associated with primary open-angle glaucoma in Caucasians from the USA. Hum Mol Genet 20: 4707–4713.
79. Mabuchi F, Sakurada Y, Kashiwagi K, Yamagata Z, Iijima H, et al. (2011) Association between SRBD1 and ELOVL5 gene polymorphisms and primary open-angle glaucoma. Invest Ophthalmol Vis Sci 52: 4626–4629.
80. Ulmer M, Li J, Yaspan BL, Ozel AB, Richards JE, et al. (2012) Genome-wide Analysis of Central Corneal Thickness in Primary Open-angle Glaucoma Cases in the NEIGHBOR and GLAUGEN consortia. Invest Ophthalmol Vis Sci.
81. Ashburner M, Ball CA, Blake JA, Botstein D, Butler H, et al. (2000) Gene ontology: tool for the unification of biology. The Gene Ontology Consortium. Nat Genet 25: 25–29.
82. Shepard AR, Jacobson N, Millar JC, Pang IH, Steely HT, et al. (2007) Glaucoma-causing myocilin mutants require the Peroxisomal targeting signal-1 receptor (PTS1R) to elevate intraocular pressure. Hum Mol Genet 16: 609–617.
83. Yang Z, Camp NJ, Sun H, Tong Z, Gibbs D, et al. (2006) A variant of the HTRA1 gene increases susceptibility to age-related macular degeneration. Science 314: 992–993.
84. Daiger SP, Rossiter BG, J, Christoffels, A; Hide, W. (1998) Data services and software for identifying genes and mutations causing retinal degeneration. IOVS 39: S295.
85. Thorleifsson G, Magnusson KP, Sulem P, Walters GB, Gudbjartsson DF, et al. (2007) Common sequence variants in the LOXL1 gene confer susceptibility to exfoliation glaucoma. Science 317: 1397–1400.
86. Kuehn MH, Kim CY, Ostojic J, Bellin M, Alward WL, et al. (2006) Retinal synthesis and deposition of complement components induced by ocular hypertension. Exp Eye Res 83: 620–628.
87. Stasi K, Nagel D, Yang X, Wang RF, Ren L, et al. (2006) Complement component 1Q (C1Q) upregulation in retina of murine, primate, and human glaucomatous eyes. Invest Ophthalmol Vis Sci 47: 1024–1029.
88. Stevens B, Allen NJ, Vazquez LE, Howell GR, Christopherson KS, et al. (2007) The classical complement cascade mediates CNS synapse elimination. Cell 131: 1164–1178.
89. Kuehn MH, Kim CY, Jiang B, Dumitrescu AV, Kwon YH (2008) Disruption of the complement cascade delays retinal ganglion cell death following retinal ischemia-reperfusion. Exp Eye Res 87: 89–95.
90. Graber JJ, Dhib-Jalbut S (2009) Protective autoimmunity in the nervous system. Pharmacol Ther 121: 147–159.
91. Morgan BP (1989) Complement membrane attack on nucleated cells: resistance, recovery and non-lethal effects. Biochem J 264: 1–14.

17

Impact of the Common Genetic Associations of Age-Related Macular Degeneration upon Systemic Complement Component C3d Levels

Tina Ristau[1], Constantin Paun[2], Lebriz Ersoy[1], Moritz Hahn[3], Yara Lechanteur[2], Carel Hoyng[2], Eiko K. de Jong[2], Mohamed R. Daha[4], Bernd Kirchhof[1], Anneke I. den Hollander[2], Sascha Fauser[1]*

1 Department of Ophthalmology, University Hospital of Cologne, Cologne, Germany, **2** Department of Ophthalmology, Radboud University Nijmegen Medical Centre, Nijmegen, the Netherlands, **3** Institute of Medical Statistics, Informatics and Epidemiology, University of Cologne, Cologne, Germany, **4** Department of Nephrology, Leiden University Nijmegen Medical Center, Leiden, the Netherlands

Abstract

Age-related macular degeneration (AMD) is a common condition that leads to severe vision loss and dysregulation of the complement system is thought to be associated with the disease. To investigate associations of polymorphisms in AMD susceptibility genes with systemic complement activation, 2655 individuals were genotyped for 32 single nucleotide polymorphisms (SNPs) in or near 23 AMD associated risk genes. Component 3 (C3) and its catabolic fragment C3d were measured in serum and AMD staging was performed using multimodal imaging. The C3d/C3 ratio was calculated and associations with environmental factors, SNPs and various haplotypes of *complement factor H* (*CFH*) genes and *complement factor B (CFB)* genes were analyzed. Linear models were built to measure the influence of genetic variants on the C3d/C3 ratio. The study cohort included 1387 patients with AMD and 1268 controls. Higher C3d/C3 ratios were found for current smoker ($p = 0.002$), higher age ($p = 1.56 \times 10^{-7}$), AMD phenotype ($p = 1.15 \times 10^{-11}$) and the two SNPs in the C3 gene rs6795735 ($p = 0.04$) and rs2230199 ($p = 0.04$). Lower C3d/C3 ratios were found for diabetes ($p = 2.87 \times 10^{-6}$), higher body mass index ($p = 1.00 \times 10^{-13}$), the SNPs rs1410996 ($p = 0.0001$), rs800292 ($p = 0.003$), rs12144939 ($p = 4.60 \times 10^{-6}$) in *CFH*, rs4151667 ($p = 1.01 \times 10^{-5}$) in *CFB* and individual haplotypes in *CFH* and *CFB*. The linear model revealed a corrected R-square of 0.063 including age, smoking status, gender, and genetic polymorphisms explaining 6.3% of the C3d/C3 ratio. After adding the AMD status the corrected R-square was 0.067. In conclusion, none of the evaluated genetic polymorphisms showed an association with increased systemic complement activation apart from two SNPs in the C3 gene. Major genetic and non-genetic factors for AMD were not associated with systemic complement activation.

Editor: Keisuke Mori, Saitama Medical University, Japan

Funding: This work was supported by the Retinovit Foundation, Germany. The funders had no role in study design, data collection and analysis, decision to publish, or preparation of the manuscript.

Competing Interests: The authors have declared that no competing interests exist.

* E-mail: sascha.fauser@uk-koeln.de

Introduction

Age-related macular degeneration (AMD) is a neurodegenerative disease causing visual impairment and blindness in the elderly population. Accumulation of drusen between Bruchs membrane and the retinal pigment epithelium characterizes the early forms while the two advanced forms show geographic atrophy and choroidal neovascularization. Risk is multifactorial including environmental and genetic factors. Genetic variation accounts for up to 71% of the disease risk [1]. Many genetic polymorphisms were found in the alternative pathway of the complement system including *complement factor H (CFH)*, *complement component 3 (C3)*, *Complement factor I (CFI)*, and *complement factor B (C2/CFB* locus) [2–8]. Complement proteins and their activation products have been identified in retinal deposits of AMD patients [3,9–11].

The alternative complement pathway is constantly activated by the spontaneous hydrolysis of a thioester bond in C3 and a tight regulation including CFH is necessary to prevent excessive activation. It is hypothesized that a dysregulation of the complement system leads to tissue damage and finally AMD.

The dysregulation of the complement system or their activation fragments were also found systemically. In AMD patients, various components of the complement system were found at increased levels such as CFB, CFD, C3a, C5a, C3d, and Ba [12,13].

While the association of genetic polymorphisms with AMD is well established, only polymorphisms in the C3 gene and few haplotypes in the CFH and CFB/C2 gene were found to be associated with complement activation products including factor C3d in two small cohorts [12,13]. The impact of other AMD susceptibility genes on the regulation of systemic complement activation remains unclear. In our study, we analyzed the association of 32 single nucleotide polymorphisms (SNPs) in or near 23 AMD risk genes with the C3d/C3 ratio as a marker for chronic complement activation in a Caucasian cohort of 2655 participants.

Table 1. Median C3d/C3 ratios for non-genetic factors.

Non-genetic factor	N (%)	Median C3d/C3 ratio (IQR)	T-test/univariate ANOVA
Female sex	1547 (58.3)	0.00424 (0.00325–0.00561)	0.90
Male sex	1108 (41.7)	0.00433 (0.00328–0.00567)	
Age 50–59 years	61 (2.3)	0.00430 (0.00337–0.00598)	1.56×10^{-7}
Age 60–69 years	879 (33.1)	0.00408 (0.00312–0.00550)	
Age 70–79 years	1140 (42.9)	0.00426 (0.00324–0.00547)	
Age 80–89 years	474 (17.9)	0.00462 (0.00356–0.00591)	
Age 90–99 years	97 (3.7)	0.00488 (0.00374–0.00705)	
No AMD	1268 (47.8)	0.00403 (0.00309–0.00536)	1.15×10^{-11}
AMD	1387 (52.2)	0.00449 (0.00348–0.00586)	
No arterial hypertension	1600 (63.6)	0.00428 (0.00328–0.00563)	0.24
Arterial hypertension	917 (36.4)	0.00425 (0.00321–0.00556)	
No diabetes	2268 (90.8)	0.00430 (0.00330–0.00567)	2.87×10^{-6}
Diabetes	231 (9.2)	0.00390 (0.00295–0.00495)	
No rheumatoid arthritis	2353 (93.5)	0.00426 (0.00327–0.00559)	0.35
Rheumatoid arthritis	164 (6.5)	0.00433 (0.00304–0.00564)	
No thyroid disease	2119 (84.2)	0.00426 (0.00326–0.00559)	0.77
Thyroid disease	398 (15.8)	0.00429 (0.00325–0.00559)	
No kidney disease	2403 (95.5)	0.00426 (0.00326–0.00559)	0.92
Kidney disease	114 (4.5)	0.00447 (0.00320–0.00572)	
No allergy	1984 (78.8)	0.00428 (0.00325–0.00562)	0.75
Allergy	533 (21.2)	0.00425 (0.00328–0.00552)	
Never smoker	1029 (43.0)	0.00431 (0.00325–0.00572)	0.002
Past smoker	1164 (48.6)	0.00415 (0.00320–0.00545)	
Current smoker	201 (8.4)	0.00451 (0.00355–0.00584)	
BMI <25	930 (40.1)	0.00464 (0.00360–0.00611)	1.00×10^{-13}
BMI 25–29	1084 (46.7)	0.00408 (0.00312–0.00531)	
BMI ≥30	308 (13.3)	0.00376 (0.00287–0.00493)	

IQR = interquartile range (1st quartile – 3rd quartile).

Methods

Study population

2655 participants from the European Genetic Database (EUGENDA, www.eugenda.org) were included in the study. The study was performed in accordance with the tenets of the Declaration of Helsinki and the Medical Research Involving Human Subjects Act (WMO) and was approved by the local ethics committee of the University Hospitals in Cologne and Nijmegen. Written informed consent was obtained from all participants.

AMD staging was performed by grading of retinal images including stereo fundus photographs (FPs), fluorescein angiograms (FAs) and spectral domain optical coherence tomograms (SDOCTs) according to the standard protocol of the Cologne Image Reading Center (CIRCL) by certified graders (TR, LE). AMD was classified by the presence of pigmentary changes together with at least 10 small drusen (<63 μm) or the presence of intermediate (63–124 μm) or large drusen (≥125 μm diameter) in the Early Treatment Diabetic Maculopathy Study (ETDRS) grid or geographic atrophy and/or choroidal neovascularisation (CNV) secondary to AMD in at least one eye.

Demographic data and non-genetic parameters including history of smoking (current/past/never), regular alcohol intake (yes/no), body mass index (BMI), arterial hypertension (yes/no), diabetes (yes/no), rheumatoid arthritis (yes/no), thyroid disease (yes/no), kidney disease (yes/no) and history of allergy (yes/no) were obtained by standardized interviewer-assisted questionnaires.

Complement component measurements and genetic analysis

Serum samples were used for C3d and C3 measurements. Serum was prepared by coagulation at room temperature. After centrifugation, the samples were stored at −80°C within 1 hour after collection. Complement component C3 and the activation fragment C3d were measured in serum samples as described previously [14]. The C3d/C3 ratio was calculated as a measure of C3 activation.

Genomic DNA was extracted from peripheral blood samples using standard procedures. Thirty-two SNPs in or near 23 AMD associated risk genes were chosen representing the majority of loci associated with AMD. Genotyping of SNPs in the *ARMS2* (rs10490924), *CFH* (rs1061170, rs800292, rs12144939, rs1410996), *CFI* (rs10033900, rs141853578), *C2* (rs9332739), *C3* (rs2230199, rs433594, rs6795735), *CFB* (rs4151667, rs641153), *CFD* (rs3826945), *LPL* (rs12678919), *LIPC* (rs10468017), *TIMP3* (rs9621532), *APOE2* (rs7412), *APOE4* (rs429358), *FADS1* (rs174547), *CETP* (rs2230199), *TLR* (rs4986790, rs3775291),

Table 2. Median C3d/C3 ratios for single nucleotid polymorphisms (SNPs).

SNP	Homozygous non-variant (n)	Heterozygous variant (n)	Homozygous variant (n)	Median C3d/C3 ratio homozygous non-variant (IQR)	Median C3d/C3 ratio heterozygous variant (IQR)	Median C3d/C3 ratio homozygous variant (IQR)	Univariate ANOVA
ARMS2	GG = 1039	GT = 825	TT = 241	0.00425	0.00416	0.00446	0.31
rs10490924				(0.00338–0.00589)	(0.00320–0.00556)	(0.00336–0.00593)	
CFH	TT = 690	TC = 967	CC = 436	0.00425	0.00418	0.00433	0.66
rs1061170				(0.00320–0.00560)	(0.00323–0.00546)	(0.00335–0.00561)	
CFH	CC = 459	CT = 453	TT = 113	0.00436	0.00404	0.00355	0.0001
rs1410996				(0.00334–0.00570)	(0.00310–0.00529)	(0.00209–0.00491)	
CFH	GG = 1177	GA = 608	AA = 95	0.00427	0.00406	0.00394	0.003
rs800292				(0.00329–0.00567)	(0.00312–0.00535)	(0.00319–0.00516)	
CFH	GG = 1290	GT = 537	TT = 64	0.00435	0.00390	0.00373	4.60×10^{-6}
rs12144939				(0.00329–0.00570)	(0.00305–0.00510)	(0.00287–0.00469)	
CFI	TT = 499	TC = 1056	CC = 547	0.00426	0.00420	0.00424	0.80
rs10033900				(0.00324–0.00570)	(0.003.24–0.00553)	(0.00325–0.00547)	
CFI	GG = 1862	GA = 10	AA = 0	0.00419	0.00485	N/A	0.18
rs141853578				(0.00321–0.00553)	(0.00415–0.00673)		
C2	CC = 927	CG = 70	GG = 0	0.00422	0.00362	N/A	0.05
rs9332739				(0.00320–0.00544)	(0.00299–0.00492)		
C3	CC = 1300	GC = 713	GG = 115	0.00415	0.00432	0.00432	0.04
rs2230199				(0.00319–0.00549)	(0.00334–0.00561)	(0.00327–0.00627)	
C3	CC = 723	CT = 900	TT = 261	0.00420	0.00420	0.00421	0.81
rs433594				(0.00320–0.00557)	(0.00323–0.00555)	(0.00328–0.00548)	
C3	GG = 1197	GA = 617	AA = 84	0.00413	0.00424	0.00448	0.04
rs6795735				(0.00317–0.00549)	(0.00334–0.00550)	(0.00333–0.00640)	
CFB	TT = 1958	TA = 160	AA = 2*	0.00428	0.00358	0.00497	1.01×10^{-5}
rs4151667				(0.00327–0.00562)	(0.00297–0.00472)	(N/A)	
CFB	GG = 1616	GA = 265	AA = 7*	0.00421	0.00414	0.00311	0.69
rs641153				(0.00324–0.00556)	(0.00314–0.00559)	(0.00223–0.00335)	
CFD	TT = 488	TC = 407	CC = 93	0.00404	0.00421	0.00413	0.95
rs3826945				(0.00320–0.00542)	(0.00319–0.00531)	(0.00308–0.00525)	
LPL	AA = 1705	AG = 388	GG = 31	0.00423	0.00423	0.00479	0.89
rs12678919				(0.00321–0.00561)	(0.00338–0.00542)	(0.00342–0.00593)	
LIPC	CC = 1057	CT = 888	TT = 144	0.00421	0.00423	0.00441	0.46
rs10468017				(0.00322–0.00546)	(0.00322–0.00562)	(0.00337–0.00558)	
TIMP3	AA = 882	AC = 77	CC = 7*	0.00411	0.00425	0.00392	0.70
rs9621532				(0.00318–0.00531)	(0.00332–0.00543)	(0.00376–0.00584)	

Table 2. Cont.

SNP	Homozygous non-variant (n)	Heterozygous variant (n)	Homozygous variant (n)	Median C3d/C3 ratio homozygous non-variant (IQR)	Median C3d/C3 ratio heterozygous variant (IQR)	Median C3d/C3 ratio homozygous variant (IQR)	Univariate ANOVA
APOE2	CC = 804	CT = 160	TT = 12	0.00420	0.00393	0.00417	0.53
rs7412				(0.00322–0.00543)	(0.00306–0.00524)	(0.00301–0.00485)	
APOE4	TT = 689	TC = 195	CC = 9*	0.00420	0.00396	0.00272	0.49
rs429358				(0.00320–0.00537)	(0.00311–0.00530)	(0.00253–0.00609)	
FADS1	TT = 995	TC = 924	CC = 209	0.00432	0.00416	0.00394	0.05
rs174547				(0.00330–0.00567)	(0.00319–0.00557)	(0.00334–0.00508)	
CETP	GG = 997	GT = 906	TT = 246	0.00420	0.00424	0.00428	0.91
rs2230199				(0.00328–0.00559)	(0.00320–0.00546)	(0.00324–0.00568)	
TLR	AA = 872	AG = 119	GG = 5	0.00419	0.00408	0.00283	0.24
rs4986790				(0.00319–0.00539)	(0.00333–0.00530)	(0.00248–0.00441)	
TLR3	CC = 497	CT = 380	TT = 86	0.00401	0.00420	0.00430	0.31
rs3775291				(0.00306–0.00561)	(0.00333–0.00513)	(0.00320–0.00594)	
SERPING	GG = 322	GA = 485	AA = 183	0.00410	0.00410	0.00428	0.56
rs2511989				(0.00317–0.00529)	(0.00322–0.00542)	(0.00316–0.00546)	
ABCA4	GG = 985	GA = 15	AA = 0	0.00418	0.00368	N/A	0.17
rs1800555				(0.00319–0.00538)	(0.00337–0.00440)		
ABCA4	GG = 975	GA = 4	AA = 0	0.00415	0.004.47	N/A	0.87
rs1800553				(0.00320–0.00538)	(0.00289–0.00659)		
ABCA4	GG = 1854	CG = 31	CC = 0	0.00419	0.00443	N/A	0.81
rs76157638				(0.00321–0.00556)	(0.00332–0.00521)		
VEGFA	AA = 629	AG = 322	GG = 42	0.00425	0.00400	0.00376	0.14
rs699946				(0.00327–0.00543)	(0.00303–0.00540)	(0.00324–0.00467)	
SPRYD7	TT = 714	TC = 220	CC = 21	0.00418	0.00433	0.00390	0.30
rs7995557				(0.00322–0.00537)	(0.00317–0.00558)	(0.00255–0.00503)	
COL8A1	GG = 1545	GT = 333	TT = 13	0.00421	0.00420	0.00502	0.73
rs13081855				(0.00322–0.00558)	(0.00321–0.00543)	(0.00342–0.00566)	
COL10A1	AA = 742	AT = 899	TT = 241	0.00424	0.00411	0.00440	0.87
rs3812111				(0.00319–0.00555)	(0.00323–0.00548)	(0.00330–0.00575)	
SLC16A8	CC = 1155	CT = 632	TT = 86	0.00421	0.00420	0.00423	0.83
rs8135665				(0.00324–0.00556)	(0.00319–0.00556)	(0.00312–0.00563)	
ADAMTS9	CC = 647	CT = 898	TT = 343	0.00425	0.00419	0.00412	0.57
rs6795735				(0.00320–0.00572)	(0.00325–0.00540)	(0.00313–0.00561)	

*Due to small number of cases excluded from univariate ANOVA analysis; IQR = interquartile range (1st quartile – 3rd quartile).

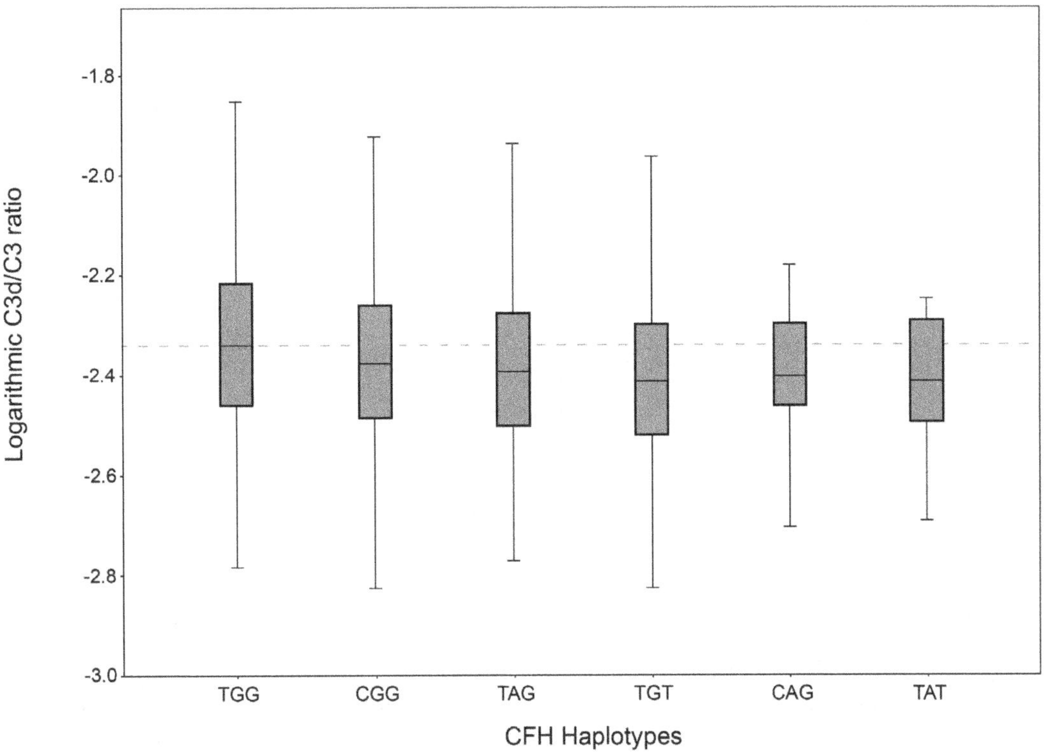

Figure 1. Logarithmic C3d/C3 ratios for haplotypes in the *CFH* gene rs1061170, rs800292 and rs12144939.

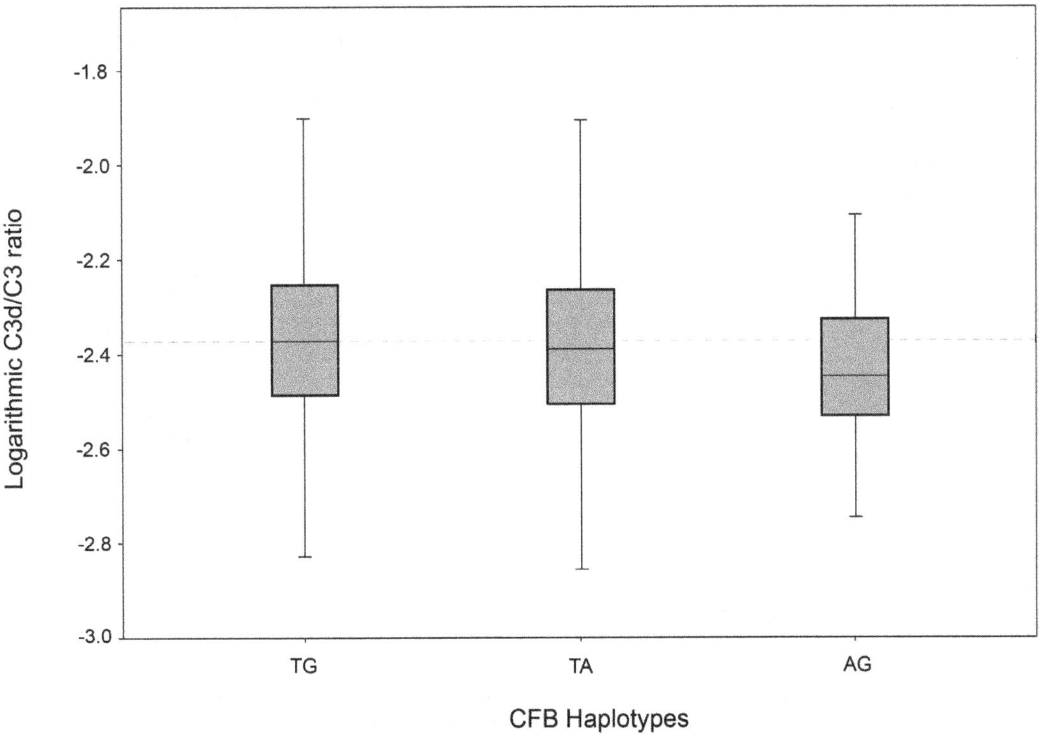

Figure 2. Logarithmic C3d/C3 ratios for haplotypes in the *CFB* gene rs4151667 and rs641153.

Table 3. Haplotypes for *CFH/CFB* and median C3d/C3 ratios.

Haplotype CFH	n	Haplotype frequency	MedianC3d/C3 ratio (IQR)	T-test
TGG	728	0.20	0.00456 (0.00345–0.00608)	-*
CGG	1544	0.42	0.00420 (0.00324–0.00550)	1.40×10^{-8}
TAG	755	0.20	0.00405 (0.00314–0.00530)	3.61×10^{-12}
TGT	620	0.17	0.00386 (0.00300–0.00504)	1.03×10^{-13}
CAG	21	0.008	0.00396 (0.00339–0.00507)	-**
TAT	18	0.005	0.00386 (0.00317–0.00513)	-**
Haplotype CFB	n	Haplotype frequency	MedianC3d/C3 ratio (IQR)	T-test
TG	3337	0.89	0.00424 (0.00325–0.00559)	-*
TA	279	0.07	0.00408 (0.00310–0.00546)	0.15
AG	152	0.04	0.00356 (0.00292–0.00471)	9.96×10^{-6}

For CFH single nucleotides polymorphisms rs1061170, rs800292, and rs12144939 and for CFB rs4151667 and rs641153 were chosen.
*T- test with comparison to reference haplotypes TGG and TG; **Due to small number of cases excluded from analysis; IQR = interquartile range (1st quartile – 3rd quartile).

SERPING (rs2511989), *ABCA4* (rs1800555, rs1800553, rs76157638), *VEGFA* (rs699946), *SPRYD7* (rs7995557), *COL8A1* (rs13081855), *COL10A1* (rs3812111), *SLC16A8* (rs8135665), *ADAMTS9-AS2* (rs6795735) genes were carried out as previously described [15].

Haplotype analysis

In order to analyze the influence of haplotypes on C3d/C3 ratios, the posterior probability of each haplotype in the CFH gene including rs1061170, rs800292 and rs12144939 and in the CFB gene including rs4151667 and rs641153 was calculated using PHASE software, version 2.1 [16,17].

Statistical analysis

All calculations were performed using SPSS software version 21.0 (IBM Software and Systems, Armonk, NY, USA). C3d/C3 ratios are given as median and interquartile range (1st quartile – 3rd quartile). Due to the skewed nature of the data, the logarithm ($\log_{10}$) of the C3d/C3 ratios was used for analysis. Associations between logarithmic C3d/C3 ratios and genetic polymorphisms, haplotypes, phenotype and environmental factors were analyzed using t-tests or univariate analysis of variance (ANOVA) depending on number of variables. Associations between AMD phenotype and genetic polymorphisms were evaluated using logistic regression analysis. Linear models were performed to illustrate the influence of the genetic factors on complement activation. P-Values <0.05 were considered statistically significant.

Results

Demographics and non-genetic factors

Mean age of the study population was 73.2±8.0 years (75.8±8.1 years for AMD patients and 70.4±6.8 years for controls, p<0.001). Demographic data, phenotype and environmental factors are summarized in Table 1. C3d/C3 ratios showed significant differences for age with increasing levels (except the youngest group from 50–59 years) and phenotype with higher values for AMD patients. A significant association was also found for diabetes, smoking, and BMI.

Associations of C3d/C3 levels with genetic polymorphisms

Significant associations of C3d/C3 levels were found in the *CFH* gene for the SNPs rs1410996, rs800292 and rs12144939, in the *CFB* gene for rs4151667 and in the *C3* gene for rs6795735 and rs2230199. In all SNPs of the *CFH* and *CFB* gene, these variants showed lower C3d/C3 ratios than the reference alleles, only variants in *C3* revealed higher values. After stratification in AMD cases and controls, associations for the major risk variants in rs1061170 (*CFHY402H*, p = 0.35 for no AMD; p = 0.55 for AMD) and rs10490924 (*ARMS2*, p = 0.75 for No AMD, p = 0.25 for AMD) with the C3d/C3 ratio could not be observed. A detailed analysis is outlined in Table 2.

For the SNPs rs1061170, rs800292 and rs12144939 in the *CFH* gene and the SNPs rs4151667 and rs641153 in the *CFB* gene, haplotypes were associated with C3d/C3 levels (Table 3). All haplotypes were associated with lower C3d/C3 levels than the reference haplotype (Figure 1 and 2).

Associations of genetic polymorphisms with AMD

Performing logistic regression analysis, protective effects were found for variants in *CFH* rs1410996, *CFH* rs800292, *CFH* rs12144939, *CFB* rs641153 and *FADS1* rs174547. Variants in *CFB rs4151667, TIMP3 rs9621532 and APOE4 rs429358* showed a trend for a protective effect on AMD without reaching statistical significance, which may be due to low minor allele frequencies or smaller effects of those SNPs.

Variants in *ARMS2* rs10490924, *CFH* rs1061170, *C3* rs2230199, *C3* rs6795735 and *CETP* rs2230199 were found to be associated with significantly higher risk for AMD (Table 4). Variants in *VEGFA rs699946, SLC16A8 rs8135665 and ADAMTS9-AS2 rs6795735* also showed a trend for a higher AMD risk without statistical significance, which also may be due to a smaller effect on AMD development for each of those SNPs compared to *ARMS2 rs10490924* or *CFH rs1061170.*

Linear Models

Linear models were composed based on univariate analysis of covariance (ANCOVA) with the logarithmic C3d/C3 ratio as dependent variable to evaluate the influence of various factors on the C3d/C3 ratio. In the first model, we included all SNPs (rs1410996, rs800292, rs12144939 in *CFH*, rs4151667 in *CFB*,

Table 4. Logistic regression analysis between AMD and single nucleotide polymorphisms SNPs+.

SNP	Heterozygous variant			Homozygous variant		
	OR	95% CI	P-value	OR	95% CI	P-value
ARMS2 rs10490924	2.32	1.90–2.84	1.00×10^{-13}	8.13	5.66–11.69	1.00×10^{-13}
CFH rs1061170	1.57	1.27–1.95	3.16×10^{-5}	3.70	2.82–4.85	1.00×10^{-13}
CFH rs1410996	0.36	0.27–0.48	5.05×10^{-12}	0.23	0.15–0.36	1.28×10^{-13}
CFH rs800292	0.61	0.49–0.75	5.38×10^{-6}	0.70	0.44–1.10	0.12
CFH rs12144939	0.57	0.47–0.71	6.71×10^{-7}	0.51	0.28–0.91	0.02
CFI rs10033900	1.07	0.85–1.35	0.59	0.99	0.76–1.28	0.93
CFI rs141853578	1.17	0.96–1.43	0.12	-*	-*	-*
C2 rs9332739	0.70	0.42–1.17	0.17	-*	-*	-*
C3 rs2230199	1.17	0.96–1.42	0.11	2.17	1.42–3.31	0.0004
C3 rs433594	0.98	0.80–1.21	0.88	0.91	0.67–1.23	0.52
C3 rs6795735	1.10	0.89–1.36	0.37	2.06	1.27–3.33	0.03
CFB rs4151667	0.74	0.52–1.05	0.08	-*	-*	-*
CFB rs641153	0.72	0.54–0.96	0.02	-*	-*	-*
CFD rs3826945	1.01	0.76–1.34	0.94	0.76	0.48–1.22	0.26
LPL rs12678919	1.02	0.80–1.29	0.89	1.11	0.51–2.43	0.79
LIPC rs10468017	0.94	0.78–1.14	0.53	0.63	0.43–0.93	0.19
TIMP3 rs9621532	0.86	0.52–1.42	0.56	-*	-*	-*
APOE2 rs7412	1.21	0.84–1.76	0.31	-*	-*	-*
APOE4 rs429358	0.84	0.60–1.17	0.30	-*	-*	-*
FADS1 rs174547	0.88	0.72–1.06	0.18	0.64	0.46–0.88	0.006
CETP rs2230199	1.39	1.15–1.70	0.001	1.38	1.02–1.87	0.04
TLR rs4986790	1.08	0.71–1.64	0.71	0.53	0.08–3.36	0.50
TLR3 rs3775291	1.00	0.75–1.34	0.99	0.78	0.48–1.27	0.32
SERPING rs2511989	1.10	0.81–1.50	0.53	0.79	0.54–1.16	0.22
ABCA4D2177 rs1800555	0.96	0.33–2.82	0.94	-*	-*	-*
ABCA4G1961 rs1800553	0.88	0.12–6.58	0.90	-*	-*	-*
ABCA4 rs76157638	2.14	0.98–4.67	0.06	-*	-*	-*
VEGFA rs699946	1.08	0.81–1.44	0.61	1.47	0.75.2.89	0.27
SPRYD7 rs7995557	1.01	0.73–1.40	0.95	0.57	0.23–1.43	0.23
COL8A1 rs13081855	1.03	0.80–1.33	0.82	0.53	0.16–1.74	0.30
COL10A1 rs3812111	1.04	0.84–1.28	0.73	1.02	0.75–1.40	0.89
SLC16A8 rs8135665	1.21	0.98–1.49	0.08	1.39	0.87–2.21	0.17
ADAMTS9-AS2 rs6795735	1.21	0.98–1.51	0.08	1.30	0.98–1.72	0.07

+Adjusted for age and gender; *analysis not performed due to small group size.

rs6795735 and rs2230199 in *C3*) that had reached statistical signifcance in the individual analysis and the two major AMD risk SNPs risk *ARMS2* rs10490924 and *CFH* rs1061170. Additionally, age, gender, and smoking status was included. The corrected R-square was 0.063. Adding the AMD status to the model, the corrected R-square was 0.067.

In the second model, *CFH* haplotypes, age, gender, and smoking status were included. The corrected R-square was 0.038.

Discussion

Dysregulation of the alternative complement pathway is thought to play a key role in AMD pathogenesis, which is also reflected by increased systemic complement levels.

In this study we analyzed the association of genetic AMD risk polymorphisms with systemic complement activation. We identified only a few variants in the *CFH*, *CFB*, and *C3* gene that showed an association with systemic complement activation, while for all other genetic polymorphisms associations were not observed.

While the association with genetic polymorphisms was weak, we found a significant association of the phenotype AMD with an increased C3d/C3 ratio which is in line with other smaller studies.[12,13] Our linear model including the AMD phenotype, the two major non-genetic risk factors age and smoking, and eight relevant SNPs could only explain 6.7% of the variation in the C3d/C3 ratio, indicating that these AMD risk polymorphisms do not explain sufficiently increased systemic complement activation found in AMD patients. The inclusion of *CFH* haplotypes in the model revealed an even lower explanation of the C3d/C3 ratio of only 3.8%.

Our analysis concentrated on C3d as a marker of chronic complement activation because it is a relatively stable protein with a long half-life. To correct for differences in the concentration of the precursor protein, we also measured C3 in the plasma.

CFH, CFB, and C3 influence the regulation of the alternative pathway of the complement system. CFH acts as the major regulator of complement activation controlling the alternative pathway in blood and on cell surfaces [18], and accelerates the decay of the alternative C3 convertase (C3bBb) [19].

CFH is also a cofactor of CFI-mediated cleavage and inactivation of C3b [20]. The formation of C3d, a polypeptide fragment generated during alternative C3 convertase cleaves C3 to C3b, is also CFH dependent [21]. Alterations in the CFH gene may change the regulating characteristics of CFH resulting in an up or down regulation of the CFH dependent elements of the alternative complement pathway. In our cohort, SNPs rs1410996, rs800292, and rs12144939 in the *CFH* gene were associated with lower C3d/C3 ratios and a lower risk for AMD, whereas the most common AMD risk variant rs1061170 was not associated with the C3d/C3 ratio even after stratification in AMD patients and controls. Additionally, *CFH* haplotypes showed lower C3d/C3 ratios in all cases compared to the reference haplotype. Therefore, *CFH* SNPs were not associated with increased systemic complement activation.

CFB is an acute phase protein involved in the alternative complement pathway as a precursor of C3 convertase. CFB is cleaved to Bb which combines with C3b to form the alternative pathway C3 convertase C3bBb. An acute phase response-mediated up-regulation may result in elevated systemic plasma levels of CFB in AMD patients and may contribute to an enhanced systemic complement activity [12,13,22]. In our study we observed lower C3d/C3 ratios for the operatively protective *CFB* variants for AMD indicating that individuals with these polymorphisms show less complement activation.

Among all analyzed SNPs, only variants in the *C3* gene were associated with higher systemic C3d/C3 ratios which aligns with the results by Hecker et al.[11] The alternative pathway of the complement system starts with spontaneous hydrolysis of C3 and variants with a higher risk for AMD seem to influence this part of the complement cascade resulting in elevated systemic complement activation. Scholl et al did not observe a correlation between genetic variants in *C3* and systemic C3d levels[12] underlining that the systemic effects of AMD susceptibility genes on complement activation are only weak.

In our study, slightly higher C3d/C3 levels were found in AMD patients. In order to not miss a combined effect of multiple SNPs, we performed linear models to illustrate the effect of the combination of SNPs on complement activation. These models could not explain the C3d/C3 ratio, showing that there have to be other systemic effects than AMD phenotype or genetic variants influencing systemic complement activation. Hecker et al also showed in a small cohort that risk haplotypes in CFH did not alter complement levels, whereas protective haplotypes reduced complement levels including C3d [12].

A limitation of our study is the analysis of only two components of the complement system, which is accompanied by several strengths including a large cohort of well-balanced AMD patients and controls, a high number of investigated SNPs and the use of multimodal imaging that avoids misclassification of phenotypes.

In summary, we showed that the major AMD risk polymorphisms in *CFH* and *ARMS2* are not associated with increased systemic complement activation as measured by the C3d/C3 ratio. Few SNPs were associated with lower levels of systemic complement activation, particularly the *CFH* and *CFB* polymorphisms that are protective against AMD. Only variants in *C3* were associated with elevated complement levels. Furthermore, a model including major genetic and non-genetic factors for AMD was not able to explain complement activation.

Author Contributions

Conceived and designed the experiments: CH ADH SF. Performed the experiments: TR LE MD ADH SF. Analyzed the data: TR CP LE MH YL BK ADH SF. Contributed reagents/materials/analysis tools: MD CH BK ADH SF. Wrote the paper: TR CP LE CH EDJ MD ADH SF.

References

1. Seddon JM, Cote J, Page WF, Aggen SH, Neale MC (2005) The US twin study of age-related macular degeneration: relative roles of genetic and environmental influences. Archives of ophthalmology 123: 321–327.
2. Edwards AO, Ritter R 3rd, Abel KJ, Manning A, Panhuysen C, et al. (2005) Complement factor H polymorphism and age-related macular degeneration. Science 308: 421–424.
3. Gold B, Merriam JE, Zernant J, Hancox LS, Taiber AJ, et al. (2006) Variation in factor B (BF) and complement component 2 (C2) genes is associated with age-related macular degeneration. Nat Genet 38: 458–462.
4. Haines JL, Hauser MA, Schmidt S, Scott WK, Olson LM, et al. (2005) Complement factor H variant increases the risk of age-related macular degeneration. Science 308: 419–421.
5. Klein RJ, Zeiss C, Chew EY, Tsai JY, Sackler RS, et al. (2005) Complement factor H polymorphism in age-related macular degeneration. Science 308: 385–389.
6. Maller JB, Fagerness JA, Reynolds RC, Neale BM, Daly MJ, et al. (2007) Variation in complement factor 3 is associated with risk of age-related macular degeneration. Nat Genet 39: 1200–1201.
7. Yates JR, Sepp T, Matharu BK, Khan JC, Thurlby DA, et al. (2007) Complement C3 variant and the risk of age-related macular degeneration. N Engl J Med 357: 553–561.
8. van de Ven JP, Nilsson SC, Tan PL, Buitendijk GH, Ristau T, et al. (2013) A functional variant in the CFI gene confers a high risk of age-related macular degeneration. Nat Genet 45: 813–817.
9. Hageman GS, Luthert PJ, Victor Chong NH, Johnson LV, Anderson DH, et al. (2001) An integrated hypothesis that considers drusen as biomarkers of immune-mediated processes at the RPE-Bruch's membrane interface in aging and age-related macular degeneration. Prog Retin Eye Res 20: 705–732.
10. Johnson PT, Betts KE, Radeke MJ, Hageman GS, Anderson DH, et al. (2006) Individuals homozygous for the age-related macular degeneration risk-conferring variant of complement factor H have elevated levels of CRP in the choroid. Proc Natl Acad Sci U S A 103: 17456–17461.
11. Nozaki M, Raisler BJ, Sakurai E, Sarma JV, Barnum SR, et al. (2006) Drusen complement components C3a and C5a promote choroidal neovascularization. Proc Natl Acad Sci U S A 103: 2328–2333.
12. Hecker LA, Edwards AO, Ryu E, Tosakulwong N, Baratz KH, et al. (2010) Genetic control of the alternative pathway of complement in humans and age-related macular degeneration. Hum Mol Genet 19: 209–215.
13. Scholl HP, Charbel Issa P, Walier M, Janzer S, Pollok-Kopp B, et al. (2008) Systemic complement activation in age-related macular degeneration. PLoS One 3: e2593.
14. Smailhodzic D, Klaver CC, Klevering BJ, Boon CJ, Groenewoud JM, et al. (2012) Risk alleles in CFH and ARMS2 are independently associated with systemic complement activation in age-related macular degeneration. Ophthalmology 119: 339–346.
15. Hawkins JR, Khripin Y, Valdes AM, Weaver TA (2002) Miniaturized sealed-tube allele-specific PCR. Hum Mutat 19: 543–553.
16. Stephens M, Smith NJ, Donnelly P (2001) A new statistical method for haplotype reconstruction from population data. Am J Hum Genet 68: 978–989.
17. Stephens M, Donnelly P (2003) A comparison of bayesian methods for haplotype reconstruction from population genotype data. Am J Hum Genet 73: 1162–1169.
18. Zipfel PF, Hallstrom T, Hammerschmidt S, Skerka C (2008) The complement fitness factor H: role in human diseases and for immune escape of pathogens, like pneumococci. Vaccine 26 Suppl 8: I67–74.
19. Khandhadia S, Cipriani V, Yates JR, Lotery AJ (2012) Age-related macular degeneration and the complement system. Immunobiology 217: 127–146.

18

Systematic Review and Meta-Analysis of the Association between Complement Factor H I62V Polymorphism and Risk of Polypoidal Choroidal Vasculopathy in Asian Populations

Zhao-Yang Wang[1,2], Keke Zhao[2], Jingwei Zheng[3], Brian Rossmiller[2], Cristhian Ildefonso[2], Manas Biswal[2], Pei-quan Zhao[1]*

1 Department of Ophthalmology, Xinhua Hospital, Shanghai Jiaotong University School of Medicine, Shanghai, China, 2 Departments of Molecular Genetics, University of Florida, Gainesville, Florida, United States of America, 3 Eye Hospital, Wenzhou Medical University, Wenzhou, Zhejiang, China

Abstract

Purpose: To investigate whether the polymorphism rs800292 (184G>A, I62V) in the complement factor H gene is associated with polypoidal choroidal vasculopathy (PCV) and the genetic difference between PCV and neovascular age-related macular degeneration (nAMD), in Asian populations.

Methods: A comprehensive literature search was performed in PubMed, Medline, Web of Science, and reference lists. A system review and meta-analysis of the association between I62V and PCV and/or nAMD were performed from 8 studies involving 5,062 subjects. The following data from individual studies were extracted and analyzed: 1) comparison of I62V polymorphisms between PCV and controls; 2) comparison of I62V polymorphisms between PCV and nAMD. Summary odds ratios (ORs) and 95% confidence intervals (CIs) were estimated using fixed-effects models. The Q-statistic test was used to assess heterogeneity, and Egger's test was used to evaluate publication bias. Sensitivity analysis and cumulative meta-analysis were also performed.

Results: The I62V polymorphism showed a significant summary OR_1 for genotype GA+GG versus homozygous genotype AA was 3.18 (95% CI, 2.51–4.04, $P<0.00001$), the OR_2 of heterozygous genotype GA versus AA was 2.29 (95% CI: 1.79–2.94, $P<0.00001$), the OR_3 of homozygous genotype GG versus AA was 4.42 (95% CI: 3.45–5.67, $P<0.00001$), and the OR_4 of allele G versus A was 2.04 (95% CI: 1.85–2.26, $P<0.00001$). Sensitivity analysis indicated the robustness of our findings, and evidence of publication bias was not observed in our meta-analysis. Cumulative meta-analysis revealed that the summary ORs were stable. There was no significant difference in every genetic model between PCV and nAMD (n = 5, $OR_1 = 0.92$, $OR_2 = 0.96$, $OR_3 = 0.90$, $OR_4 = 0.94$).

Conclusions: Our analysis provides evidence that the I62V polymorphism is associated with an increased risk of PCV. The variant of I62V could be a promising genetic biomarker of PCV in Asian populations.

Editor: Michael G. Anderson, University of Iowa, United States of America

Funding: This study was supported by Project of the National Natural Science Funds of China (No. 81371040, 81070760 and No. 81100677), and Shanghai Rising-Star Program (No. 12QA1402200). The funders had no role in study design, data collection and analysis, decision to publish, or preparation of the manuscript.

Competing Interests: The authors have declared that no competing interests exist.

* E-mail: zhaokekewzy@hotmail.com

These authors contributed equally to this work.

Introduction

Polypoidal choroidal vasculopathy (PCV) is a hemorrhagic and exudative macular disorder that is characterized by inner branching choroidal networks with surrounding polypoidal dilatation of the choroidal vessels, which can be clearly demonstrated by indocyanine green angiography [1].

PCV can occur in any gender or race, but it is more commonly seen in Asians than in Caucasians, accounting for 24.5% of patients with findings suggestive of neovascular age-related macular degeneration (nAMD) in the Chinese population [2], for 24.6% in the Korean population [3], for 54.7% in the Japanese population [4], but for only about 4–9.8% in Caucasians. [1].

PCV is categorized by some experts as a subtype of nAMD, [4,5] but others consider it as a different disease entirely. [3,6–8] Clinically, PCV shares several common manifestations with nAMD, such as subretinal exudation and hemorrhage involving the macular region. However, important differences have been noted that patients with PCV are younger and more likely Asians. Their eyes are lack of drusen, often occurrence with serosanguinous maculopathy or hemorrhagic pigment epithelial detachment. They show different responses to photodynamic therapy and

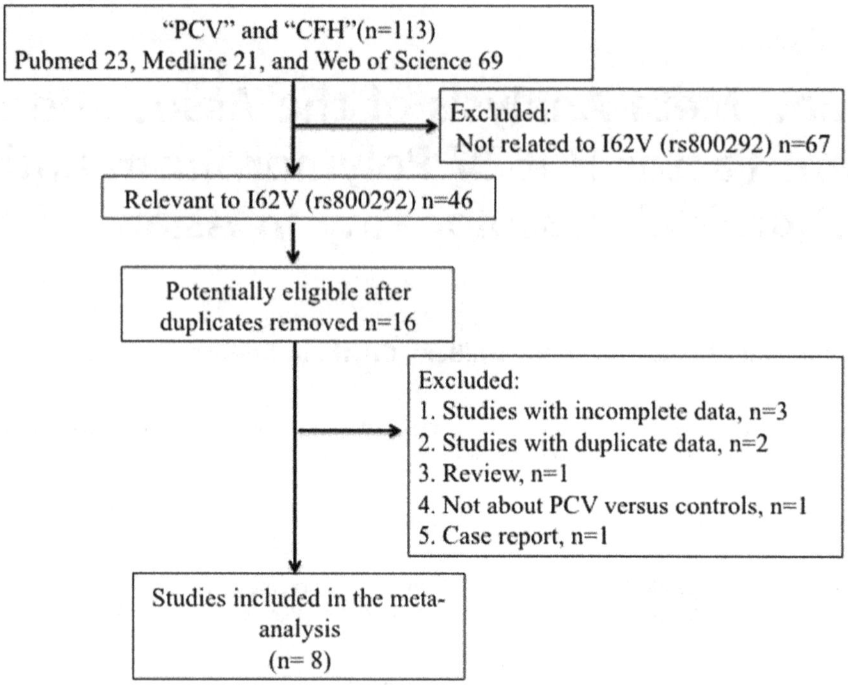

Figure 1. The literature search process. Flow diagram depicts the screening process of retrieved articles, including the reason for and number of exclusions. CFH = complement factor H; PCV = polypoidal choroidal vasculopathy.

therapy involving anti-vascular endothelial growth factor (VEGF) agents.

There are also significant differences in angiographic and optical coherence tomography features between PCV and nAMD. Histopathological studies suggest differences in the anatomical details of the associated vascular abnormalities in the retina and choroids and the relative role of VEGF. These similarities and differences have been a subject of much interest and debate regarding whether the vascular abnormality in PCV represents neovascularization or a phenotype distinct from choroidal neovascularization (CNV). [9].

The etiology of PCV remains largely unknown. It is known as a multifactorial disease due to multiple environmental risk factors and genetic factors or to the interactions between these. The phenotypic similarities between PCV and nAMD lead to the hypothesis that genes involved in AMD may also play a role in

Table 1. Main Characteristics of the Studies Included in the Meta-Analysis.

First Author	Published Year	Ethnic	Totlal (N)			Average Age(yrs)			Gender Ratio(M/F)			Study Type
			PCV	nAMD	Control	PCV	nAMD	Control	PCV	nAMD	Control	
Miki[21]	2013	Japanese	175	NA	150	74.2±7.5 72.1±7.1	NA	72.1±5.6	147/28	NA	116/34	Case control
Zhang[22]	2013	Chinese	250	157	204	65±8.6	67±9.2	69±9.0	166/84	101/56	124/80	Cohort
Ueda-Arakawa[23]	2013	Japanese	87*	97*	NA	71.5±8.4	74.8±8.3	NA	70/17	76/21	NA	Case control
Chantaren[24]	2012	Thai	97	NA	102	62.9±8.9	NA	62.2±7.6	48/49	NA	50/52	Case control
Tanaka[25]	2011	Japanese	381	253	277	69.9±.9.1	73.7±7.5	72.9±8.7	271/110	188/65	111/166	Case control
Hayashi[26]	2010	Japanese	518*	408*	1351*	75.1±8.5	77.7±8.4	51.2±16.3	381/137	293/115	722/629	Case control
Goto[27]	2009	Japanese	100*	100*	190*	72.7±8.3	74.6±8.8	72.2±8.5	81/19	73/27	86/104	Case control
Lee[28]	2008	Singapore Chinese	72	NA	93	63.8±7.6	NA	67.2±4.6	46/26	NA	40/53	Case control

NA = not available; nAMD = neovascular age-related macular degeneration; PCV = polypoidal choroidal vasculopathy.
*The number of cases or controls was changed in the next meta-analysis, but the reason was not given.

Table 2. Allele and Genotype Distribution of the I62V Polymorphism.

First Author	PCV	Genotype				G Allele	nAMD	Genotype				G Allele	Control	Genotype				G Allele	HWE
	(N)	GG	GA	AA	A/G	Frequency (%)	(N)	GG	GA	AA	A/G	Frequency (%)	(N)	GG	GA	AA	A/G	Frequency (%)	P value
Miki[21]	175	100	65	10	85/265	75.71	NA	NA	NA	NA	NA	NA	150	54	63	33	129/ 171	57.00	0.08
Zhang[22]	250	131	107	12	131/ 369	73.80	157	92	52	13	78/ 236	75.16	204	75	85	44	173/ 235	57.60	0.04
Ueda-Arakawa[23]	80	51	22	7	36/ 124	77.50	87	56	25	6	37/ 137	78.74	NA	NA	NA	NA	NA	NA	NA
Chantaren[24]	97	46	47	4	55/ 139	71.65	NA	NA	NA	NA	NA	NA	102	29	59	14	87/ 117	57.35	0.06
Tanaka[25]	381	210	150	21	192/ 570	74.80	253	147	93	13	119/ 387	76.48	277	100	141	36	213/ 341	61.55	0.21
Hayashi[26]	511	290	182	39	260/ 762	74.56	400	228	148	24	196/ 604	75.50	1338	456	649	233	1115/ 1561	58.33	0.94
Goto[27]	95	47	43	5	53/ 137	72.11	96	47	46	3	52/ 140	72.92	188	60	92	36	212/ 164	56.38	0.94
Lee[28]	72	41	27	4	35/ 109	75.69	NA	NA	NA	NA	NA	NA	93	36	41	16	73/ 113	60.75	0.47

HWE = HardyeWeinberg equilibrium; NA = not available; nAMD = neovascular age-related macular degeneration; PCV = polypoidal choroidal vasculopathy.

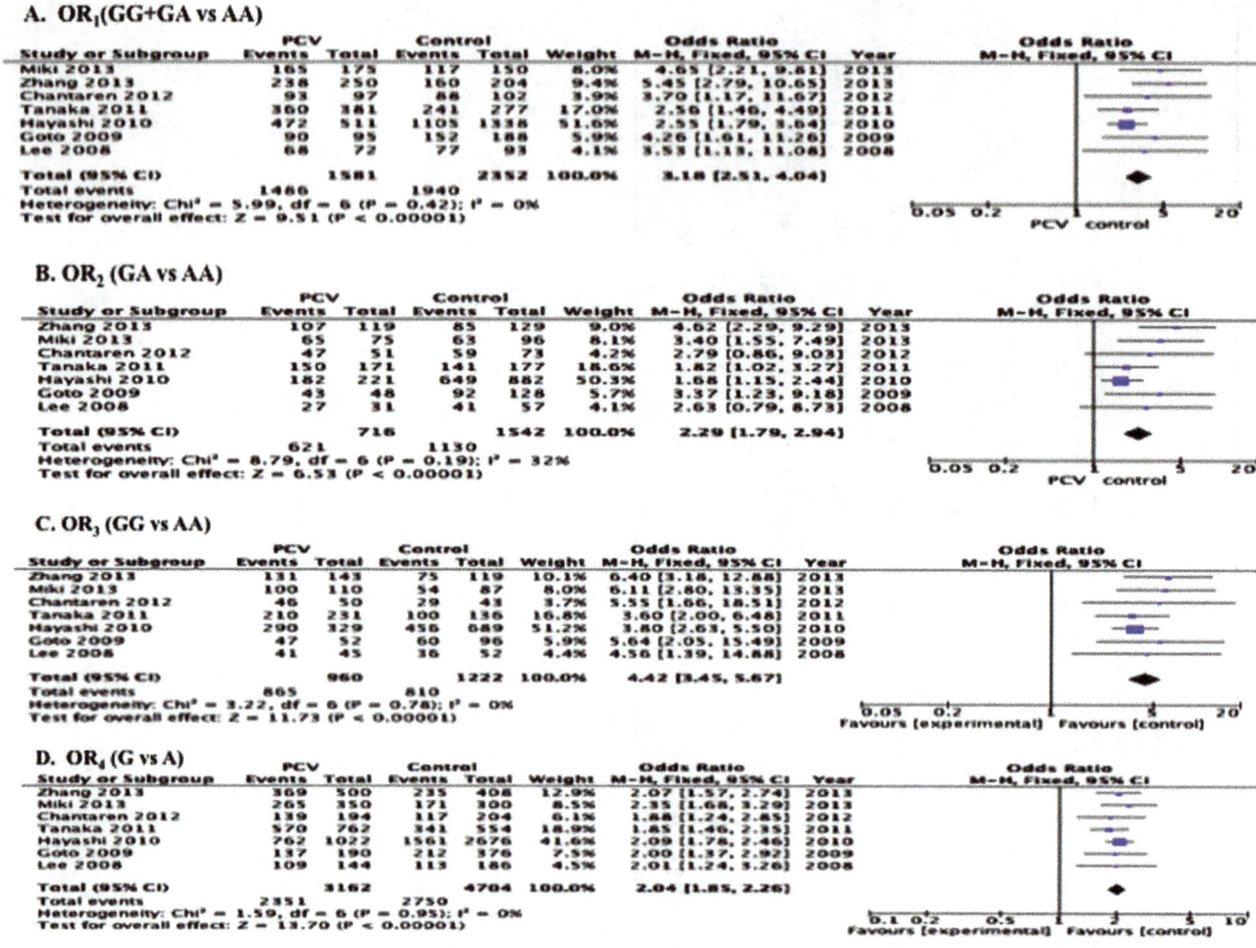

Figure 2. Forest plots of meta-analysis of the association between I62V polymorphism and PCV. Odds ratios (black *squares)* and 95% confidence intervals (bars) are given for each study. Also shown are the *diamonds* of the summary ORs based on the Mantel–Haenszel fixed-effects model (M-H Overall). CI = confidence interval; OR = odds ratio. A: OR_1(GG+GA vs AA); B: OR_2 (GA vs AA); C: OR_3 (GG vs AA); D: OR_4 (G vs A).

PCV. [9] Therefore, investigators have now focused on comparing these two entities to discover if these two different phenotypes can be attributed to genetic differences that may reveal different underlying pathogenic mechanisms. Several candidate genes such as complement factor H (CFH), high temperature required factor A1 (HTRA1), and age-related maculopathy susceptibility 2 (ARMS2) have been reported to increase the risk of AMD and PCV development. [10–12] The CFH I62V coding variant (rs800292) on chromosome 1q32 has been extensively studied via genetic and molecular approaches, which provide strong statistical evidence for disease association and a plausible biologic context supporting this variant as an attractive candidate for a causal polymorphism leading to the development of AMD and PCV. [13–15] However, the population heterogeneity and relatively small sizes studies warrant confirmation of the association of I62V with PCV across different studies in different populations. Here we conducted a meta-analysis of previous studies representing an assessment of the association between the

Table 3. Meta-analysis compared the allelic frequencies of I62V between PCV and nAMD.

		Sample Size			Test of Association	Test of Heterogeneity	
Polymorphism	Studies(N)	PCV	nAMD	Statistical Method	OR (95% CI)	P Value	$I^{2\%}$
(GA+GG) vs AA	5	1317	993	Odds Ratio (M-H, Fixed, 95% CI)	0.92 [0.65, 1.30]	0.48	0
GA vs AA	5	588	423	Odds Ratio (M-H, Fixed, 95% CI)	0.96 [0.67, 1.38]	0.27	22
GG vs AA	5	813	629	Odds Ratio (M-H, Fixed, 95% CI)	0.90 [0.63, 1.27]	0.69	0
G vs A	5	2634	1986	Odds Ratio (M-H, Fixed, 95% CI)	0.94 [0.82, 1.07]	1	0

CI = confidence interval; M-H = Mantel–Haenszel model; nAMD = neovascular age-related macular degeneration; OR = odds ratio; PCV = polypoidal choroidal vasculopathy.

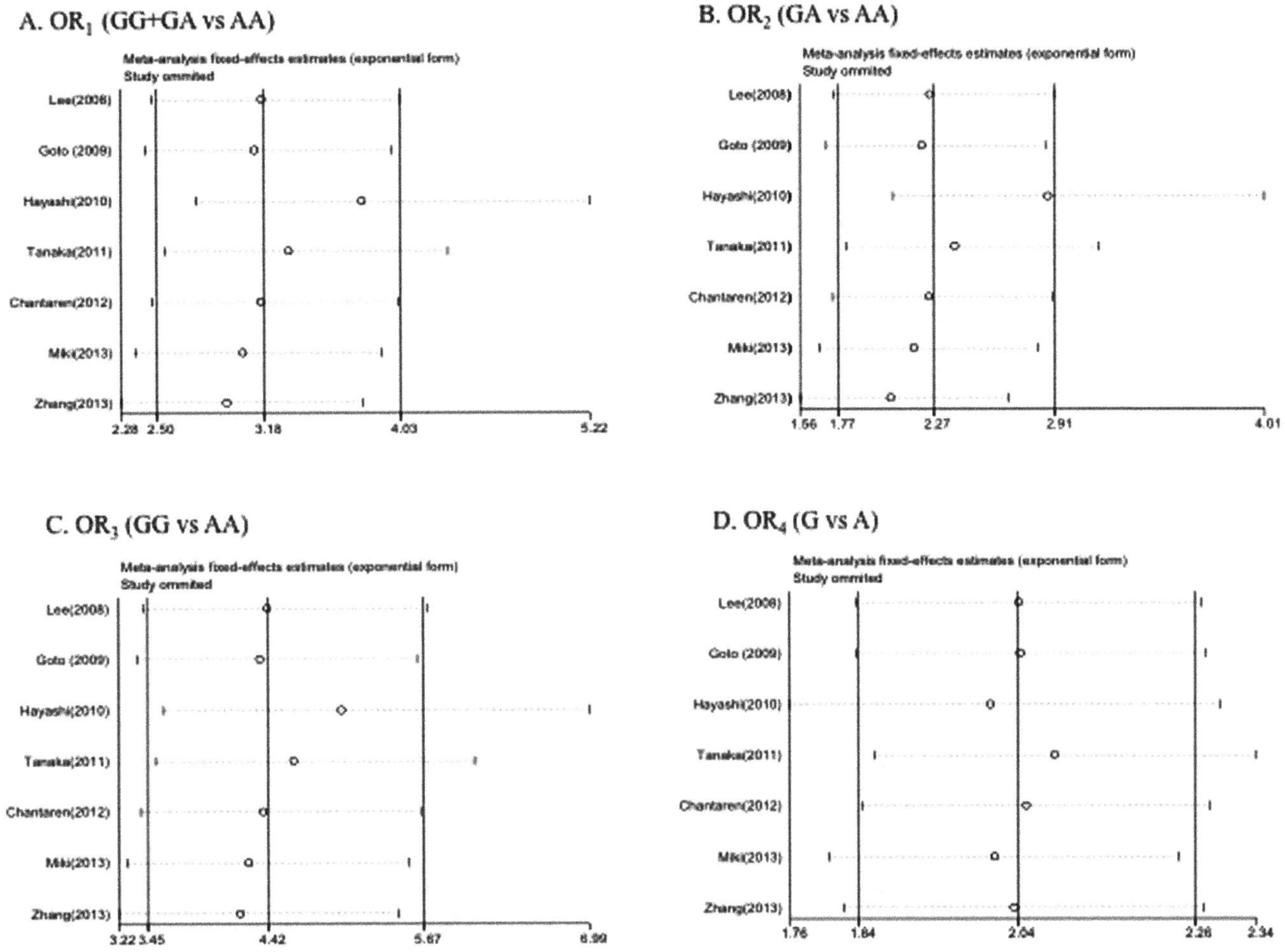

Figure 3. Results of Leave-One-Out Sensitivity Analysis. The horizontal axis shows the omitted study. The horizontal axis represents the odds ratio. Every circle indicates the pooled OR when the left study is omitted in this meta-analysis. The two ends of every broken line represent the respective 95% confidence interval. A: OR_1(GG+GA vs AA); B: OR_2 (GA vs AA); C: OR_3 (GG vs AA); D: OR_4 (G vs A).

CFH I62V variant and PCV and/or nAMD, comprising a total of 5,062 subjects, to more reliably compare the genetic effect of CFH I62V between PCV and nAMD.

Materials and Methods

Identification and Eligibility of Relevant Studies

This meta-analysis was conducted according to the PRISMA guidelines. [16] We searched PubMed, Medline and Web of Science using the following search terms: ("polypoidal choroidal vasculopathy" OR "PCV") and ("CFH" OR "complement factor H"), and other alternative names (I62V, Val62Ile,184G>A, rs800292). All related articles should have been published before Aug 31, 2013 and without any language limitation.

Studies were included only if they fulfill all of the following five criteria: (1) All patients had a complete ophthalmic examination, including fundus photography, and fluorescent or indocyanine green angiography (ICG). The diagnostic criteria of PCV was based on these clinical features and ICG showing a branching vascular network terminating in polypoidal swelling. The diagnostic criteria of nAMD based on the clinical features and grading were classified using a standard grid suggested by the International Age-related Maculopathy Epidemiologic Study Group for age-related maculopathy. (2) Study design was limited to case-control study, cohort study, or population-based epidemiologic survey, not a review, case report, or editorial comment. (3) The major study objective was to evaluate the association between CFH I62V polymorphism and PCV and/or nAMD. (4) Raw data of allele or genotype frequencies or counts available. Allele was A/G, and the genotypes covered AA, AG, and GG. (5) For studies published by the same group on the same gene and markers, only the most recent report or the report with the largest sample size was included for analysis.

Data Extraction

Two reviewers (Z.Y.W. and K.K.Z.) independently extracted the data and evaluated the quality. The following variables were extracted from each study: the name of the first author, year of publication, ethnicity, phenotype of cases evaluated, sample size, mean age and sex ratio of study participants, and allele and genotype distributions in cases and controls. If publications listed allele and genotype counts stratified according to the PCV sub-phenotype, they were combined into one case group.

Independent review and resolution by a third reviewer (P.Q.Z.) was sought if the two reviewers disagreed.

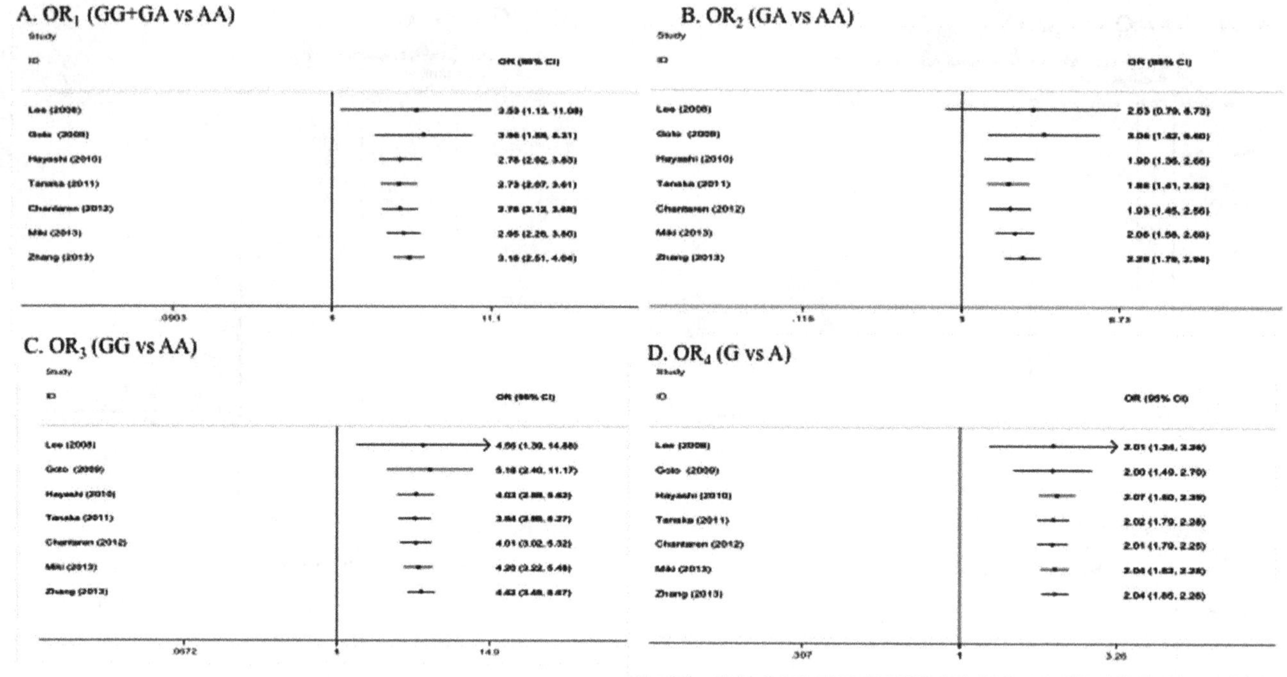

Figure 4. Cumulative meta-analysis of the association between I62V polymorphism and PCV. Every circle represents the pooled OR when studies accumulated over time, and the horizontal line represents the 95% confidence interval of pooled OR. A: OR_1(GG+GA vs AA); B: OR_2 (GA vs AA); C: OR_3 (GG vs AA); D: OR_4 (G vs A).

Statistical Analysis

Hardy-Weinberg Equilibrium (HWE) was tested by the exact test to compare the observed genotype frequencies with the expected genotype frequencies within the control subjects. [17] To investigate the associations of I62V polymorphism with PCV, the allele and genotype frequencies of the SNPs between PCV and controls were compared. To determine whether PCV and nAMD have different genetic risks, the allele frequencies of the SNPs were compared between patients with PCV and nAMD in the studies that included both disorders. The following four odds ratios (ORs) and their 95% confidence intervals (95% CIs) were calculated in each study: OR_1 for (GG+GA) versus AA, OR_2 for GA versus AA, OR_3 for GG versus AA, and OR_4 for allele G versus A.

Between-study heterogeneity was assessed by the Q-statistic test and I^2 statistic. [18,19] A P value <0.1 was considered statistically significant for the Q-statistic test. [18] I^2 ranges between 0% and 100% (where a value of 0% represents no heterogeneity) and larger values represent increasing heterogeneity. The fixed-effects estimates were described in the text for originally homogenous or post hoc homogenized datasets. If there was evidence of between-study heterogeneity, random-effects estimates were described. [18,19].

To assess the publication bias and small-study bias, a funnel plot of the data was applied. In addition, Egger's test was used to detect publication bias. [20] A leave-one-out sensitivity analysis was performed by iteratively removing 1 study at a time to confirm that our findings were not driven by any single study. Cumulative meta-analysis was performed to evaluate the accumulation of evidence on the association between CFH I62V and PCV. The results of individual studies were pooled using the software Review Manager (version 5.2, the Cochrane Collaboration, Oxford, England; available at: http://ims.cochrane.org/revman. Accessed June 30, 2013). All other statistical analysises were performed using Stata software (version 11.0; Stata Corporation, College Station, TX). All tests were 2-tailed. A P value <0.05 was considered statistically significant except for the test of between-study heterogeneity.

Results

Eligibility of Studies

A total of 113 relevant studies were identified by our initial search, of which 8 studies were eligible for inclusion in the review. [21–28] Two of these studies did not have genotype information, but authors kindly provided supplementary information. [22,23] Figure 1 shows the flow chart of the selection process used to identify the studies concerned. Table 1 lists the studies included in the meta-analysis together with summary characteristics of study subjects. The combined sample size for this meta-analysis was 5,062, which included 1,680 PCV patients, 1,015 nAMD patients and 2,367 controls. The average ages ranged from 63.8 to 75.7 years in PCV groups, 67.0 to 77.7 years in nAMD groups and 51.2 to 72.2 years in control groups. Gender ratios (male/female) in the 3 groups varied from 0.98 (48/49) to 5.28 (147/28) in PCV groups, 1.80 (101/56) to 3.62 (76/21) in nAMD groups, and from 0.67 (111/166) to 3.41 (116/34) in control groups. All studies, except 1 study [22] was cohort design, were case–control designs with subjects of Asian ancestry, 5 studies were conducted in Japan, 1 study was conducted in China, 1 study was conducted in Singapore, 1 study was conducted in Thailand (Table 1).

Quantitative Synthesis

Allele and genotype distributions for the I62V polymorphism from individual studies are shown in Table 2. Except one study not observing HWE [22], and one study without a control group [23], all other studies observed HWE and were included in pooling (Table 2).

We initially performed a meta-analysis based on different genetic models between PCV and Control groups. In the fixed-effects model, the pooled OR_1 for the risk allele (GA+GG) versus AA was 3.18 (95% CI, 2.51–4.04, *P<0.00001*), pooled OR_2 for GA versus AA was 2.29 (95% CI: 1.79–2.94, *P<0.00001*), pooled OR_3 for GG versus AA was 4.42 (95% CI: 3.45–5.67, *P<0.00001*), and pooled OR_4 for the risk allele G versus A was 2.04 (95% CI: 1.85–2.26, *P<0.00001*) (Figure 2). The heterogeneity tests of these 4 comparisons are also shown in Figure 2.

We also calculated four summary ORs between PCV group and nAMD group. No significant difference between PCV and nAMD ($n=5$, $OR_1=0.92$, $OR_2=0.96$, $OR_3=0.90$, $OR_4=0.94$) was found in each genetic model (Table 3).

Sensitivity Analysis and Cumulative Meta-Analysis

To evaluate the robustness of the association results, we performed a leave-one-out sensitivity analysis by iteratively removing one study at a time and recalculating the summary OR. The summary ORs remained stable (Figure 3), indicating that our results were not driven by any single study and that similar results could be obtained after excluding the two study not observing the HWE.

The cumulative meta-analysis revealed that the summary ORs were very high in the first two studies but did not vary much after the third study (Figure 4).

Publication Bias

We assessed publication bias using Egger's test. No statistically significant evidence of publication bias was detected for the OR_1 ($P=0.12$), OR_2 ($P=0.10$), OR_3 ($P=0.11$) and OR_4 ($P=0.82$).

Discussion

The reliable assessment of the association between *CFH* I62V and PCV has been hindered in low frequency of variant alleles and small sample sizes in studies. To overcome these barriers, we performed a systematic meta-analysis to summarize the evidence to date regarding the association between CFH I62V and PCV, representing a pooled total of 6 case-control and 1 cohort studies between PCV and Control, 5 case-control studies between PCV and nAMD, involving 5,062 subjects.

Our meta-analysis focused on the association between the CFH I62V polymorphism and PCV risk specifically. The results indicate a strong association between CFH I62V and PCV with no evidence of publication bias. The ORs of all comparisons supported the view that I62V is a risk factor for PCV in Asian populations, and these results also showed that the G allele might be a PCV-causing locus and that the GG homozygote genotype (4.4-fold) had a stronger effect than the GA heterozygote genotype (2.3-fold) with a significant dose response correlation. In individuals carrying at least one copy of the risk allele, disease risk was increased by 3.2-fold.

In addition, sensitivity analyses by iteratively removing one study at a time including one study not observing HWE [22] and one study without control group [23] with the leave-one-out sensitivity analysis showed similar and consistent result, thus indicating the robustness of our findings.

CFH is a critical negative regulator of the alternative pathway of the complement system. It binds to C3b, promotes the decay of C3 convertase, and serves as a cofactor for the factor I–mediated proteolytic inactivation of C3b, resulting in the inhibition of the complement cascade. [29] The CFH gene is found on the 1q32 region. Although the pathogenetic mechanism of CFH leading to PCV is still unclear, the I62V coding variant (rs800292) in CFH has been extensively studied via genetic and molecular approaches, which provide strong statistical evidence for disease association and a plausible biologic context supporting this variant as an attractive candidate for a causal polymorphism leading to the development of AMD and PCV. [13–15] Recently, one meta-analysis, reported by Yuan et al [30], demonstrated that the I62V polymorphism is significantly associated with AMD in Asian populations but there is no link in Caucasian populations. In the current study, we provide evidence that the I62V polymorphism is associated with an increased risk of PCV. There was no significant difference in every genetic model between PCV and nAMD ($n=5$, $OR_1=0.92$, $OR_2=0.96$, $OR_3=0.90$, $OR_4=0.94$) in our study.

Our meta-analysis did not found any heterogeneity in each of the OR. To minimize the bias of our research, we did not use the option of language limitation on PubMed, Medline, or Web of Science, and all previous studies that met our criteria were included. The study must be published in peer-reviewed journals; second, we collected the nAMD data in our studies, excluding the data of dry AMD and other type of wet AMD, such as Retinal angiomatous proliferation; third, all studies which fulfill the inclusion criteria were conducted with subjects of Asian ancestry, 5 studies were conducted in Japan, 1 study was conducted in China, 1 study was conducted in Singapore, 1 study was conducted in Thailand. We didn't find any evidence or study about CFH I62V and PCV with subjects of Caucasian, Africa and other populations based upon our search strategy. Chen et al [31] also reported that the polymorphisms at CFH, LOC387715, HTRA1, and C2 were found to be significantly associated with PCV, which was similar to our conclusions. But in their research the number of included studies was 5, which were all included in our study.

Several limitations of this meta-analysis should be acknowledged. First, there were a limited number of original studies, and all reports were on Eastern Asians. There were no reports on research involving Caucasian, Africa or other populations. These conclusions remain to be confirmed by further research. Second, because the allele and genotype data were not available in several studies, [13,32,33] our meta-analysis may have not included all the studies that have been published. Third, by studying CFH I62V polymorphism and other CFH polymorphisms (e.g., Y402H, C3 and CFB) in this population, it may be useful to understand the effect of these variations on the onset and progression of PCV.

In conclusion, our analysis provides evidence that the CFH I62V polymorphism is associated with an increased risk of PCV in the Asian population. We found that Asian patients with the CFH I62V variant might have a higher risk of developing PCV compared with controls. Our results expand the number of confirmed PCV susceptibility loci for Asian populations and provide a better understanding of the genetic architecture underlying disease susceptibility. The potential for preclinical prediction in future genetic testing may advance by combined evaluation of inherited susceptibility with previously established loci. Further investigations are necessary to confirm the roles of the CFH I62V polymorphism reported in a limited number of original studies. Genetic analysis might provide timely preclinical prediction, prevention, and treatment for PCV.

Author Contributions

Conceived and designed the experiments: ZYW PQZ KKZ. Performed the experiments: KKZ ZYW. Analyzed the data: JZ ZYW KKZ. Contributed reagents/materials/analysis tools: BR CI MB. Wrote the paper: ZYW BR CI MB.

References

1. Koh AH; Expert PCV Panel, Chen LJ, Chen SJ, Chen Y, et al. (2013) Polypoidal choroidal vasculopathy: evidence-based guidelines for clinical diagnosis and treatment. Retina 33: 686–716.
2. Liu Y, Wen F, Huang S, Luo G, Yan H, et al. (2007) Subtype lesions of neovascular age-related macular degeneration in Chinese patients. Graefes Arch Clin Exp Ophthalmol 245: 1441–5.
3. Byeon SH, Lee SC, Oh HS, Kim SS, Koh HJ, et al. (2008) Incidence and clinical patterns of polypoidal choroidal vasculopathy in Korean patients. Jpn J Ophthalmol 52: 57–62.
4. Maruko I, Iida T, Saito M, Nagayama D, Saito K (2007) Clinical characteristics of exudative age-related macular degeneration in Japanese patients. Am J Ophthalmol 144: 15–22.
5. Takahashi K, Ishibashi T, Ogur Y, Yuzawa M (2008) [Classification and diagnostic criteria of age-related macular degeneration]. Nippon Ganka Gakkai Zasshi 112: 1076–1084.
6. Lim TH, Laude A, Tan CS (2010) Polypoidal choroidal vasculopathy: an angiographic discussion. Eye (Lond) 24: 483–490.
7. Okubo A, Sameshima M, Uemura A, Kanda S, Ohba N (2002) Clinicopathological correlation of polypoidal choroidal vasculopathy revealed by ultrastructural study. Br J Ophthalmol 86: 1093–8.
8. Sho K, Takahashi K, Yamada H, Wada M, Nagai Y, et al. (2003) Polypoidal choroidal vasculopathy: incidence, demographic features, and clinical characteristics. Arch Ophthalmol 121: 1392–1396.
9. Laude A, Cackett PD, Vithana EN, Yeo IY, Wong D, et al. (2010) Polypoidal choroidal vasculopathy and neovascular age-related macular degeneration: same or different disease? Prog Retin Eye Res 29: 19–29.
10. Lima LH, Schubert C, Ferrara DC, Merriam JE, Imamura Y, et al. (2010) Three major loci involved in age-related macular degeneration are also associated with polypoidal choroidal vasculopathy. Ophthalmology 117: 1567–70.
11. Gotoh N, Yamada R, Nakanishi H, Saito M, Iida T, et al. (2008) Correlation between CFH Y402H and HTRA1 rs11200638 genotype to typical exudative age-related macular degeneration and polypoidal choroidal vasculopathy phenotype in the Japanese population. Clin Experiment Ophthalmol 36: 437–42.
12. Bessho H, Honda S, Kondo N, Negi A (2011) The association of age-related maculopathy susceptibility 2 polymorphisms with phenotype in typical neovascular age-related macular degeneration and polypoidal choroidal vasculopathy. Mol Vis 17: 977–82.
13. Sakurada Y, Kubota T, Imasawa M, Mabuchi F, Tateno Y, et al (2011) Role of complement factor H I62V and age-related maculopathy susceptibility 2 A69S variants in the clinical expression of polypoidal choroidal vasculopathy. Ophthalmology 118: 1402–7.
14. Mori K, Horie-Inoue K, Gehlbach PL, Takita H, Kabasawa S, et al. (2010) Phenotype and genotype characteristics of age-related macular degeneration in a Japanese population. Ophthalmology 117: 928–38.
15. Kondo N, Honda S, Kuno S, Negi A (2009) Coding variant I62V in the complement factor H gene is strongly associated with polypoidal choroidal vasculopathy. Ophthalmology 116: 304–10.
16. Moher D, Liberati A, Tetzlaff J, Altman DG (2009) Preferred reporting items for systematic reviews and meta-analyses: the PRISMA statement. BMJ 339: b2535.
17. Wigginton JE, Cutler DJ, Abecasis GR (2005) A note on exact tests of Hardy-Weinberg equilibrium. Am J Hum Genet 76: 887–93.
18. Ioannidis JP, Patsopoulos NA, Evangelou E (2007) Heterogeneity in meta-analyses of genome-wide association investigations. PLoS ONE 2: e841.
19. Higgins JP, Thompson SG, Deeks JJ, Altman DG (2003) Measuring inconsistency in meta-analyses. BMJ 327: 557–60.
20. Egger M, Davey Smith G, Schneider M, Minder C (1997) Bias in meta-analysis detected by a simple, graphical test. BMJ 315: 629–34.
21. Miki A, Honda S, Kondo N, Negi A (2013) The Association of Age-related Maculopathy Susceptibility 2 (ARMS2) and Complement Factor H (CFH) Variants with Two Angiographic Subtypes of Polypoidal Choroidal Vasculopathy. Ophthalmic Genet 34: 146–50.
22. Zhang X, Li M, Wen F, Zuo C, Chen H, et al. (2013) Different impact of high-density lipoprotein-related genetic variants on polypoidal choroidal vasculopathy and neovascular age-related macular degeneration in a Chinese Han population. Exp Eye Res 108: 16–22.
23. Ueda-Arakawa N, Ooto S, Nakata I, Yamashiro K, Tsujikawa A, et al. (2013) Prevalence and genomic association of reticular pseudodrusen in age-related macular degeneration. Am J Ophthalmol 155: 260–269.e2.
24. Chantaren P, Ruamviboonsuk P, Ponglikitmongkol M, Tiensuwan M, Promso S (2012) Major single nucleotide polymorphisms in polypoidal choroidal vasculopathy: a comparative analysis between Thai and other Asian populations. Clin Ophthalmol. 6: 465–71.
25. Tanaka K, Nakayama T, Yuzawa M, Wang Z, Kawamura A, et al. (2011) Analysis of candidate genes for age-related macular degeneration subtypes in the Japanese population. Mol Vis 17: 2751–8.
26. Hayashi H, Yamashiro K, Gotoh N, Nakanishi H, Nakata I, et al. (2010) CFH and ARMS2 variations in age-related macular degeneration, polypoidal choroidal vasculopathy, and retinal angiomatous proliferation. Invest Ophthalmol Vis Sci. 51: 5914–9.
27. Goto A, Akahori M, Okamoto H, Minami M, Terauchi N, et al. (2009) Genetic analysis of typical wet-type age-related macular degeneration and polypoidal choroidal vasculopathy in Japanese population. J Ocul Biol Dis Infor 2: 164–175.
28. Lee KY, Vithana EN, Mathur R, Yong VH, Yeo IY, et al. (2008) Association analysis of CFH, C2, BF, and HTRA1 gene polymorphisms in Chinese patients with polypoidal choroidal vasculopathy. Invest Ophthalmol Vis Sci 49: 2613–9.
29. Rodríguez de Córdoba S, Esparza-Gordillo J, Goicoechea de Jorge E, Lopez-Trascasa M, Sánchez-Corral P (2004) The human complement factor H: functional roles, genetic variations and disease associations. Mol Immunol 41: 355–67.
30. Yuan D, Yang Q, Liu X, Yuan D, Yuan S, et al. (2013) Complement factor H Val62Ile variant and risk of age-related macular degeneration: a meta-analysis. Mol Vis 19: 374–83.
31. Chen H, Liu K, Chen LJ, Hou P, Chen W, Pang CP (2012) Genetic associations in polypoidal choroidal vasculopathy: a systematic review and meta-analysis. Mol Vis18: 816–29.
32. Liu K, Chen LJ, Tam PO, Shi Y, Lai TY, et al. (2013) Associations of the C2-CFB-RDBP-SKIV2L locus with age-related macular degeneration and polypoidal choroidal vasculopathy. Ophthalmology 120: 837–43.
33. Nakata I, Yamashiro K, Yamada R, Gotoh N, Nakanishi H, et al. (2012) Significance of C2/CFB variants in age-related macular degeneration and polypoidal choroidal vasculopathy in a Japanese population. Invest Ophthalmol Vis Sci53: 794–8.

19

Elevated High-Density Lipoprotein Cholesterol and Age-Related Macular Degeneration: The Alienor Study

Audrey Cougnard-Grégoire[1,2*], Marie-Noëlle Delyfer[1,2,3], Jean-François Korobelnik[1,2,3], Marie-Bénédicte Rougier[3], Mélanie Le Goff[1,2], Jean-François Dartigues[1,2], Pascale Barberger-Gateau[1,2], Cécile Delcourt[1,2]

1 Université de Bordeaux, Bordeaux, France, **2** INSERM (Institut National de la Santé Et de la Recherche Médicale), ISPED (Institut de Santé Publique d'Épidémiologie et de Développement), Centre INSERM U897-Epidemiologie-Biostatistique, Bordeaux, France, **3** Centre Hospitalier Universitaire (CHU) de Bordeaux, Service d'Ophtalmologie, Bordeaux, France

Abstract

Background: Lipid metabolism and particularly high-density lipoprotein (HDL) may be involved in the pathogenic mechanism of age-related macular degeneration (AMD). However, conflicting results have been reported in the associations of AMD with plasma HDL and other lipids, which may be confounded by the recently reported associations of AMD with HDL-related genes. We explored the association of AMD with plasma lipid levels and lipid-lowering medication use, taking into account most of HDL-related genes associated with AMD.

Methods: The Alienor study is a population-based study on age-related eye diseases performed in 963 elderly residents of Bordeaux (France). AMD was graded from non mydriatic color retinal photographs in three exclusive stages: no AMD (n = 430 subjects, 938 eyes); large soft distinct drusen and/or large soft indistinct drusen and/or reticular drusen and/or pigmentary abnormalities (early AMD, n = 176, 247); late AMD (n = 40, 61). Associations of AMD with plasma lipids (HDL, total cholesterol (TC), Low-density lipoprotein (LDL), and triglycerides (TG)) were estimated using Generalized Estimating Equation logistic regressions. Statistical analyses included 646 subjects with complete data.

Results: After multivariate adjustment for age, sex, educational level, smoking, BMI, lipid-lowering medication use, cardiovascular disease and diabetes, and for all relevant genetic polymorphisms (ApoE2, ApoE4, CFH Y402H, ARMS2 A69S, LIPC rs10468017, LIPC rs493258, LPL rs12678919, ABCA1 rs1883025 and CETP rs3764261), higher HDL was significantly associated with an increased risk of early (OR = 2.45, 95%CI: 1.54–3.90; P = 0.0002) and any AMD (OR = 2.29, 95%CI: 1.46–3.59; P = 0.0003). Association with late AMD was far from statistical significance (OR = 1.58, 95%CI: 0.48–5.17; p = 0.45). No associations were found for any stage of AMD with TC, LDL and TG levels, statin or fibrate drug use.

Conclusions: This study suggests that elderly patients with high HDL concentration may be at increased risk for AMD and, further, that HDL dysfunction might be implicated in AMD pathogenesis.

Editor: Demetrios Vavvas, Massachusetts Eye & Ear Infirmary, Harvard Medical School, United States of America

Funding: Laboratoires Théa (Clermont-Ferrand, France), Fondation Voir et Entendre (Paris, France), Laboratoires Théa participated in the design of the study, but no sponsor participated in the collection, management, statistical analysis and interpretation of the data, nor in the preparation, review or approval of the present manuscript.

Competing Interests: ACG, none; JFK, Laboratoires Théa, Alcon, Allergan, Carl Zeiss Meditec, Bayer, Novartis; MND, Laboratoires Théa, Novartis; MBR, Allergan, Bausch Lomb, Laboratoires Théa, Biogen, Novartis; MLG, none; JFD, Novartis, IPSEN, Merck Serono, Lundbeck; PBG, Lesieur, Bausch & Lomb, Aprifel, Danone Institute, Canadian Association of Gerontology, the Jean Mayer Human Nutrition Research Center on Aging, Tufts University, Alzheimer's Association, Groupe Lipides et Nutrition, Institut Pasteur, Conseil Re´gional d'Aquitaine, Vifor Pharma, Danone, Institut Carnot LISA and Groupe Lipides et Nutrition; CD, Laboratoires The´a, Bausch&Lomb, Novartis.

* E-mail: Audrey.Cougnard-Gregoire@isped.u-bordeaux2.fr

Introduction

Age-related macular degeneration (AMD) is the leading cause of blindness in high-income countries, and the third global cause of blindness in the world [1]. This disease affects 2.5 million subjects in Europe [2] and 1.75 million in the USA [3]. While the pathophysiology of AMD remains elusive, a number of risk factors, such as smoking, nutrition and several genetic polymorphisms have been evidenced [4]. The early stage of AMD is characterized by the presence of large and soft drusen (extracellular deposits, seen as yellow spots on the retina) and/or of pigmentary abnormalities. The later stages involve atrophy of the retinal pigment epithelium (RPE) (dry form) or the development of choroidal neovascularization (wet form).

With advancing age, there is a deposit of lipid particles in normal Bruch's membrane (BrM) leading to the creation of a lipid wall, external to the RPE basal lamina, impairing nutrient exchange between the choriocapillaris and the RPE and compromising retinal function [5–8]. The observation that the location of the lipid wall was the same as and precedes the basal linear deposits and drusen suggested its contribution to drusen formation

[6,8]. Indeed, lipids (both esterified and unesterified cholesterol, and phosphatidylcholine) represent at least 40% of the volume of drusen [6,9,10].

Furthermore, within the genomic era, several lipid-related genes have been reported to be associated with AMD. The E4 allele of the Apolipoprotein E gene (ApoE4) is associated with a reduced risk for AMD, while the ApoE2 increases the risk for AMD [11,12]. ApoE plays a key role in cholesterol metabolism [13] and is associated with macular pigment optical density [14]. Other genes present particularly in the high-density lipoprotein cholesterol (HDL) pathway as the hepatic lipase gene (LIPC) [15–22], the lipoprotein lipase gene (LPL) [15,17,18], the cholesterol ester transferase gene (CETP) [16,17,21] and the ABC-binding cassette A1 (ABCA1) gene [15–18,21] have been shown to be associated with AMD in genome-wide association (GWAS) studies and have been confirmed in several epidemiological studies [21,23], including the Alienor study [22].

These findings have led to the hypothesis that lipid metabolism and particularly HDL is involved in the pathogenic mechanism of AMD [6,9,24]. However, conflicting results have been reported with regard to the associations of AMD with serum HDL concentration. An increasing number of studies reported higher risk for AMD among subjects with elevated HDL [25–31], few others reported a reduced risk [32–34] and some others reported no significant associations [35–38].

Other associations between serum lipids such as total cholesterol (TC), low-density lipoprotein (LDL) and triglycerides (TG), and AMD have also been investigated with still conflicting findings. In 1992, the Eye Disease Case Control Study Group, reported a significant 4-fold increased risk for exudative AMD with the highest serum cholesterol concentration [39]. Since then, only five studies reported a significant increased risk of AMD with high level of total cholesterol [23,33,40–42], while 13 reported no significant association [26,27,30,32,34–38,43–46], and two an inverse relationship [47,48].

Recently, Ebrahimi *et al* suggested that before excluding the role of systemic lipids in AMD, the role of plasma lipids in the context of genotype could be examined to identify predisposition in a subset of patients at risk for AMD due to genotype and plasma lipid levels [24].

Thus, the aim of this study was to explore the association between plasma lipid levels, lipid-lowering drug use and AMD, taking into account most of HDL-related genes associated with AMD, in the framework of a population-based study.

Subjects and Methods

Study Purpose

The Alienor (Antioxydants, LIpids Essentiels, Nutrition et maladies OculaiRes) Study is a population-based study aimed at assessing the associations of age-related eye diseases (AMD, glaucoma, cataract, dry eye syndrome) with nutritional factors (in particular antioxidants, macular pigment, and fatty acids), determined from plasma measurements and estimations of dietary intake [49]. It also takes into account other major determinants of eye disease, including gene polymorphisms, lifestyle and vascular factors.

Study Sample

Subjects of the Alienor Study were recruited from an ongoing population-based study (Three-City [3C] Study) on the vascular risk factors for dementia [50]. The 3C Study included 9294 subjects aged 65 years and older from three French cities (Bordeaux, Dijon, Montpellier), among whom 2104 were recruited in Bordeaux. Subjects were contacted individually from the electoral rolls. They were initially recruited in 1999 to 2001 and were followed-up about every 2 years since baseline (Figure 1). Data collected at each examination included cognitive testing with diagnoses of dementia and assessment of vascular risk factors. In addition, fasting blood and DNA samples were collected at baseline and kept frozen at −80°C.

The Alienor Study consisted in an eye examination, which was proposed to all participants of the third follow-up (2006–2008) of the 3C cohort in Bordeaux. Among the 1450 alive participants re-examined in 2006 to 2008, 963 (66.4%) participated in the Alienor Study, and 487 (33.6%) declined participation. Detailed characteristics of participants and nonparticipants have been published elsewhere [49].

This research followed the tenets of the Declaration of Helsinki. Participants gave written consent for participation in the study. The design of the Alienor Study has been approved by the Ethical Committee of Bordeaux (Comite de Protection des Personnes Sud-Ouest et Outre-Mer III) in May 2006.

Eye Examination

The eye examination took place in the Department of Ophthalmology of the University Hospital of Bordeaux, France. It included a recording of ophthalmological history, measures of visual acuity, refraction, two 45° nonmydriatic color retinal photographs (one centered on the macula, the other centered on the optic disc), measures of intraocular pressure and central corneal thickness, and break-up time test. A self-completed questionnaire on risk factors specific to the eye and dry eye symptoms was completed at home and brought back on the day of the eye examination.

Retinal photographs were performed using a nonmydriatic retinograph (TRC NW6S; Topcon, Tokyo, Japan) and were interpreted in duplicate by two specially trained technicians. Inconsistencies between the two interpretations were adjudicated by a retina specialist for classification of AMD and other retinal diseases and by a glaucoma specialist for classification of glaucoma. All cases of late AMD, other retinal diseases, and glaucoma were reviewed and confirmed by specialists.

Classification of AMD

Retinal photographs were interpreted according to the international classification [51] and to a modification of the grading scheme used in the Multi-Ethnic Study of Atherosclerosis for drusen size, location, and area [52]. Late AMD was defined by the presence of neovascular AMD or geographic atrophy within the grid (3000 μm from the foveola). Neovascular AMD included serous or hemorrhagic detachment of the retinal pigment epithelium (RPE) or sensory retina, subretinal or sub-RPE hemorrhages, and fibrous scar tissue. Geographic atrophy was defined as a discrete area of retinal depigmentation, 175 μm in diameter or larger, characterized by a sharp border and the presence of visible choroidal vessels. Five cases of late AMD had no gradable photographs and were classified by ophthalmological history of AMD and AMD therapy (in particular, antiangiogenic agents and photodynamic therapy) and confirmed by their treating ophthalmologist. Early AMD was defined by the presence of soft distinct drusen and/or soft indistinct drusen and/or reticular drusen and/or pigmentary abnormalities. Soft distinct and soft indistinct drusen were larger than 125 μm in diameter and had, respectively, uniform density and sharp edges or decreasing density from the center outward and fuzzy edges. Pigmentary abnormalities were defined as areas of hyperpigmentation and/or hypopigmentation (without visibility of choroidal vessels). Eyes

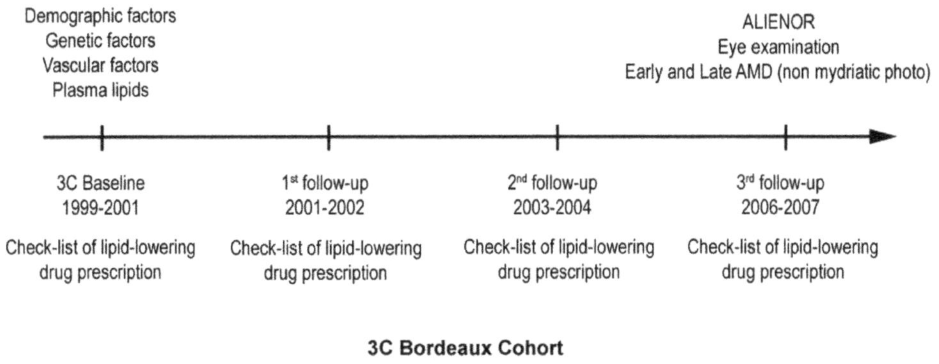

Figure 1. Design of the Alienor study. Abbreviations: AMD: age-related macular degeneration.

were classified according to 3 exclusive groups: no AMD, early AMD, late AMD.

Plasma Lipids Measurements

Plasma measurements were determined from fasting blood samples collected at the 3C baseline visit (1999–2001) into heparinized evacuated tubes and centrifuged at 1000 g for 10 min. Plasma lipids (TC, LDL, HDL, and TG) were measured at the Biochemistry Laboratory of the University Hospital of Dijon.

Lipid Lowering Medications

The clinical baseline (from 1999 to 2001) and follow-up examinations (1st follow-up examination from 2001 to 2002; 2nd follow-up examination from 2003 to 2004 and 3rd follow-up examination from 2006 to 2007) included an inventory of all drugs used during the preceding month. Medical prescriptions and, where feasible, the medications themselves were seen by the interviewer. The name of the medication was recorded, and all drugs were subsequently coded according to the French translation of the world health organization (WHO) anatomical therapeutic chemical (ATC) classification [53]. Three classes of lipid-lowering medications were defined according to the ATC classification: 1) Statins (ATC codes: C10AA; C10BA; C10BX); 2) Fibrates (ATC codes: C10AB); 3) Others (ATC codes: C10AC; C10AD; C10AX). Lipid-lowering medication use was defined as the use of at least one of the preceding classes of drugs between the baseline and the last follow-up.

Other Variables

The following potential confounders have been selected based on literature results reporting significant associations of AMD or serum lipid concentrations with age, gender, educational level, smoking, body mass index (BMI), hypertension, cardiovascular disease, diabetes, Complement Factor H (CFH) Y402H (rs1061170), Age-Related Maculopathy Susceptibility 2 (ARMS2, rs10490924) A69S, apolipoproteins E2 (ApoE2) and E4 (ApoE4), LIPC (rs10468017), LIPC (rs493258), LPL (rs12678919), ABCA1 (rs1883025) and CETP (rs3764261) polymorphisms.

Data were collected during a face-to-face interview using a standardized questionnaire administered by a trained psychologist or nurse. At baseline, general data included: demographic characteristics, educational level and smoking. BMI (kg/m^2) was calculated as weight/height^2 using weight and height measured at baseline. Two separate measures of blood pressure in a seated position were performed in all participants. The first blood pressure measurement was recorded at the beginning of the interview and the second one at the end, using a digital electronic tensiometer (OMRON M4, France). The average systolic blood pressure (SBP) was the average of these two SBP measures. The same calculation was made for the average diastolic blood pressure (DBP). Hypertension was defined as average SBP≥140 mmHg and/or average DBP≥90 mmHg and/or antihypertensive medication use at baseline examination.

Genetic polymorphisms were determined by the Lille Génopôle, from the DNA samples collected at baseline (1999–2001). The included genetic factors have been shown to be very strong predictors of risk for AMD and/or cardiovascular disease in previous studies, including the Alienor Study [19,54–56].

Statistical Analyses

Associations of baseline demographic, behavioural, anthropometric, medical and genetic characteristics with plasma lipid concentrations, statin and fibrate drug use were examined with Student test, Analysis of variance (ANOVA), and Chi-square test, as appropriate.

Associations of early and late AMD with plasma lipid variables, statin and fibrate drug use were estimated using logistic Generalized Estimating Equation (GEE) models, taking into account the data from both eyes and their intra-individual correlation. [57] In all analyses, subjects without any AMD were considered as the reference group.

GEE models for plasma lipids, statin and fibrate drug use were adjusted first for age and gender only (Model 1); in Model 2 we performed additional adjustment for educational level (no education or primary school or short secondary school *vs.* long secondary school or high school or university), smoking (never, 1 to less than 20 pack-years, 20 pack-years or more), BMI (kg/m^2, < 25, [25–30], ≥30), hypertension, cardiovascular disease, diabetes (Fasting glycemia ≥6.1 mmol/L or nonfasting glycemia ≥ 11.0 mmol/l or antidiabetic medication) and for lipid-lowering medications (at one examination or more), for plasma lipid concentrations; and for HDL, LDL and TG, only for statin and fibrate drug use. Finally, Model 3 was adjusted with all previous variables and genetic risk factors (ApoE2, ApoE4, CFH Y402H, ARMS2 A69S, LIPC rs10468017, LIPC rs493258, LPL rs12678919, ABCA1 rs1883025 and CETP rs3764261 polymorphisms).

Potential interactions between plasma lipid levels and lipid-lowering medication use and between plasma lipid levels and genetic polymorphisms were assessed. Lipid-lowering medications use and genetic polymorphisms were introduced in the models one by one. We withdrew interaction terms when not statistically significant (P>0.05).

False positive results are a critical concern when a number of association tests are performed. To address this issue, we applied Bonferroni correction to correct for multiple testing.

All statistical analyses were performed using SAS version 9.2 (SAS Institute Inc, Cary, NC; procedure GENMOD for the GEE analysis).

Results

Among the 963 subjects of the ALIENOR study, subjects were aged 80.2 years on average and the proportion of women was 61.9%. Among the 963 subjects, 84 (8.7%) subjects had ungradable photographs in both eyes and 54 (5.6%) had missing data for plasma lipid measurement and/or lipid-lowering drug use. Thus the statistical analyses were conducted on 825 subjects (85.7%) corresponding to 1595 eyes.

Table 1 presents the plasma lipid concentrations and lipid lowering drug use of the ALIENOR subjects according to AMD status. HDL was higher in early and late AMD cases, while there were no differences for TC, LDL or TG. No associations were found for use of statin or fibrates.

Tables 2 and 3 present the associations of plasma lipids and lipid lowering medications with genetic polymorphisms. After Bonferroni correction (P = 0.0055), subjects with at least one Apo E2 allele had lower mean level of TC and LDL and higher mean level of TG than those with no Apo E2 allele. Subjects with at least one Apo E4 allele used significantly more statins than subjects with no ApoE4 allele. For CETP rs3764261, subjects with AA genotype had significantly higher mean level of HDL than subjects with CC or AC genotypes. No associations were found between ApoE4, CFH Y402H, ARMS2 A69S, LIPC rs493258, LIPC rs10468017, ABCA1 rs1883025 polymorphisms and plasma lipid levels. No associations were found between CFH Y402H, ARMS2 A69S, LIPC rs493258, LIPC rs10468017, LPL, ABCA1 and CETP polymorphisms and statin and fibrate drug use.

Associations with baseline demographic, behavioural and anthropometric characteristics and plasma lipid concentrations are presented in Table S1 in File S1. After Bonferroni correction (P = 0.0083), TC and HDL were significantly higher in women, never smokers and subjects with lower BMI. TG was significantly higher in smokers and subjects with higher BMI. No associations were found for LDL, Statin and Fibrates use (Table S1 in File S1). With regard to medical characteristics at baseline, after Bonferroni correction (P<0.017), TC and LDL were significantly higher in the absence of cardiovascular disease, HDL was higher in the absence of cardiovascular disease, hypertension or diabetes, and TG was higher in the presence of cardiovascular disease, hypertension or diabetes (Table S2 in File S1). Statin use was significantly associated with the presence of cardiovascular disease, hypertension and diabetes, and having higher levels of LDL and TG and lower level of HDL. No such associations were found for use of fibrates (Tables S2 and S3 in File S1).

Table 4 presents association of AMD with plasma lipids levels, statin and fibrate drug use. After adjustment for age and sex (model 1) and Bonferroni correction (P = 0.0125), higher HDL was significantly associated with an increased risk of early and any AMD (OR ranging from 1.77–1.84 per 1 mmol/L, P values ranging from 0.0008–0.003). HDL was associated with late AMD (OR = 2.41, P = 0.04) with a P value<0.05, but did not remained significant after Bonferroni correction. No associations were found for any stage of AMD with TC, LDL and TG concentrations, or statin and fibrate drug use.

After further adjustment for educational level, smoking, BMI, lipid-lowering medication use, cardiovascular disease and diabetes,

Table 1. Plasma lipid levels and statin and fibrate drug use according to AMD status, in subjects of the Alienor study (N = 825).

	TC (mM)	LDL (mM)	HDL (mM)	TG (mM)	Statin*		Fibrates†	
					No (N = 507)	Yes (N = 318)	No (N = 663)	Yes (N = 162)
	Mean (SD)	Mean (SD)	Mean (SD)	Mean (SD)	N (%)	N (%)	N (%)	N (%)
AMD								
None (N = 540)	5.78 (0.95)	3.66 (0.83)	1.56 (0.38)	1.24 (0.59)	331 (65.3)	209 (65.72)	441 (66.52)	99 (61.11)
Early AMD (N = 238)	5.81 (0.98)	3.62 (0.85)	1.66 (0.41)	1.17 (0.51)	145 (28.6)	93 (29.25)	183 (27.60)	55 (33.95)
Late AMD (N = 47)	5.72 (1.17)	3.48 (0.96)	1.69 (0.45)	1.21 (0.66)	31 (6.1)	16 (5.03)	39 (5.88)	8 (4.94)
P value‡	*P = 0.83*	*P = 0.36*	*P = 0.0009*	*P = 0.26*	*P = 0.80*		*P = 0.27*	

Abbreviations: AMD: age-related macular degeneration; TC: Total cholesterol; TG: Triglycerides;
*Use of statin at one examination or more;
†Use of fibrate at one examination or more;
‡ANOVA were performed to compare the difference in distribution of plasma lipid levels between AMD stages; χ^2 tests were performed to compare the differences in statin and fibrates drug uses between AMD stages.

Table 2. Plasma lipid levels according to genetic characteristics in subjects of the Alienor study (N = 825).

	TC (mM)	LDL (mM)	HDL (mM)	TG (mM)
	Mean (SD)	Mean (SD)	Mean (SD)	Mean (SD)
ApoE2 (N = 815)				
No allele E2 (N = 711)	5.83 (1.00)	3.70 (0.86)	1.58 (0.39)	1.20 (0.53)
At least 1 allele E2 (N = 104)	5.53 (0.78)	3.26 (0.66)	1.64 (0.40)	1.37 (0.77)
*P value**,†	*0.004*	*<0.0001*	*0.15*	*0.004*
ApoE4 (N = 815)				
No allele E4 (N = 670)	5.78 (0.98)	3.62 (0.85)	1.60 (0.39)	1.22 (0.57)
At least 1 allele E4 (N = 145)	5.84 (0.96)	3.71 (0.83)	1.58 (0.39)	1.20 (0.58)
*P value**,†	*0.48*	*0.23*	*0.54*	*0.72*
LPL rs12678919 (N = 714)				
A A (N = 531)	5.76 (0.97)	3.62 (0.86)	1.57 (0.39)	1.25 (0.59)
A G (N = 170)	5.80 (0.97)	3.70 (0.81)	1.57 (0.37)	1.16 (0.49)
G G (N = 13)	5.37 (0.80)	3.10 (0.63)	1.83 (0.43)	0.97 (0.51)
*P value**,†	*0.32*	*0.04*	*0.06*	*0.04*
CETP rs3764261 (N = 719)				
C C (N = 377)	5.74 (0.97)	3.66 (0.86)	1.51 (0.34)	1.26 (0.61)
A C (N = 287)	5.77 (0.99)	3.59 (0.84)	1.63 (0.41)	1.20 (0.53)
A A (N = 55)	5.90 (0.93)	3.59 (0.78)	1.81 (0.43)	1.12 (0.43)
*P value**,†	*0.50*	*0.60*	*<0.0001*	*0.14*
LIPC rs493258 (N = 736)				
C C (N = 215)	5.79 (0.99)	3.65 (0.86)	1.56 (0.39)	1.28 (0.63)
T C (N = 352)	5.76 (0.94)	3.63 (0.84)	1.58 (0.37)	1.21 (0.53)
T T (N = 169)	5.76 (1.03)	3.60 (0.84)	1.61 (0.41)	1.22 (0.58)
*P value**,†	*0.95*	*0.84*	*0.43*	*0.39*
LIPC rs10468017 (N = 723)				
C C (N = 375)	5.75 (0.98)	3.64 (0.87)	1.57 (0.38)	1.21 (0.57)
T C (N = 289)	5.77 (0.96)	3.61 (0.83)	1.60 (0.38)	1.23 (0.52)
T T (N = 59)	5.76 (1.07)	3.57 (0.88)	1.61 (0.45)	1.28 (0.73)
*P value**,†	*0.98*	*0.81*	*0.50*	*0.64*
ABCA1 rs1883025 (N = 736)				
C C (N = 390)	5.79 (1.02)	3.63 (0.87)	1.61 (0.39)	1.22 (0.53)
C T (N = 290)	5.75 (0.93)	3.62 (0.83)	1.56 (0.38)	1.24 (0.62)
T T (N = 57)	5.70 (0.87)	3.63 (0.74)	1.49 (0.37)	1.28 (0.62)
*P value**,†	*0.70*	*0.98*	*0.07*	*0.73*
CFH Y402H (N = 802)				
T T (N = 362)	5.74 (0.93)	3.60 (0.81)	1.59 (0.39)	1.21 (0.56)
T C (N = 346)	5.82 (0.99)	3.67 (0.85)	1.61 (0.41)	1.19 (0.52)
C C (N = 94)	5.82 (1.11)	3.63 (0.99)	1.59 (0.38)	1.31 (0.65)
*P value**,†	*0.51*	*0.53*	*0.81*	*0.17*
ARMS2 A69S (N = 736)				
G G (N = 475)	5.79 (0.96)	3.60 (0.81)	1.59 (0.39)	1.21 (0.56)
G T (N = 234)	5.75 (0.98)	3.67 (0.85)	1.61 (0.41)	1.19 (0.52)
T T (N = 27)	5.56 (1.18)	3.63 (0.99)	1.59 (0.38)	1.31 (0.65)
*P value**,†	*0.46*	*0.53*	*0.81*	*0.17*

Abbreviations: TC: Total cholesterol; TG: Triglycerides;
*ANOVA or Student t-tests were performed for means comparison;
†Statistically significant p-value <0.0055 (Bonferroni corrected, P = 0.05/9 = 0.0055).

Table 3. Statin and fibrate drug use according to genetic characteristics in subjects of the Alienor study (N = 825).

	Statin*		**Fibrates†**	
	No (N = 507)	**Yes (N = 318)**	**No (N = 663)**	**Yes (N = 162)**
	N (%)	**N (%)**	**N (%)**	**N (%)**
ApoE2 (N = 815)	(N = 500)	(N = 315)	(N = 656)	(N = 159)
No allele E2 (N = 711)	427 (85.4)	284 (90.2)	569 (86.7)	142 (89.3)
At least 1 allele E2 (N = 104)	73 (14.6)	31 (9.8)	87 (13.3)	17 (10.7)
P value‡,§	*0.05*		*0.38*	
ApoE4 (N = 815)	(N = 500)	(N = 315)	(N = 656)	(N = 159)
No allele E4 (N = 670)	432 (86.4)	238 (75.6)	544 (82.9)	126 (79.2)
At least 1 allele E4 (N = 145)	68 (13.6)	77 (24.4)	112 (17.1)	33 (20.8)
P value‡,§	*<0.0001*		*0.28*	
LPL rs12678919 (N = 714)	(N = 437)	(N = 277)	(N = 580)	(N = 134)
A A (N = 531)	323 (73.9)	208 (75.1)	430 (74.1)	101 (75.4)
A G (N = 170)	105 (24.0)	65 (23.5)	139 (24.0)	31 (23.1)
G G (N = 13)	9 (2.1)	4 (1.4)	11 (1.9)	2 (1.5)
P value‡,§	*0.82*		*0.93*	
CETP rs3764261 (N = 719)	(N = 440)	(N = 279)	(N = 585)	(N = 134)
C C (N = 377)	225 (51.1)	152 (54.5)	309 (52.8)	68 (50.8)
A C (N = 287)	177 (40.2)	110 (39.4)	228 (39.0)	59 (44.0)
A A (N = 55)	38 (8.6)	17 (6.1)	48 (8.2)	7 (5.2)
P value‡,§	*0.40*		*0.36*	
LIPC rs493258 (N = 736)	(N = 452)	(N = 284)	(N = 599)	(N = 137)
C C (N = 215)	130 (28.8)	85 (29.9)	184 (30.7)	31 (22.6)
T C (N = 352)	217 (48.0)	135 (47.5)	280 (46.7)	72 (52.5)
T T (N = 169)	105 (23.2)	64 (22.5)	135 (22.5)	34 (24.8)
P value‡,§	*0.94*		*0.17*	
LIPC rs10468017 (N = 723)	(N = 443)	(N = 280)	(N = 588)	(N = 135)
C C (N = 375)	230 (51.9)	145 (51.8)	311 (52.9)	64 (47.4)
T C (N = 289)	175 (39.5)	114 (40.7)	228 (38.8)	61 (45.2)
T T (N = 59)	38 (8.6)	21 (7.5)	49 (8.3)	10 (7.4)
P value‡,§	*0.86*		*0.39*	
ABCA1 rs1883025 (N = 736)	(N = 452)	(N = 284)	(N = 599)	(N = 137)
C C (N = 390)	247 (54.6)	143 (50.3)	315 (52.6)	75 (54.8)
C T (N = 290)	173 (38.3)	116 (40.8)	238 (39.7)	51 (37.2)
T T (N = 57)	32 (7.1)	25 (8.8)	46 (7.7)	11 (8.0)
P value‡,§	*0.46*		*0.86*	
CFH Y402H (N = 802)	(N = 494)	(N = 308)	(N = 643)	(N = 159)
T T (N = 362)	226 (45.7)	136 (44.2)	284 (44.2)	78 (49.1)
T C (N = 346)	218 (41.6)	128 (41.6)	281 (43.7)	65 (40.9)
C C (N = 94)	50 (14.3)	44 (14.3)	78 (12.1)	16 (10.1)
P value‡,§	*0.20*		*0.50*	
ARMS2 A69S (N = 736)	(N = 452)	(N = 284)	(N = 599)	(N = 117)
G G (N = 475)	291 (64.4)	184 (64.8)	390 (65.1)	85 (62.0)
G T (N = 234)	141 (31.2)	93 (32.7)	185 (30.9)	49 (35.8)
T T (N = 27)	20 (4.4)	7 (2.5)	24 (4.0)	3 (2.2)
P value‡,§	*0.37*		*0.37*	

* Use of statin at one examination or more;

†Use of fibrate at one examination or more;

‡χ^2 tests were performed for frequency comparison;

§Statistically significant p-value <0.0055 (Bonferroni corrected, P = 0.05/9 = 0.0055).

Table 4. Associations of AMD with plasma lipids levels in the Alienor study (odds-ratios (OR) and [95% confidence interval (CI)] for 1 mmol/L increase).

			Model 1* (N = 1595 eyes)			Model 2† (N = 1518 eyes)			Model 3‡ (N = 1246 eyes)		
		None	Any AMD	Early AMD	Late AMD	Any AMD	Early AMD	Late AMD	Any AMD	Early AMD	Late AMD
			(n = 410)	(n = 336)	(n = 74)	(n = 376)	(n = 307)	(n = 69)	(n = 308)	(n = 247)	(n = 61)
TC		ref	1.02	1.03	1.00	0.99	0.99	1.01	1.03	1.03	0.99
			[0.88–1.17]	[0.89–1.19]	[0.69–1.46]	[0.86–1.15]	[0.85–1.15]	[0.69–1.50]	[0.88–1.21]	[0.88–1.21]	[0.68–1.45]
	P value§		*0.81*	*0.71*	*0.98*	*0.93*	*0.88*	*0.94*	*0.69*	*0.70*	*0.97*
LDL		ref	0.93	0.96	0.86	0.91	0.92	0.86	0.93	0.93	0.88
			[0.79–1.10]	[0.81–1.13]	[0.57–1.30]	[0.77–1.08]	[0.77–1.10]	[0.55–1.36]	[0.78–1.12]	[0.78–1.12]	[0.59–1.32]
	P value§		*0.40*	*0.60*	*0.47*	*0.28*	*0.36*	*0.53*	*0.47*	*0.47*	*0.55*
HDL		ref	1.84	1.77	2.41	1.83	1.71	2.58	2.29	2.45	1.58
			[1.29–2.63]	[1.22–2.57]	[1.03–5.64]	[1.25–2.70]	[1.15–2.54]	[0.95–7.05]	[1.46–3.59]	[1.54–3.90]	[0.48–5.17]
	P value§		*0.0008*	*0.003*	*0.04*	*0.002*	*0.008*	*0.06*	*0.0003*	*0.0002*	*0.45*
TG		ref	0.87	0.85	0.92	0.86	0.83	0.96	0.85	0.79	1.30
			[0.67–1.13]	[0.65–1.11]	[0.49–1.71]	[0.64–1.14]	[0.62–1.11]	[0.47–1.97]	[0.62–1.17]	[0.56–1.12]	[0.48–3.52]
	P value§		*0.30*	*0.24*	*0.78*	*0.28*	*0.21*	*0.90*	*0.33*	*0.19*	*0.61*

Abbreviations: AMD: age-related macular degeneration; TC: Total cholesterol; TG: Triglycerides;
*adjusted for age and gender;
†adjusted for age, gender, educational level, smoking, BMI, hypertension, hypolipidemic drug, cardiovascular disease, and diabetes;
‡adjusted for age, gender, educational level, smoking, BMI, hypertension, hypolipidemic drug, cardiovascular disease, diabetes, ApoE2, ApoE4, CFH Y402H, ARMS2 A69S, LIPC(rs10468017), LIPC(rs493258) LPL, ABCA1 and CETP polymorphisms;
§Statistically significant p-value <0.0125 (Bonferroni corrected, $P = 0.05/4 = 0.0125$).

higher HDL remained significantly associated with an increased risk of early (OR = 1.71, P = 0.008) or any AMD (OR = 1.83, P = 0.002) and tended to be associated with increased risk of late AMD, but did not reach statistical significance (OR = 2.58, P = 0.06) especially after Bonferroni correction. No associations were found for any stage of AMD with TC, LDL and TG levels and statin and fibrate drug use.

After further adjustment for all relevant genetic polymorphisms (apoE2, ApoE4, CFH Y402H, ARMS2 A69S, LIPC rs10468017, LIPC rs493258, LPL rs12678919, ABCA1 rs1883025 and CETP rs3764261), higher HDL remained significantly associated with an increased risk of early (OR = 2.45, P = 0.0002) or any AMD (OR = 2.29, P = 0.0003). Association with late AMD was far from statistical significance (OR = 1.58, p = 0.45). No associations were found for any stage of AMD with TC, LDL and TG levels and statin and fibrate drug use (Table 5).

No significant interactions were found between plasma lipid levels and genetic polymorphisms, or between plasma lipid levels and lipid-lowering medication use, with regard to the risk for AMD, suggesting that genetic background and use of lipid-lowering medication do not modify the association of plasma lipid levels with AMD (data not shown).

Discussion

In the present study, after full adjustment, elevated HDL was significantly associated with an increased risk of any and early AMD, independent of many potential confounders, including the major genetic polymorphisms involved in the risk for AMD. Results for late AMD were in the same direction, but far from statistical significance. No associations were found for any stage of AMD with other plasma lipids as well as statin or fibrate drug use.

Our results are consistent with findings of several previous studies which did not adjust for genetic polymorphisms. In cross-sectional studies, high HDL concentration was associated with early AMD in the Beaver Dam study [28]; with soft drusen in the POLA study [26] and with AMD in the Oklahoma Indians population AMD [25]. In a case-control study, Hyman *et al* reported a positive association between HDL and neovascular AMD (OR of highest quintile vs. lowest quintile serum HDL, 2.3; 95%CI, 1.1–4.7) [27]. In the prospective Rotterdam study, HDL was associated with an increased incidence of any AMD [31]. In the Beaver Dam study, higher HDL at baseline was associated with the 10 year incidence of geographic atrophy (RR per 10 mg/dl HDL cholesterol, 1.29; 95% CI, 1.05–1.58; P = 0.01) [30].

Data from other studies have been inconsistent regarding the association between HDL and AMD. In the Blue Mountains Eye Study, there was no significant cross-sectional association of HDL with geographic atrophy (OR: 0.82; 95%CI: 0.19–3.46), or exudative macular degeneration (OR: 1.73; 95%CI: 0.83–3.62) [37], whereas elevated HDL was associated with a decreased 5-years incidence of late AMD (RR per standard deviation increase, 0.74; 95% CI, 0.56–0.99) [34]. In the Beaver Dam study Offspring study, higher HDL was associated with lower risk of early AMD (OR per 5 mg.dl:0.91, 95%CI: 0.83–0.998) [32]. In a case control study, Nowak *et al* found a significant decrease of HDL concentration in AMD patients in comparison with controls, supported by the findings of Reynolds *et al.* where elevated HDL was associated with a reduced risk of late AMD (P<0.05), especially for the neovascular form (P = 0.03) [23,33]. The pooled data from the Beaver Dam, the Blue Mountains and the Rotterdam studies showed no significant associations between HDL and incident AMD [38]. The cross sectional study of the Singapore Malay Eye Study (SiMES) found no significant

Table 5. Associations of AMD with statin and fibrate drug use in the Alienor study (odds-ratios (OR) and [95% confidence interval (CI)] for 1 mmol/L increase).

	None	Model 1* (N = 1595 eyes)			Model 2† (N = 1518 eyes)			Model 3‡ (N = 1246 eyes)		
		Any AMD	Early AMD	Late AMD	Any AMD	Early AMD	Late AMD	Any AMD	Early AMD	Late AMD
		(n = 410)	(n = 336)	(n = 74)	(n = 376)	(n = 307)	(n = 69)	(n = 308)	(n = 247)	(n = 61)
Statin use‖	ref	0.99	1.01	0.78	1.05	1.10	0.68	1.16	1.22	0.72
		[0.75–1.32]	[0.75–1.36]	[0.41–1.49]	[0.77–1.44]	[0.79–1.53]	[0.33–1.38]	[0.80–1.70]	[0.82–1.81]	[0.31–1.70]
P value#		*0.96*	*0.95*	*0.45*	*0.75*	*0.57*	*0.29*	*0.43*	*0.33*	*0.46*
Fibrates useβ	ref	1.24	1.32	0.97	1.26	1.36	0.95	1.44	1.50	1.32
		[0.89–1.73]	[0.93–1.86]	[0.43–2.15]	[0.89–1.80]	[0.94–1.96]	[0.41–2.24]	[0.96–2.17]	[0.98–2.29]	[0.50–3.52]
P value#		*0.20*	*0.11*	*0.93*	*0.20*	*0.10*	*0.92*	*0.08*	*0.06*	*0.58*

Abbreviations: AMD: age-related macular degeneration;
*adjusted for age and gender;
†adjusted for age, gender, educational level, smoking, BMI, hypertension, HDL, LDL, triglycerides, cardiovascular disease, and diabetes;
‡adjusted for age, gender, educational level, smoking, BMI, hypertension, HDL, LDL, triglycerides, cardiovascular disease, diabetes, ApoE2, ApoE4, CFH Y402H, ARMS2 A69S, LIPC(rs10468017), LIPC(rs493258) LPL, ABCA1 and CETP polymorphisms;
‖Use of statin at one examination or more;
#Statistically significant p-value <0.025 (Bonferroni corrected, P = 0.05/2 = 0.025);
βUse of fibrate at one examination or more.

associations between HDL and early (OR per mmol/l: 1.14; 95%CI: 0.72–1.82) or late AMD (OR per mmol/l: 0.42; 95%CI: 0.10–1.80) [35]. Similarly, a meta-analysis did not report significant associations between HDL and late AMD for prospective cohort studies (RR: 1.00; 95%CI: 0.97–1.02) as well as cross sectional studies (OR: 1.06; 95%CI: 0.80–1.39) or case-control study (RR: 3.35; 95%CI: 0.92–12.23) [36].

In the present study, no statistically significant associations of AMD with TC, LDL or TG were found. Findings on cholesterol have been inconsistent in the literature. Some studies reported that elevated total cholesterol concentration was associated with an increased risk of AMD [23,33,39–42]. In contrast, few studies found a significant inverse relation between total serum cholesterol and AMD [47,48] while numerous other studies reported no significant association [26,27,30,32,35,36,43–45]. Few studies reported an increased risk of AMD with high level of LDL [23,33,38,58] and TG [58].

We found no association between statin or fibrate drug use and AMD. In the literature, the association between the use of cholesterol-lowering medications and AMD has been intensively studied. Again, the results have been inconsistent. Several studies suggested a protective effect of statins use on the AMD risk [59–66] while many others reported either no protective effect [26,40,67–75] or even further a potential deleterious role [76,77]. Finally, recent reviews reported that available data on RCT or prospective studies are insufficient to conclude that statins exhibit any role in preventing or delaying the onset or progression of AMD [78,79].

The reasons underlying these inconsistencies are not clearly understood. A difficulty in the interpretation of the positive relationship between elevated HDL and AMD is that plasma lipids concentrations may not reflect tissue-specific effects. Indeed, results obtained with multiple biochemical, histochemical, and ultrastructural methods, mainly performed by Cristina Curcio's team, suggest that RPE secretes apolipoprotein B (ApoB)-lipoprotein particles of unusual composition into BrM, where they accumulate with age eventually forming a lipid wall that is a precursor of basal linear deposit [9,24]. In addition, an accumulation of oxidized ApoB100 lipoproteins in BrM, drusen and basal deposits have been observed in AMD. In atherosclerosis, the oxidation of ApoB100 lipoproteins lead to mainly innate immune system-mediated inflammation which initiates a cascade of pathological events ending with the formation of atherosclerotic plaques [24]. Thus, the oxidized ApoB100 in BrM have been suggested to initiate inflammation, innate immune response and drusen formation sharing with the "response to retention" hypothesis of atherosclerosis [24]. In this hypothesis, the retention of cholesterol-rich, atherogenic lipoproteins provokes a cascade of responses that lead to disease in a previously non-lesional artery. Similarly, it has been suggested that in AMD, the retention of a sub-endothelial apolipoprotein B may lead to the formation of AMD lesion [24]. However, this theory does not exclude the potential contribution of lipoprotein synthesized in the liver or in intestine transported by bloodstream [10].

The increasing number of studies associating high HDL with increased risk for AMD suggests the possibility of a real relationship between high HDL and AMD, which might be due to a dysfunction of HDL. Recent findings on strategies to reduce cardiovascular risk turned attention to HDL quality (the HDL functional capability such as anti-oxidative, anti-inflammatory, anti-apoptotic, anti-infectious or anti-thrombotic functions of HDL) rather than quantity. Some studies suggested that plasma HDL concentrations do not predict functionality and composition of HDL [80] and may be a potential factor of conflicting results in the literature [81]. Indeed, HDL are highly heterogeneous in structure (density, size, charge and protein) and biologic function [80]. The anti-oxidant and anti-inflammatory activities of HDL can become ineffective due to inflammation and other factors such as myeloperoxidase-mediated oxidation. Consequently, HDL may turn into dysfunctional, pro-inflammatory and pro-oxidant particles that promote LDL oxidation and impair cholesterol efflux and reverse cholesterol transport [80,81]. Thus, recent studies suggested that testing functionality, composition (such as concentration of HDL subfractions) and anti-inflammatory properties of HDL will be better markers than testing plasma HDL concentration for identifying subjects at risk for coronary heart disease [81,82]. Briefly, HDL subclasses can be classified by their density (HDL2, HDL3), their size (2a, 2b, 3a, 3b, 3c) their charge (pre-β, α, pre-α) and their main apolipoprotein content (apoA-I or both apoA1 and apoA-II) [81]. Under dyslipidaemic conditions, changes in HDL subfraction levels and functions are currently observed. HDL2 and more particularly HDL2b seem to be more predictive of coronary heart disease risk than HDL or HDL3 [81]. Accordingly, it has been reported that, HDL2b levels are lower in subjects with coronary artery disease compared to healthy subjects and inversely related to disease severity and progression of coronary lesions. Furthermore, the concentration of pre-β-particles has been found to increase in subjects with coronary artery and heart diseases and with myocardial infarction. Inversely, the levels of large α1- and pre-α particles have been reported to decrease in subjects with coronary heart disease in comparison with healthy subjects [81]. To our knowledge, no such studies have been conducted in the field of AMD.

One strength of the present study is that major potential confounding factors were taken into account, including socio-demographic status, factors related to vascular diseases, use of lipid-lowering medications and the major genetic polymorphisms. Indeed, regarding genetic polymorphism, GWAS studies of AMD identified new loci that were associated with blood lipids and particularly HDL levels [83,84]. Most of the variants discovered affected blood lipid levels and are also associated with coronary artery disease [84]. In the present study, the association of AMD with HDL remained significant after taking these polymorphisms into account and no interactions of HDL concentration with genetic polymorphisms were identified.

One limitation of our study could come from the representativeness of the sample. The Alienor subsample tends to over-represent younger subjects and high socioeconomic status, among subjects participating to the 3C Study [49]. The individuals included in this study may accordingly be healthier and present different lifestyles, mainly concerning their diet and physical activity, in comparison with the general population. The distribution of vascular characteristics or the prevalence of eye diseases may have been affected due to these differences. However, participants from the 3C Study which were included in the Alienor study were not different from those who were not included for most parameters of interest in our study [49]. Moreover, as described previously [49], the age- and gender-specific prevalence rates of AMD in the Alienor study were similar to those observed in other studies performed in Europe [2,85] and other industrialized countries [3]. Data collection was performed in the same way in all individuals irrespective of their AMD stage and photograph graders had no access to data related to plasma lipids, or any other cardiovascular or genetic characteristics. Consequently, we can assume that the error was not differential and was unlikely to have biased the estimation of any of the associations of AMD with vascular parameters.

Another limitation of our study is the relatively small number of late AMD cases, which may have induced insufficient statistical power for detecting some associations with serum lipids concentrations (in particular for HDL, which presented a tendency to an increased risk for late AMD, but did not reach statistical significance).

Lastly, a potential limitation is the high number of comparisons performed. Therefore, we cannot exclude that some of the observed associations were due to chance finding. However, we adjusted for this by using Bonferroni correction with many associations remaining highly significant. In addition our findings are mostly consistent with previous studies in this field.

In conclusion, our results suggest that elderly patients with high HDL concentration may be at increased risk for AMD. This association might reflect HDL dysfunction in AMD. In accordance with the field of cardiovascular diseases, epidemiological studies are needed on the associations of AMD with HDL subfractions and functions, in order to better understand the potential role of lipid metabolism, and in particular of cholesterol reverse transport, in AMD.

Author Contributions

Conceived and designed the experiments: MND JFK MBR JFD PBG CD. Performed the experiments: MND JFK MBR JFD PBG CD. Analyzed the data: ACG MLG CD. Contributed reagents/materials/analysis tools: MND JFK MBR JFD PBG CD. Wrote the paper: ACG CD. Revised the manuscript for important intellectual content: MND JFK MBR MLG JFD PBG CD.

References

1. Resnikoff S, Pascolini D, Etya'ale D, Kocur I, Pararajasegaram R, et al. (2004) Global data on visual impairment in the year 2002. Bull World Health Organ 82: 844–851.
2. Augood CA, Vingerling JR, de Jong PT, Chakravarthy U, Seland J, et al. (2006) Prevalence of age-related maculopathy in older Europeans: the European Eye Study (EUREYE). Arch Ophthalmol 124: 529–535.
3. Friedman DS, O'Colmain BJ, Munoz B, Tomany SC, McCarty C, et al. (2004) Prevalence of age-related macular degeneration in the United States. Arch Ophthalmol 122: 564–572.
4. Lim LS, Mitchell P, Seddon JM, Holz FG, Wong TY (2012) Age-related macular degeneration. Lancet 379: 1728–1738.
5. Bretillon L, Acar N, Seeliger MW, Santos M, Maire MA, et al. (2008) ApoB100,LDLR−/− mice exhibit reduced electroretinographic response and cholesteryl esters deposits in the retina. Invest Ophthalmol Vis Sci 49: 1307–1314.
6. Curcio CA, Johnson M, Rudolf M, Huang JD (2011) The oil spill in ageing Bruch membrane. Br J Ophthalmol 95: 1638–1645.
7. Fliesler SJ, Bretillon L (2010) The ins and outs of cholesterol in the vertebrate retina. J Lipid Res 51: 3399–3413.
8. Kishan AU, Modjtahedi BS, Martins EN, Modjtahedi SP, Morse LS (2011) Lipids and age-related macular degeneration. Surv Ophthalmol 56: 195–213.
9. Curcio CA, Johnson M, Huang JD, Rudolf M (2010) Apolipoprotein B-containing lipoproteins in retinal aging and age-related macular degeneration. J Lipid Res 51: 451–467.
10. Wang L, Clark ME, Crossman DK, Kojima K, Messinger JD, et al. (2010) Abundant lipid and protein components of drusen. PLoS One 5: e10329.
11. Souied EH, Benlian P, Amouyel P, Feingold J, Lagarde JP, et al. (1998) The epsilon4 allele of the apolipoprotein E gene as a potential protective factor for exudative age-related macular degeneration. Am J Ophthalmol 125: 353–359.
12. Thakkinstian A, Bowe S, McEvoy M, Smith W, Attia J (2006) Association between apolipoprotein E polymorphisms and age-related macular degeneration: A HuGE review and meta-analysis. Am J Epidemiol 164: 813–822.
13. Mahley RW, Rall SC, Jr. (2000) Apolipoprotein E: far more than a lipid transport protein. Annu Rev Genomics Hum Genet 1: 507–537.
14. Loane E, McKay GJ, Nolan JM, Beatty S (2010) Apolipoprotein E genotype is associated with macular pigment optical density. Invest Ophthalmol Vis Sci 51: 2636–2643.
15. Chen W, Stambolian D, Edwards AO, Branham KE, Othman M, et al. (2010) Genetic variants near TIMP3 and high-density lipoprotein-associated loci influence susceptibility to age-related macular degeneration. Proc Natl Acad Sci U S A 107: 7401–7406.
16. Conley YP, Thalamuthu A, Jakobsdottir J, Weeks DE, Mah T, et al. (2005) Candidate gene analysis suggests a role for fatty acid biosynthesis and regulation of the complement system in the etiology of age-related maculopathy. Hum Mol Genet 14: 1991–2002.
17. Kanda A, Chen W, Othman M, Branham KE, Brooks M, et al. (2007) A variant of mitochondrial protein LOC387715/ARMS2, not HTRA1, is strongly associated with age-related macular degeneration. Proc Natl Acad Sci U S A 104: 16227–16232.
18. Neale BM, Fagerness J, Reynolds R, Sobrin L, Parker M, et al. (2010) Genome-wide association study of advanced age-related macular degeneration identifies a role of the hepatic lipase gene (LIPC). Proc Natl Acad Sci U S A 107: 7395–7400.
19. Scholl HP, Fleckenstein M, Charbel Issa P, Keilhauer C, Holz FG, et al. (2007) An update on the genetics of age-related macular degeneration. Mol Vis 13: 196–205.
20. Yates JR, Sepp T, Matharu BK, Khan JC, Thurlby DA, et al. (2007) Complement C3 variant and the risk of age-related macular degeneration. N Engl J Med 357: 553–561.
21. Yu Y, Reynolds R, Fagerness J, Rosner B, Daly MJ, et al. (2011) Association of variants in the LIPC and ABCA1 genes with intermediate and large drusen and advanced age-related macular degeneration. Invest Ophthalmol Vis Sci 52: 4663–4670.
22. Merle BM, Maubaret C, Korobelnik JF, Delyfer MN, Rougier MB, et al. Association of HDL-related loci with age-related macular degeneration and plasma lutein and zeaxanthin: the Alienor Study. PLoS One in press.
23. Reynolds R, Rosner B, Seddon JM (2010) Serum lipid biomarkers and hepatic lipase gene associations with age-related macular degeneration. Ophthalmology 117: 1989–1995.
24. Ebrahimi KB, Handa JT (2011) Lipids, lipoproteins, and age-related macular degeneration. J Lipids 2011: 802059.
25. Butt AL, Lee ET, Klein R, Russell D, Ogola G, et al. (2011) Prevalence and risks factors of age-related macular degeneration in Oklahoma Indians: the Vision Keepers Study. Ophthalmology 118: 1380–1385.
26. Delcourt C, Michel F, Colvez A, Lacroux A, Delage M, et al. (2001) Associations of cardiovascular disease and its risk factors with age-related macular degeneration: the POLA study. Ophthalmic Epidemiol 8: 237–249.
27. Hyman L, Schachat AP, He Q, Leske MC (2000) Hypertension, cardiovascular disease, and age-related macular degeneration. Age-Related Macular Degeneration Risk Factors Study Group. Arch Ophthalmol 118: 351–358.
28. Klein R, Klein BE, Franke T (1993) The relationship of cardiovascular disease and its risk factors to age-related maculopathy. The Beaver Dam Eye Study. Ophthalmology 100: 406–414.
29. Klein R, Klein BE, Jensen SC (1997) The relation of cardiovascular disease and its risk factors to the 5-year incidence of age-related maculopathy: the Beaver Dam Eye Study. Ophthalmology 104: 1804–1812.
30. Klein R, Klein BE, Tomany SC, Cruickshanks KJ (2003) The association of cardiovascular disease with the long-term incidence of age-related maculopathy: the Beaver Dam Eye Study. Ophthalmology 110: 1273–1280.
31. van Leeuwen R, Klaver CC, Vingerling JR, Hofman A, van Duijn CM, et al. (2004) Cholesterol and age-related macular degeneration: is there a link? Am J Ophthalmol 137: 750–752.
32. Klein R, Cruickshanks KJ, Nash SD, Krantz EM, Nieto FJ, et al. (2010) The prevalence of age-related macular degeneration and associated risk factors. Arch Ophthalmol 128: 750–758.
33. Nowak M, Swietochowska E, Marek B, Szapska B, Wielkoszynski T, et al. (2005) Changes in lipid metabolism in women with age-related macular degeneration. Clin Exp Med 4: 183–187.
34. Tan JS, Mitchell P, Smith W, Wang JJ (2007) Cardiovascular risk factors and the long-term incidence of age-related macular degeneration: the Blue Mountains Eye Study. Ophthalmology 114: 1143–1150.
35. Cackett P, Wong TY, Aung T, Saw SM, Tay WT, et al. (2008) Smoking, cardiovascular risk factors, and age-related macular degeneration in Asians: the Singapore Malay Eye Study. Am J Ophthalmol 146: 960–967 e961.
36. Chakravarthy U, Wong TY, Fletcher A, Piault E, Evans C, et al. (2010) Clinical risk factors for age-related macular degeneration: a systematic review and meta-analysis. BMC Ophthalmol 10: 31.
37. Smith W, Mitchell P, Leeder SR, Wang JJ (1998) Plasma fibrinogen levels, other cardiovascular risk factors, and age-related maculopathy: the Blue Mountains Eye Study. Arch Ophthalmol 116: 583–587.
38. Tomany SC, Wang JJ, Van Leeuwen R, Klein R, Mitchell P, et al. (2004) Risk factors for incident age-related macular degeneration: pooled findings from 3 continents. Ophthalmology 111: 1280–1287.

39. The Eye Disease Case-Control study-Goup(1992) Risk factors for neovascular age-related macular degeneration. The Eye Disease Case-Control Study Group. Arch Ophthalmol 110: 1701–1708.
40. Hogg RE, Woodside JV, Gilchrist SE, Graydon R, Fletcher AE, et al. (2008) Cardiovascular disease and hypertension are strong risk factors for choroidal neovascularization. Ophthalmology 115: 1046–1052 e1042.
41. Mitchell P, Wang JJ, Foran S, Smith W (2002) Five-year incidence of age-related maculopathy lesions: the Blue Mountains Eye Study. Ophthalmology 109: 1092–1097.
42. Ulas F, Balbaba M, Ozmen S, Celebi S, Dogan U (2013) Association of dehydroepiandrosterone sulfate, serum lipids, C-reactive protein and body mass index with age-related macular degeneration. Int Ophthalmol.
43. Buch H (2005) Fourteen-year incidence of age-related maculopathy and cause-specific prevalence of visual impairment and blindness in a Caucasian population: the Copenhagen City Eye Study. Acta Ophthalmol Scand 83: 400–401.
44. Blumenkranz MS, Russell SR, Robey MG, Kott-Blumenkranz R, Penneys N (1986) Risk factors in age-related maculopathy complicated by choroidal neovascularization. Ophthalmology 93: 552–558.
45. Sanders TA, Haines AP, Wormald R, Wright LA, Obeid O (1993) Essential fatty acids, plasma cholesterol, and fat-soluble vitamins in subjects with age-related maculopathy and matched control subjects. Am J Clin Nutr 57: 428–433.
46. Tsang NC, Penfold PL, Snitch PJ, Billson F (1992) Serum levels of antioxidants and age-related macular degeneration. Doc Ophthalmol 81: 387–400.
47. Klein R, Clegg L, Cooper LS, Hubbard LD, Klein BE, et al. (1999) Prevalence of age-related maculopathy in the Atherosclerosis Risk in Communities Study. Arch Ophthalmol 117: 1203–1210.
48. Klein R, Klein BE, Marino EK, Kuller LH, Furberg C, et al. (2003) Early age-related maculopathy in the cardiovascular health study. Ophthalmology 110: 25–33.
49. Delcourt C, Korobelnik JF, Barberger-Gateau P, Delyfer MN, Rougier MB, et al. (2010) Nutrition and age-related eye diseases: the ALIENOR (Antioxydants, Lipides Essentiels, Nutrition et maladies OculaiRes) Study. Journal Nutr Health Aging 14(10): 854–861.
50. 3C Study Group(2003) Vascular factors and risk of dementia: design of the Three-City Study and baseline characteristics of the study population. Neuroepidemiology 22: 316–325.
51. Bird AC, Bressler NM, Bressler SB, Chisholm IH, Coscas G, et al. (1995) An international classification and grading system for age-related maculopathy and age-related macular degeneration. The International ARM Epidemiological Study Group. Surv Ophthalmol 39: 367–374.
52. Klein R, Klein BE, Knudtson MD, Wong TY, Cotch MF, et al. (2006) Prevalence of age-related macular degeneration in 4 racial/ethnic groups in the multi-ethnic study of atherosclerosis. Ophthalmology 113: 373–380.
53. Centre National Hospitalier d'Information sur le Médicament(CNHIM). Theriaque Web site. Available: https://www.theriaque.org. Accessed February 1, 2013.
54. Baird PN, Richardson AJ, Robman LD, Dimitrov PN, Tikellis G, et al. (2006) Apolipoprotein (APOE) gene is associated with progression of age-related macular degeneration (AMD). Hum Mutat 27: 337–342.
55. Delcourt C, Delyfer MN, Rougier MB, Amouyel P, Colin J, et al. (2011) Associations of Complement Factor H and smoking with early age-related macular degeneration: the ALIENOR study. Invest Ophthalmol Vis Sci.
56. Seddon JM, Francis PJ, George S, Schultz DW, Rosner B, et al. (2007) Association of CFH Y402H and LOC387715 A69S with progression of age-related macular degeneration. JAMA 297: 1793–1800.
57. Zeger SL, Liang KY, Albert PS (1988) Models for longitudinal data: a generalized estimating equation approach. Biometrics 44: 1049–1060.
58. Davari MH, Gheitasi H, Yaghobi G, Heydari B (2012) Correlation between Serum Lipids and Age-related Macular Degeneration: A Case-Control Study. J Res Health Sci 13: 98–101.
59. Hall NF, Martyn CN (2002) Could statins prevent age-related macular degeneration? Expert Opin Pharmacother 3: 803–807.
60. McCarty CA, Mukesh BN, Guymer RH, Baird PN, Taylor HR (2001) Cholesterol-lowering medications reduce the risk of age-related maculopathy progression. Med J Aust 175: 340.
61. Wilson HL, Schwartz DM, Bhatt HR, McCulloch CE, Duncan JL (2004) Statin and aspirin therapy are associated with decreased rates of choroidal neovascularization among patients with age-related macular degeneration. Am J Ophthalmol 137: 615–624.
62. McGwin G, Jr., Owsley C, Curcio CA, Crain RJ (2003) The association between statin use and age related maculopathy. Br J Ophthalmol 87: 1121–1125.
63. Friedman E, Rigas IK, Makar K (2005) The relationship of statin use to the development of age-related macular degeneration. IOVS 46: 199.
64. McGwin G, Jr., Xie A, Owsley C (2005) The use of cholesterol-lowering medications and age-related macular degeneration. Ophthalmology 112: 488–494.
65. Tan JS, Mitchell P, Rochtchina E, Wang JJ (2007) Statins and the long-term risk of incident age-related macular degeneration: the Blue Mountains Eye Study. Am J Ophthalmol 143: 685–687.
66. Drobek-Slowik M, Karczewicz D, Safranow K, Jakubowska K, Chlubek D (2008) [Use of statins as a form of protection against age-related macular degeneration (AMD)]. Klin Oczna 110: 50–54.
67. Klein R, Klein BE, Jensen SC, Cruickshanks KJ, Lee KE, et al. (2001) Medication use and the 5-year incidence of early age-related maculopathy: the Beaver Dam Eye Study. Arch Ophthalmol 119: 1354–1359.
68. Klein R, Klein BE, Tomany SC, Danforth LG, Cruickshanks KJ (2003) Relation of statin use to the 5-year incidence and progression of age-related maculopathy. Arch Ophthalmol 121: 1151–1155.
69. van Leeuwen R, Vingerling JR, Hofman A, de Jong PT, Stricker BH (2003) Cholesterol lowering drugs and risk of age related maculopathy: prospective cohort study with cumulative exposure measurement. BMJ 326: 255–256.
70. Smeeth L, Cook C, Chakravarthy U, Hubbard R, Fletcher AE (2005) A case control study of age related macular degeneration and use of statins. Br J Ophthalmol 89: 1171–1175.
71. McGwin G, Jr., Modjarrad K, Hall TA, Xie A, Owsley C (2006) 3-hydroxy-3-methylglutaryl coenzyme a reductase inhibitors and the presence of age-related macular degeneration in the Cardiovascular Health Study. Arch Ophthalmol 124: 33–37.
72. Klein R, Knudtson MD, Klein BE (2007) Statin use and the five-year incidence and progression of age-related macular degeneration. Am J Ophthalmol 144: 1–6.
73. Kaiserman N, Vinker S, Kaiserman I (2009) Statins do not decrease the risk for wet age-related macular degeneration. Curr Eye Res 34: 304–310.
74. Maguire MG, Ying GS, McCannel CA, Liu C, Dai Y (2009) Statin use and the incidence of advanced age-related macular degeneration in the Complications of Age-related Macular Degeneration Prevention Trial. Ophthalmology 116: 2381–2385.
75. Shalev V, Sror M, Goldshtein I, Kokia E, Chodick G (2011) Statin use and the risk of age related macular degeneration in a large health organization in Israel. Ophthalmic Epidemiol 18: 83–90.
76. Etminan M, Brophy JM, Maberley D (2008) Use of statins and angiotensin converting enzyme inhibitors (ACE-Is) and the risk of age-related macular degeneration: nested case-control study. Curr Drug Saf 3: 24–26.
77. VanderBeek BL, Zacks DN, Talwar N, Nan B, Stein JD (2013) Role of statins in the development and progression of age-related macular degeneration. Retina 33: 414–422.
78. Peponis V, Chalkiadakis SE, Bonovas S, Sitaras NM (2010) The controversy over the association between statins use and progression of age-related macular degeneration: a mini review. Clin Ophthalmol 4: 865–869.
79. Gehlbach P, Li T, Hatef E (2012) Statins for age-related macular degeneration. Cochrane Database Syst Rev 3: CD006927.
80. G HB, Rao VS, Kakkar VV (2011) Friend Turns Foe: Transformation of Anti-Inflammatory HDL to Proinflammatory HDL during Acute-Phase Response. Cholesterol 2011: 274629.
81. Eren E, Yilmaz N, Aydin O (2012) High Density Lipoprotein and it's Dysfunction. Open Biochem J 6: 78–93.
82. Fisher EA, Feig JE, Hewing B, Hazen SL, Smith JD (2012) High-density lipoprotein function, dysfunction, and reverse cholesterol transport. Arterioscler Thromb Vasc Biol 32: 2813–2820.
83. Kathiresan S, Willer CJ, Peloso GM, Demissie S, Musunuru K, et al. (2009) Common variants at 30 loci contribute to polygenic dyslipidemia. Nat Genet 41: 56–65.
84. Teslovich TM, Musunuru K, Smith AV, Edmondson AC, Stylianou IM, et al. (2010) Biological, clinical and population relevance of 95 loci for blood lipids. Nature 466: 707–713.
85. Vingerling JR, Dielemans I, Hofman A, Grobbee DE, Hijmering M, et al. (1995) The prevalence of age-related maculopathy in the Rotterdam Study. Ophthalmology 102: 205–210.

Synthesis and Propagation of Complement C3 by Microglia/Monocytes in the Aging Retina

Matt Rutar[1]*, Krisztina Valter[1,2], Riccardo Natoli[1,2], Jan M. Provis[1,2]

1 The John Curtin School of Medical Research, The Australian National University (ANU), Canberra, Australian Capital Territory, Australia, **2** ANU Medical School, The Australian National University (ANU), Canberra, Australian Capital Territory, Australia

Abstract

Introduction: Complement activation is thought to contribute to the pathogenesis of age-related macular degeneration (AMD), which may be mediated in part by para-inflammatory processes. We aimed to investigate the expression and localization of C3, a crucial component of the complement system, in the retina during the course of aging.

Methods: SD rats were born and reared in low-light conditions, and euthanized at post-natal (P) days 100, 450, or 750. Expression of C3, IBA1, and Ccl- and Cxcl- chemokines was assessed by qPCR, and *in situ* hybridization. Thickness of the ONL was assessed in retinal sections as a measure of photoreceptor loss, and counts were made of C3-expressing monocytes.

Results: C3 expression increased significantly at P750, and correlated with thinning of the ONL, at P750, and up-regulation of GFAP. *In situ* hybridization showed that C3 was expressed by microglia/monocytes, mainly from within the retinal vasculature, and occasionally the ONL. The number of C3-expressing microglia increased significantly by P750, and coincided spatiotemporally with thinning of the ONL, and up-regulation of Ccl- and Cxcl- chemokines.

Conclusions: Our data suggest that recruited microglia/monocytes contribute to activation of complement in the aging retina, through local expression of C3 mRNA. C3 expression coincides with age-related thinning of the ONL at P750, although it is unclear whether the C3-expressing monocytes are a cause or consequence. These findings provide evidence of activation of complement during natural aging, and may have relevance to cellular events underling the pathogenesis of age-related retinal diseases.

Editor: Erica Lucy Fletcher, The University of Melbourne, Australia

Funding: Funding provided by Australian Research Council Centres of Excellence Program Grant (CE0561903). The funders had no role in study design, data collection and analysis, decision to publish, or preparation of the manuscript.

Competing Interests: The authors have declared that no competing interests exist.

* E-mail: matt.rutar@anu.edu.au

Introduction

Aging involves the gradual accumulation of changes associated with a heightened vulnerability to various diseases [1,2]. Age-related macular degeneration (AMD) is a leading cause of blindness in people aged over 65 [3], with estimated worldwide prevalence of 30 to 50 million [4] which is expected to increase substantially in coming decades [5]. Involvement of inflammatory processes in the pathogenesis of AMD has been steadily accruing for many years [6,7,8,9,10,11]. In recent times, identification of involvement of the complement system has firmly placed inflammation as a key factor influencing the onset and progression of AMD [12,13].

The complement system is a component of the innate immune response providing a rapid host defence against a range of immunological challenges, and aiding in the maintenance of homeostasis (Reviewed in [14,15]). Despite this beneficial function, a pathogenic role of the complement system in AMD has been revealed through a string of seminal gene association studies. These identified a significant association between the Y402H sequence variant in the regulatory gene complement factor H (CFH) with the incidence of AMD [16,17,18,19], along with other susceptibility variants in complement pathway genes C2 [12,20], CFB [12,20], and the central component C3 [21,22,23,24,25] in later studies. However, a number of key aspects of the disease process remain unclear, including the cellular events that synthesise and promote complement activity in the retina (reviewed in [12]).

Recently, the concept of para-inflammation – a state of low-grade chronic inflammation – has gained considerable attention as a factor in the development of age-related diseases [26,27]. Para-inflammation is thought to occur in tissues under noxious stress, including accumulation of free radicals during aging [1], and acts as an immunological mechanism to maintain tissue homeostasis [26]. However, this response is not stable and in aging persistent factors may promote a chronic dysregulation of para-inflammation, leading to pathology [26,28]. As such, para-inflammation in the aging retina may play a role in the pathology of age-related retinopathies such as AMD [26,28]. Significantly, expression of various complement components, including C3, has been shown to increase with age in mice [28], although the cellular mechanisms which mediate the elevation of complement in aging are presently unknown [28].

In previous studies we have used a rat model of retinal light damage to gain an understanding of how the retina responds to damage, specifically the expression and localisation of inflammatory mediators from complement and chemokine pathways [29,30,31,32]. These investigations have shown – for the first time – that retinal monocytes/microglia synthesise C3 and deposit it in the outer retina during damage [30]. In the current study, we aim to describe the normal aging process in rats of the same strain as used in our light damage model, in order to clarify the factors which may promote chronic complement synthesis. Our results show that C3 mRNA is expressed by microglia/monocytes in the retina which gradually increase in number over the course of normal aging. This coincides spatiotemporally with thinning of the ONL at P750 and up-regulation of chemokines with age, although the casual role C3-expressing monocytes/microglia in these processes is unclear. These data inform our understanding of complement activity in the context of normal aging of the retina in our model, and may also provide insight into the complement-related processes in diseases such as AMD.

Methods

Rearing Conditions, Tissue Collection and Processing

The study was approved by the Animal Experimentation Ethics Committee (AEEC) of the Australian National University (R.BSB.05.10). All experiments conducted were in accordance with the ARVO Statement for the Use of Animals in Ophthalmic and Vision Research. Sprague-Dawley (SD) rats were born and reared in low-light conditions (5 lux) for 100, 450, or 750 post-natal days (P), with food and water provided *ad libitum.*

At the appropriate age, animals were euthanized by overdose of barbiturate administered by an intraperitoneal injection (60 mg/kg bodyweight, Valabarb; Virbac, Australia) which also included 2% lidocaine (Troy Laboratories, NSW, Australia) to minimize animal suffering. The left eye from each animal was marked at the superior surface for orientation then enucleated and processed for cryosectioning, while the retina from right eye was excised through a corneal incision and prepared for RNA extraction. Eyes collected for cryosectioning were quickly immersion-fixed in 4% paraformaldehyde in 0.1 M PBS (pH 7.3) for 3 hours at room temperature, then processed as described previously [31], and cryosectioned at 16 µm. Retinas for RNA extraction were immediately immersed in chilled RNAlater solution (Ambion, Austin, TX), then stored in accordance with the manufacturer's instructions. The RNA samples were then extracted and analysed following a previously established methodology [29,33].

Quantitative Real Time Polymerase Chain Reaction (qPCR)

Quantitative PCR was used to measure expression of C3, 6 chemokines, and two house-keeping genes (Table 1). First-strand cDNA synthesis was performed as described previously [29]. Gene amplification was measured using commercially available Taq-Man hydrolysis probes (Applied Biosystems, Foster City, CA), the details of which are provided in Table 1. The hydrolysis probes were applied in accordance with a previously established qPCR protocol [29]. The fold change was determined using the $\Delta\Delta C_q$ method where the expression of the target gene was normalised relative to the expression of two reference genes – glyceraldehyde-3-phosphate dehydrogenase (GAPDH), and Actin beta (Actb). Previous studies have shown that expression of GAPDH and Actb does not change with respect to age in either the retina or brain [34,35]. Amplification specificity of each primer pair was assessed using gel electrophoresis.

ONL Thickness Measurements

Thickness of the ONL was used to measure photoreceptor loss in each age group. ONL thickness was measured in 1 mm increments along the full-length of retinal cryosections cut in the para-saggital plane (superio-inferior), close to the vertical meridian. The DNA-specific dye bisbenzamide (Calbiochem, La Jolla, CA) was used to visualize the cellular layers. ONL thickness was calculated as the ratio of ONL thickness to the distance between the outer- and inner- limiting membranes (OLM-ILM), to take into account any obliquely cut sections or regions. The total ONL ratio from each retina is the average of 3 retina sections at comparable locations.

In situ Hybridisation

To investigate localisation of C3 mRNA transcripts, a digoxygenin-conjugated riboprobe to C3 was generated for *in situ* hybridisation on cryosections of retinal tissue, as described in a previous study conducted by our group [30]. Synthesis of the C3 riboprobe and *In situ* hybridisation were performed in accordance with methodology described previously [36]; the C3 riboprobe was hybridised overnight at 57°C, and then washed in saline sodium citrate (pH 7.4) at 60°C. The bound probe was visualised with NBT/BCIP (Nitro blue tetrazolium/5-Bromo-4-chloro-3-indolyl

Table 1. Taqman® probes used.

Gene Symbol	Gene Name	Catalogue	Entrez Gene ID
Actb	Actin, beta	Rn00667869_m1	NM_031144.2
C3	Complement component 3	Mm00437858_m1	NM_009778.2
Ccl2	Chemokine (C-C motif) ligand 2	Rn01456716_g1	NM_031530.1
Ccl3	Chemokine (C-C motif) ligand 3	Rn00564660_m1	NM_013025.2
Ccl4	Chemokine (C-C motif) ligand 4	Rn00587826_m1	NM_053858.1
Ccl7	Chemokine (C-C motif) ligand 7	Rn01467286_m1	NM_001007612.1
Cxcl10	Chemokine (C-X-C motif) ligand 10	Rn01413889_g1	NM_139089.1
Cxcl11	Chemokine (C-X-C motif) ligand 11	Rn00788262_g1	NM_182952.2
Gapdh	Glyceraldehyde-3-phosphate dehydrogenase	Rn99999916_s1	NM_017008.3
Gfap	Glial fibrillary acidic protein	Rn00566603_m1	NM_017009.2

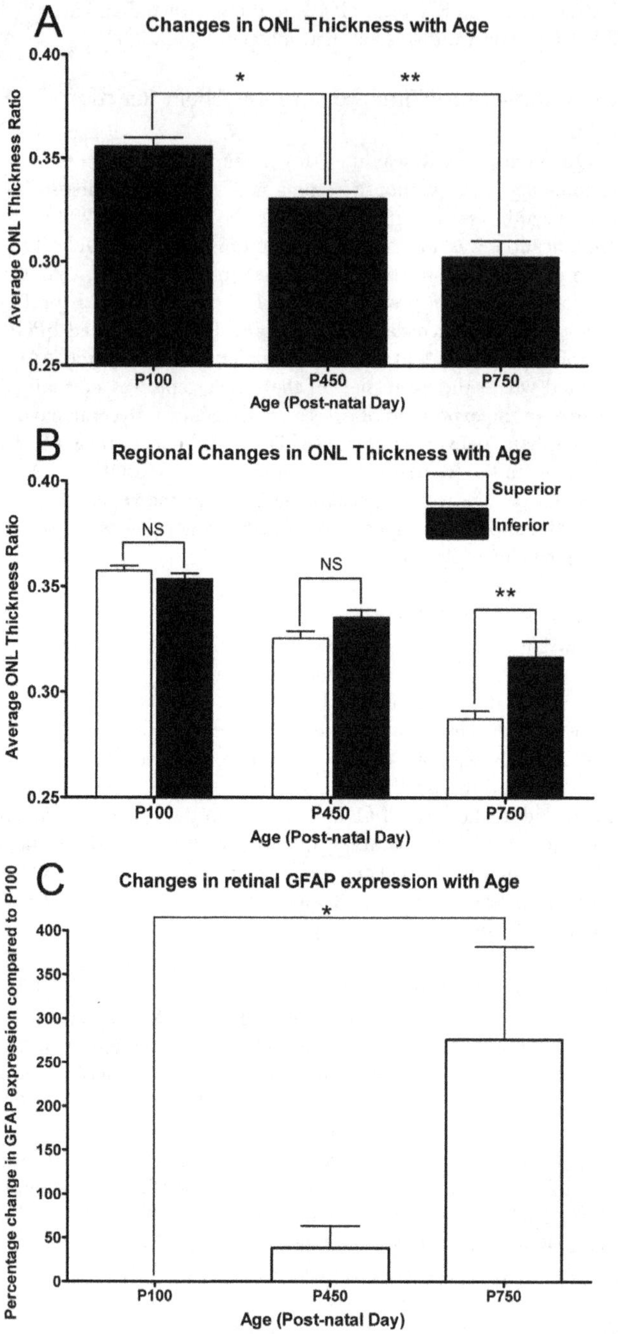

Figure 1. Quantification of ONL thickness and GFAP expression with respect to age. A: The thickness of the ONL decreased progressively throughout the aging time course, and was markedly reduced by P750 ($P<0.05$). **B:** Regional variation in ONL thickness was not observed at P100 and P450 age-groups across the vertical meridian ($P>0.05$). At P750, the greater thinning was observed in the superior retina than the inferior (<0.05). **C:** The expression of GFAP was found to increase at P450, however this was not significant compared to P100 ($P>0.05$). At P750 a 276% increase was observed in the expression of GFAP, compared to P100 ($P<0.05$). P100 n = 3, P450 n = 3, P750 n = 3; error bars represent SEM. '*' denotes a significant change using ANOVA with Tukey's post-test where $P<0.05$, '**' denotes $P<0.01$.

phosphate), which was followed by a counterstain using standard immunohistochemical labelling for either IBA1 or isolectin B_4 (described further in 'immunohistochemistry') as required.

Immunohistochemistry

Cryosections from each treatment group were used for immunohistochemical analysis, using an antibody against IBA1 (1:500, Cat# 019-19741; Wako, Osaka, Japan). Blood vessels were visualised using an isolectin B_4 stain, conjugated to FITC (1:100, Cat# L2895; Sigma-Aldrich, St. Louis, MO). Immunohistochemistry was performed using methodology previously described [29]. Immunofluorescence was viewed using a Zeiss laser scanning microscope, and acquired using PASCAL software (Zeiss, v4.0). Images were enhanced for publication using Adobe Photoshop software, which was standardised between images.

Quantification of C3-expressing Cells

Counts of C3-expressing cells were performed on retinal cryosections stained for C3 using *in situ* hybridisation (as described above); identification of these C3-expressing cells as monocytes/microglia was confirmed in a previous investigation by our group [30]. Counts of C3-expressing cells were carried out along the full-length of retinal sections cut in the para-saggital plane (supero-inferior) close to the vertical meridian, in adjacent fields measuring 1 mm across. The counts of C3-expressing cells were grouped according to their localisation in either the retinal vasculature, ONL, or choroidal vasculature. The total number of C3-expressing cells from each retina is the average of 3 sections at comparable locations.

Statistical Analysis

Statistical analysis was performed using the one-way ANOVA with Tukey's multiple comparison post-test, or the unpaired Student's t-test. For each analysis, differences with a P value <0.05 were considered statistically significant.

Results

Quantification of ONL Thickness and GFAP Expression with Age

The average thickness of the ONL gradually reduced throughout the aging timecourse (Figure 1A). ONL thickness decreased significantly by P450, compared to animals aged P100 ($P<0.05$). At P750, the ONL was significantly thinner than both P450 and P100 age-groups ($P<0.05$). Additionally, there was regional variation in the rate of ONL thinning, between superior and inferior retina, as a function of age (Figure 1B). At P450 superior retina shows a trend towards being thinner than inferior retina, but the difference is not significant ($P>0.05$). However, in P750 animals, the superior portion of the retina was significantly thinner than inferior retina ($P<0.05$).

We also detected modulation of the stress-marker GFAP over the aging timecourse (Figure 1C). Expression of GFAP increased significantly to 276% by P750 compared to P100 ($P<0.05$). Although the expression of GFAP at P450 also showed a tentative increase compared to P100, this proved to be highly inconsistent, and was not significant in relation to either P100 or P750 age groups.

Differential Expression and Localisation of C3 in the Retina

Using qPCR, the differential expression of C3 in the retina was assessed over the age timecourse (Figure 2). The expression of C3 did not change appreciably between animals aged P100, and those aged P450 (8.3%, $P>0.05$). At P750 however, the expression of C3 was significantly increased, reaching a differential expression of 264.3%, relative to animals aged P100 ($P<0.05$).

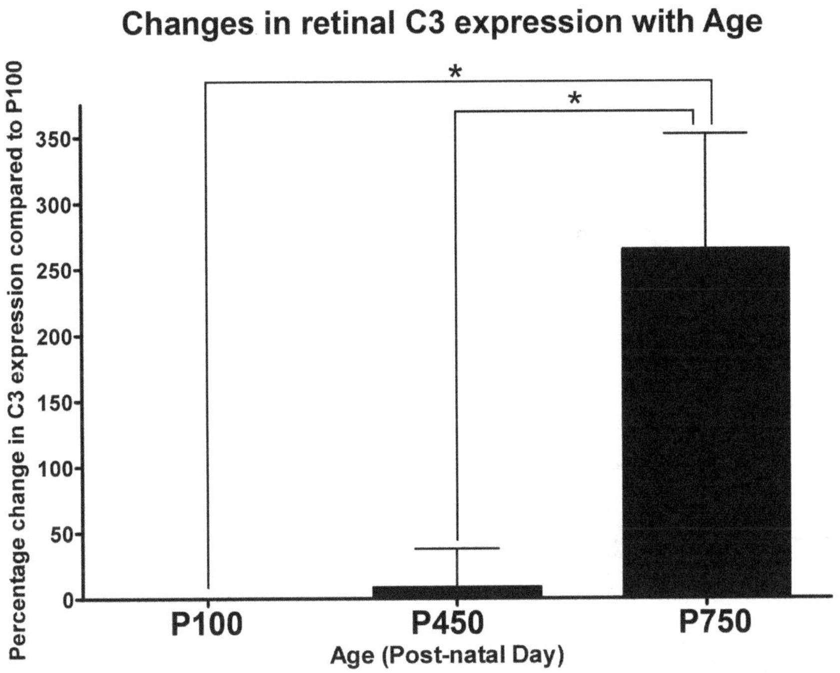

Figure 2. Expression of C3 in the neural retina by qPCR over the aging timecourse. No appreciable difference was observed in the expression of C3 between P100 and P450 age groups (P>0.05). By P750 there was a robust 264.3% increase in the expression of C3, compared to P100 and P450 (P<0.05). P100 n = 3, P450 n = 3, P750 n = 3; error bars represent SEM. '*' denotes a significant change using ANOVA with Tukey's post-test where P<0.05.

Localisation of C3 expression in the retina was assessed with *in situ* hybridisation over the aging timecourse (Figures 3, 4 and 5). *In situ* hybridisation was preferred over immunohistochemistry for this purpose, since the propensity of C3 protein to be deposited on activating surfaces may lead to false-positive observations. C3 mRNA was expressed in the aging retina by cells immunoreactive for the monocyte/microglia marker IBA1 (Figure 5A–I), consistent with our previous findings in a light-induced model of retinal degeneration [30]. Staining for C3 mRNA was evident within the cytoplasm of cells, which was often clustered in small process-like ramifications (Figure 5A–C, G–I; Arrows). Few C3-expressing cells were detected at P100, close to zero per retina (Figure 3, histogram); this was not significantly changed at P450 (0.6 per retina, P>0.05). However, by P750 the number of C3-expressing cells had significantly increased to 11.6 per retina, P<0.05 (Figure 3A–H, and histogram). The distribution of C3-expressing cells in superior and inferior retina is shown in Figure 4, histogram A. In P100 and P450 animals C3-expressing cells were evenly distributed across superior and inferior retina. At P750 however, C3-expressing cells were far more numerous in the superior portion of the retina than the inferior (9.7 and 2.1 respectively, P< 0.05).

The increased numbers of C3-expressing cells were mainly associated with the retinal vasculature (P<0.05) (Figure 4, histogram B), although there was also a modest increase in C3-expressing cells the ONL and subretinal space (P<0.05, Figure 4, histogram B). In general, C3-expressing cells were not observed in the choroid; rather, C3-expressing cells were mainly located in-and-around the retinal blood vessels at P750, in a pattern consistent with vascular cuffing (Figure 3A–C, D–E, F–G). C3-expressing cells were also detected at P750 in the optic nerve (Figure 6A, D–E) and at the optic nerve head (Figure 6B–C), in the ciliary body in association with the pars plicata (Figure 6G) and at the border of the pars plana and retina (Figure 6H, I–J).

Expression of Ccl- and Cxcl- Chemokines in the Retina

In general, expression of Ccl2, Ccl3, Ccl4, Ccl7 (Figure 7A), and Cxcl10, Cxcl11 (Figure 7B) did not change significantly in P450 animals, compared those aged P100 (P>0.05), with the exception of Cxcl11 (43.7%, P<0.05). While there was some evidence of an increase in Ccl2 expression at P450 (134.9%), it was variable between animals and not statistically significant (P>0.05). By P750 however, significant increases expression of all Ccl- and Cxcl- chemokines examined was detected compared to P100 (P> 0.05), the most highly upregulated being Ccl2 (195.6%) and Cxcl10 (665.0%).

Discussion

The current study contributes to an understanding of complement activation in normal aging of the retina through several key aspects. Primarily, we show using in situ hybridisation, that IBA1-positive microglia/monocytes are a source of C3 mRNA in the aging retina, and are found associated primarily with the retinal vasculature as well as in the ONL at P750. We also find IBA1-positive C3-expressing cells beyond the retinal margins within the ciliary body, and in the optic nerve head in the aged retinas. In addition, we show that increased numbers of C3-expressing cells coincide spatiotemporally with increased expression of chemokines (Ccl- and Cxcl-), up-regulation of GFAP, and follow the initial thinning of the ONL. However, the role of C3-expressing monocytes/microglia in relation to these features of the aging process remains unclear.

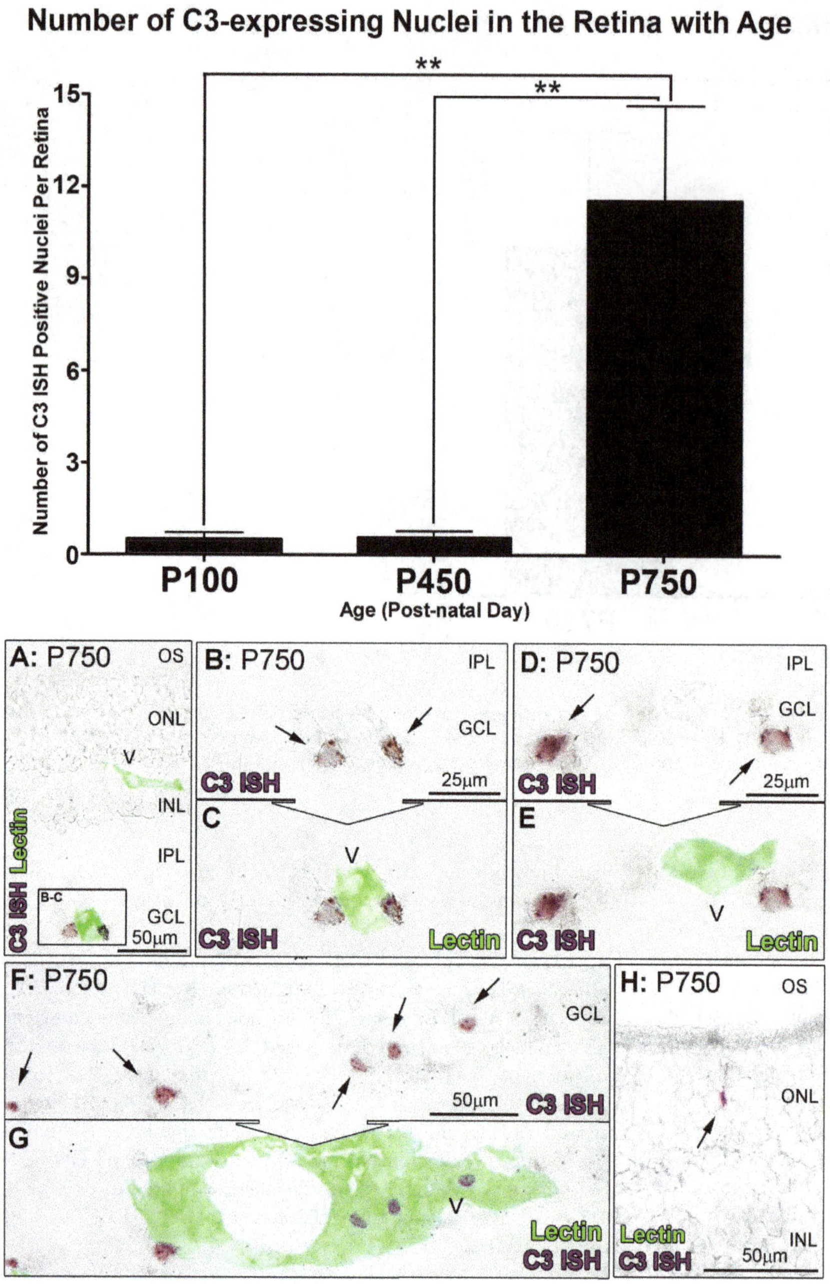

Figure 3. ***In situ* hybridisation for C3 mRNA in the retina with respect to age. A–F:** Representative images show *In situ* hybridisation for C3 mRNA (purple) and vessels (lectin staining, green) in the retina. In retinas from P750, expression of C3 was apparent in cells (A, C, E, arrows) closely associated with vessels from the retinal vasculature stained with lectin (B, D, E). **H:** Staining for C3 was also occasionally observed among cells situated in the ONL (arrow). **Histogram:** Quantification of C3-expressing cells per retina showed no significant change at P450 compared to P100 (0.6 per retina, $P>0.05$). At P750, C3-expressing cells increased significantly ($P<0.05$) to 11.6 per retina compared to both P100 and P450 groups. P100 n = 3, P450 n = 3, P750 n = 3; error bars represent SEM. '*' denotes a significant change using ANOVA with Tukey's post-test where $P<0.05$, '**' denotes $P<0.01$. V, retinal blood vessel; INL, inner nuclear layer; IPL, inner plexiform layer; GCL, ganglion cell layer; ONL, outer nuclear layer; OS, outer segments.

Complement Activity and Normal Aging of the Retina

Several investigations have previously described increased expression of complement components mRNAs – including C3– in the retinas of mice aged 20–24 months, compared to those aged 3 months [28,37]. In this study we show, for the first time, that a source of C3 mRNA in the aging retina is from increased numbers of IBA1-immunoreactive microglia/monocytes located in the retinal vasculature and in the ONL. We find that these cells accumulate preferentially in superior retina at P750 at the site of maximal thinning of the ONL, and in spatiotemporal correlation with the location of the *area centralis* of the rat retina (see [31,38]) – a homologue of the human macula. Similarly, age-related thinning of the ONL, and up-regulation of GFAP have been characterised in several human studies [39,40,41]. These findings from the normally aging rat retina are also consistent with our previous findings from younger rats of the same strain using a retinal light-

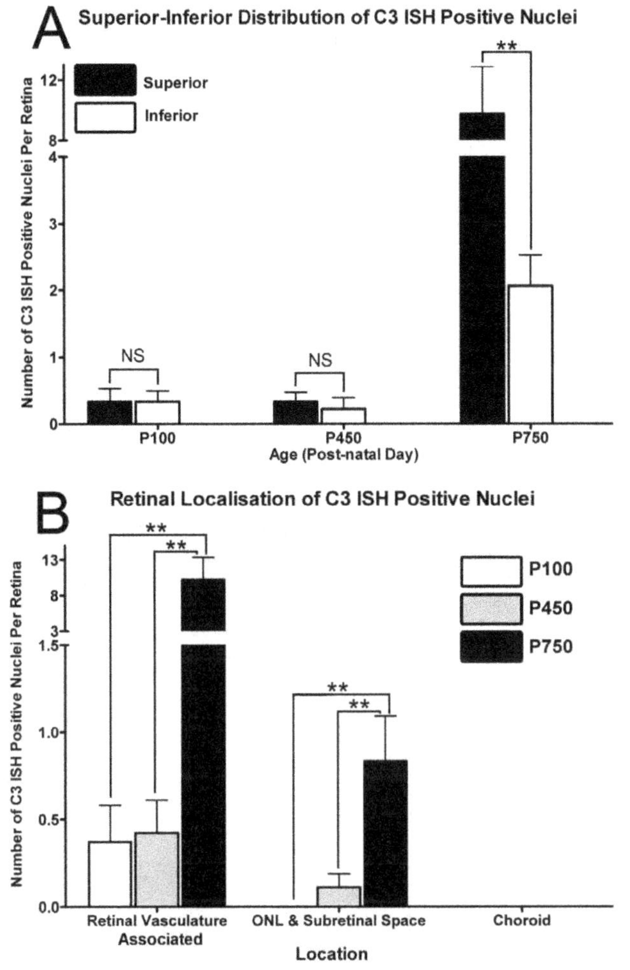

Figure 4. Distribution of *In situ* hybridisation for C3 mRNA in the over the aging timecourse. A: C3-expressing cells were evenly distributed across superior and inferior retina P100 and P450 animals ($P>0.05$). At P750, C3-expressing cells were more numerous in the superior portion of the retina than the inferior (9.7 and 2.1 respectively, $P<0.05$). **B:** Increases in C3-expressing cells were predominately associated with the retinal vasculature at P750 ($P<0.05$), with more modest increases apparent in the ONL and subretinal space over the same period ($P<0.05$). P100 n = 3, P450 n = 3, P750 n = 3; error bars represent SEM. '*' denotes a significant change using ANOVA with Tukey's post-test where $P<0.05$, '**' denotes $P<0.01$.

damage model, in which C3-expressing monocytes appear in the superior retina at the locus of damage [30]. It should be noted however that the number of animals in the current study was relatively small, which is primarily attributed to the difficulties in rearing a large cohort to an advanced age such as P750. Nevertheless, the data are sufficiently robust and significant, and are in agreement with previous findings [28].

C3 is a key complement component that drives activation of all three pathways (reviewed in [15]). While activation of complement has beneficial properties including promoting the clearance of debris [14,42,43,44], immune complexes [15,45,46,47], and apoptotic cells [48,49,50,51], it may also exacerbate degeneration if activated in an inappropriate manner. Such activation is implicated in various neurodegenerative disorders, as well as ischemia- and trauma-related injuries (reviewed in [44,52,53]). In the retina, recent experimental evidence indicates that copious synthesis of C3 is detrimental, in that a C3-expressing adenovirus transfected into mice retinas promotes degeneration of RPE and photoreceptors [54]. Such degeneration may be accelerated by the ablation of CFH, which spurs increased deposition of C3 in the outer retina of aged mice, as well as reduced retinal function [55]. Whether the accumulation of C3-expressing cells, as observed here, are a causative factor in the age-related thinning of the ONL, or a stress-related consequence of this phenomenon, is unclear. Nevertheless, increased synthesis of C3 by an accumulation of microglia/monocytes with age is likely to contribute to a propensity for increased complement activity in the retinal environment.

Origins of C3-expressing Cells in the Aging Retina

The origin of the C3-expressing microglia/monocytes, and the avenue of their accumulation in the retina, remains uncertain. In this study we observe C3-expressing cells in and around the retinal vasculature, and at the both the ciliary margin and in the optic nerve. In particular, this distribution is consistent with recruitment of non-intrinsic, bone-marrow (BM)-derived monocytes into the retina, in findings garnered from several studies. Chimeric mice stressed by either *N*-methyl-*N*-nitrosourea (MNU) injection, retinal detachment, or light damage, have observed that BM-derived cells migrate into the retina along the retinal vasculature via the ciliary margin and optic disc, and are recruited to the ONL and subretinal space at the locus of damage [56,57]. This distribution is also consistent with our understanding of the development of microglial populations in the retina [58]. Taken together, the striking similarity of these findings do suggest that *at least some* C3-expressing cells may be recruited BM-derived cells. However, we cannot discount the possibility that the C3-expressing cells include resident microglia, in which C3-expression has been induced by a parainflammatory environment. Further studies are needed to confirm these observations, using chimeras, parabiosis, or methods of monocyte depletion.

It is possible that escalation of complement activation in the aging retina, as indicated by increased C3 expression in the current study, is driven by aberrant para-inflammatory processes stimulated by the aging retinal environment (reviewed in [26]). Oxidative stress is a commonly accepted consequence of aging, and increases in markers such as oxidative low density lipoprotein and dinitrophenylated proteins have been observed in the retinas of aged mice [26]. Moreover, several investigations have demonstrated that complement activation may be stimulated by oxidative by-products. Mice immunized with the oxidative damage by-product CEP develop retinal degeneration and show increased deposition of complement C3 in the outer retina [59,60]. Studies have also shown that RPE cultures exposed to photo-oxidative stress or oxidized photoreceptor outer segments have reduced expression of the complement regulatory gene CFH [61,62]. Activation and deposition of complement may also be stimulated in microglia by increases in age-related deposits such as lipofuscin (reviewed in [63]). Recent evidence *in vitro* suggests that accumulation of lipofuscin/A2E in microglial cells promotes activation of complement, by simultaneously reducing synthesis of the complement inhibitor CFH while increasing expression of CFB [64].

Increases in C3-expressing monocytes/microglia in the aging retina are also likely to be stimulated by the increased expression of chemokines in the aging retina. Our data show that expression of both Ccl- and Cxcl- chemokines is up-regulated by P750, and is correlated with increases in C3-expressing cells. Previous micro-array analysis of aged retinas have also reported increased expression of the chemokines Ccl2, Ccl3, and Ccl12 in 20

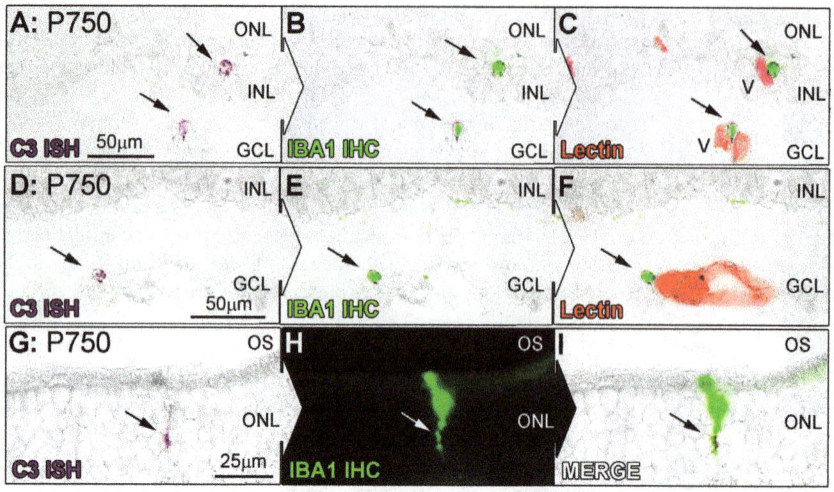

Figure 5. Co-immunolabeling of C3-expressing cells (purple) for IBA1 (green) at P750. A–I: Representative images at P750 show *In situ* hybridisation for C3 mRNA, IBA1 immunoreactivity, and lectin staining (red) for retinal vasculature in the retina. C3 staining (A, D, arrows) was found to correlate strongly with IBA1-immunoreactive microglia/monocytes (B, E, arrows), which were in close association with both superficial and deep retinal vasculature (C, F, arrows). C3-expressing cells in the ONL (G, arrow) also showed specificity for IBA1-immunreactive microglia at the ONL/OS margin (H,I, arrows). V, retinal blood vessel; INL, inner nuclear layer; GCL, ganglion cell layer; ONL, outer nuclear layer; OS, outer segments.

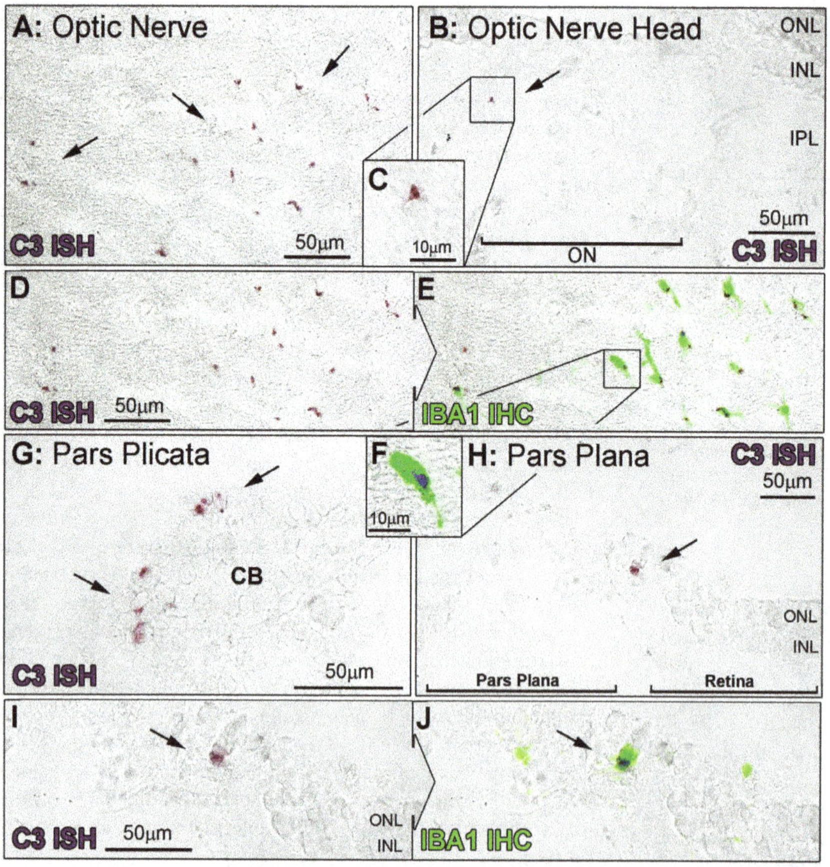

Figure 6. ***In situ*** **hybridisation for C3-expressing cells in the optic nerve and ciliary body.** Representative images demonstrate *In situ* hybridisation for C3 mRNA (purple) and IBA1-immunoreactive microglia/monocytes (green) at the optic nerve (A-F) and ciliary body (G-J), at P750. **A–F:** An abundance of C3-expressing cells were evident in section of the optic nerve tissue (A, arrows), and were immunoreactive for IBA1 (D–F). C3-expressing cells were also occasionally found emerging from the optic nerve head (B–C, arrow). **G–J:** At P750, C3-expressing cells were observed within the ciliary body, including the pars plicata (G, arrows) and the pars plana, particularly at the retinal margin (H, arrow). These cells were also immunoreactive for IBA1 (I–J). CB, ciliary body; V, retinal blood vessel; INL, inner nuclear layer; IPL, inner plexiform layer; ONL, outer nuclear layer.

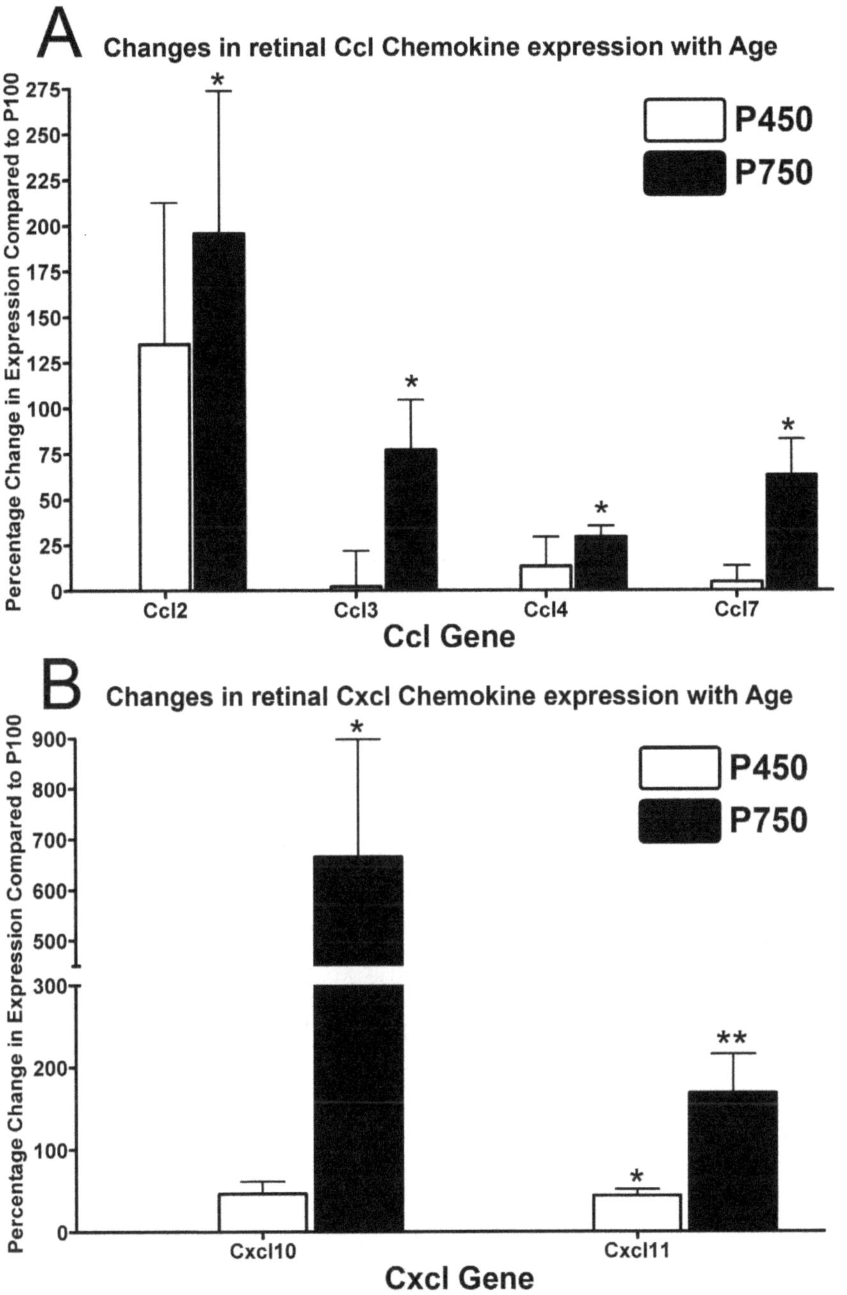

Figure 7. Expression of Ccl- (A) and Cxcl- (B) chemokines in the neural retina by qPCR over the aging timecourse. A: The expression of Ccl2, Ccl3, Ccl4, Ccl7 did not change appreciably in animals aged P450 ($P>0.05$), while a significant up-regulation was observed in P750 animals for all Ccl- genes ($P<0.05$), compared to P100; a large increase in Ccl2 expression was observed at P450, although this was not significant ($P>0.05$). **B:** At P450, there was a small increase in expression of Cxcl11 ($P<0.05$), but not Cxdc10 ($P>0.05$). By P750 there was a considerable increase in the expression of both Cxcl- genes compared to P100, particularly Cxcl10 ($P<0.05$). P100 n = 4, P450 n = 4, P750 n = 4; error bars represent SEM. '*' denotes a significant change using ANOVA with Tukey's post-test where $P<0.05$, '**' denotes $P<0.01$.

month-old mice compared to those aged 3-months [28]. We have recently shown that in the light-induced model of retinal degeneration, suppression of Ccl2 expression with a targeted small-interfering RNA (siRNA) inhibits recruitment of IBA1-positive monocytes/microglia, and reduces photoreceptor death in the retina [32]. Moreover, ablation of Ccl2 impairs the recruitment of BM-derived microglia/monocytes in retinas of in chimeric mice, where subclinical damage and parainflammation are induced by γ-ray irradiation [65].

Relevance to Human Aging and AMD

Advancing age is the most consistent risk factors for AMD (reviewed in [66]). The findings of current study, and others [26], suggest that advancing age and para-inflammation predisposes the retina towards a pro-inflammatory and pro-complement environment, which in turn contributes to the pathogenesis of AMD. The cellular events leading to propagation of complement in the retina are not well understood (reviewed in [12,67]) although it is well established that polymorphisms in a range of complement-related genes are associated with risk of AMD (reviewed in [12]). Moreover, recent findings from a large-scale gene expression study show that human donor eyes with any form of AMD have increased levels of expression of complement genes, including C3 [68]. The present findings from aging rat retina are consistent with those analyses [62], in that both show increases in C3 expression in the neural retina, while the current investigation further identifies monocytes/microglia as a source of this expression in the aging retina.

It is well established that recruitment of microglia/monocytes to the macula is strongly associated with all forms of AMD pathology [10,11,69,70,71,72], and studies in experimental neovascular 'wet' AMD show that inhibition of monocyte recruitment reduces in the size of the neovascular lesion, compared to controls [73,74]. Recent studies utilising AMD donor tissue have demonstrated that monocyte-recruiting chemokines, including Ccl2 and Cxcl10, are up-regulated in all forms of the disease [68]. Moreover, evidence from Sennlaub and colleagues indicates that elevated levels of Ccl2 in atrophic AMD lesions are accompanied by an influx of $Ccr2^{+}$ monocytes [75]. This association is further confirmed in animal models, where suppression of Ccl2 reduces the extent of cell death in both experimental neovascularisation [76] and light-induced degeneration [32,75]. Our current findings, in conjunctions with others [28], also show similar up-regulation of Ccl- and Cxcl-chemokines during normal retinal aging.

Conclusion

Our findings suggest that the expression of C3 increases in the aging rat retina, due to the local synthesis of C3 by monocytes/microglia, and further implicate complement in the progression of retinal degeneration. While low levels of complement activation in the retina may be beneficial to the maintenance of retinal homeostasis, in circumstances of chronic para-inflammation it seems that over-activation may contribute to chronic stress and degeneration. This interpretation is consistent with findings showing that polymorphism in the C3 regulator CFH is associated with increased risk of AMD. Synthesis of C3 by microglia/macrophages and their increasing presence in the degenerating retina implicates them in complement activation in retinal aging. Consequently, modulation of microglial activation may be useful strategy to control detrimental propagation of complement in the aging retina, and in turn retinal degenerations such as AMD.

Author Contributions

Conceived and designed the experiments: MR KV JP. Performed the experiments: MR RN. Analyzed the data: MR JP. Contributed reagents/materials/analysis tools: MR KV RN JP. Wrote the paper: MR JP.

References

1. Harman D (1981) The aging process. Proc Natl Acad Sci U S A 78: 7124–7128.
2. Bonnel S, Mohand-Said S, Sahel JA (2003) The aging of the retina. Exp Gerontol 38: 825–831.
3. Ambati J, Ambati BK, Yoo SH, Ianchulev S, Adamis AP (2003) Age-related macular degeneration: etiology, pathogenesis, and therapeutic strategies. Surv Ophthalmol 48: 257–293.
4. Ambati J (2011) Age-related macular degeneration and the other double helix. The Cogan Lecture. Invest Ophthalmol Vis Sci 52: 2165–2169.
5. Rein DB, Wittenborn JS, Zhang X, Honeycutt AA, Lesesne SB, et al. (2009) Forecasting age-related macular degeneration through the year 2050: the potential impact of new treatments. Arch Ophthalmol 127: 533–540.
6. Penfold PL, Madigan MC, Gillies MC, Provis JM (2001) Immunological and aetiological aspects of macular degeneration. Prog Ret Eye Res 20: 385–414.
7. Penfold PL, Provis JM, Billson FA (1987) Age-related macular degeneration: ultrastructural studies of the relationship of leucocytes to angiogenesis. Graefes Arch Clin Exp Ophthalmol 225: 70–76.
8. Penfold PL, Killingsworth MC, Sarks SH (1985) Senile macular degeneration: the involvement of immunocompetent cells. Graefes Arch Clin Exp Ophthalmol 223: 69–76.
9. Penfold P, Killingsworth M, Sarks S (1984) An ultrastructural study of the role of leucoytes and fibroblasts in the breakdown of Bruch's membrane. Aust J Ophthalmol 12: 23–31.
10. Gupta N, Brown KE, Milam AH (2003) Activated microglia in human retinitis pigmentosa, late-onset retinal degeneration, and age-related macular degeneration. Exp Eye Res 76: 463–471.
11. Cherepanoff S, McMenamin P, Gillies MC, Kettle E, Sarks SH (2009) Bruch's membrane and choroidal macrophages in early and advanced age-related macular degeneration. Br J Ophthalmol 94: 918–925.
12. Anderson DH, Radeke MJ, Gallo NB, Chapin EA, Johnson PT, et al. (2010) The pivotal role of the complement system in aging and age-related macular degeneration: hypothesis re-visited. Prog Retin Eye Res 29: 95–112.
13. Donoso LA, Kim D, Frost A, Callahan A, Hageman G (2006) The role of inflammation in the pathogenesis of age-related macular degeneration. Surv Ophthalmol 51: 137–152.
14. Paidassi H, Tacnet-Delorme P, Garlatti V, Darnault C, Ghebrehiwet B, et al. (2008) C1q binds phosphatidylserine and likely acts as a multiligand-bridging molecule in apoptotic cell recognition. J Immunol 180: 2329–2338.
15. Walport MJ (2001) Complement. Second of two parts. N Engl J Med 344: 1140–1144.
16. Edwards AO, Ritter R, 3rd, Abel KJ, Manning A, Panhuysen C, et al. (2005) Complement factor H polymorphism and age-related macular degeneration. Science 308: 421–424.
17. Klein RJ, Zeiss C, Chew EY, Tsai JY, Sackler RS, et al. (2005) Complement factor H polymorphism in age-related macular degeneration. Science 308: 385–389.
18. Hageman GS, Anderson DH, Johnson LV, Hancox LS, Taiber AJ, et al. (2005) A common haplotype in the complement regulatory gene factor H (HF1/CFH) predisposes individuals to age-related macular degeneration. Proc Natl Acad Sci U S A 102: 7227–7232.
19. Haines JL, Hauser MA, Schmidt S, Scott WK, Olson LM, et al. (2005) Complement factor H variant increases the risk of age-related macular degeneration. Science 308: 419–421.
20. Jakobsdottir J, Conley YP, Weeks DE, Ferrell RE, Gorin MB (2008) C2 and CFB genes in age-related maculopathy and joint action with CFH and LOC387715 genes. PLoS One 3: e2199.
21. Spencer KL, Olson LM, Anderson BM, Schnetz-Boutaud N, Scott WK, et al. (2008) C3 R102G polymorphism increases risk of age-related macular degeneration. Hum Mol Genet 17: 1821–1824.
22. Park KH, Fridley BL, Ryu E, Tosakulwong N, Edwards AO (2009) Complement component 3 (C3) haplotypes and risk of advanced age-related macular degeneration. Invest Ophthalmol Vis Sci 50: 3386–3393.
23. Maller JB, Fagerness JA, Reynolds RC, Neale BM, Daly MJ, et al. (2007) Variation in complement factor 3 is associated with risk of age-related macular degeneration. Nat Genet 39: 1200–1201.
24. Yates JR, Sepp T, Matharu BK, Khan JC, Thurlby DA, et al. (2007) Complement C3 variant and the risk of age-related macular degeneration. N Engl J Med 357: 553–561.
25. Despriet DD, van Duijn CM, Oostra BA, Uitterlinden AG, Hofman A, et al. (2009) Complement component C3 and risk of age-related macular degeneration. Ophthalmology 116: 474–480 e472.
26. Xu H, Chen M, Forrester JV (2009) Para-inflammation in the aging retina. Prog Retin Eye Res 28: 348–368.
27. Medzhitov R (2008) Origin and physiological roles of inflammation. Nature 454: 428–435.
28. Chen M, Muckersie E, Forrester JV, Xu H (2010) Immune activation in retinal aging: a gene expression study. Invest Ophthalmol Vis Sci 51: 5888–5896.
29. Rutar M, Natoli R, Valter K, Provis JM (2011) Early focal expression of the chemokine Ccl2 by Müller cells during exposure to damage-inducing bright continuous light. Invest Ophthalmol Vis Sci 52 (5): 2379–2388.
30. Rutar M, Natoli R, Valter K, Provis JM (2011) Analysis of complement expression in light-induced retinal degeneration: Synthesis and deposition of C3 by microglia/macrophages is associated with focal photoreceptor degeneration. Invest Ophthalmol Vis Sci 52 (8): 5347–5358.
31. Rutar M, Provis JM, Valter K (2010) Brief exposure to damaging light causes focal recruitment of macrophages, and long-term destabilization of photoreceptors in the albino rat retina. Curr Eye Res 35: 631–643.
32. Rutar MV, Natoli RC, Provis JM (2012) Small interfering RNA-mediated suppression of Ccl2 in Muller cells attenuates microglial recruitment and photoreceptor death following retinal degeneration. J Neuroinflammation 9: 221.
33. Natoli R, Provis J, Valter K, Stone J (2008) Gene regulation induced in the C57BL/6J mouse retina by hyperoxia: a temporal microarray study. Mol Vis 14: 1983–1994.

34. Yoshida S, Yashar BM, Hiriyanna S, Swaroop A (2002) Microarray analysis of gene expression in the aging human retina. Invest Ophthalmol Vis Sci 43: 2554–2560.
35. Slagboom PE, de Leeuw WJ, Vijg J (1990) Messenger RNA levels and methylation patterns of GAPDH and beta-actin genes in rat liver, spleen and brain in relation to aging. Mech Ageing Dev 53: 243–257.
36. Cornish EE, Madigan MC, Natoli R, Hales A, Hendrickson AE, et al. (2005) Gradients of cone differentiation and FGF expression during development of the foveal depression in macaque retina. Vis Neurosci 22: 447–459.
37. Ma W, Cojocaru R, Gotoh N, Gieser L, Villasmil R, et al. (2013) Gene expression changes in aging retinal microglia: relationship to microglial support functions and regulation of activation. Neurobiol Aging 34: 2310–2321.
38. Rapp L, Naash M, Wiegand R, et al. (1985) Morphological and biochemical comparisons between retinal regions having differing susceptibility to photoreceptor degeneration. In: LaVail MM, Hollyfield JG, Anderson RE, editors. Retinal Degeneration: Experimental and Clinical Studies: Liss Alan R Inc. 421–437.
39. Gartner S, Henkind P (1981) Aging and degeneration of the human macula. 1. Outer nuclear layer and photoreceptors. Br J Ophthalmol 65: 23–28.
40. Gao H, Hollyfield JG (1992) Aging of the human retina. Differential loss of neurons and retinal pigment epithelial cells. Invest Ophthalmol Vis Sci 33: 1–17.
41. Wu KHC, Madigan MC, Billson F, Penfold PL (2003) Differential expression of GFAP in early v late AMD: a quantitative analysis. Br J Ophthalmol 87: 1159–1166.
42. Sim RB, Kishore U, Villiers CL, Marche PN, Mitchell DA (2007) C1q binding and complement activation by prions and amyloids. Immunobiology 212: 355–362.
43. Gasque P (2004) Complement: a unique innate immune sensor for danger signals. Mol Immunol 41: 1089–1098.
44. Gasque P, Dean YD, McGreal EP, VanBeek J, Morgan BP (2000) Complement components of the innate immune system in health and disease in the CNS. Immunopharmacology 49: 171–186.
45. Davies KA, Schifferli JA, Walport MJ (1994) Complement deficiency and immune complex disease. Springer Semin Immunopathol 15: 397–416.
46. Botto M (1998) C1q knock-out mice for the study of complement deficiency in autoimmune disease. Exp Clin Immunogenet 15: 231–234.
47. Navratil JS, Korb LC, Ahearn JM (1999) Systemic lupus erythematosus and complement deficiency: clues to a novel role for the classical complement pathway in the maintenance of immune tolerance. Immunopharmacology 42: 47–52.
48. Korb LC, Ahearn JM (1997) C1q binds directly and specifically to surface blebs of apoptotic human keratinocytes: complement deficiency and systemic lupus erythematosus revisited. J Immunol 158: 4525–4528.
49. Taylor PR, Carugati A, Fadok VA, Cook HT, Andrews M, et al. (2000) A hierarchical role for classical pathway complement proteins in the clearance of apoptotic cells in vivo. J Exp Med 192: 359–366.
50. Trouw LA, Blom AM, Gasque P (2008) Role of complement and complement regulators in the removal of apoptotic cells. Mol Immunol 45: 1199–1207.
51. Gullstrand B, Martensson U, Sturfelt G, Bengtsson AA, Truedsson L (2009) Complement classical pathway components are all important in clearance of apoptotic and secondary necrotic cells. Clin Exp Immunol 156: 303–311.
52. Ricklin D, Lambris JD (2013) Complement in immune and inflammatory disorders: pathophysiological mechanisms. J Immunol 190: 3831–3838.
53. Brennan FH, Anderson AJ, Taylor SM, Woodruff TM, Ruitenberg MJ (2012) Complement activation in the injured central nervous system: another dual-edged sword? J Neuroinflammation 9: 137.
54. Cashman SM, Desai A, Ramo K, Kumar-Singh R (2011) Expression of complement component 3 (C3) from an adenovirus leads to pathology in the murine retina. Invest Ophthalmol Vis Sci 52: 3436–3445.
55. Coffey PJ, Gias C, McDermott CJ, Lundh P, Pickering MC, et al. (2007) Complement factor H deficiency in aged mice causes retinal abnormalities and visual dysfunction. Proc Natl Acad Sci U S A 104: 16651–16656.
56. Joly S, Francke M, Ulbricht E, Beck S, Seeliger M, et al. (2009) Cooperative phagocytes: resident microglia and bone marrow immigrants remove dead photoreceptors in retinal lesions. Am J Pathol 174: 2310–2323.
57. Kaneko H, Nishiguchi KM, Nakamura M, Kachi S, Terasaki H (2008) Characteristics of bone marrow-derived microglia in the normal and injured retina. Invest Ophthalmol Vis Sci 49: 4162–4168.
58. Diaz-Araya CM, Provis JM, Penfold PL, Billson FA (1995) Development of microglial topography in human retina. J Comp Neurol 363: 53–68.
59. Hollyfield JG (2010) Age-related macular degeneration: the molecular link between oxidative damage, tissue-specific inflammation and outer retinal disease: the Proctor lecture. Invest Ophthalmol Vis Sci 51: 1275–1281.
60. Hollyfield JG, Bonilha VL, Rayborn ME, Yang X, Shadrach KG, et al. (2008) Oxidative damage-induced inflammation initiates age-related macular degeneration. Nat Med 14: 194–198.
61. Chen M, Forrester JV, Xu H (2007) Synthesis of complement factor H by retinal pigment epithelial cells is down-regulated by oxidized photoreceptor outer segments. Exp Eye Res 84: 635–645.
62. Lau LI, Chiou SH, Liu CJ, Yen MY, Wei YH (2011) The effect of photo-oxidative stress and inflammatory cytokine on complement factor H expression in retinal pigment epithelial cells. Invest Ophthalmol Vis Sci 52: 6832–6841.
63. Kennedy CJ, Rakoczy PE, Constable IJ (1995) Lipofuscin of the retinal pigment epithelium: a review. Eye (Lond) 9 (Pt 6): 763–771.
64. Ma W, Coon S, Zhao L, Fariss RN, Wong WT (2012) A2E accumulation influences retinal microglial activation and complement regulation. Neurobiol Aging.
65. Chen M, Zhao J, Luo C, Pandi SP, Penalva RG, et al. (2012) Para-inflammation-mediated retinal recruitment of bone marrow-derived myeloid cells following whole-body irradiation is CCL2 dependent. Glia 60: 833–842.
66. Klein R (2005) Epidemiology of Age-related macular degeneration. In: Penfold P, Provis J, editors. Macular Degeneration. Berlin: Springer-Verlag.
67. Karagianni N, Adamis AP The case for complement and inflammation in AMD: open questions. Adv Exp Med Biol 703: 1–7.
68. Newman AM, Gallo NB, Hancox LS, Miller NJ, Radeke CM, et al. (2012) Systems-level analysis of age-related macular degeneration reveals global biomarkers and phenotype-specific functional networks. Genome Med 4: 16.
69. Patel M, Chan CC (2008) Immunopathological aspects of age-related macular degeneration. Semin Immunopathol 30: 97–110.
70. Ezzat MK, Hann CR, Vuk-Pavlovic S, Pulido JS (2008) Immune cells in the human choroid. Br J Ophthalmol 92: 976–980.
71. Penfold PL, Killingsworth MC, Sarks SH (1986) Senile macular degeneration. The involvement of giant cells in atrophy of the retinal pigment epithelium. Invest Ophthalmol Vis Sci 27: 364–271.
72. Wong J, Madigan M, Billson F, Penfold P (2001) Quantification of leukocyte common antigen (CD45) expression in macular degeneration. Invest Ophthalmol Vis Sci 42: S227.
73. Espinosa-Heidmann DG, Suner IJ, Hernandez EP, Monroy D, Csaky KG, et al. (2003) Macrophage depletion diminishes lesion size and severity in experimental choroidal neovascularization. Invest Ophthalmol Vis Sci 44: 3586–3592.
74. Sakurai E, Anand A, Ambati BK, van Rooijen N, Ambati J (2003) Macrophage depletion inhibits experimental choroidal neovascularization. Invest Ophthalmol Vis Sci 44: 3578–3585.
75. Sennlaub F, Auvynet C, Calippe B, Lavalette S, Poupel L, et al. (2013) CCR2(+) monocytes infiltrate atrophic lesions in age-related macular disease and mediate photoreceptor degeneration in experimental subretinal inflammation in Cx3cr1 deficient mice. EMBO Mol Med 5: 1775–1793.
76. Luhmann UF, Robbie S, Munro PM, Barker SE, Duran Y, et al. (2009) The drusenlike phenotype in aging Ccl2-knockout mice is caused by an accelerated accumulation of swollen autofluorescent subretinal macrophages. Invest Ophthalmol Vis Sci 50: 5934–5943.

21

IKK2 Inhibition Attenuates Laser-Induced Choroidal Neovascularization

Huayi Lu[1,3], Qingxian Lu[1,2], Subhash Gaddipati[1,2], Ramesh Babu Kasetti[1], Wei Wang[1], Manolis Pasparakis[4], Henry J. Kaplan[1], Qiutang Li[1,2]*

1 Departments of Ophthalmology and Visual Sciences, University of Louisville School of Medicine, Louisville, Kentucky, United States of America, **2** James Graham Brown Cancer Center, University of Louisville School of Medicine, Louisville, Kentucky, United States of America, **3** Second Hospital of Jilin University, Changchun, Jilin Province, P.R. China, **4** Institute for Genetics, University of Cologne, Cologne, Germany

Abstract

Choroidal neovascularization (CNV) is aberrant angiogenesis associated with exudative age-related macular degeneration (AMD), a leading cause of blindness in the elderly. Inflammation has been suggested as a risk factor for AMD. The IKK2/NF-κB pathway plays a key role in the inflammatory response through regulation of the transcription of cytokines, chemokines, growth factors and angiogenic factors. We investigated the functional role of IKK2 in development of the laser-induced CNV using either *Ikk2* conditional knockout mice or an IKK2 inhibitor. The retinal neuronal tissue and RPE deletion of IKK2 was generated by breeding *Ikk2*$^{-/flox}$ mice with *Nestin-Cre* mice. Deletion of *Ikk2* in the retina caused no obvious defect in retinal development or function, but resulted in a significant reduction in laser-induced CNV. In addition, intravitreal or retrobulbar injection of an IKK2 specific chemical inhibitor, TPCA-1, also showed similar inhibition of CNV. Furthermore, *in vitro* inhibition of IKK2 in ARPE-19 cells significantly reduced heat shock-induced expression of NFKBIA, IL1B, CCL2, VEGFA, PDGFA, HIF1A, and MMP-2, suggesting that IKK2 may regulate multiple molecular pathways involved in laser-induced CNV. The *in vivo* laser-induced expression of VEGFA, and HIF1A in RPE and choroidal tissue was also blocked by TPCA-1 treatment. Thus, IKK2/NF-κB signaling appears responsible for production of pro-inflammatory and pro-angiogenic factors in laser-induced CNV, suggesting that this intracellular pathway may serve as an important therapeutic target for aberrant angiogenesis in exudative AMD.

Editor: Jing Chen, Children's Hospital Boston, United States of America

Funding: This work was supported by National Institutes of Health grants EY019891 and EY021584 and Ernest & Elizabeth Althose Special Scholar Award to Qiutang Li from Research to Prevent Blindness. The funders had no role in study design, data collection and analysis, decision to publish, or preparation of the manuscript.

Competing Interests: The authors have declared that no competing interests exist.

* E-mail: q.li@louisville.edu

Introduction

Age-related macular degeneration (AMD) is the most common cause of irreversible blindness in humans over 55, and affects 10 to 15 million people in the USA [1]. Many factors contribute to AMD development, including age, genetic predisposition and environmental factors, such as smoking and possibly diet [2]. There are two forms of AMD, i.e., dry (non-exudative) and wet (exudative). Dry AMD is most common accounting for 90% of the disease and marked by a slow progressive degeneration of both retinal pigment epithelium (RPE) and overlying photoreceptors within the macula. In contrast, wet AMD is characterized by aberrant angiogenesis within the subretinal space, referred to as choroidal neovascularization (CNV) or within the retina, referred to as retinal angiomatous proliferation (RAP), and usually causes severe and rapid vision loss [2]. FDA-approved drugs for the treatment of wet AMD include Lucentis (Ranibizumab), Eylea (Aflibercept), and Macugen (Pegaptanib), all of which target VEGF to slow the growth of abnormal blood vessels and reverse the increased vascular permeability associated with new vessel formation [3–5]. These drugs, as well as Avastin (Bevacizumab), have been shown to be effective in the treatment of many patients with wet AMD but they require frequent intravitreal injections and resistance to anti-VEGF monotherapy in wet AMD is also apparent. Therefore, development of new therapeutic approaches or combination therapies is needed.

The cause of CNV is still under intense investigation and inflammation appears to be an important component. Drusen, a clinical feature associated with AMD and choroidal neovascularization, contains C-reactive protein, complement factors (C3a and C5a), and matrix metalloproteases [6]. Macrophages, lymphocytes and other inflammatory cell types are found in subfoveal CNV membranes [7]. Genetic polymorphism in complement factor H, a complement-inactivating factor, as well as other complement genes has a strong association with AMD [8–10]. These observations suggest that inhibition of inflammation may be a logical approach to prevent or delay the onset of AMD.

Mounting evidence indicates that NF-κB signaling plays a key role in controlling innate and adaptive immunity [11]. The NF-κB family consists of 5 structurally related proteins including p100, p105, relA, relB and c-Rel. In resting cells, NF-κB dimers are retained in the cytoplasm through association with inhibitory IκB proteins, such as IκBα. IκB stability is controlled by the IKK complex. There are two IκB kinases in the complex, namely, IKK1 and IKK2, with IKK2 being the major control for NF-κB activation; lack of this kinase blocks NF-κB activity and, in turn, the pro-inflammatory response [12,13]. Activation of IKK2 causes IκB phosphorylation that leads to ubiquitin-dependent protein degradation, and thus, releases IκB-bounded NF-κB from the cytoplasm. Nuclear localization of NF-κB activates the transcription of many cytokine, chemokine, and growth factors genes [13].

We hypothesize that oxidative stress and hypoxia during aging induce sustained IKK-NF-κB activation and chronic inflammation in the RPE and choroid, leading to up-regulation of angiogenic factors and aberrant neovascularization (Fig.1). To assess the functional role of IKK2 in aberrant angiogenesis, we investigated the effect of *Ikk2* gene deletion or chemical inhibition of IKK2 activity on development of laser-induced CNV, a murine model of wound healing accompanied by oxidative stress and inflammation [14,15]. Since total *Ikk2* knockout mice die *in utero* between E12.5 and E14.5 due to liver apoptosis, we generated conditional knockout mice by breeding the $Ikk2^{-/flox}$ mice with *Nestin-Cre* mice to create deletion of *Ikk2* in the RPE and retinal neurons. Deletion of functional IKK2 in the retina did not affect normal retinal development or function, but significantly reduced laser-induced CNV. Similarly, intravitreal or retrobulbar injection of an IKK2 specific chemical inhibitor, 2-[(aminocarbonyl)amino]-5-(4-fluorophenyl)-3-thiophenecarboxamide (TPCA-1), caused a similar reduction in CNV. Both *in vitro* and *in vivo* experiments showed that TPCA-1 treatment inhibited injury-induced expression of multiple genes, suggesting that the anti-angiogenic effect of IKK2 inhibition involved multiple molecular pathways. Our data showed that NF-κB signaling, through regulation of pro-inflammatory and pro-angiogenic factors, played an important role in the development of laser-induced CNV. We propose that the IKK2/NF-κB pathway may serve as a novel therapeutic target in the prevention or treatment of wet AMD.

Materials and Methods

Ethics statement

All animal experiments (Protocol: 12010) were approved by Institutional Animal Care and Use Committee, the Animal Care Committee at the University of Louisville, and were conducted in accordance with the guidelines of Association for Research in Vision and Ophthalmology on the use of animals in research.

Animals

The $Ikk2^{+/-}$ mice and $Ikk2^{flox/flox}$ mice were generated and described previously [12,16]_ENREF_32_ENREF_27. The $Nestin\text{-}Cre^{+}$ transgenic mice (stock # 003771) [17], the *mT/mG* (membrane-Tomato/membrane-Green) homozygous transgenic mice (stock # 007676) [18], and the wild type control C57BL6J mice (stock # 000664) were purchased from the Jackson Laboratory. Compound lines of the $Ikk2^{-/flox}/Nestine\text{-}Cre^{+/-}$ and control $Ikk2^{+/flox}/Nestine\text{-}Cre^{+/-}$ mice, were generated by crossing $Ikk2^{+/-}/Nestin\text{-}Cre^{+/+}$ with $Ikk2^{flox/flox}$ mouse lines. The $Nestin\text{-}Cre^{+/-}/mT/mG^{+/-}$ and *control* $mT/mG^{+/-}$ mice were generated through the cross-breeding of the $Nestin\text{-}Cre^{+/-}$ mice to the $mT/mG^{+/+}$ homozygous transgenic mice. All animals were maintained and used in accordance with the guidelines of Association for Research in Vision and Ophthalmology on the use of animals in research and according to the guidelines of the Animal Care Committee at the University of Louisville.

Laser treatment

The laser-induced neovascularization was performed on mice at ages between 6–10 weeks. The pupils were dilated with a single drop mixture of 0.06% tropicamide and 0.3% phenylephrine hydrochloride. Two minutes later, the mice were anaesthetized with intraperitoneal injection of Ketamine-Xylazine solution (Ketamine at 15 mg/mL saline and Xylazine at 6 mg/mL saline) at 0.05 mL per 10 g body weight. Diode laser burns applied with a Novus Spectra ophthalmic laser (Lumenis, Inc., Santa Clara, CA) mounted on a slit lamp (Model SL-M; Zeiss, Inc., Tokyo, Japan) generated four lesions symmetrically surrounding the optic nerve of each eye. A coverslip coated with 2.5% hypromellose ophthalmic demulcent solution was held on the mouse cornea, which served to subtract the optics of the cornea and lens for optimal view of the retina and spots of the laser lesions [19]. The laser variables included a 50 µm spot size, 0.05 second-duration, and power at 250 mW. The power used was assessed by the ability to produce a blister indicating rupture of the Bruch's membrane. Laser spots were evaluated by fluorescein angiography and dextran green or isolectin IB4 staining for the presence of CNV at days 7 and 10 after laser treatment.

Retrobulbar injection

Under deep anesthesia, mouse was placed on its side, and a beveled G33 needle was inserted at an approximately 45° angle into the eye, from lateral to the medial canthus, through the conjunctiva membrane. The needle was positioned behind the globe of the eye in the retrobulbar sinus after piercing through the conjunctiva. The mice received unilateral retrobulbar injection of 20 µL of 10 mM IKK2 inhibitor TPCA1 in PBS containing 20% dimethyl sulfoxide (DMSO). Retrobulbar injection of 20 µL vehicle buffer (PBS/20% DMSO) served as control.

Intravitreal injection

Right after laser injury, the mouse eye was decompressed by inserting a 30G needle through the conjunctiva and sclera at

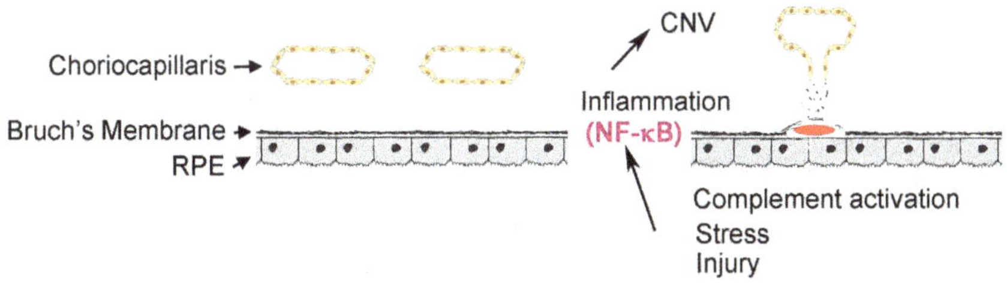

Figure 1. Schematic diagram shows targeting strategy by inhibiting IKK2/NF-κB pathway to prevent choroidal neovascularization (CNV) in AMD. Chronic inflammation and oxidative stress caused by pathologic changes, tissue damage or local components activation in subretinal space induce expression and secretion of cytokines, growth factors and extracellular matrix molecules by RPE, which in turn initiate CNV. NF-κB is a key transcription factor necessary for inflammatory and stress responses. Inhibition of NF-κB activation by IKK2 inhibitor is postulated to prevent chronic inflammation- and oxidative stress-induced CNV formation.

1 mm behind the limbus. Microinjector UMP3 equipped with Nanofil syringe 100 μL and 33G blunt needle (Word precision instruments, Sarasota, FL) was used for injection. The needle was positioned firmly when the operator felt a slightly resistance and then 2 μL of solution was slowly injected in 10 seconds. The topical Ocuflox drops were applied after procedure to prevent infection.

Optokinetic reflex (OKR) measurements

Visual function was assessed using a non-invasive OptoMotry© optokinetic testing system (CerebralMechanics, Lethbridge, AB, Canada), following the procedures described and validated previously [20,21]. Briefly, mice standing unrestrained on the central platform tracked a rotating grating with reflexive head movement behavior. Testing was initiated by projecting a grating of low spatial frequency [0.042 cycles/degree (c/d)], rotating at 12 degrees/second at maximum 100% contrast, i.e. the bars of the gratings are maximally black and the background is maximally white. Spatial frequency of the grating was increased until the animal no longer responded. The threshold of maximum spatial frequency that the mouse could track is a correlate of visual acuity. OKR could detect visual function for each eye separately. OKR response to the rotation of the gradient in a clockwise direction is dependent upon the left eye, whereas rotation in a counterclockwise direction is dependent upon the right eye.

Fluorescein angiography

In vivo fundus fluorescein angiography of CNV was conducted using a retinal camera (model TRC 50X; Topcon America Corp., Paramus, NJ) with Canon 5D digital imaging hardware. The pupil dilation and anesthesia were performed as describe above. Fluorescein fundus images were taken at 3–6 min after intraperitoneal injection of 0.3–0.5 mL of 100 mg/mL Fluorescein (10% w/v). Lesion sizes were graded on the spatial comparison between the fluorescein leakage area and the optic nerve disc area [22], 0: no leakage; 1: the area of fluorescein leakage was equal to disc area, 2: the area of fluorescein leakage was approximately double to the disc area.

Fluorescein-labeled dextran staining and isolectin IB4 staining to evaluate CNV area

Under deep anesthesia, the mouse right atrium was cut and the blood immediately was washed for 3 min with 0.5 mL/min of PBS through the left ventricle with assistance of a perfusion pump, and followed by syringe injection of 1.5 mL PBS containing 50 mg/mL fluorescein-labeled dextran (FITC-dextran, 2 million average molecular weight, Sigma-Aldrich, St. Louis, MO), and then perfusion-fixed with 4% paraformaldehyde (PFA) for 6 min. The eyes were removed and immerse-fixed in 4% PFA at 4°C for overnight. After rinsed in PBS, cornea, lens, and the neurosensory retina were carefully removed from the eyecup. Five radial cuts were made from the edge of the eyecup to the equator; the RPE/choroid/sclera complex was flat-mounted in 50% glycerol containing PBS with the sclera facing down on a glass slide. A laser spot with green vessels was scored as CNV-positive, and a laser spot lacking green vessels was scored CNV-negative. The flat-mounted retina was imaged at 5× magnification using a Zeiss Axio Imager M2 system equipped with Apotome, and attached to both AxioCam and AxioVision cameras. The free hand selection tool was used to delineate the boundaries of CNV complexes and the total area of each lesion across all sections was measured and expressed in square micrometers (μm^2) to determine maximum CNV complex area. The sum of CNV area in each eye was compared among different animals and experimental conditions.

For isolectin IB4 staining, laser injured eyes were enucleated and fixed at 4°C with ice-cold 4% paraformaldehyde in PBS for overnight. The anterior segment, lens, and retina were removed, and the remaining eye cups with attached RPE layer were washed with PBS and incubated for overnight at room temperature with1:100 dilution of 1 mg/mL solution of AlexaFluor 594 conjugated isolectin IB4 (Invitrogen, Oregon, USA) [23]. After incubation, the eye cups were washed with PBS, the sclera-choroid/RPE complexes with radial cut were flat mounted for fluorescence microscopy right after the staining. The area of fluorescence was quantified as described above.

Histological studies

The eyes were dissected from euthanized mice and fixed immediately in 4% PFA for overnight at 4°C, and then subjected to either paraffin embedding or OCT embedding for Cryostat sectioning. Seven μm of paraffin-embedded sections was cut and de-paraffinized prior to staining with hematoxylin and eosin (H&E). The mean thickness of the CNV membrane was obtained by examining the serial sections of whole eyes and using the maximum thickness measurements of each of the four lesion sites per eye. Frozen tissue sections from the *Nestin-Cre*$^{+/-}$/*mT/mG*$^{+/-}$ and control *mT/mG*$^{+/-}$ mice were examined for the switch from red fluorescence to green fluorescence using Zeiss Axio Imager M2 system equipped with ApoTome, and attached with AxioCam and AxioVision cameras. The cell layers of the inner nuclear layer and outer nuclear layer were counted by random sampling 10 sagittal sections from each eye.

Western blot analysis

Skin, brain and retina tissues from *Ikk2*$^{-/fl}$/*Nestine-Cre*$^{+/-}$ and WT (*Ikk2*$^{+/fl}$) control mice were collected and homogenized in cold immunoprecipitation assay buffer (20 mM Tris-HCl, pH 7.4, 100 mM NaCl, and 0.2% each of deoxycholate, Triton X-100, and Nonidet P-40) containing 1× complete protease-inhibitor mixture (Roche Diagnostics, Indianapolis, IN). Equal amounts of whole-cell lysates were separated on 10% sodium dodecyl sulfate polyacrylamide gel (SDS-PAGE) and transferred to a nitrocellulose membrane. For immunoblotting, the mouse anti-IKK2 antibody (Biosource AH00362, 1:100 dilution), and mouse anti-β-actin (1:1000, cat #A2228, Sigma, St. Louis, MO) were used as primary antibodies. The horseradish peroxidase-conjugated goat-anti-mouse secondary antibody and an enhanced chemiluminescence (ECL) system (Amersham Pharmacia, Piscataway, NJ) were used to visualize the signals. For immunobloting of IκBα and α-tubulin in the ARPE-19 cells pre-treated with TPCA-1 and TNFα, rabbit anti-IκBα antibody (1:250 dilution, Santa Cruz Biotechnology, Inc, sc-371) and mouse anti-α-tubulin antibody (1:500 dilution, Sigma, T9026) were used. For thermal injured ARPE-19 cells, rabbit-anti-NF-κB p65 antibody (1:200 dilution, Santa Cruz Biotechnology, Inc., sc-372) and rabbit-anti-NF-κB p65 (Ser536) antibody (1:500 dilution, Cell Signaling Technology, Inc., Cat #3033) were used.

RNA isolation and Quantitative (q)-PCR

The total RNA from the spleens, brains and retinas of *Ikk2*$^{-/flox}$/*Nestine-Cre*$^{+/-}$ and WT control mice were extracted using TRIzol reagent (Invitrogen). The total RNA from the RPE/Choroid/Sclera tissues of laser injury eyes was extracted using TRIzol reagent (Invitrogen) after removing the anterior segment, vitreous, and retina. The A260/A280 ratio of all RNA samples was >2.0 as measured by Nanodrop. Double-stranded cDNA was reverse-transcribed using random primers and SuperScript VILO cDNA synthesis kit (Invitrogen). Real time qPCR by a SYBR green-based PCR method was performed on a MX3005p system (Agilent Technologies, Inc., Santa Clara, CA), with a program of a 10-minute initial hot-start activation of Taq polymerase at 95°C, followed by 40 cycles of amplification (95°C for 10 seconds, 56°C for 5 seconds, and 72°C for 10 seconds). The comparative CT (threshold cycle) method normalized to β-actin was used to analyze relative changes in gene expression. The primers for human NFKBIA (IκBα) (ID 10092619a1), IL1B (Il1β) (ID 27894305b1), CCL2 (ID 4506841a1), VEGFA (ID 30172564a1), PDGFA (ID 15208658a1), HIF1A (ID 4504385a1), MMP2 (11342666a2), mouse Hif1a (ID 7363433a1), and Hmox1 (6754212a1) were designed based on the online PrimerBank database (Harvard Medical School, Boston, MA). The qPCR primer sequences for human ACTB (beta-actin), mouse Actb(beta-actin) and mouse Ikbkb (Ikk2) have been published elsewhere [24,25]. The detailed primer information is listed in Table 1.

TNFα induced IκBα degradation and TPCA-1 treatment on ARPE-19 cells

ARPE-19 cell, a human RPE cell line, was cultured according to supplier's instruction (ATCC, catalog CRL-2302, Manassas, VA). When reaching 90% confluence in 3.5 cm plates, the cells were pretreated with TPCA-1 (Tocris Bioscience, Ellisville, Missouri) at 0, 2, 20 and 200 μM for 30 minutes, and then added with TNFα at 10 ng/mL for additional 15 or 30 minutes. Control samples are treated with TPCA-1 only. Protein lysates were subjected to Western blotting for detection of IκBα degradation.

Table 1. List of primers used for qPCR.

Gene	Primer sequence
Mouse *Ikbkb*	F-5′-GGAGTACTGCCAAGGAGGAGAT-3′ R-5′-ACAGGCTGCCAGTTAGGGAGGAAG-3′
Mouse *Actb*	F-5′-CCAGTTGGTAACAATGCCATGT-3′ R-5′-TGT ATG CTA TAC GAA GTT AT-3′
human *ACTB*	F-5′-AACTCCATCATGAAGTGTGACG-3′ R-5′-GATCCACATCTGCTGGAAGG-3′
human *NFKBIA*	F-5′-CTCCGAGACTTTCGAGGAAATAC-3′ R-5′-GCCATTGTAGTTGGTAGCCTTCA-3′
human *IL1B*	F-5′-ATGATGGCTTATTACAGTGGCAA-3′ R-5′-GTCGGAGATTCGTAGCTGGA-3′
Human *CCL2*	F-5′-CAGCCAGATGCAATCAATGCC-3′ R-5′-TGGAATCCTGAACCCACTTCT-3′
Human *VEGFA*	F-5′-CAACATCACCATGCAGATTATGC-3′ R-5′-GCTTTCGTTTTTGCCCCTTTC-3′
Human *PDGFA*	F-5′-CCAGCGACTCCTGGAGATAGA-3′ R-5′-CTTCTCGGGCACATGCTTAGT-3′
Human *HIF1A*	F-5′-GGCGCGAACGACAAGAAAAAG-3′ R-5′-CCTTATCAAGATGCGAACTCACA-3′
Human *MMP2*	F-5′-GCCCCAGACAGGTGATCTTG-3′ R-5′-GCTTGCGAGGGAAGAAGTTGT-3′
mouse *Vegfa*	F-5′-ACAGCACAGCAGATGTGAATGCAG-3′ R-5′-TTACACGTCTGCGGATCTTGGACA-3′
mouse *Hif1a*	F-5′-ACCTTCATCGGAAACTCCAAAG-3′ R-5′-CTGTTAGGCTGGGAAAAGTTAGG-3′
mouse *Hmox1*	F-5′-AAGCCGAGAATGCTGAGTTCA-3′ R-5′-GCCGTGTAGATATGGTACAAGGA-3′

Thermal injury experiments

The confluent ARPE-19 cells cultured on 3.5 cm plates were pretreated with or without 5 μM TPCA1 (Tocris Bioscience, Ellisville, Missouri) for 30 minutes prior to thermal injury. The thermal injury experiments were carried out by replacing the medium in cell plates with 10 mL HEPES-buffered saline pre-warmed at 55°C for 5 seconds before changed back to normal culture medium at 37°C in the presence or absence of 5 μM TPCA1. Cells were harvested at 10, 30, 60, 120 minutes after heat shock for protein preparation and the total RNA for qPCR was isolated using TRIzol reagents at 4 hours after heat shock.

Luciferase assay

293/NF-κB-Luc cells (Cat # RC0014, Affymetrix, Inc., Santa Clara, CA) were plated in poly-lysine coated 96-well plates. The cells at 90% confluence were pretreated with 0, 1, 2.5, 5, 10 μM TPCA1 for 30 minutes, then stimulated with 10 ng/mL TNFα (PeproTech Inc., Rocky Hill, NJ) in the presence of indicated amount of TPCA-1 (Tocris Bioscience, Ellisville, Missouri) for 5 hours, and followed by protein lysate collection and luciferase assay. TPCA-1 and TNFα untreated sample used as controls. Luciferase assays were performed using Luciferase assay kit (E1910, Promega, Madison, WI) following the manufacturer's protocol.

MTT cell viability assay

The HEK293T and ARPE-19 cells were cultured in poly-lysine coated and uncoated 96-well plates, respectively. The cells at 60–70% confluence were treated in the following 3 conditions, i.e., 50 μM TPCA1 alone, 10 ng/mL TNFα alone or in combination of both TPCA-1 and TNFα after a 30 minutes pretreatment of 50 μM TPCA1. Cell without any drug treatment served as controls. The cell viability after 12 hours of drug treatment was measured by a MTT assay. Briefly, 0.2 mL of 3-[4,5-dimethylthiazol-2-yl]-2,5-diphenyltetrazolium bromide (MTT) at 5 mg/mL in PBS was added to each well and the cells were incubated at 37°C for 4 hours. After the medium was removed, the purple formazan precipitate was solubilized in 200 μL DMSO. Absorbance was measured at 560 nm with background subtraction at 670 nm. Measurements were made in triplicate and the error bars represent the standard deviation. The Student's two-tailed *t*-test was used to determine statistical significance.

Flow cytometry

Flow cytometry was performed as described previously [26]. Briefly, the single cell suspensions were prepared from thymus, spleen, and bone marrow of the mice at 7 days after receiving a single retrobulbar injection of 20 μL of 10 mM (56 μg) TPCA-1 in PBS or control vehicle, and passed through 70-μm nylon mesh (Fisher Scientific). After lysis of RBCs using ACK buffer (0.83% ammonium chloride, 0.1% potassium bicarbonate, 0.037% EDTA [pH 7.2]), Fc receptors were blocked with anti-CD16/32 antibody (Ab) before staining. To stain cell surface antigens, 10^6 cells in 50 μL of staining buffer (1×PBS containing 3% BSA and 0.1% sodium azide) were incubated at 4°C for 30 minutes with fluorochrome-conjugated mAbs, and analyzed on a four-color BD FACSCalibur (BD Biosciences), the data was analyzed with CellQuestPro 5.1.1 software (BD Biosciences). Antibodies used for staining were as follows: rat anti-mouse CD16/32 blocking Ab (clone 2.4G2) was obtained from BD Biosciences (San Diego, CA); and rat anti-mouse TCR-β-FITC (H57-597), CD8a-PE (53-6.7), CD4-APC (GK1.5), B220-PE (RA3-6B2), IgD-APC (11-26), IgM-FITC (eB121-15F9), CD11b-APC (M1/70), Ly6C-PE (HK1.4),

Ly6G-FITC (RB6-8C5), 7-amino-actinomycin D (7-AAD), and PE-conjugated rat IgG2a or IgG2b isotype Ab controls were purchased from eBiosciences (San Diego, CA).

Statistical analysis

The quantitative data were presented as means ± standard deviation (SD). CNV spot number, area, and choroidal neovascular membranes between the mutant and WT groups or drug treated and vehicle-treated controls were compared by performing a two-tail Student's t-test on raw data. P-values of less than 0.05 were considered to be significant.

Results

IKK2 is not essential for normal retinal development and function

To examine the functional role of IKK2 in development of laser-induced CNV, we generated conditional *Ikk2* mutant mice by breeding *Ikk2*$^{-/flox}$ mice carrying one *Ikk2* mutant allele and the *Ikk2-flox* allele [27] with the mouse line expressing *Cre* recombinase under control of the *Nestin* promoter (Fig. 2A). To directly visualize the neuronal and RPE deletion of the loxP-flanked sequence in the eye by the *Nestin* promoter-driven *Cre* recombinase, we first bred *Nestin-Cre* mice into *mT/mG* (membrane-Tomato/membrane-Green) dual color fluorescent Cre-reporter mice. GFP expression is blocked in these mice by a loxP flanked red fluorescent protein (tdTomato) expression cassette in non-Cre cells, but allowed in cells expressing Cre after the Cre-mediated deletion of the loxP flanked tdTomato expression cassette. This double-fluorescent system allows direct visualization of Cre positive (green) and Cre negative (red) cells in the retina. Our data clearly showed that Nestin-Cre caused a selective loxP flanked genomic recombination in retinal neurons and RPE cells but not in choroidal tissue (Fig. 2B). Very few red colored cells were detected in the neurosensory retina, indicating that the Nestin-Cre mediated recombination was highly efficient (Fig. 2C). Significant reduction of *Ikk2* expression at the mRNA and protein level was detected in the retina and brain, but not skin, by RT-PCR and Western blotting after Nestin-Cre mediated deletion of the loxP-flanked *Ikk2* allele (Fig. 2D). These results indicated that *Ikk2* was efficiently knocked out in the RPE and retinal neurons in the *Ikk2*$^{-/flox}$/*Nestin-Cre*$^{+}$ mice.

After confirmation of the conditional knockout of the *Ikk2* gene in retinal neurons and RPE cells, we first evaluated retinal development and found no overt morphological defect in the *Ikk2*$^{-/flox}$/*Nestin-Cre*$^{+}$ retina by light microscopy (Fig. 3A and 3B). Both WT and *Ikk2*$^{-/flox}$/*Nestin-Cre*$^{+}$ retinas showed approximately 9–10 rows of nuclei in the outer nuclear layer (ONL) and 5 rows of nuclei in the inner nuclear layer (INL). The average ONL cell layers for WT and mutant mice were 9.8+0.32 and 9.6+0.48, respectively (Fig. 3C). The average INL cell layers for WT and mutant mice were 4.6+0.48 and 4.5+0.5, respectively. There were no significant differences in OKR spatial frequency thresholds [38] between *Ikk2*$^{-/flox}$/*Nestin-Cre*$^{+}$ and WT control mice, suggesting normal visual acuity in *Ikk2*$^{-/flox}$/*Nestin-Cre*$^{+}$ mice (Fig. 3D). These results indicate that IKK2 is not essential for normal retinal development or function.

Loss of *Ikk2* inhibits laser-induced CNV

To determine whether the absence of *Ikk2* influences choroidal neovascularization *in vivo*, we adopted a laser-induced CNV model [19], and evaluated the incidence of fluorescein leakage on fluorescent angiograms (FA) performed on the *Ikk2*$^{-/flox}$/*Nestine-Cre*$^{+}$ (*Ikk2*$^{-/-}$) retina on day 7 after laser treatment, compared to laser-induced CNV in control WT and *Ikk2*$^{+/flox}$/*Nestine-Cre*$^{+}$ (*Ikk2*$^{+/-}$) mice (Fig. 4A–C). Fluorescein fundus images were taken 3–6 minutes after intraperitoneal injection of 0.3 mL of 100 mg/mL Fluorescein (10% w/v). During this period, the size of fluorescein leakage spots was relatively stable and the area of each fluorescent spot was measured and expressed as arbitrary unit in relevant to the area of the optic nerve disc (Figure S1 in File S1). Newly formed microvessels with clear evidence of fluorescein leakage were observed in 63% of the laser-induced lesions in WT and *Ikk2*$^{+/flox}$/*Nestine-Cre*$^{+}$ mice, compared to 35% in *Ikk2*$^{-/flox}$/*Nestine-Cre*$^{+}$ mice. The average score of fluorescein leakage was reduced from 2.5 in WT mice and 2.4 in *Ikk2*$^{+/flox}$/*Nestine-Cre*$^{+}$ mice to 1.2 in *Ikk2*$^{-/flox}$/*Nestine-Cre*$^{+}$ mice (Fig. 4D).

CNV formation was further visualized by AlexaFluor 594-labeled isolectin IB4 staining (Fig. 4E–G). Although there was no significant difference in CNV area between WT and heterozygous *Ikk2*$^{+/flox}$/*Nestine-Cre*$^{+}$ mice (Fig. 4H), complete knockout of both *Ikk2* alleles in the retina of *Ikk2*$^{-/flox}$/*Nestin-Cre*$^{+}$ mice resulted in a 5-fold reduction in the size of CNV lesions compared to control mice (Fig. 4H). Furthermore, the thickness of the neovascular membrane was quantified by examining serial sections and using the maximum thickness measurements as indicated as in Fig.4I–J; an 80% reduction was observed in *Ikk2*$^{-/flox}$/*Nestin-Cre*$^{+}$ mice compared to *Ikk2*$^{+/flox}$/*Nestine-Cre*$^{+}$ mice (Fig. 4I–K). These data showed that there was a significant reduction in the size and thickness of the CNV complex in *Ikk2*$^{-/flox}$/*Nestin-Cre*$^{+}$ mice, suggesting that IKK2 plays a critical role in aberrant angiogenesis.

IKK2 chemical inhibitors reduce laser-induced CNV

To explore the therapeutic potential of IKK2 inhibitors in treating CNV, we next tested the effects of a potent (IC_{50} = 17.9 nM) and selective IKK-2 inhibitor, 2-[(aminocarbonyl)amino]-5-(4-fluorophenyl)-3-thiophenecarboxamide (TPCA-1) _ENREF_49[28], on laser-induced CNV. One eye of each mouse was treated with laser burns, followed by a single retrobulbar or intravitreal injection of either TPCA-1 or the control vehicle. As shown in figure 5A, a single retrobulbar injection of 20 μL TPCA-1 at 1, 5, 10, or 20 mM, resulted in a dose-dependent reduction in laser-induced CNV, with 5 mM being the minimum concentration to show an inhibitory effect (Fig. 5A). The average area of CNV spots in the TPCA-1 treated eyes was significantly reduced, especially in both the 10 mM (56 μg) and 20 mM (112 μg) groups, being approximately one third of the CNV area in control eyes (Fig. 5A). Clinical examination of the retina and OKR (on days 6 and 21) post retrobulbar injection of 20 μl TPCA-1 was normal (Fig. 5B, Figure S2 in File S1). Importantly, mice injected with control solvent either retrobulbarly or intravitreally showed no significant difference in laser-induced CNV in WT mice, indicating that the surgical procedure itself did not affect the incidence of laser-induced CNV (Fig. 5C, vehicle vs. WT). We observed that retrobulbar injection achieved a similar inhibitory effect as intravitreal injection, although the retrobulbar route required a larger injection volume (20 μl of 10 mM TPCA-1 compared to 2 μl of 10 mM TPCA-1) (Fig. 5C). We also observed that the inhibitory effect of retrobulbar injected 10 mM TPCA-1 was comparable to intravitreal anti-mouse VEGF 164 polyclonal antibody (R&D System, Cat#AF-493-NA) with regard to CNV size (Fig. 5E).

We noticed that the laser burn causes a continuous influx of inflammatory cells into the injury site with the peak at 3 days post-laser, the same time interval required for the onset of neovascularization [29]. To test if TPCA-1 will inhibit CNV development after neovascularization has started, we gave TPCA-1 3 days after the laser burn. A similar inhibitory effect on CNV was observed

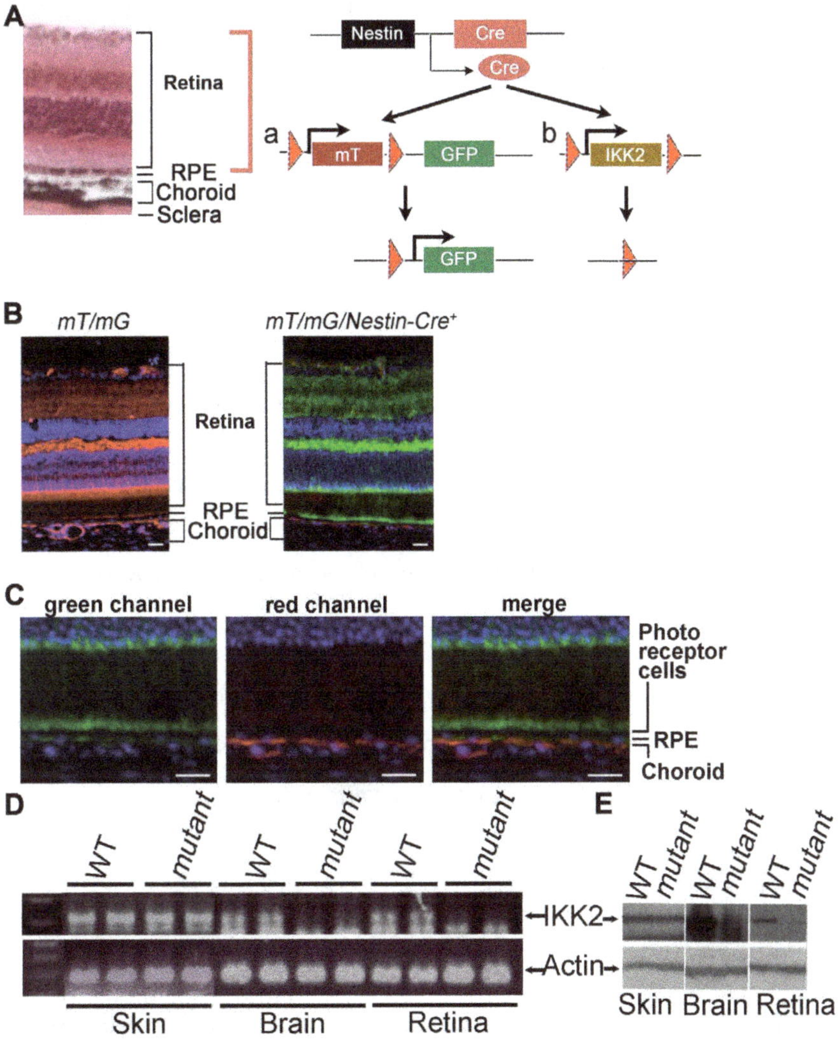

Figure 2. IKK2 is deleted in the RPE and retinal neurons in *$Ikk2^{-/flox}$/Nestin-Cre^{+}* mice. (A) Nestin-promoter-driven Cre mediated specific deletion of the LoxP flanked genomic sequence was tested on mT/mG/Nestin-Cre^{+} mice (a) and performed on *$Ikk2^{-/flox}$/Nestin-Cre^{+}* mice (b). The *mT/mG* (membrane-Tomato/membrane-Green) mouse strain contains a Cre-reporter transgene knocked into the Rosa26 locus. When bred with the *nestin-Cre* mice, the Cre recombinase mediated the genomic deletion of the LoxP (solid triangles)-flanked tdTomato (red) STOP cassette and in turn led to expression of the downstream membrane-targeted enhanced green fluorescent protein (GFP). A similar nestin-Cre mediated homologous recombination to obtain a neuronal and RPE deletion of *Ikk2* in retina was designed by breeding the *$Ikk2^{-/flox}$* mouse carrying one *Ikk2* mutant allele and one *Ikk2*-flox allele with the mouse line expressing *Cre* recombinase under control of *Nestin* promoter (*Nestin-Cre*). The hematoxylin- and eosin-stained wild type mouse eye section on left show anatomy of retina, choroid, and sclera. (B, C) The RPE and neuronal retinal cell deletion of the LoxP-flanked tdTomato STOP cassette mediated by *Nestin-Cre* was confirmed by the red-to-green fluorescent color conversion on the retinas of the *mT/mG/Nestin-Cre^{+}* cre reporter mice, whereas the adjacent choroid tissue did not show such red-to-green change, as shown at lower (B) and higher (C) magnification images. Red cells represent cre-negative cells, while green cells are cre-positive cells. (D) Reverse transcription PCR showed that *Ikk2* mRNA was eliminated in both retina and brain, but not in the control tissue, i.e., the skin of the *$Ikk2^{-/flox}$/Nestin-Cre^{+}* mice. (E) Western clot analysis showed that the IKK2 protein was absent in the retina and brain, but not in the skin of the *$Ikk2^{-/flox}$/Nestin-Cre^{+}* mice. Size bar = 20 μm in B and C.

with either retrobulbar or intravitreal injection (Fig. 5D). These data show that the IKK2 inhibitor, TPCA-1, can inhibit CNV whether administered prior to or after the onset of angiogenesis, suggesting that IKK2 is critical for the expression of trophic factor(s) important for aberrant neovascularization.

Local administration of TPCA-1 shows no systemic toxicity

It has been previously shown that systemic administration of the IKK2 inhibitor ML120B for four days caused depletion of bone marrow B cells and thymocytes due to increased TNF-α-mediated apoptosis of lymphocytes [30]. Similar toxicity was observed in mice in which lethally irradiated hosts were transplanted with either IKK2- or p65-deficient fetal liver cells [31,32]. In order to assess the potential toxicity of retrobulbar TPCA-1 we used flow cytometry to analyze systemic lymphoid tissues. A single retrobulbar injection of 56 μg TPCA-1 for 7 days did not alter the proportion of $CD4^{+}/CD8^{+}$ double and single positive T cells in both spleen and thymus (Fig. 6A–B). TPCA-1 treated mice showed no obvious alteration in mature ($IgD^{high}IgM^{low}$) or immature ($IgD^{low}IgM^{high}$) $B220^{+}$ B-cell populations in the spleen (Fig. 6C), or in mature recirculating ($B220^{+}IgD^{high}IgM^{int}$), transitional immature ($B220^{+}IgM^{high}IgD^{int}$), immature ($B220^{+}IgM^{high}IgD^{-}$) or precursor ($B220^{+}IgM^{-}IgD^{-}$) B cells in the bone marrow either

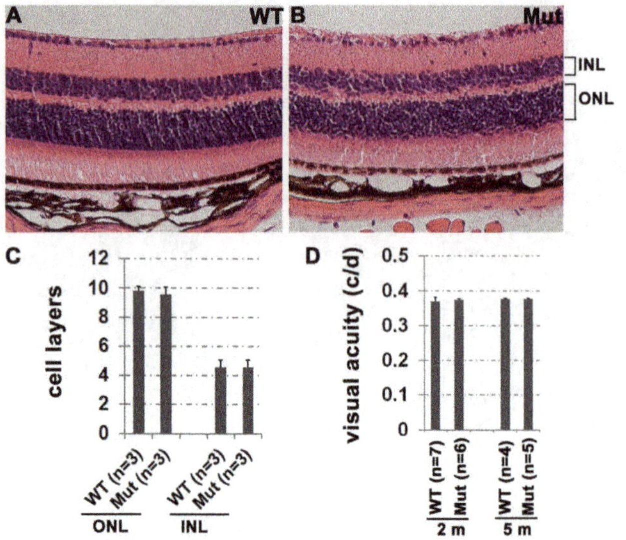

Figure 3. IKK2 is not required for retina development and function. (A, B) The paraffin-embedded retinal sections from the wild type control (WT) (A) and *Ikk2*$^{-/flox}$*/Nestin-Cre*$^{+}$ (Mut) (B) mice at age of 2 month old were stained by hematoxylin and eosin (H&E) method. (C) The quantitative comparison of the cell layers in the outer nuclear layer (ONL) and inner nuclear layer (INL) between WT (n = 3 mice) and Mut (n = 3 mice) mice at 2 month old. (D) Visual acuity was tested on wild type (WT) control and *Ikk2*$^{-/flox}$*/Nestin-Cre*$^{+}$ (Mut) mice at the age of 2 and 5 month old by OKR. Error bars indicate standard deviation.

(Fig. 6D). There was also no significant difference noticed in the monocyte populations in the spleen of TPCA-1 treated mice - i.e. neutrophil (CD11b^{+}Ly6G^{+}/Ly6C^{int}), monocyte (CD11b^{+}Ly6G^{-}/Ly6C^{+}) and mature macrophage (CD11b^{+}Ly6G^{-}/Ly6C^{-}) cells (Fig. 6E). Staining of CD11b and CD4 positive cells with 7AAD showed no increase in cell death (Fig. 6F). Thus, our data suggested that periocular (i.e. retrobulbar) administration of the IKK2 inhibitor, TPCA-1, did not cause systemic toxicity to the immune system. In addition, histological examination showed no noticeable morphological changes or tissue toxicity in the liver and spleen of the TPCA-1 treated mice (Fig. 6G).

It is well documented that NF-κB inhibition enhances TNFα-induced apoptosis in HEK293T cells. Similarly, TPCA-1 significantly reduced the viability of HEK293 cells, and the addition of TNFα increased cell death (Fig. 6H left panel), suggesting TPCA-1 sensitized HEK293T cells to TNFα induced apoptosis. We then asked whether TPCA-1 was also able to affect ARPE-19 cell viability. In contrast to HEK293T cell, TPCA-1 showed no toxicity for ARPE-19 cells (Fig. 6H, right panel), even at the higher concentration of 50 μM which specifically blocked NF-κB activation in both HEK293T and ARPE-19 cells (Fig. 7A–B).

TPCA-1 attenuates thermal injury-induced expression of angiogenic factors

Given that activation of IKK-NF-κB signaling induced expression of growth factors and chemokines associated with angiogenesis [33], we investigated whether TPCA-1 inhibited laser-induced CNV through down-regulation of other inflammatory and angiogenic factors that promoted neovascularization. It is well known that TNF-α activates the IKK-NF-κB signal transduction pathway, leading to transcriptional activation of downstream target genes. To determine an optimal inhibitory dose for TPCA-1 to block NF-κB activation, we first performed a dose-dependent inhibition assay in HEK293T cells using a commercially available κB luciferase assay system (Promega). The κB-luciferase activity induced by TNFα was significantly inhibited by TPCA-1 at 1 μM, and was dose dependent and reaching a peak at the highest dosage used in this assay (10 μM, approximately a 7-fold reduction) (Fig. 7A). We next examined the inhibitory effect of TPCA-1 on ARPE-19 cells by visualizing TNFα-induced IκBα degradation on Western blots. In general, TNFα activates IKK2 which phosphorylates its downstream IκBα serine residues at 32 and 36, leading to ubiquitin-dependent degradation of this inhibitory protein. Degradation of IκBα releases the NF-κB dimer into the nucleus to activate downstream transcriptional targets [34]. When ARPE-19 cells were treated with 10 ng/mL TNFα, endogenous IκBα protein was rapidly degraded within 15 minutes (Fig. 7B). In contrast, pre-incubation of the cells with 20 μM and 200 μM TPCA-1 completely blocked TNFα-induced IκBα degradation (Fig. 7B).

We next explored the inhibitory effect of TPCA-1 on NF-κB activation induced by heat shock to mimic the laser injury [35]. Human ARPE-19 cells were pretreated with or without 5 μM TPCA-1 for 30 minutes and were quickly shocked by heat at 55°C for 5 seconds; they were then cultured in the presence or absence of 5 μM TPCA-1 for various times. The phosphorylation of NF-κB p65 subunit at Ser536, which mediates IκB release and DNA binding, was analyzed by Western blotting. Heat shock induced a slight increase in p65 phosphorylation at Ser 536, starting at 30 minutes after heating; however, such heat shock-induced p65 phosphorylation was significantly reduced in the presence of TPCA-1, suggesting that TPCA-1 blocked the heat shock-induced NF-κB activation (Fig. 7C). Furthermore, to examine whether TPCA-1 affected heat shock-induced gene expression, we heat-shocked ARPE-19 cells at 55°C for 5 seconds. Total RNA was isolated from those cells at 4 hrs and subjected to qPCR analysis of downstream target genes. As shown in figure 7D and 7E, heat shock significantly induced expression of NFKBIA, IL1B, CCL2, VEGF-A, PDGFA, HIF1A, and MMP-2, all of which have been shown to be regulated by NF-κB signaling and participate in regulation of angiogenesis. Notably, TPCA-1 significantly blocked the activation of these downstream genes (Fig. 7D and 7E). Next, we confirmed that mRNA expression of Vegfa and Hif1a was induced by the laser injury and that their expression was suppressed by TPCA-1 *in vivo* (Fig. 7F). In addition, the induced heme oxygenase enzyme HO-1 isoform (Hmox1), a sensor of cellular oxidative stress, was also significantly induced by laser injury and its response was also blocked by TPCA-1, suggesting that NF-κB/IKK2 regulates laser induced CNV formation through multiple pathways including inflammation, hypoxia, and oxidative stress (Fig. 7F). Our results suggest that IKK2 inhibition by its specific inhibitor TPCA-1 is able to block laser-induced CNV through the IKK-NF-κB signaling pathway, and in turn, the transcription of its downstream target genes that promote neovascularization.

Discussion

Abnormal growth of choroidal blood vessels into the subretinal space (i.e. CNV) is a major cause of severe vision loss in AMD. The most effective current treatment for CNV is intravitreal injection of antibodies that block the action of VEGF [2]. Because over 60% of AMD patients with CNV do not have improved vision after anti-VEGF antibody treatment, other alternative treatments are being sought. Inflammation has been linked to the development of CNV and NF-κB is a master regulator of inflammation. Therefore, we explored the effect of inhibiting the

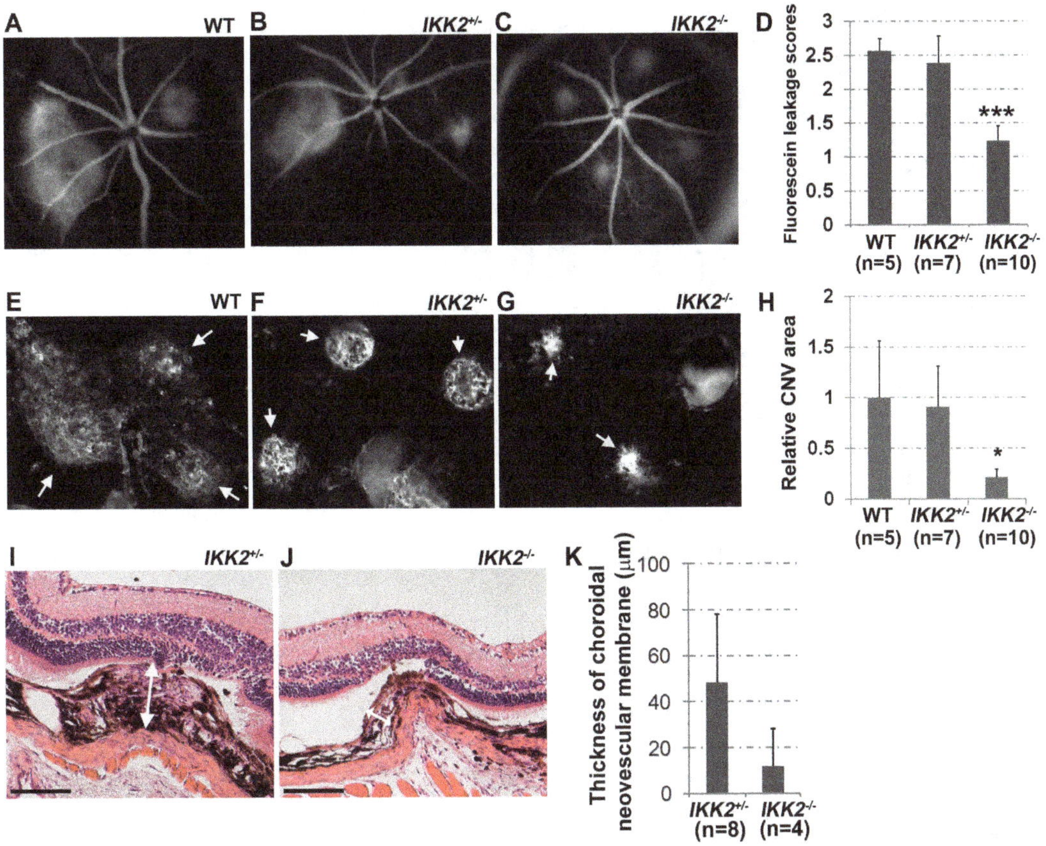

Figure 4. Induction of the laser-induced CNV is inhibited in the *Ikk2$^{-/flox}$/Nestine-Cre^{+}* mice. The development of CNV after laser photocoagulation was quantified by scoring the fluorescence leakage and isolectin IB4 stain areas and measuring the thickness of choroidal neovascular membrane. (A–C) Fundus photographs and fluorescein angiogram (A–C) were taken from the wild type (WT), *Ikk2$^{+/flox}$/Nestine-Cre^{+}* (*Ikk2$^{+/-}$*), and *Ikk2$^{-/flox}$/Nestine-Cre^{+}* (*Ikk2$^{-/-}$*) mouse eyes that had been treated with laser injury for 7 days. The development of CNV was quantified by scoring the relative average size of fluorescence leakage in each animal (D) comparing to optic disk size. N = number of mice. (E–G) The images of Alexa Fluor 568 conjugated isolectin IB4 stained CNVs were taken from the indicated mouse eyes at 7 days post-laser injury. Arrows indicate the CNV identified by isolectin IB4 staining. (H) The summary of the mean CNV area from each genotypic animal was shown as relative to that induced in the WT eyes. N = number of mice. (I and J) Representative H&E stained eye sections show the neovascular membrane networks originating from the choroicapillaries passing through the broken Bruch's membrane. The white arrows with two arrowheads show the thickness of choroidal neovascular membrane. The scale bar represents 50 µm in length. (K) Quantification of the thickness of the choroidal neovascular membrane. Error bars indicate standard deviation. Two-tail T-test: * $p<0.05$, *** $p<0.005$. n indicates the number of laser-injured spots.

NF-κB signaling pathway in an experimental model of CNV induced by laser injury to the retina. We observed in the present study that inhibition of IKK2/NF-κB activation by the pharmaceutical IKK2 inhibitor TPCA-1 or using *Ikk2* conditional knockout mice dramatically inhibited laser-induced CNV.

Clinical evidence shows that in many patients VEGF is critical for endothelial cell proliferation and angiogenesis that leads to CNV. VEGF consists of several isomers (VEGF-A, VEGF-B, VEGF-C, and VEGF-D) that have a different ability to promote angiogenesis [36,37]. Increased levels of the VEGF protein has been detected in RPE cells of CNV membranes in AMD [7,38–41]; in basal laminar deposits of surgically excised CNV membranes; in vitreous samples of patients with neovascular retinopathies [7,39,40]. In addition, VEGF is known as a vascular permeability factor that can increase blood vessel leakage by interrupting endothelial layer tight junctions. Multiple anti-VEGF drugs are beneficial in inhibiting CNV and restoring visual function. The production of VEGF and PDGF, and the activation of multiple pro-inflammatory gene products (e.g. CCL2, ICAM-1, IL1B and IL-8) are regulated by the transcription nuclear factor NF-κB [42–46]. Thus, inhibition of the NF-κB pathway by pharmaceutical intervention may open a novel approach to prevent CNV [22].

Mounting evidence indicates that NF-κB also functions as a regulator of angiogenesis promoting tumor growth by upregulating the expression of angiogenic factors, such as IL-8, CCL2 and VEGF [47,48]. It has been documented that NF-κB is involved in the upregulation of VEGF mRNA in multiple cancer cell lines [49]. Although the VEGF promoter contains a region with putative NF-κB binding sites, deletion of these binding sites had little effect on VEGF expression, suggesting that direct binding of NF-κB to the VEGF promoter may not be required for its expression [50]. However, it was recently proposed that NF-κB modulates VEGF transcription though HIF1A, a key transcription factor for VEGF during hypoxia [16,51], and a recent study showed that transcriptional activation of the Hif1a gene by IKK2-activated NF-κB precedes HIF1A protein accumulation both *ex vivo* and *in vivo* [52]. Mice lacking *Ikk2* subjected to hypoxia revealed a pronounced defect in Hif1a mRNA expression and protein accumulation, as well as defective induction of HIF1A targeted genes, including VEGF [52].

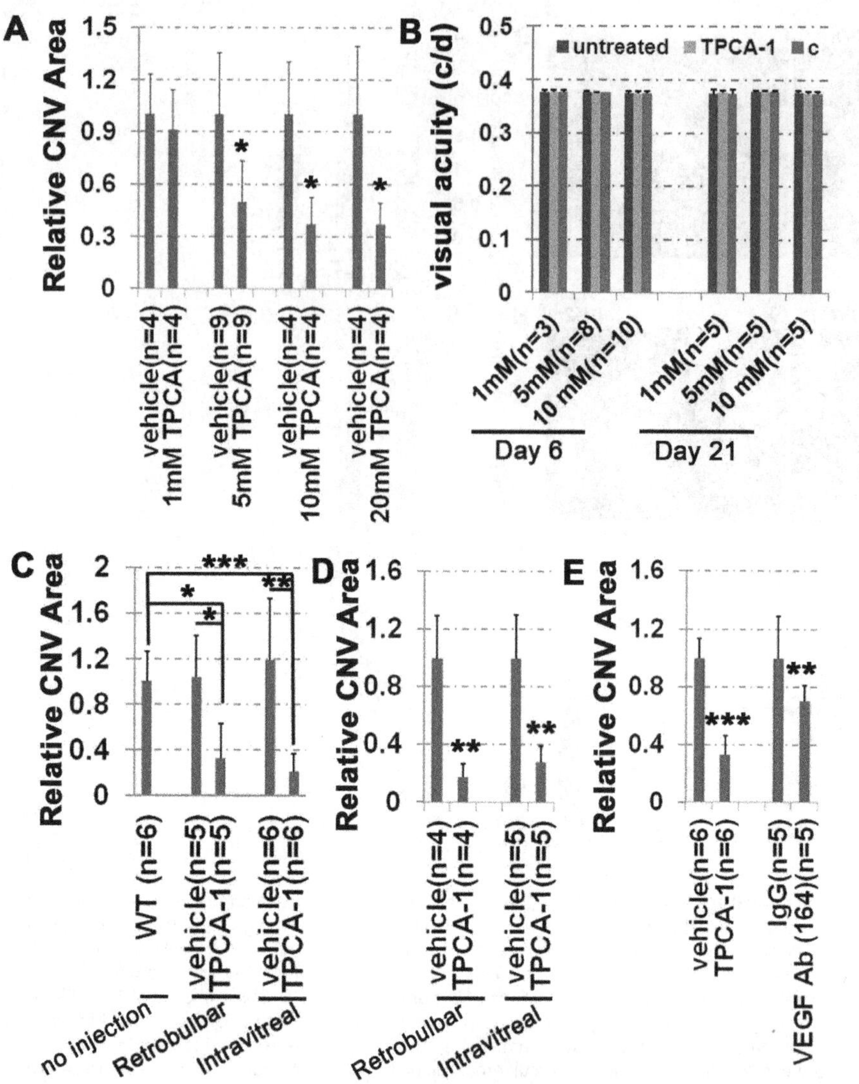

Figure 5. IKK2 chemical inhibitor TPCA-1 significantly reduces the laser-induced CNV formation. (A) The size measurements on the laser induced vascular sprouting in the eyes injected with 20 μL TPCA-1 or control vehicle (PBS/20% DMSO). 20 μL of IKK2 chemical inhibitor TPCA-1 at indicated concentration was retrobulbarly injected immediately after the laser injury. CNVs were visualized by FITC-dextran staining 7 days after laser injury and quantified as area size relative to CNV area in the control mice injected with vehicle solution. (B) Visual function was measured by OKR tests performed on the laser-injured and TPCA-1 treated mice on day-6 and -21 post laser injury. The mice received a retrobulbar injection of 20 μL TPCA-1 at the concentrations indicated under the X-axis of the graph in one eye right after laser injury. "Untreated" represents the results from the eyes without any injection. "TPCA-1" represents the visual acuity from the eyes retrobulbarly injected with 20 μL TPCA-1. "c" represents the combined visual acuity test results from both TPCA-1 treated and untreated eyes. (C) The size of CNV area developed in the laser-induced and TPCA-1 treated eyes was normalized to the size of CNV area in the laser-induced WT eyes that had not been given any injection after laser injury. The TPCA-1 treatment was given once to the mice via either retrobulbar (20 μL 10 mM TPCA-1 or control vehicle) or intravitreal (2 μL 10 mM TPCA-1 or control vehicle) injection immediately after laser injury and, seven days later, the FITC-dextran stained images were taken and calculated. (D) The size of CNV area developed in the laser-induced and TPCA-1 treated eyes was normalized to the size of CNV area in the laser-induced, and control solvent vehicle injected eyes. The TPCA-1 treatment was given once to the mice via either retrobulbar (20 μL 10 mM TPCA-1 or control vehicle) or intravitreal (2 μL 10 mM TPCA-1 or control vehicle) injection at 3 days after laser injury. The images were taken and calculated at 7 days after laser injury. (E) Comparison of the relative sizes of CNV area in the laser-injured mice that had been treated with either retrobulbar injection of 20 μL of 10 mM TPCA-1 or intravitreal injection of 2 μL of 2 μg/μL mouse VEGF 164 affinity purified polyclonal antibody. They were normalized to the size of CNV area in the laser-injured mice that had been treated with control solvent vehicle and IgG isotype control antibody, respectively. Error bars indicate standard deviation. Two-tail T-test: * $p<0.05$; ** $p<0.01$, *** $p<0.005$. "n" indicates the number of mice used at each condition.

We hypothesize that injury or inflammation in the laser injured retina may induce aberrant angiogenesis through the release of angiogenic factors that are regulated directly by NF-κB similar to that demonstrated for tumor cells [52–59]. We observed that TPCA-1, a selective inhibitor of IKK2, led to significant suppression of several pro-angiogenic molecules including IL1B, CCL2, VEGFA, PDGFA, HIF1A, and MMP-2 (Fig. 7). Furthermore, we also observed the inhibition of laser-induced CNV in genetic mouse mutants in which *Ikk2* was selectively deleted in RPE cells and retinal neurons but not in the vascular endothelium.

Inhibition of the NF-κB activation pathway has gained increasing interest in the treatment of several diseases including asthma, chronic obstructive pulmonary disease, and inflammation-associated cancer [60,61] because of its anti-inflammatory effects.

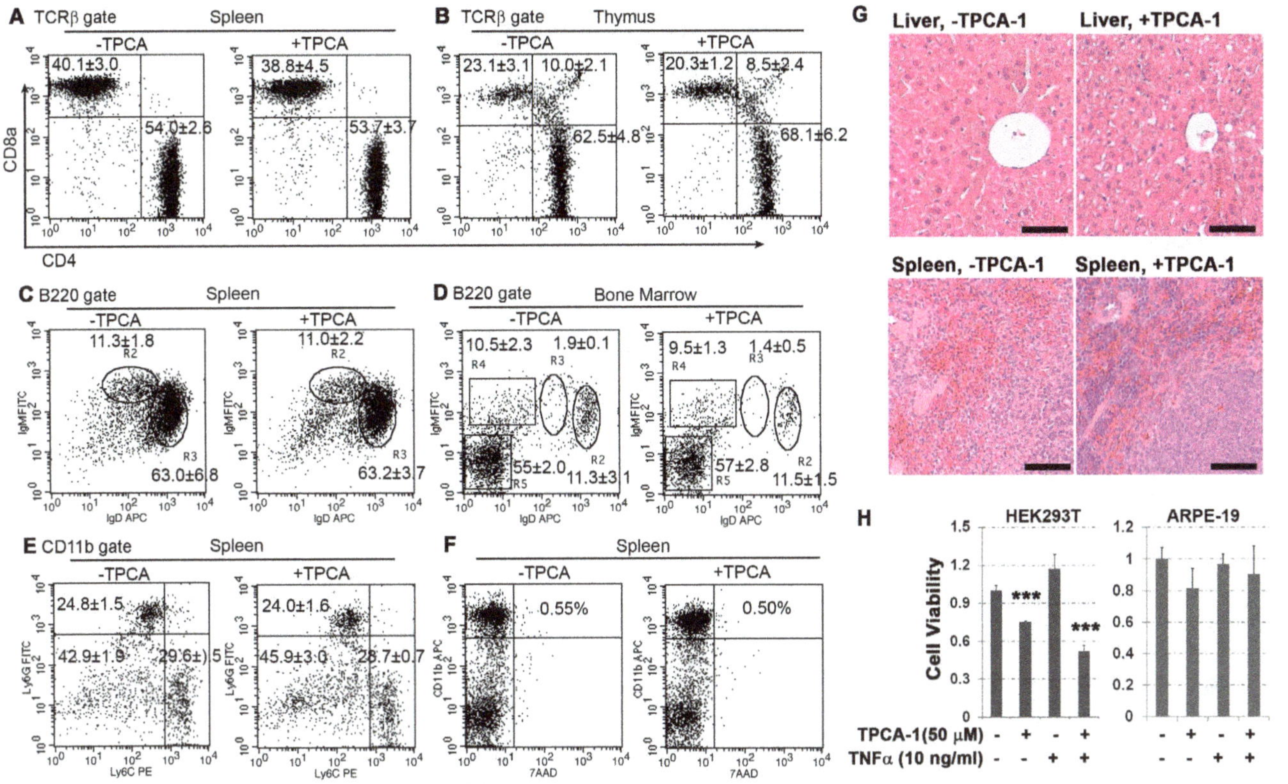

Figure 6. Retrobulbar administration of TPCA-1 causes no obvious toxicity to blood cells. (A–F) Flow cytometric analyses of blood cell population. Single cell suspension was prepared from spleen, thymus and bone marrow of the mice at 7 days after laser-injury followed immediately by a single retrobulbar injection of 56 μg TPCA-1 in 20 μL vehicle solution (PBS/20% DMSO) or control vehicle only in 20 μL. The representative plots are shown and numerical values represent the average (±SD, n>5). Statistics were performed using ProStat 5.5 program, and showing no significant difference in all the groups. $P \leq 0.05$ is considered as significant. (A, B) The $CD4^+$ and $CD8a^+$ T cells from the TCRβ-gated populations in spleen (A) and thymus (B) were calculated and plotted. (C, D) Spleen (C) and bone marrow (D) cells were isolated from TPCA-1 treated (+) and untreated (−) mice and stained with anti-B220, anti-IgM, and anti-IgD antibodies. Data in (C) show the percentile of mature ($IgD^{high}IgM^{low}$) and immature ($IgD^{low}IgM^{high}$) B cells in the B220-gated splenocytes, and data in (D) show the percentages of mature recirculating (R2, $IgD^{high}IgM^{int}$), transitional immature (R3, $IgM^{high}IgD^{int}$), immature (R4, $IgM^{high}IgD^-$) and precursor (R5, IgM^-IgD^-) B cell populations in the B220-gated bone marrow cells. (E) Spleen cells were isolated from TPCA-1 treated (+) and untreated (−) mice and stained with anti-CD11b, anti-Ly6C and anti-Ly6G antibodies. The numerical values are shown as the average of neutrophil ($Ly6G^+/Ly6C^{int}$), monocyte ($Ly6G^-/Ly6C^+$) and mature macrophage ($Ly6G^-/Ly6C^-$) from the CD11b gate in the spleens. (F) Spleen cells were stained with 7AAD to detect dead cells. The numerical values are shown as the average of the $CD11b^+$ $7AAD^+$ populations in splenic lymphoid cells. (G) Hematoxylin and eosin (H&E) histological staining was performed to evaluate toxicity to liver and spleen at 7 days after treatment. The scale bar represents 50 μm in length. (H) Relative cell viability of HEK293T cells (left panel) and ARPE-19 cells (right panel) was shown at 12 hours after being cultured with 50 μM TPCA-1 or 10 ng/mL TNFα or combination of both. The cells were pretreated with 50 μM TPCA-1 for 30 minutes prior to addition of 10 ng/mL TNFα for combination treatment. Cell viability was measured using MTT assay. Data are represented as the mean±SD from three independent experiments. Asterisk indicates Two-tail T-test: *** $p<0.005$.

IKK2, the proximal kinase leading to NF-κB activation, is an excellent target for inhibition of this pathway [13]. However, oral and systemic delivery of these inhibitors has been shown to be toxic to bone marrow and epithelial cells [30,62–64]. Therefore, local delivery of this drug to the eye is an attractive therapeutic alternative. Our data showed that retrobulbar injection of 56 μg TPCA-1 inhibited laser-induced CNV in mice and had no detrimental effect to liver, spleen and bone marrow derived cells (Fig. 6A–G), as well as skin epithelium (data not shown). Consistent with a previous report [65], IKK2 inhibition by TPCA-1 did not cause ARPE-19 cell death even with TNFα induction (Fig. 6H). In addition, neither genetic deletion of *Ikk2* gene nor periocular administration of TPCA-1 showed an adverse effect on retinal histology or visual function (Fig. 3 and Fig. 5B).

Anti-VEGF therapy for CNV results in significant vision gain in approximately one-third of patients with wet AMD mostly due to its anti-permeability effect but not the inhibition of aberrant angiogenesis [66–68]. In search of better treatments, a multi-targeted therapeutic approach has been proposed and a recent clinical study using anti-PDGF and anti-VEGF combination therapy in wet AMD has reported improved visual outcome compared with anti-VEGF monotherapy [69_ENREF_69]. Targeting multiple signaling pathways involved in CNV may be a better option to improve therapeutic results. As a key regulator of several factors promoting inflammation and angiogenesis, IKK2/NF-κB inhibition is a rational therapeutic strategy. Another advantage of IKK2/NF-κB inhibition therapy over anti-VEGF monotherapy is the targeting of an earlier phase of angiogenesis by inhibiting inflammation. In summary, we have demonstrated that periocular injection of TPCA-1, a selective IKK2 inhibitor, is able to reduce the development of laser-induced CNV by blocking activation of the NF-κB signal pathway that is important for expression of multiple inflammatory and angiogenic factors. Our results suggest that IKK2 inhibition could be a potential novel approach to prevent or reduce CNV formation.

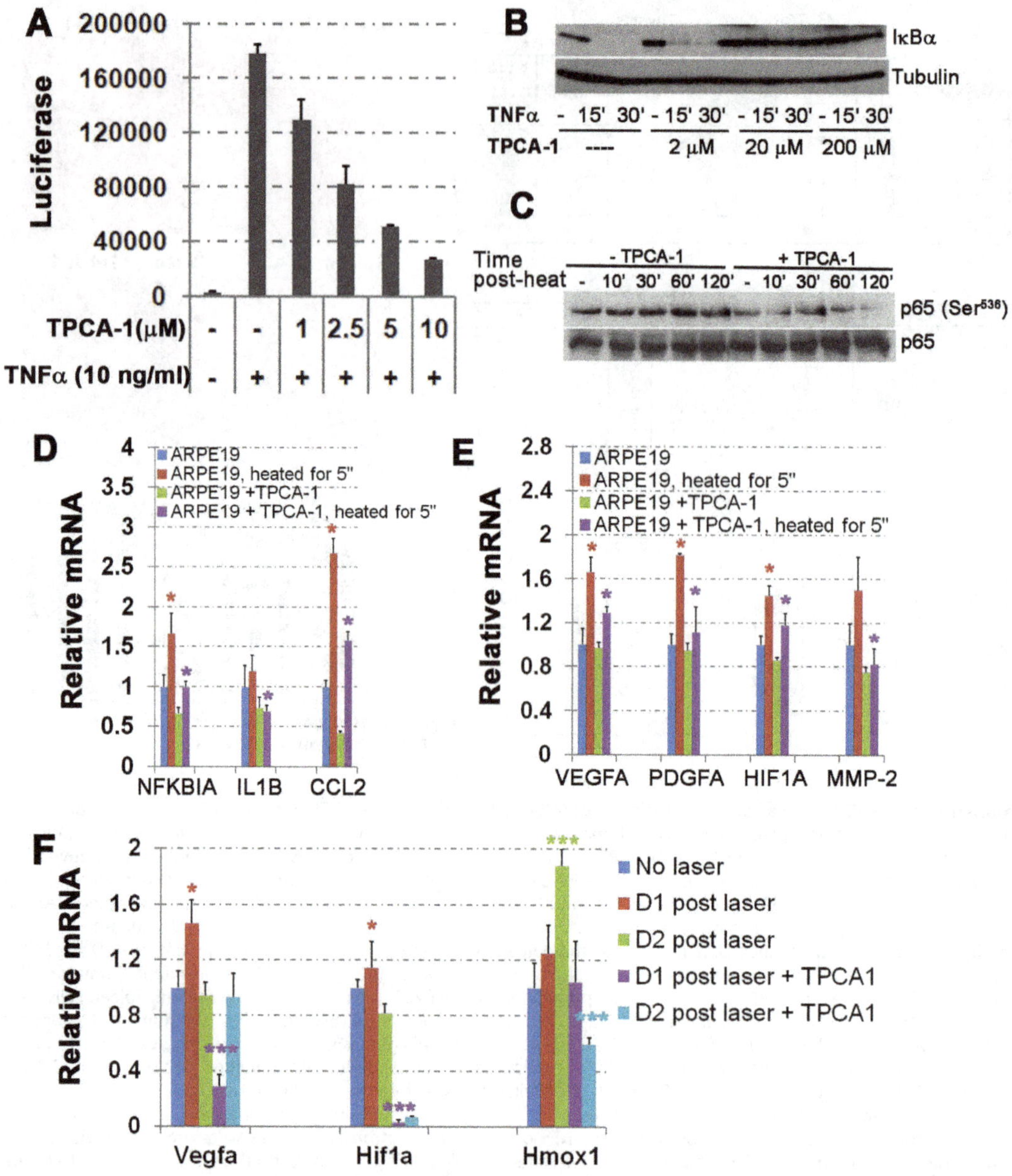

Figure 7. TPCA-1 inhibits NF-κB signaling pathway and the thermal injury-induced angiogenesis-associated factors. (A) TPCA-1 inhibits the TNFα-induced κB-Luciferase activity in a dosage dependent manner. 293T cells containing κB-Luciferase reporter were pretreated with or without TPCA1 for 30 minutes, then stimulated with 10 ng/mL TNFα to induce κB-Luciferase expression in the presence of the indicated amount of TPCA-1 for 5 hours, and followed by cell lysis and luciferase assay. (B) TPCA-1 inhibits TNFα-induced IκBα degradation in a dosage dependent manner. ARPE-19 cells were pretreated with TPCA-1 at indicated concentration for 30 minutes prior to addition of 10 ng/mL of TNFα for 15 and 30 minutes in the presence of the same amount of TPCA-1. Protein lysates were analyzed for the levels of IκBα and tubulin (as a loading control) by Western blotting. (C) TPCA-1 treatment inhibits the thermal injury-induced p65 phosphorylation at serine 536 amino acid residue. The ARPE-19 cells at 80% confluence in the complete DMEM/F-20 medium were pretreated with 5 μM TPCA-1 for 30 minutes and followed by heat shock for 5 seconds with addition of 10 mL HEPES-buffered saline preheated at 55°C; and then the heating medium was immediately replaced with normal complete DMEM/F-20 medium containing 5 μM TPCA-1 and further cultured at 37°C for 10, 30, 60, and 120 minutes before the protein lysates were collected. Western blotting was used to detect the total NF-κB p65 protein and the activated form of NF-κB p65 phosphorylated at Serine 536. (D and E) TPCA-1 treatment reduces thermal injury-induced and NF-κB dependent transcription of signaling protein, cytokine and chemokine, such as IκBα, IL1B and CCL2 (D), as well as of those associated with angiogenesis, such as VEGF-A, PDGFA, HIF-1A, and MMP-2 (E) in ARPE-19 cells. Cells were treated similarly as described in C. Four hours after the thermal treatment, RNAs were isolated for qPCR analysis. Relative mRNA levels were normalized to β-actin first, and then the fold increase or decrease by heat shock. Cells were treated with heat shock at the presence or absence of TPCA-1 or treated with TPCA-1 without heat shock were compared to control cells without heat shock and TPCA treatment. Error bars indicate standard deviation. Two-tail T-test: * $p<0.05$, n = 3. The red * indicates the comparison between the heat shocked cells and control cells. The purple * indicates the comparison between the heat shocked cells at the presence or absence of TPCA-1. (F) Relative mRNA level of Vegfa, Hif1a, and Hmox1 was shown in the RPE/Choroid/Sclera tissues collected from laser injured eyes treated with or without TPCA-1. Mice received the retrobulbar injection of 56 μg TPCA-1 or vehicle solution and the RNA samples were prepared from RPE/Choroid/Sclera tissues at day 1 and day 2 post injury. Each RNA sample was pooled from 4 eyes in the same condition and the control sample is from the eyes without laser injury. Red and green * show the significant difference between the indicated sample and control sample without laser injury. Purple and light blue *** show the significant difference between the laser injured samples at the presence or absence of TPCA-1. Error bars indicate standard deviation. Two-tail T-test: * $p<0.05$, *** $p<0.005$, n = 3.

Supporting Information

File S1 Contains: Figure S1 Fluorescein angiography of laser induced CNV and size grading for fluorescein leakage. (A) Lesion sizes were graded based on the relative comparison to the optic nerve disk area. (B–C) Lesion sizes in the same eye were graded at 3 and 6 minutes after intraperitoneal injection of fluorescein. Figure S2 Fundus photography before and after retrobulbar injection. (A–A1) the fundus images of a mouse eye before and after retrobulbar injection of 50 μL of PBS/20% DMSO. (B–B1) the fundus images of another eye before and after retrobulbar injection of 50 μL of PBS/20% DMSO.

Acknowledgments

Authors thank Research to Prevent Blindness, Inc, New York, N.Y. for departmental support, and Guirong Liu for tissue processing in the histology core of the Department of Ophthalmology and Visual Sciences.

Author Contributions

Conceived and designed the experiments: HL Q. Lu WW HJK Q. Li. Performed the experiments: HL Q. Lu SG RBK Qli. Analyzed the data: HL Q. Lu SG RBK WW HJK Q. Li. Contributed reagents/materials/ analysis tools: Q. Lu MP Q. Li. Wrote the paper: Q. Lu HJK Q. Li.

References

1. Haines JL, Spencer KM, Pericak-Vance MA (2007) Bringing the genetics of macular degeneration into focus. Proc Natl Acad Sci U S A 104: 16725–16726.
2. Rattner A, Nathans J (2006) Macular degeneration: recent advances and therapeutic opportunities. Nat Rev Neurosci 7: 860–872.
3. Brown DM, Kaiser PK, Michels M, Soubrane G, Heier JS, et al. (2006) Ranibizumab versus verteporfin for neovascular age-related macular degeneration. N Engl J Med 355: 1432–1444.
4. Gragoudas ES, Adamis AP, Cunningham ET, Jr., Feinsod M, Guyer DR (2004) Pegaptanib for neovascular age-related macular degeneration. N Engl J Med 351: 2805–2816.
5. Rosenfeld PJ, Brown DM, Heier JS, Boyer DS, Kaiser PK, et al. (2006) Ranibizumab for neovascular age-related macular degeneration. N Engl J Med 355: 1419–1431.
6. Lommatzsch A, Hermans P, Muller KD, Bornfeld N, Bird AC, et al. (2008) Are low inflammatory reactions involved in exudative age-related macular degeneration? Morphological and immunhistochemical analysis of AMD associated with basal deposits. Graefes Arch Clin Exp Ophthalmol 246: 803–810.
7. Grossniklaus HE, Miskala PH, Green WR, Bressler SB, Hawkins BS, et al. (2005) Histopathologic and ultrastructural features of surgically excised subfoveal choroidal neovascular lesions: submacular surgery trials report no. 7. Arch Ophthalmol 123: 914–921.
8. Seddon JM, Gensler G, Milton RC, Klein ML, Rifai N (2004) Association between C-reactive protein and age-related macular degeneration. JAMA 291: 704–710.
9. Hageman GS, Anderson DH, Johnson LV, Hancox LS, Taiber AJ, et al. (2005) A common haplotype in the complement regulatory gene factor H (HF1/CFH) predisposes individuals to age-related macular degeneration. Proc Natl Acad Sci U S A 102: 7227–7232.
10. Haines JL, Hauser MA, Schmidt S, Scott WK, Olson LM, et al. (2005) Complement factor H variant increases the risk of age-related macular degeneration. Science 308: 419–421.
11. Li Q, Verma IM (2002) NF-kappaB regulation in the immune system. Nat Rev Immunol 2: 725–734.
12. Li Q, Van Antwerp D, Mercurio F, Lee KF, Verma IM (1999) Severe liver degeneration in mice lacking the IkappaB kinase 2 gene. Science 284: 321–325.
13. Hacker H, Karin M (2006) Regulation and function of IKK and IKK-related kinases. Sci STKE 2006: re13.
14. Yang XM, Wang YS, Zhang J, Li Y, Xu JF, et al. (2009) Role of PI3K/Akt and MEK/ERK in mediating hypoxia-induced expression of HIF-1alpha and VEGF in laser-induced rat choroidal neovascularization. Invest Ophthalmol Vis Sci 50: 1873–1879.
15. Grossniklaus HE, Kang SJ, Berglin L (2010) Animal models of choroidal and retinal neovascularization. Prog Retin Eye Res 29: 500–519.
16. Semenza GL (2001) HIF-1, O(2), and the 3 PHDs: how animal cells signal hypoxia to the nucleus. Cell 107: 1–3.
17. Tronche F, Kellendonk C, Kretz O, Gass P, Anlag K, et al. (1999) Disruption of the glucocorticoid receptor gene in the nervous system results in reduced anxiety. Nat Genet 23: 99–103.
18. Muzumdar MD, Tasic B, Miyamichi K, Li L, Luo L (2007) A global double-fluorescent Cre reporter mouse. Genesis 45: 593–605.
19. Bora PS, Hu Z, Tezel TH, Sohn JH, Kang SG, et al. (2003) Immunotherapy for choroidal neovascularization in a laser-induced mouse model simulating exudative (wet) macular degeneration. Proc Natl Acad Sci U S A 100: 2679–2684.
20. Prusky GT, Alam NM, Beekman S, Douglas RM (2004) Rapid quantification of adult and developing mouse spatial vision using a virtual optomotor system. Invest Ophthalmol Vis Sci 45: 4611–4616.
21. Franco LM, Zulliger R, Wolf-Schnurrbusch UE, Katagiri Y, Kaplan HJ, et al. (2009) Decreased visual function after patchy loss of retinal pigment epithelium induced by low-dose sodium iodate. Invest Ophthalmol Vis Sci 50: 4004–4010.
22. Hu W, Criswell MH, Ottlecz A, Cornell TL, Danis RP, et al. (2005) Oral administration of lumiracoxib reduces choroidal neovascular membrane development in the rat laser-trauma model. Retina 25: 1054–1064.
23. Connor KM, Krah NM, Dennison RJ, Aderman CM, Chen J, et al. (2009) Quantification of oxygen-induced retinopathy in the mouse: a model of vessel loss, vessel regrowth and pathological angiogenesis. Nat Protoc 4: 1565–1573.
24. Neuvians TP, Gashaw I, Sauer CG, von Ostau C, Kliesch S, et al. (2005) Standardization strategy for quantitative PCR in human seminoma and normal testis. J Biotechnol 117: 163–171.
25. Luedde T, Assmus U, Wustefeld T, Meyer zu Vilsendorf A, Roskams T, et al. (2005) Deletion of IKK2 in hepatocytes does not sensitize these cells to TNF-induced apoptosis but protects from ischemia/reperfusion injury. J Clin Invest 115: 849–859.
26. Ye F, Han L, Lu Q, Dong W, Chen Z, et al. (2011) Retinal self-antigen induces a predominantly Th1 effector response in Axl and Mertk double-knockout mice. J Immunol 187: 4178–4186.
27. Pasparakis M, Courtois G, Hafner M, Schmidt-Supprian M, Nenci A, et al. (2002) TNF-mediated inflammatory skin disease in mice with epidermis-specific deletion of IKK2. Nature 417: 861–866.
28. Podolin PL, Callahan JF, Bolognese BJ, Li YH, Carlson K, et al. (2005) Attenuation of murine collagen-induced arthritis by a novel, potent, selective small molecule inhibitor of IkappaB Kinase 2, TPCA-1 (2-[(aminocarbonyl)amino]-5-(4-fluorophenyl)-3-thiophenecarboxamide), occurs via reduction of proinflammatory cytokines and antigen-induced T cell Proliferation. J Pharmacol Exp Ther 312: 373–381.
29. Liu J, Jha P, Lyzogubov VV, Tytarenko RG, Bora NS, et al. (2011) Relationship between complement membrane attack complex, chemokine (C–C motif) ligand 2 (CCL2) and vascular endothelial growth factor in mouse model of laser-induced choroidal neovascularization. J Biol Chem 286: 20991–21001.
30. Nagashima K, Sasseville VG, Wen D, Bielecki A, Yang H, et al. (2006) Rapid TNFR1-dependent lymphocyte depletion in vivo with a selective chemical inhibitor of IKKbeta. Blood 107: 4266–4273.
31. Grossmann M, Metcalf D, Merryfull J, Beg A, Baltimore D, et al. (1999) The combined absence of the transcription factors Rel and RelA leads to multiple hemopoietic cell defects. Proc Natl Acad Sci U S A 96: 11848–11853.
32. Senftleben U, Li ZW, Baud V, Karin M (2001) IKKbeta is essential for protecting T cells from TNFalpha-induced apoptosis. Immunity 14: 217–230.
33. Sakamoto K, Maeda S, Hikiba Y, Nakagawa H, Hayakawa Y, et al. (2009) Constitutive NF-kappaB activation in colorectal carcinoma plays a key role in angiogenesis, promoting tumor growth. Clin Cancer Res 15: 2248–2258.
34. Karin M, Ben-Neriah Y (2000) Phosphorylation meets ubiquitination: the control of NF-[kappa]B activity. Annu Rev Immunol 18: 621–663.
35. Dinh HK, Zhao B, Schuschereba ST, Merrill G, Bowman PD (2001) Gene expression profiling of the response to thermal injury in human cells. Physiol Genomics 7: 3–13.
36. Ferrara N, Gerber HP, LeCouter J (2003) The biology of VEGF and its receptors. Nat Med 9: 669–676.
37. Penn JS, Madan A, Caldwell RB, Bartoli M, Caldwell RW, et al. (2008) Vascular endothelial growth factor in eye disease. Prog Retin Eye Res 27: 331–371.
38. Kliffen M, Sharma HS, Mooy CM, Kerkvliet S, de Jong PT (1997) Increased expression of angiogenic growth factors in age-related maculopathy. Br J Ophthalmol 81: 154–162.
39. Lopez PF, Sippy BD, Lambert HM, Thach AB, Hinton DR (1996) Transdifferentiated retinal pigment epithelial cells are immunoreactive for vascular endothelial growth factor in surgically excised age-related macular degeneration-related choroidal neovascular membranes. Invest Ophthalmol Vis Sci 37: 855–868.
40. Aiello LP, Avery RL, Arrigg PG, Keyt BA, Jampel HD, et al. (1994) Vascular endothelial growth factor in ocular fluid of patients with diabetic retinopathy and other retinal disorders. N Engl J Med 331: 1480–1487.
41. Adamis AP, Shima DT, Yeo KT, Yeo TK, Brown LF, et al. (1993) Synthesis and secretion of vascular permeability factor/vascular endothelial growth factor by human retinal pigment epithelial cells. Biochem Biophys Res Commun 193: 631–638.

42. Ryuto M, Ono M, Izumi H, Yoshida S, Weich HA, et al. (1996) Induction of vascular endothelial growth factor by tumor necrosis factor alpha in human glioma cells. Possible roles of SP-1. J Biol Chem 271: 28220–28228.
43. Shono T, Ono M, Izumi H, Jimi SI, Matsushima K, et al. (1996) Involvement of the transcription factor NF-kappaB in tubular morphogenesis of human microvascular endothelial cells by oxidative stress. Mol Cell Biol 16: 4231–4239.
44. Yoshida S, Ono M, Shono T, Izumi H, Ishibashi T, et al. (1997) Involvement of interleukin-8, vascular endothelial growth factor, and basic fibroblast growth factor in tumor necrosis factor alpha-dependent angiogenesis. Mol Cell Biol 17: 4015–4023.
45. Levine L, Lucci JA, 3rd, Pazdrak B, Cheng JZ, Guo YS, et al. (2003) Bombesin stimulates nuclear factor kappa B activation and expression of proangiogenic factors in prostate cancer cells. Cancer Res 63: 3495–3502.
46. Yu HG, Yu LL, Yang Y, Luo HS, Yu JP, et al. (2003) Increased expression of RelA/nuclear factor-kappa B protein correlates with colorectal tumorigenesis. Oncology 65: 37–45.
47. Ono M (2008) Molecular links between tumor angiogenesis and inflammation: inflammatory stimuli of macrophages and cancer cells as targets for therapeutic strategy. Cancer Sci 99: 1501–1506.
48. Aggarwal BB, Shishodia S, Sandur SK, Pandey MK, Sethi G (2006) Inflammation and cancer: how hot is the link? Biochem Pharmacol 72: 1605–1621.
49. Shibata A, Nagaya T, Imai T, Funahashi H, Nakao A, et al. (2002) Inhibition of NF-kappaB activity decreases the VEGF mRNA expression in MDA-MB-231 breast cancer cells. Breast Cancer Res Treat 73: 237–243.
50. Ramanathan M, Pinhal-Enfield G, Hao I, Leibovich SJ (2007) Synergistic up-regulation of vascular endothelial growth factor (VEGF) expression in macrophages by adenosine A2A receptor agonists and endotoxin involves transcriptional regulation via the hypoxia response element in the VEGF promoter. Mol Biol Cell 18: 14–23.
51. Schofield CJ, Ratcliffe PJ (2004) Oxygen sensing by HIF hydroxylases. Nat Rev Mol Cell Biol 5: 343–354.
52. Rius J, Guma M, Schachtrup C, Akassoglou K, Zinkernagel AS, et al. (2008) NF-kappaB links innate immunity to the hypoxic response through transcriptional regulation of HIF-1alpha. Nature 453: 807–811.
53. Koch AE, Halloran MM, Haskell CJ, Shah MR, Polverini PJ (1995) Angiogenesis mediated by soluble forms of E-selectin and vascular cell adhesion molecule-1. Nature 376: 517–519.
54. Taylor BS, de Vera ME, Ganster RW, Wang Q, Shapiro RA, et al. (1998) Multiple NF-kappaB enhancer elements regulate cytokine induction of the human inducible nitric oxide synthase gene. J Biol Chem 273: 15148–15156.
55. Stetler-Stevenson WG (1999) Matrix metalloproteinases in angiogenesis: a moving target for therapeutic intervention. J Clin Invest 103: 1237–1241.
56. Yasuda M, Shimizu S, Ohhinata K, Naito S, Tokuyama S, et al. (2002) Differential roles of ICAM-1 and E-selectin in polymorphonuclear leukocyte-induced angiogenesis. Am J Physiol Cell Physiol 282: C917–925.
57. Zhou A, Scoggin S, Gaynor RB, Williams NS (2003) Identification of NF-kappa B-regulated genes induced by TNFalpha utilizing expression profiling and RNA interference. Oncogene 22: 2054–2064.
58. Sainson RC, Johnston DA, Chu HC, Holderfield MT, Nakatsu MN, et al. (2008) TNF primes endothelial cells for angiogenic sprouting by inducing a tip cell phenotype. Blood 111: 4997–5007.
59. van Beijnum JR, Buurman WA, Griffioen AW (2008) Convergence and amplification of toll-like receptor (TLR) and receptor for advanced glycation end products (RAGE) signaling pathways via high mobility group B1 (HMGB1). Angiogenesis 11: 91–99.
60. Gupta SC, Sundaram C, Reuter S, Aggarwal BB (2010) Inhibiting NF-kappaB activation by small molecules as a therapeutic strategy. Biochim Biophys Acta 1799: 775–787.
61. Arkan MC, Greten FR (2011) IKK- and NF-kappaB-mediated functions in carcinogenesis. Curr Top Microbiol Immunol 349: 159–169.
62. Mankan AK, Canli O, Schwitalla S, Ziegler P, Tschopp J, et al. (2011) TNF-alpha-dependent loss of IKKbeta-deficient myeloid progenitors triggers a cytokine loop culminating in granulocytosis. Proc Natl Acad Sci U S A 108: 6567–6572.
63. Greten FR, Arkan MC, Bollrath J, Hsu LC, Goode J, et al. (2007) NF-kappaB is a negative regulator of IL-1beta secretion as revealed by genetic and pharmacological inhibition of IKKbeta. Cell 130: 918–931.
64. Wullaert A, Bonnet MC, Pasparakis M (2011) NF-kappaB in the regulation of epithelial homeostasis and inflammation. Cell Res 21: 146–158.
65. Yang P, McKay BS, Allen JB, Jaffe GJ (2004) Effect of NF-kappa B inhibition on TNF-alpha-induced apoptosis in human RPE cells. Invest Ophthalmol Vis Sci 45: 2438–2446.
66. Brown DM, Kaiser PK, Michels M, Soubrane G, Heier JS, et al. (2006) Ranibizumab versus verteporfin for neovascular age-related macular degeneration. N Engl J Med 355: 1432–1444.
67. Rosenfeld PJ, Brown DM, Heier JS, Boyer DS, Kaiser PK, et al. (2006) Ranibizumab for neovascular age-related macular degeneration. N Engl J Med 355: 1419–1431.
68. Regillo CD, Brown DM, Abraham P, Yue H, Ianchulev T, et al. (2008) Randomized, double-masked, sham-controlled trial of ranibizumab for neovascular age-related macular degeneration: PIER Study year 1. Am J Ophthalmol 145: 239–248.
69. Ophthotech's Novel Anti-PDGF Combination Agent Fovista Demonstrated Superior Efficacy Over Lucentis Monotherapy in Large Controlled Wet AMD Trial. (2012) Princeton, NJ: BusinessWire; June 13.

22

Interleukin-17 Retinotoxicity Is Prevented by Gene Transfer of a Soluble Interleukin-17 Receptor Acting as a Cytokine Blocker: Implications for Age-Related Macular Degeneration

Daniel Ardeljan[1,2], Yujuan Wang[1,3], Stanley Park[1,4], Defen Shen[1], Xi Kathy Chu[1], Cheng-Rong Yu[5], Mones Abu-Asab[6], Jingsheng Tuo[1], Charles G. Eberhart[7], Timothy W. Olsen[8], Robert F. Mullins[9], Gary White[10], Sam Wadsworth[10], Abraham Scaria[10], Chi-Chao Chan[1]*

1 Immunopathology Section, Laboratory of Immunology, National Eye Institute, National Institutes of Health, Bethesda, Maryland, United States of America, **2** School of Medicine, Johns Hopkins University, Baltimore, Maryland, United States of America, **3** Zhongshan Ophthalmic Center, Sun Yat-sen University, Guangzhou, China, **4** Howard Hughes Medical Institute, Chevy Chase, Maryland, United States of America, **5** Molecular Immunology Section, Laboratory of Immunology, National Eye Institute, National Institutes of Health, Bethesda, Maryland, United States of America, **6** Histology Core, Laboratory of Immunology, National Eye Institute, National Institutes of Health, Bethesda, Maryland, United States of America, **7** Department of Pathology, Johns Hopkins University, Baltimore, Maryland, United States of America, **8** Department of Ophthalmology, Emory University, Atlanta, Georgia, United States of America, **9** Department of Ophthalmology and Visual Sciences, University of Iowa Carver College of Medicine, Iowa City, Iowa, United States of America, **10** Genzyme Corporation, Framingham, Massachusetts, United States of America

Abstract

Age-related macular degeneration (AMD) is a common yet complex retinal degeneration that causes irreversible central blindness in the elderly. Pathology is widely believed to follow loss of retinal pigment epithelium (RPE) and photoreceptor degeneration. Here we report aberrant expression of interleukin-17A (IL17A) and the receptor IL17RC in the macula of AMD patients. *In vitro*, IL17A induces RPE cell death characterized by the accumulation of cytoplasmic lipids and autophagosomes with subsequent activation of pro-apoptotic Caspase-3 and Caspase-9. This pathology is reduced by siRNA knockdown of *IL17RC*. IL17-dependent retinal degeneration in a mouse model of focal retinal degeneration can be prevented by gene therapy with adeno-associated virus vector encoding soluble IL17 receptor. This intervention rescues RPE and photoreceptors in a MAPK-dependent process. The IL17 pathway plays a key role in RPE and photoreceptor degeneration and could hold therapeutic potential in AMD.

Editor: James T. Rosenbaum, Oregon Health & Science University, United States of America

Funding: The National Eye Institute Intramural Research Program & Genzyme funded the work. The funder Genzyme provided support in the form of salaries for authors GW, SW, and AS, but did not have any additional role in the study design, data collection and analysis, decision to publish, or preparation of the manuscript.

Competing Interests: The authors would also like to make explicit their collaboration with Genzyme Corp. Three of the co-authors, GW, SW, and AS are employees of Genzyme, who funded their salaries. GW and AS are listed as inventors on a patent application held by the company. Patent application name: "Composition and Methods for Inhibiting Interleukin Pathways" and number WO 2009042162. There are no further patents, products in development or marketed products to declare.

* E-mail: chanc@nei.nih.gov

Introduction

Age-related macular degeneration (AMD) is the leading cause of central irreversible blindness in people age 55 and older [1,2]. The disease is characterized earliest by the appearance of extracellular material (drusen) in macular Bruch's membrane and external to the retinal pigment epithelium (RPE). Many patients develop one of two phenotypes: geographic atrophy (GA or "dry AMD") characterized by atrophy of RPE and photoreceptors, or neovascular AMD (nAMD or "wet AMD") characterized by choroidal neovascularization (CNV). AMD risk factors include aging, smoking, and genetics, particularly a common polymorphism in complement factor H. RPE damage is an inciting event believed to be the primary pathological insult leading to photoreceptor atrophy [3]. The specific mechanism is largely unknown.

Growing clinical suspicion is emerging for involvement of interleukin-17A (IL17A) in AMD. Complement component C5a, found in AMD patient serum and in drusen [4–6], induces IL17A secretion from $CD4^{+}$ T cells [7]. IL17A in the serum and hypomethylation of the *IL17RC* promoter in twins with discordant AMD status has been shown [7,8]. Subsequently, we noted that the anti-inflammatory agent TSG-6 halted $Ccl2^{-/-}/Cx3cr1^{-/-}/Crb1^{rd8}$ (DKO/*rd8*) retinal degeneration and found that treated retinas expressed less *Il17a* [9]. IL17A has been shown to drive autoimmune diseases including rheumatoid arthritis and experimental autoimmune uveitis [10].

Since AMD patients present without systemic inflammation, we hypothesized that local IL17 signaling was retinotoxic in AMD. We first characterized the expression of IL17A and IL17RC in the AMD retina and then determined the cytokine's effect on RPE viability *in vitro*. Finally, we knocked down IL17 signaling in a mouse model of focal retinal degeneration (DKO/*rd8*) [11,12] using an adeno-associated viral vector encoding a soluble IL17 receptor.

Results

Aberrant Levels of IL17A and IL17RC in the AMD Macula

We isolated RNA from microdissected macular lesions of 107 paraffin-embedded eyes from 67 advanced stage AMD donors (35 GA, 72 nAMD) and 17 eyes from 10 age-matched control donors collected over the past 50 years from Johns Hopkins and NEI. Only 41 (38.3%) of AMD eyes (9 GA, 32 nAMD) and 8 (47.1%) of control eyes yielded quantifiable results. We also detected transcripts in sub-macular choroid button of 9 control and 17 AMD donor eyes.

Macular *IL17A* expression averaged from 14- to 20-fold higher in AMD vs. normal tissue (Figure 1A–B). Macular *IL17RC* averaged from 47- to 93-fold higher in AMD vs. normal tissue (Figure 1C). Twenty-seven AMD and four normal retinas were assayed in the periphery, but *IL17A* was below the detectable threshold for the qRT-PCR assay in all specimens. *IL17RC* was detectable in 3 (11.1%) AMD peripheral samples, and among these 3 samples, *IL17RC* averaged 20-fold higher in the macula vs. periphery (Figure 1D). *IL17F*, an *IL17A* homologue that has some functional overlap [13], was undetectable in all samples.

Due to the ~40% yield obtained from the paraffin-embedded slides, we validated our findings using 10 fresh eyes (5 normal, 5 AMD). These AMD donors had early/intermediate AMD pathologies. The macular tissues were paraformaldehyde fixed, cytoprotected, and snap frozen, and thus in significantly better condition for assaying mRNA expression. All samples yielded measurable results. Respectively, *IL17A* and *IL17RC* expression averaged 8.2- and 6.2-fold higher in AMD vs. normal (Figure 1E–F).

Enhanced diffuse immunoreactivity of both IL17A and IL17RC was observed in GA and nAMD (Figure 1G). IL17A immunoreactivity was slightly greater in the macula as compared to the periphery (Figure 1H), but retinal IL17RC was evenly distributed. These results indicate significant aberrant expression of *IL17A* and *IL17RC* mRNA within AMD lesions.

IL17A is Cytotoxic to ARPE-19

Degenerative changes to RPE were evaluated in the ARPE-19 cell line. IL17A challenge activated pro-apoptotic Caspase-9 and Caspase-3 (Figure 2A). The pathology of ARPE-19 encompassed lipid accumulations, autophagosomes, mitochondrial damage, nuclear pyknosis, and necrosis (Figure 2B). Viability was assessed by the enzymatic redox of MTT, a mitochondrial reaction requiring NADPH-dependent oxidoreductases, to distinguish cell-type effects of IL17A. IL17A reduced ARPE-19 viability by 25% at 1 ng/ml, whereas COS-7 were relatively unaffected until 100 times that amount was added (Figure 2C). ARPE-19 cells expressed significantly higher levels of IL17RA and IL17RC (Figure 2D), suggesting that ARPE-19 may be more sensitive to IL17A than are COS-7 due to differences in receptor expression.

IL17RC siRNA Rescues ARPE-19 from IL17A Challenge

In order to determine whether receptor expression could modulate IL17A cytotoxicity, we knocked down *IL17RC* with siRNA. ARPE-19 were transfected with control (ctrl) or *IL17RC* siRNA prior to IL17A challenge. *IL17RC* siRNA, but not ctrl siRNA, reduced *IL17RC* expression (Figure 3A). *IL17RC* siRNA, but not ctrl siRNA, prevented IL17A-mediated reductions in viability (Figure 3B) and markedly reduced activation of Caspase-9 and Caspase-3 (Figure 3C). We concluded that downregulating receptor expression could prevent IL17-mediated cytotoxicity.

sIL17R Ameliorates Retinal Degeneration in DKO/rd8 Mice via MAPK

We hypothesized that IL17A neutralization could prevent retinal degeneration in DKO/*rd8*. *Il17a* expression in the retina is approximately 30-fold greater in DKO/*rd8* compared to WT at 2 months of age (Figure 4A). To inhibit IL17 in the retina, we administered intravitreal AAV2 vectors encoding soluble IL17 receptor (sIL17R, Figure S1A–B) into right eyes and empty vector (EV) into left eyes of 40 DKO/*rd8* mice over two independent trials and followed them for 2 months. AAV2 vectors preferentially transfect retinal ganglion cells and secreted proteins are detected throughout the entirety of the retina [14,15]. Injection of AAV2.sIL17R resulted in sIL17R protein expression, no change in retinal *Il17a* transcripts, and a near-significant reduction in *Il6* (Figure S1C–E), supporting sIL17R expression in AAV2.sIL17R- but not in AAV2.EV-treated eyes.

Intervention with sIL17R prevented retinopathy: (i) lesions were fewer by fundoscopy (Figure 4B, Figure S2A–B); (ii) A2E concentration–a lipofuscin fluorophore generated from the visual cycle flux of all-trans-retinal and a biomarker of RPE damage [16]–was reduced (Figure 4C); (iii) photoreceptor atrophy was prevented (Figure 4D, Table S1); (iv) RPE were preserved, evidenced by the lack of vacuolation, lipofuscin, glycogen deposits, undigested photoreceptor outer segments, and mitochondrial atrophy compared to RPE in EV-treated eyes (Figure 4E). The data supports our previous finding that correlated successful anti-inflammatory therapy with reduced *Il17a* expression in DKO/*rd8* retina [9].

We wanted to confirm that sIL17R dampened IL17 signal transduction. IL17A binds to hetero- or homodimers of IL17RA and IL17RC, inducing transcription of pro-inflammatory cytokines via Akt, MAPKs (ERK1/2 and p38), and NF-κB [17–19]. We analyzed Erk1/2, p38, and Akt phosphorylation *ex vivo* after challenge with recombinant murine Il17a. Protein lysates were extracted from 12 DKO/*rd8* retinas, 6 expressing EV and 6 expressing sIL17R. Neurosensory retinas were co-incubated with Il17a for 0, 5, or 15 minutes (Figure 4F). There was a 50% reduction in background MAPK and Akt phosphorylation in sIL17R versus EV tissue. Il17a induced p38 and Erk1/2 phosphorylation but was blocked by sIL17R intervention. Akt was not induced in the EV retina, suggesting that Akt had no direct input from Il17a in this tissue. We evaluated NF-κB induction in EV versus sIL17R retinas yet observed no difference in cellular localization (Figure S3). These data corroborate the efficacy of sIL17R and suggest a MAPK-dependent mechanism in the IL17-laden retina.

Discussion

IL17 was aberrantly expressed in AMD macular lesions compared to non-diseased maculas from controls. This was also true when comparing macular with peripheral expression within AMD retinas. Using a combination of cell and animal studies, we found that IL17 signaling is damaging to cultured RPE and to the retina in a mouse model.

IL17A challenge of ARPE-19 cells reduced cell viability, activated caspase effector proteins, and induced ultrastructural pathology commonly seen in RPE of AMD eyes. Curiously, there was no clear dose-dependent relationship between IL17A concentration and cell viability. Over the course of 5–7 independent experiments using 4–5 replicates per treatment,

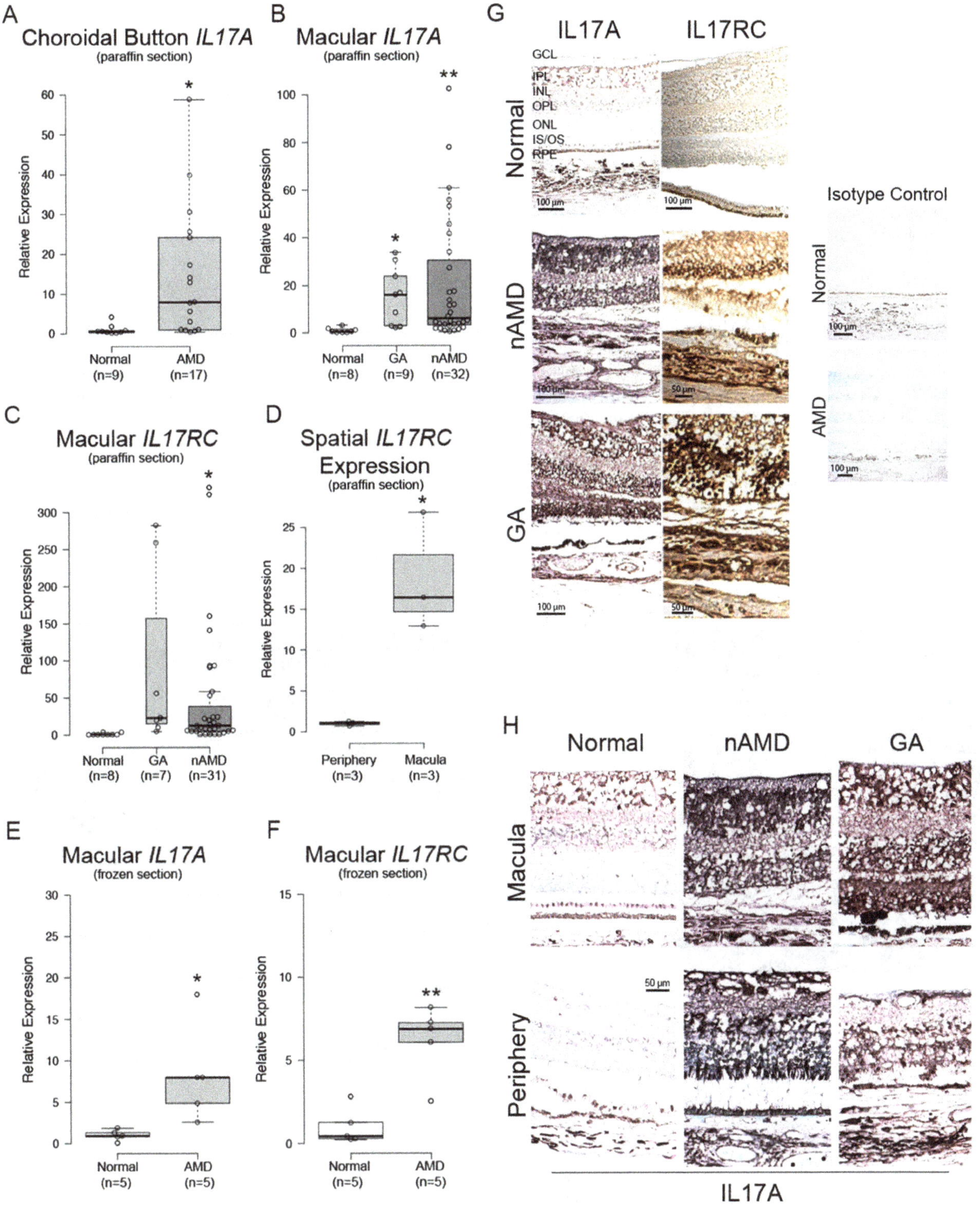

Figure 1. *IL17A* and *IL17RC* expression in AMD tissue. *IL17A* mRNA expression in paraffin-embedded (A) sub-macular choroid button and (B) macula. (C) *IL17RC* mRNA expression in paraffin-embedded macula. (D) *IL17RC* mRNA expression in macula vs. periphery of 3 donors. (E, F) Macular *IL17A* and *IL17RC* mRNA were verified in paraformaldehyde-fixed fresh frozen tissue. (G) Immunohistochemical detection of IL17A and IL17RC in paraffin-embedded macular sections. Isotype controls lacked primary antibodies. (H) Comparison of macular and peripheral IL17A immunostains. For box plots: center lines show the medians; box limits indicate the 25th and 75th percentiles as determined by R software; whiskers extend 1.5 times the interquartile range from the 25th and 75th percentiles, outliers are represented by dots; width of the boxes is proportional to the square root of the sample size; data points are plotted as open circles; sample numbers are indicated beneath each column. GA = geographic atrophy; nAMD = neovascular AMD; GCL = ganglion cell layer; IPL = inner plexiform layer; INL = inner nuclear layer; OPL = outer plexiform layer; ONL = outer nuclear layer; IS/OS = inner/outer segment; RPE = retinal pigment epithelium. *: $P<0.05$; **: $P<0.005$; ***: $P<0.0001$.

IL17A nonetheless consistently reduced the viability of ARPE-19 compared to untreated cells. In the case of COS-7, similar reductions were only observed once the cells were co-incubated with a dose 100 times more concentrated than ARPE-19. Using two-way ANOVA to test the validity of these results based upon the two independent variables (here: cell type and IL17A dose), it was significantly different with regard to the viability effects due to changing cell type, but not IL17A dosage. This indicated that ARPE-19 cells and COS-7 cells do indeed respond differently when co-incubated with the cytokine. The effects on viability are nonetheless resolved when examining by TEM. It as this level of detail that various pathological ultrastructures are consistent with changes observed in RPE of AMD lesions: lipid deposits highly reminiscent of the lipofuscin accretions commonly observed in aged RPE and which may potentiate AMD pathophysiology [20]; autophagosomes which are observed in AMD [21]; mitochondrial damage; and nuclear pyknosis and necrosis. Furthermore, siRNA knockdown of IL17RC was sufficient to rescue ARPE-19 viability in the presence of IL17A associated with significant reductions in caspase activation.

The ultimate goal of the present study was to evaluate the therapeutic potential of IL17A knockdown in a preclinical retinal degeneration model. Our lab has generated a mouse model of focal retinal degeneration that undergoes progressive retinal degeneration beginning as early as 2–3 weeks after birth. Despite controversy in recent years [22], the retinal pathology of DKO/*rd8* can be described by two distinct lesions: 1.) "AMD-like" degeneration of RPE and subsequently inner and outer segments of photoreceptors and 2.) "dystrophic/dysplastic" *rd8*-associated lesions affecting inner and outer nuclear layer (INL and ONL) neurons and outer plexiform layer (OPL). AMD-like lesions are associated with dysregulation of the complement system, the RPE, and retinal microglia [23–25], all of which are key immunological factors in AMD pathophysiology. Moreover, the elevation of A2E, a biomarker of AMD is measured in DKO/*rd8* eyes [30,33].

Mice of the C57BL/6N strain (in this study referred to as "WT"), which all possess the $Crb1^{rd8}$ allele, do not uniformly exhibit signs of retinal dystrophy, as evidenced by wide variations in ophthalmic phenotype within the strain across different research institutions [26]. Furthermore, a $Ccl2^{-/-}/Cx3cr1^{-/-}$ strain lacking $Crb1^{rd8}$ possesses AMD-like lesions caused by age and light-stress [27]. However, DKO/*rd8* is not identical to AMD, especially when noting that anatomically mice lack the macula. Nonetheless, in addition to the above-noted histologic and immunologic features, DKO/*rd8* shares clear IL17 immunopathological features with AMD (Figure 4A).

In DKO/*rd8*, IL17 inhibition using sIL17R, a dominant-negative IL17A inhibitor, was prospectively retinoprotective. This model has a particular allure given the ability to negate all effects due to population variance (even within inbred strains variance is

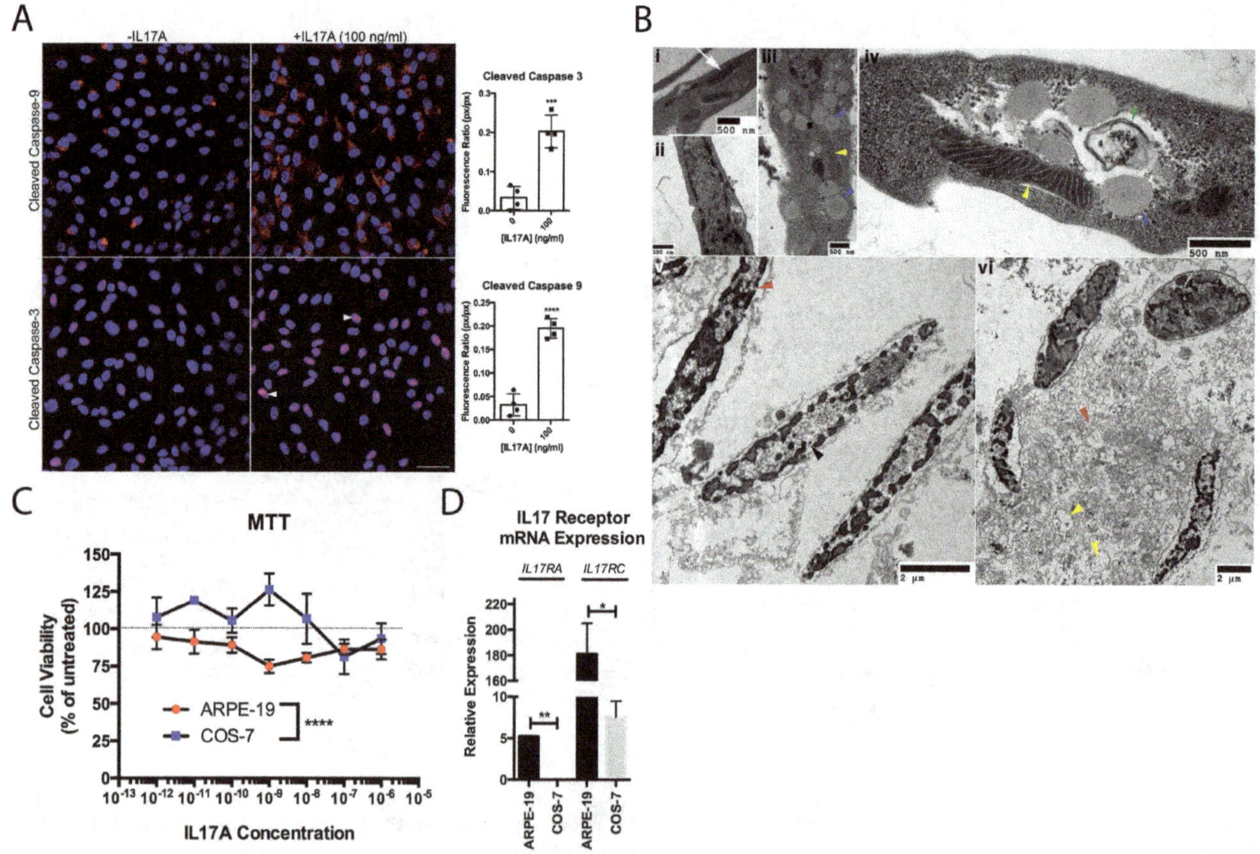

Figure 2. IL17A is cytotoxic to ARPE-19. (A) Confocal microscopy of ARPE-19 treated 48h with IL17A. Nuclear signal of cleaved Caspase-3 (arrowheads). Blue = DAPI. Scale bar = 50 μm. Graphical representation of confocal data presented to the right of the panel. (B) ARPE-19 ultrastructure cultured without (i–ii) and with (iii–vi) 10 ng/ml IL17A for 48h. Indicated are healthy mitochondria (i, white arrow), lipid deposits (iii, iv, blue arrowheads), autophagosomes (iv, green arrowhead), mitochondrial damage (iii, iv, vi, yellow arrowheads), pyknotic nuclear clumps (v, black arrowhead), and cytoplasmic necrosis (vi, red arrowhead). (C) ARPE-19 vs. COS-7 viability after 48h treatment with IL17A. (D) Relative expression of IL17 receptors in ARPE-19 vs. COS-7. Data are presented as mean ± SEM. *: P<0.05, **: P<0.01, ***: P<0.001; ****: P<0.0001.

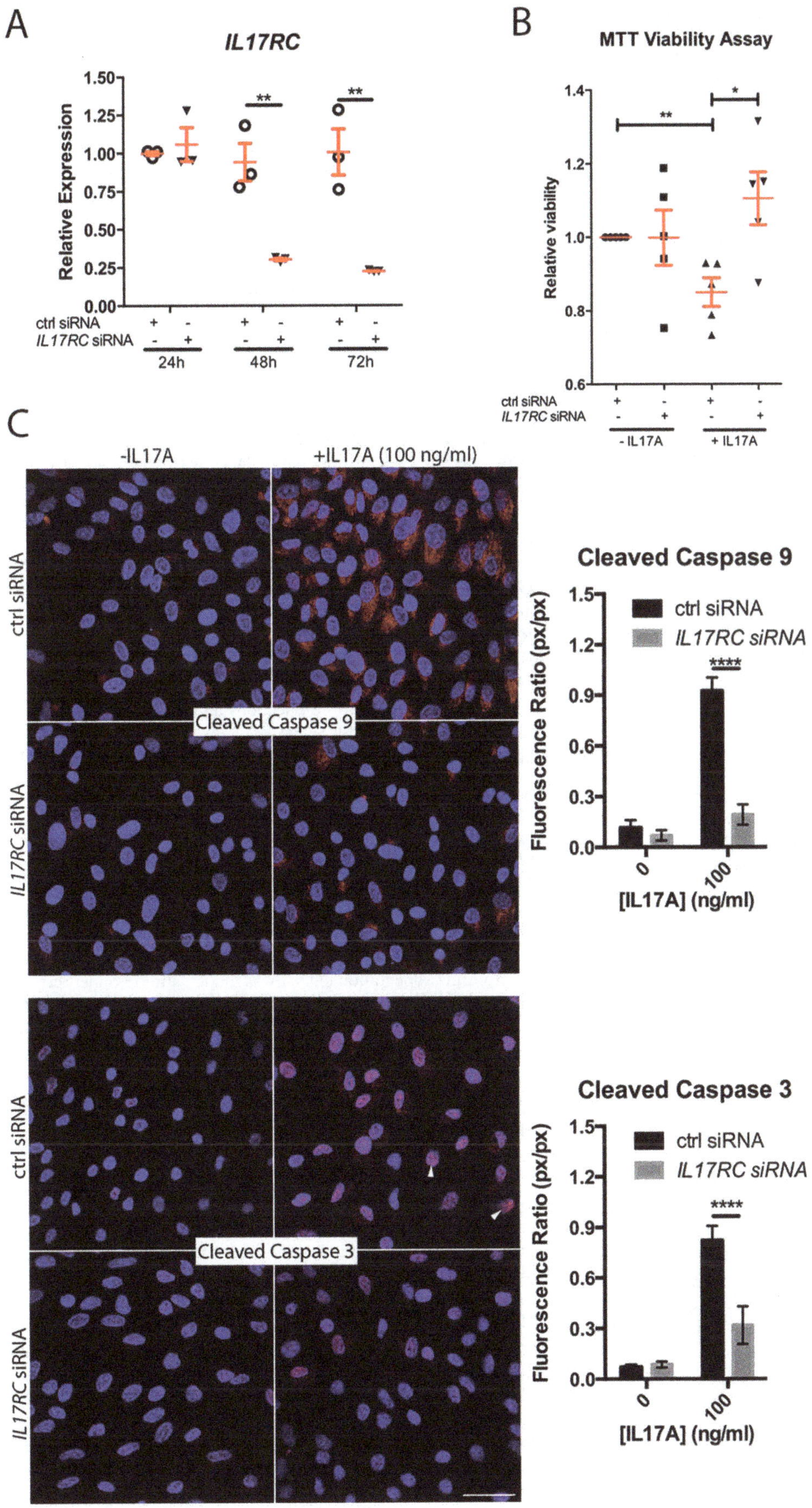
A
IL17RC
Relative Expression
1.50
1.25
1.00
0.75
0.50
0.25
0.00
**
**
ctrl siRNA
IL17RC siRNA
24h
48h
72h
B
MTT Viability Assay
Relative viability
1.4
1.2
1.0
0.8
0.6
**
*
ctrl siRNA
IL17RC siRNA
- IL17A
+ IL17A
C
-IL17A
+IL17A (100 ng/ml)
ctrl siRNA
IL17RC siRNA
Cleaved Caspase 9
Cleaved Caspase 3
Cleaved Caspase 9
Fluorescence Ratio (px/px)
ctrl siRNA
IL17RC siRNA
****
[IL17A] (ng/ml)
Cleaved Caspase 3
Fluorescence Ratio (px/px)
ctrl siRNA
IL17RC siRNA
****
[IL17A] (ng/ml)

Figure 3. *IL17RC* siRNA prevents IL17A-induced pathology. (A) *IL17RC* knockdown by 0.04 μM siRNA. *IL17RC* was measured by qPCR at 24h, 48h, and 72h post-transfection relative to a universal mRNA standard. (B) Relative viability of ctrl or *IL17RC* siRNA-transfected ARPE-19 with 100 ng/ml IL17A. (C) Confocal microscopy of ctrl or *IL17RC* siRNA-transfected ARPE-19 treated with or without IL17A. Nuclear localization of Caspase-3 (arrowheads). Graphical representation of the Caspase:DAPI ratio are indicated to the right of the images. Blue = DAPI. Scale bar = 50 μm. *: P<0.05; **: P<0.005; ****: P<0.0001. Data are presented as mean ± SEM.

observed [26]) by using the contralateral eye as an internal control [28]. Consequently, between-eye comparisons revealed significant improvements in clinical lesion score, reductions in A2E burden, rescue of retinal architecture histologically and prevention of RPE ultrastructural pathology. Although it is likely that the multiple cell types found within the retina utilize the MAPK signaling cascades towards various ends, it is reassuring to have observed that sIL17R intervention blocked signal transduction via Erk1/2 and p38, a result in line with IL17 signal transduction. Additionally, together with the finding of enhanced ERK1/2 phosphorylation in GA AMD tissue and that Erk1/2 inhibition rescued RPE degeneration in a mouse model [29], these data strengthen the notion that MAPK-mediated IL17 signals are involved in retinal degeneration. Interestingly, sIL17R reduced *Il17rc* retinal transcripts (Figure S2C–D), which, together with the observation that IL17A induces *IL17RA* and *IL17RC in vitro* [30], suggests a positive feedback loop may amplify IL17 signals in susceptible tissues.

Recent efforts have drawn attention to the inflammasome machinery, particularly interleukin-18 (IL-18), as an inciting factor in AMD [31,32]. Accumulation of toxic *Alu* RNA following loss of DICER1 within RPE activates the NLRP3 inflammasome and consequently IL-18, thus inducing RPE degeneration and contributing to GA pathogenesis [31]. IL-18 and IL-1β, the latter being an inflammasome-induced pro-inflammatory cytokine that is also aberrantly expressed in AMD lesions, have together been shown to induce IL17A [33,34]. Furthermore, A2E accumulating over time within RPE can serve as a catalyst for IL-1β production via activation of the NLRP3 inflammasome [35]. Consequently, the evolving story of inflammasome activation and IL-18 activity to explain AMD pathology is appealing [36,37]. However, despite detrimental effects in a mouse model of GA, IL-18 was protective in mouse models of CNV [38]. Given these seemingly contradictory effects, understanding the downstream effectors of the inflammasome machinery is essential towards elucidating possible pathologic drivers and identifying therapeutic targets in AMD [39].

IL17A remains one promising downstream effector of IL-18/IL-1β. Data from our lab show that RPE challenged with NLRP3 secrete IL-18 and IL-1β, and form autophagosomes [40,41]. Inflammasome-derived IL-18/IL-1β can promote IL17 production from Th17 cells and γδ T cells in a process that is regulated by autophagy [41]. The possibility of ocular resident and/or other cells as the IL17A source in the eyes with AMD requires further investigation given the paucity of observed lymphocytes in AMD lesions [42]. The IL17 pathway is thus poised at the intersection of AMD pathogenesis associated with complement-laden drusen accumulation and inflammasome activation in the macula. The present study indicates that IL17A signaling is both cytotoxic and retinotoxic and should be further considered as a potential therapeutic target in AMD.

Materials and Methods

Human Tissue

Tissue investigation was conducted according to Declaration of Helsinki principles and approved by the NIH IRB. Eyes were obtained from the NIH clinical center and Johns Hopkins Wilmer Eye Institute (107 eyes from 67 advanced stage AMD donors and 10 eyes from normal donors), Minnesota Eye Bank (9 normal and 17 AMD), and University of Iowa (5 normal and 5 AMD). Donors signed consent forms from each institution and protocols were approved by each institution's IRB, as appropriate.

Cell Culture

ARPE-19 and COS-7 cells (ATCC, Manassas, VA, USA) were used. ARPE-19 were cultured at 37°C with 5% CO_2 in 10% Fetal Bovine Serum (FBS) DMEM/F12 Ham's and COS-7 were cultured in 10% FBS/DMEM. Cells were serum-starved without antibiotics for 24 h and treated for 48 h with recombinant IL17A (R&D Systems, Minneapolis, MN).

Animals

Ccl2$^{-/-}$/*Cx3cr1*$^{-/-}$/*Crb1*^{rd8} mice were generated from the C57BL/6N (*Crb1*^{rd8}) background. Where necessary, C57BL/6N are referred to as "WT." At 4–5 weeks of age, 1.0×10^9 DNase-Resistant Particles (DRPs) of AAV2.sIL17R were injected into right eyes and 1.0×10^9 DRPs of AAV2.EV were injected into left eyes of 40 mice in 2 independent trials and followed for 8 weeks. Six mice received the same injections and were used for Western blots. We complied with the Association for Research in Vision and Ophthalmology statement for the use of animals and the NEI's Institutional Animal Care and Use Committee approved protocols.

Quantitative Reverse-transcriptase PCR (qRT-PCR)

Human tissues were paraffin-embedded or fresh frozen and RNA was extracted using the Paradise RNA isolation kit (Applied Biosystems, Foster City, CA). For cell and animal studies, total RNA was extracted using Trizol (Qiagen, Hilden, Germany) and chloroform/isopentanol. cDNA was made with the SuperScript II kit (Invitrogen). SYBR Green (Qiagen) primers were used for human *IL17A*, human *IL17RC*, mouse *Il17a*, and mouse *Il17rc*. The TaqMan Gene expression assay (Applied Biosystems) was used for human *IL8* and mouse *Il6*. All data were normalized to the *beta-actin* mRNA level. Expression fold-change was calculated by $2^{-\Delta\Delta CT}$.

Immunohistochemistry

Paraffin-embedded human eye sections were deparaffinized, rehydrated, and fixed in acetone. Primary antibodies: IL17A (polyclonal rabbit anti-human IgG, 1:100 dilution, Catalog #13082-1-AP, Proteintech, Chicago, IL) IL17RC (polyclonal rabbit anti-human IgG, 1:100 dilution, Catalog #sc-99937, Santa Cruz Biotechnology, Santa Cruz, CA). Secondary antibody: biotin conjugated, goat anti-rabbit IgG (Vector Laboratories, Burlingame, CA). Chromagen: 3,3′-diaminobenzidine (Biocare Medical, Concord, CA). Slides were counterstained with 1% methyl green. For westerns, primary antibodies include phospho- and total-Erk1/2, phospho- and total-Akt, phospho- and total-p38, and GAPDH (Cell Signaling Technology).

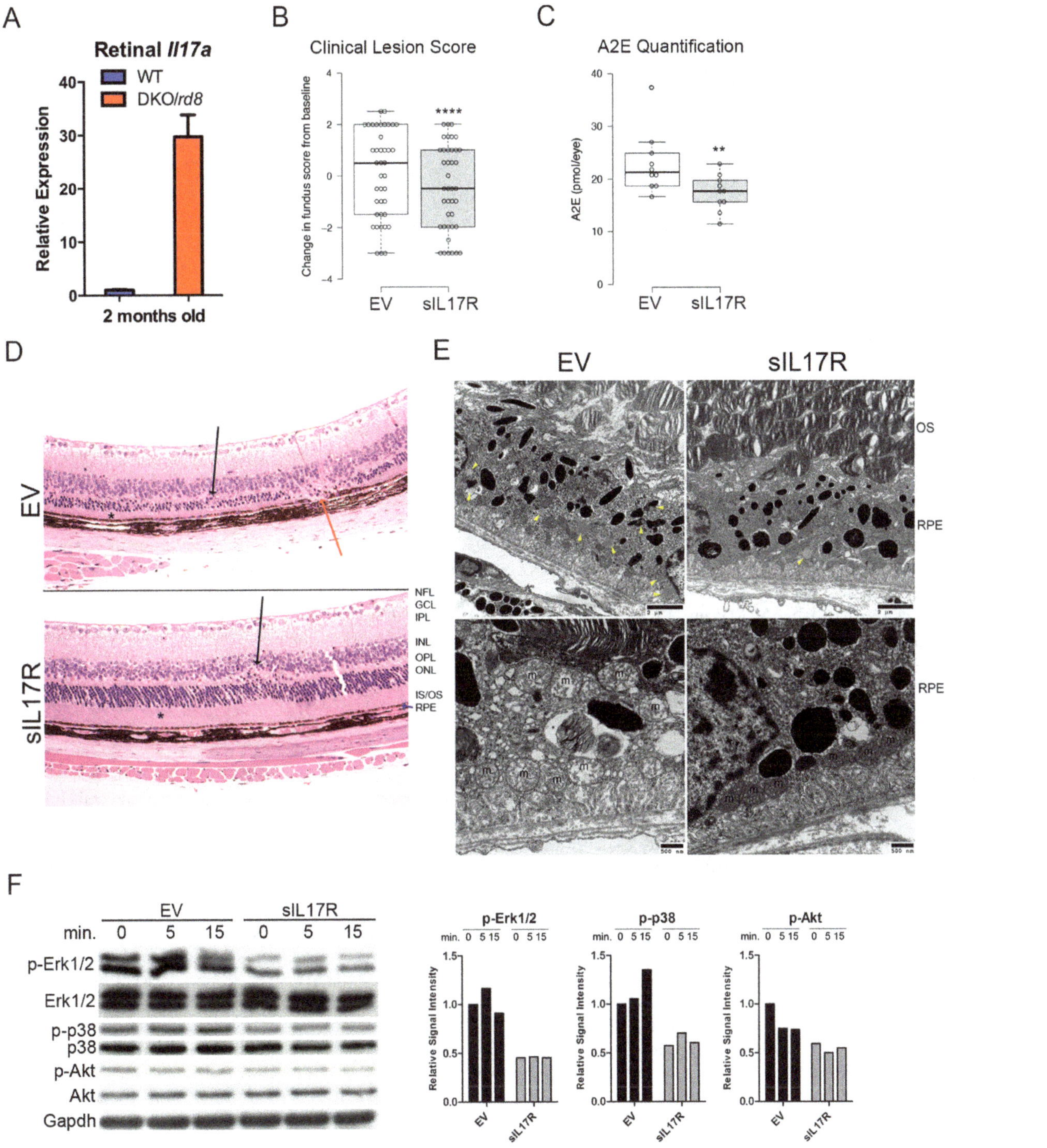

Figure 4. sIL17R prevents retinotoxicity in DKO/*rd8*. (A) Retinal *Il17a* transcripts as a function of animal age. (B) Fundoscopic results 2 months post-intervention. (C) A2E quantification. For box plots: center lines show the medians; box limits indicate the 25th and 75th percentiles as determined by R software; whiskers extend 1.5 times the interquartile range from the 25th and 75th percentiles, outliers are represented by dots; width of the boxes is proportional to the square root of the sample size; data points are plotted as open circles. (D) Histopathological findings: sIL17R preserved photoreceptor IS/OS thickness compared to EV (asterisks) and maintained thickness of the ONL. EV retinas showed RPE degeneration (red arrow). Dystrophic *rd8* lesions are indicated (black arrows). (E) Abundant lipofuscin in EV but not in sIL17R RPE (yellow arrowheads, upper left and right). Mitochondria (m) are damaged and disorganized within EV RPE (lower left) but are viable and organized in sIL17R RPE (lower right). EV RPE show extensive vacuolization, undigested OS and poor basal infoldings (lower left). (F) Western blot of downstream Il17 signaling. EV and sIL17R neuroretinas were treated with 50 ng/ml Il17a for 0, 5, or 15 min *ex vivo*. Relative Signal Intensities are presented of phosphorylated proteins relative to total protein to the right of the blots. NFL = nerve fiber layer; GCL = ganglion cell layer; IPL = inner plexiform layer; INL = inner nuclear layer; OPL = outer plexiform layer; ONL = outer nuclear layer; IS/OS = inner/outer segment; RPE = retinal pigment epithelium *: $P<0.05$; **: $P<0.005$; ****: $P<0.00001$.

MTT Assay

ARPE-19 or COS-7 cells were plated in quadruplicate on 96-well plates (2×10^4 cells/well). Cells were serum-starved for 24h then treated for 48h with IL17A. Cells were incubated 4h in 0.5 mg/ml MTT dissolved in DMEM/F12. DMSO was added. Absorption was measured at 570 nm (Synergy II plate reader; Gen5 software; BioTek, Winooski, VT) and normalized to that of untreated cells.

siRNA Transfection

IL17RC small interfering or nonspecific control siRNA RNA (Santa Cruz Biotechnology, Santa Cruz, CA, USA) were transfected at a concentration of 0.04 µM into ARPE-19 cells using transfection reagent according to the manufacturer's protocol. Transfected cells were serum-starved in media without antibiotics for 24h and treated for 48h with 100 ng/ml IL17A before RNA extraction, immunofluorescence, or MTT assay.

Soluble Vector Construction and Characterization

Soluble IL17R/9gly/CH3 was cloned into plasmid pCBA(2) [43], which contains hybrid chicken beta-actin (CBA) promoter and bovine growth hormone polyadenylation signal sequence (BGH poly A). The expression cassette was transferred to pre-viral plasmid vector pAAVSP70 containing AAV2 inverted terminal repeats [44]. The recombinant vector AAV2.sIL17R was produced by triple transfection of 293 cells with pAAVSP70.-sIL17R and helper plasmids p5repΔCMVcap [45] and pHelper (Stratagene, La Jolla, CA, USA). In empty vector (AAV2.EV), a 3.8 kb intron from alpha-1-antitrypsin replaced sIL17R. Vectors were purified from cell lysates with an iodixanol step gradient and HiTrap Heparin column (GE Healthcare Life Sciences, Piscataway, NJ, USA) on an ÅKTA FPLC system (GE Healthcare Life Sciences, Piscataway, NJ) [45,46]. Viral vector titers were determined using a TaqMan RT-PCR assay (ABI Prism 7700; Applied Biosystems, Foster City, CA, USA) with primers specific for BGH poly A.

For sIL17R binding to IL17A, ELISA plates were coated with 100 µg/ml human IL17A or mouse IL17A overnight, then blocked with 1% BSA. Serial two-fold dilutions of sIL17R were added in triplicate to the plate and incubated for 1 h at 37°C. Unbound receptor was washed from the plate in an ELISA plate washer. 100 µl biotinylated anti-IL17RA (1 µg/ml) was added to each well and incubated 1 h at room temperature and excess antibody was washed away. Each well was incubated with streptavidin-HRP conjugate and washed. Bound HRP was measured by incubation with TMBD substrate for 20 minutes followed by addition of acid stop solution. OD were measured at 450 nm.

sIL17R ELISA

Eyes were removed from euthanized mice and stored at −70°C until the assay. The vitreous humor and the retinas were dissected from frozen eyes and homogenized in 200 µL of lysis buffer provided in the ELISA kit. Undiluted homogenates were clarified by centrifugation and assayed for IL17R levels using the human IL17R Duoset kit (R&D Systems).

Animal Fundoscopy

Fundoscopy was performed before injection and 2 months post-injection. An endoscope with parallel illumination and observation channels was connected to a Nikon D90 digital camera. Mice received intraperitoneal injection of ketamine (1.4 mg/mouse) and xylazine (0.12 mg/mouse) for systemic anesthesia and topical 1% tropicamide ophthalmic solution (Alcon Inc, Fort Worth, TX) for pupil dilation. Grading of the fundoscopic lesions (Table 1) was conducted by a masked observer.

A2E Extraction and Quantification

A2E ([2,6-dimethyl-8-(2,6,6-trimethyl-1-cyclohexen-1-yl)-1E,3E,5E,7E-octatetra-enyl]-1-(2-hydroxyethyl)-4-[4-methyl-6(2,6,6-trimethyl-1-cyclohexen-1-yl) 1E,3E,5E,7E-hexatrienyl]-pyridinium) was extracted with chloroform/methanol as previously described [47]. A2E detection and quantification was performed by liquid-chromatography mass spectrometry using a QTRAP 2000 linear ion trap tandem mass spectrometer (Applied Biosystems/MDS SCIEX, Concord, Ontario, Canada) with an Agilent 1100 LC system (Agilent, Wilmington, DE). A gradient of 80% to 98% methanol was used to separate A2E on a C18 column (Zorbax; Agilent) at a flow-rate of 0.3 ml/min. A2E was quantified using external A2E standards.

Histopathology

Eyes were fixed for 30 min in 4% (v/v) gluteraldehyde followed by 10% (v/v) formalin for 1 h. Fixed eyes were embedded in methacrylate and serially sectioned in the vertical pupillary optic nerve plane. Each eye was cut into four sections and stained with hematoxylin and eosin, then analyzed under a light microscope. For transmission electron microscopy, mouse eyes were fixed in 2.5% gluteraldehyde and 0.5% osmium tetroxide, dehydrated, and embedded into Spurr's epoxy resin. 90 nm sections were made and double-stained with uranyl acetate and lead citrate, and viewed using a JEOL JEM 1010 transmission electron microscope.

Western Blot

Neurosensory retinas were isolated from 6 DKO/*rd8* mice two weeks after AAV2.sIL17R and AAV2.EV injection. Retinas were cultured 2 h *ex vivo* at 37°C and 5% CO_2 in 1% BSA in PBS.

Table 1. Clinical scores of the disease.

Progression	+1	>10% increase in retinal lesion number
	+2	>50% increase in size of ≥1/3 of lesions
	+3	>5 fused lesions or appearance of >2 chorioretinal scars
	+4	diffuse chorioretinal scars
Regression	−1	>10% decrease in retinal lesion number
	−2	>50% decrease in size of ≥1/3 of lesions
	−3	>50% disappearance of retinal lesions
	−4	total disappearance of retinal lesions

Retinas were treated with 50 ng/ml recombinant mouse Il17a (R&D Systems) for 0, 5, or 15 min. Protein lysates were isolated in RIPA and complete protein lysis buffer, homogenized using a P200 pipette, and kept on ice 30 min with occasional vortexing. Following centrifugation (16,000 rpm, 30 min, 4°C), we measured protein concentration using the BCA assay (Pierce, Rockford, IL). 10% polyacrylamide gels (Invitrogen) were loaded with 10 µg protein/lane and ran at 125 V for 1 h. Transfer was performed onto a nitrocellulose membrane (Invitrogen) at 300 mA for 1 h at 4°C. Membranes were blocked in 5% BSA for 1 h and incubated with primary antibody overnight at 4°C on a shaker. Membranes were incubated with the secondary antibody goat anti-rabbit conjugated to HRP (1:10,000) for 45 min at room temperature. Membranes were exposed using SuperSignal West Dura (Pierce).

Confocal Microscopy

Cells or frozen mouse eye sections were fixed in 4% paraformaldehyde for 15 min, washed in PBS, and blocked in ICC buffer with 5% goat or rabbit serum for 30 min at 4°C. Primary antibody incubation occurred overnight at 4°C. Secondary antibody incubation lasted 1 h at room temperature. Slides were mounted in Vectashield fluorescent media (Vector Labs) and imaged with an Olympus FV1000 Confocal Scanning Scope. Primary antibodies: Cleaved Caspase-3 diluted 1:200 (Cell Signaling Technology, Danvers, MA), Cleaved Caspase-9 diluted 1:100 (Santa Cruz), and NF-κB p65 diluted 1:50 (Cell Signaling Technology). Secondary antibodies: goat anti-rabbit IgG (1:400), rabbit anti-goat IgG (1:400), and rabbit anti-mouse IgG (1:400). DAPI (1:1000) marked nuclei.

Statistics

GraphPad was used for statistical tests. Cell and patient qRT-PCR data was evaluated using the unpaired T-test. MTT assays were compared using two-way ANOVA. For mean fluorescence quantification, the ratios of secondary antibody (red signal) to DAPI (blue signal) were compared by two-way ANOVA. For mouse qRT-PCR, clinical fundus scores, and A2E, the paired T-test was used. $P<0.05$ determined statistical significance.

Supporting Information

Figure S1 AAV2.sIL17R vector design and efficacy. (A) AAV2.sIL17R domains. (B) sIL17R binding data for mouse and human cytokine presented. (C) ELISA quantification of sIL17R protein in mouse retina 2 months post-injection. qRT-PCR measurement of retinal (D) *Il17a* and (E) *Il6* mRNA. *: P<0.05; n.s. = not significant.

Figure S2 sIL17R vector attenuates retinal lesions by clinical and molecular evaluation. (A) Representative fundus images comparing baseline to 2 months post-injection of EV or sIL17R vector with lesion score indicated to the right. (B) Intra-mouse pairwise comparison of lesion scores, EV vs. sIL17R (80 eyes total from 40 mice); all points to the right of the red line indicate that the sIL17R-treated eye faired better than its contralateral counterpart. Lower *Il17rc* transcript expression in sIL17R vs. EV retinas 2 months post-injection by qRT-PCR (C) and end-stage gel (D).

Figure S3 Cellular Localization of NF-κB in DKO/*rd8*. Confocal microscopy of immunolabeled frozen eye sections from EV and sIL17R eyes 2 months post-intervention. INL = inner nuclear layer, ONL = outer nuclear layer.

Table S1 Histopathologic results. Clinical and histologic descriptions of all mice used in the study.

Acknowledgments

We would like to thank Jayakrishna Ambati (University of Kentucky) and Lois Smith (Harvard Medical School) for their critical review of the manuscript. We gratefully acknowledge the NIH Histology Core for their services regarding routine histology and immunohistochemistry.

Author Contributions

Conceived and designed the experiments: DA CCC. Performed the experiments: DA YW SP DFS XKC MAA JT GW CCC. Interpreted the data: DA CRY JT CCC. Contributed reagents/materials/analysis tools: CGE TWO RFM SW AS CCC. Wrote the paper: DA.

References

1. The Eye Diseases Prevalence Research Group (2004) Causes and Prevalence of Visual Impairment Among Adults in the United States. Arch Ophthalmol 122: 477–485.
2. Coleman HR, Chan CC, Ferris FL III, Chew EY (2008) Age-related macular degeneration. Lancet 372: 1835–1845.
3. Curcio CA, Medeiros NE, Millican CL (1996) Photoreceptor loss in age-related macular degeneration. Invest Ophthalmol Vis Sci 37: 1236–1249.
4. Hecker LA, Edwards AO, Ryu E, Tosakulwong N, Baratz KH, et al. (2010) Genetic control of the alternative pathway of complement in humans and age-related macular degeneration. Hum Mol Genet 19: 209–215.
5. Reynolds R, Hartnett ME, Atkinson JP, Giclas PC, Rosner B, et al. (2009) Plasma complement components and activation fragments: associations with age-related macular degeneration genotypes and phenotypes. Invest Ophthalmol Vis Sci 50: 5818–5827.
6. Scholl HP, Charbel Issa P, Walier M, Janzer S, Pollok-Kopp B, et al. (2008) Systemic complement activation in age-related macular degeneration. PLoS One 3: e2593.
7. Liu B, Wei L, Meyerle C, Tuo J, Sen HN, et al. (2011) Complement Component C5a Promotes Expression of IL-22 and IL-17 from Human T cells and its Implication in Age-related Macular Degeneration. J Transl Med 9: 1–12.
8. Wei L, Liu B, Tuo J, Shen D, Chen P, et al. (2012) Hypomethylation of the IL17RC promoter associates with age-related macular degeneration. Cell Rep 2: 1151–1158.
9. Tuo J, Cao X, Shen D, Wang Y, Zhang J, et al. (2012) Anti-inflammatory recombinant TSG-6 stabilizes the progression of focal retinal degeneration in a murine model. J Neuroinflammation 9: 59–67.
10. Luger D, Silver PB, Tang J, Cua D, Chen Z, et al. (2008) Either a Th17 or a Th1 effector response can drive autoimmunity: conditions of disease induction affect dominant effector category. J Exp Med 205: 799–810.
11. Chan CC, Ross RJ, Shen D, Ding X, Majumdar Z, et al. (2008) Ccl2/Cx3cr1-deficient mice: an animal model for age-related macular degeneration. Ophthalmic Res 40: 124–128.
12. Tuo J, Bojanowski CM, Zhou M, Shen D, Ross RJ, et al. (2007) Murine ccl2/cx3cr1 deficiency results in retinal lesions mimicking human age-related macular degeneration. Invest Ophthalmol Vis Sci 48: 3827–3836.
13. Ishigame H, Kakuta S, Nagai T, Kadoki M, Nambu A, et al. (2009) Differential roles of interleukin-17A and -17F in host defense against mucoepithelial bacterial infection and allergic responses. Immunity 30: 108–119.
14. Pechan P, Rubin H, Lukason M, Ardinger J, DuFresne E, et al. (2009) Novel anti-VEGF chimeric molecules delivered by AAV vectors for inhibition of retinal neovascularization. Gene Ther 16: 10–16.
15. Mori K, Gehlbach P, Yamamoto S, Duh E, Zack DJ, et al. (2002) AAV-mediated gene transfer of pigment epithelium-derived factor inhibits choroidal neovascularization. Invest Ophthalmol Vis Sci 43: 1994–2000.
16. Ben-Shabat S, Parish CA, Hashimoto M, Liu J, Nakanishi K, et al. (2001) Fluorescent pigments of the retinal pigment epithelium and age-related macular degeneration. Bioorg Med Chem Lett 11: 1533–1540.
17. Gaffen SL (2009) Structure and signalling in the IL-17 receptor family. Nat Rev Immunol 9: 556–567.
18. Gaffen SL (2011) Recent advances in the IL-17 cytokine family. Curr Opin Immunol 23: 613–619.

19. Chen Y, Kijlstra A, Yang P (2011) IL-17A stimulates the production of inflammatory mediators via Erk1/2, p38 MAPK, PI3K/Akt, and NF-kappaB pathways in ARPE-19 cells. Mol Vis 17: 3072–3077.
20. Ardeljan D, Chan CC (2013) Aging is not a disease: distinguishing age-related macular degeneration from aging. Prog Retin Eye Res 37: 68–89.
21. Klettner A, Kauppinen A, Blasiak J, Roider J, Salminen A, et al. (2013) Cellular and molecular mechanisms of age-related macular degeneration: from impaired autophagy to neovascularization. Int J Biochem Cell Biol 45: 1457–1467.
22. Mattapallil MJ, Wawrousek EF, Chan CC, Zhao H, Roychoudhury J, et al. (2012) The Rd8 mutation of the Crb1 gene is present in vendor lines of C57BL/6N mice and embryonic stem cells, and confounds ocular induced mutant phenotypes. Invest Ophthalmol Vis Sci 53: 2921–2927.
23. Ross RJ, Zhou M, Shen D, Fariss RN, Ding X, et al. (2008) Immunological protein expression profile in Ccl2/Cx3cr1 deficient mice with lesions similar to age-related macular degeneration. Exp Eye Res 86: 675–683.
24. Shen D, Cao X, Zhao L, Tuo J, Wong WT, et al. (2011) Naloxone ameliorates retinal lesions in Ccl2/Cx3cr1 double-deficient mice via modulation of microglia. Invest Ophthalmol Vis Sci 52: 2897–2904.
25. Chu XK, Wang Y, Ardeljan D, Tuo J, Chan CC (2013) Controversial view of a genetically altered mouse model of focal retinal degeneration. Bioengineered 4: 130–135.
26. Simon MM, Greenaway S, White JK, Fuchs H, Gailus-Durner V, et al. (2013) A comparative phenotypic and genomic analysis of C57BL/6J and C57BL/6N mouse strains. Genome Biol 14: R82.
27. Chen M, Hombrebueno JR, Luo C, Penalva R, Zhao J, et al. (2013) Age- and light-dependent development of localised retinal atrophy in CCL2(−/−) CX3CR1(GFP/GFP) mice. PLoS One 8: e61381.
28. Popp N, Chu XK, Shen D, Tuo J, Chan CC (2013) Evaluating Potential Therapies in a Mouse Model of Focal Retinal Degeneration with Age-related Macular Degeneration (AMD)-Like Lesions. J Clin Exp Ophthalmol 4: 1000296.
29. Dridi S, Hirano Y, Tarallo V, Kim Y, Fowler BJ, et al. (2012) ERK1/2 activation is a therapeutic target in age-related macular degeneration. Proc Natl Acad Sci U S A 109: 13781–13786.
30. Chu XK, Wang Y, Shen D, Ogilvy AJ, Li R, et al. (2013) Adult human RPE has greater susceptibility to IL17A-induced degeneration than fetal human RPE. ARVO Abstr 1780. Seattle, WA.
31. Tarallo V, Hirano Y, Gelfand BD, Dridi S, Kerur N, et al. (2012) DICER1 loss and Alu RNA induce age-related macular degeneration via the NLRP3 inflammasome and MyD88. Cell 149: 847–859.
32. Kaneko H, Dridi S, Tarallo V, Gelfand BD, Fowler BJ, et al. (2011) DICER1 deficit induces Alu RNA toxicity in age-related macular degeneration. Nature 471: 325–330.
33. Dungan LS, Mills KH (2011) Caspase-1-processed IL-1 family cytokines play a vital role in driving innate IL-17. Cytokine 56: 126–132.
34. Lalor SJ, Dungan LS, Sutton CE, Basdeo SA, Fletcher JM, et al. (2011) Caspase-1-processed cytokines IL-1beta and IL-18 promote IL-17 production by gammadelta and CD4 T cells that mediate autoimmunity. J Immunol 186: 5738–5748.
35. Anderson OA, Finkelstein A, Shima DT (2013) A2E induces IL-1ss production in retinal pigment epithelial cells via the NLRP3 inflammasome. PLoS One 8: e67263.
36. Campbell M, Doyle SL (2013) An eye on the future of inflammasomes and drug development in AMD. J Mol Med (Berl) 91: 1059–1070.
37. Marneros AG (2013) NLRP3 Inflammasome Blockade Inhibits VEGF-A-Induced Age-Related Macular Degeneration. Cell Rep 4: 945–958.
38. Doyle SL, Campbell M, Ozaki E, Salomon RG, Mori A, et al. (2012) NLRP3 has a protective role in age-related macular degeneration through the induction of IL-18 by drusen components. Nat Med 18: 791–798.
39. Rosenbaum JT (2012) Eyeing macular degeneration–few inflammatory remarks. N Engl J Med 367: 768–770.
40. Wang Y, M A-A, Shen D, Chu XK, Ogilvy AJ, et al. (2013) NLRP3 inflammasome activation in human retinal pigment epithelium under inflammation and oxidative stress. ARVO Abstr #149. Seattle, WA.
41. Mills KH, Dungan LS, Jones SA, Harris J (2013) The role of inflammasome-derived IL-1 in driving IL-17 responses. J Leukoc Biol 93: 489–497.
42. Penfold PL, Killingsworth MC, Sarks SH (1985) Senile macular degeneration: the involvement of immunocompetent cells. Graefes Arch Clin Exp Ophthalmol 223: 69–76.
43. Xu L, Daly T, Gao C, Flotte TR, Song S, et al. (2001) CMV-beta-actin promoter directs higher expression from an adeno-associated viral vector in the liver than the cytomegalovirus or elongation factor 1 alpha promoter and results in therapeutic levels of human factor X in mice. Hum Gene Ther 12: 563–573.
44. Ziegler RJ, Lonning SM, Armentano D, Li C, Souza DW, et al. (2004) AAV2 vector harboring a liver-restricted promoter facilitates sustained expression of therapeutic levels of alpha-galactosidase A and the induction of immune tolerance in Fabry mice. Mol Ther 9: 231–240.
45. Vincent KA, Piraino ST, Wadsworth SC (1997) Analysis of recombinant adeno-associated virus packaging and requirements for rep and cap gene products. J Virol 71: 1897–1905.
46. Zolotukhin S, Potter M, Zolotukhin I, Sakai Y, Loiler S, et al. (2002) Production and purification of serotype 1, 2, and 5 recombinant adeno-associated viral vectors. Methods 28: 158–167.
47. Karan G, Lillo C, Yang Z, Cameron DJ, Locke KG, et al. (2005) Lipofuscin accumulation, abnormal electrophysiology, and photoreceptor degeneration in mutant ELOVL4 transgenic mice: a model for macular degeneration. Proc Natl Acad Sci U S A 102: 4164–4169.

Foveal Morphology Affects Self-Perceived Visual Function and Treatment Response in Neovascular Age-Related Macular Degeneration

Yousif Subhi[1,2], Gitte Ø. Henningsen[1], Charlotte T. Larsen[1], Mette S. Sørensen[1], Torben L. Sørensen[1,2]*

1 Clinical Eye Research Unit, Department of Ophthalmology, Copenhagen University Hospital Roskilde, Roskilde, Denmark, **2** University of Copenhagen, Copenhagen, Denmark

Abstract

Objectives: To investigate the relationship between foveal morphology and self-perceived visual function in patients with neovascular age-related macular degeneration (AMD) and whether foveal characteristics are associated with Ranibizumab treatment response on the self-perceived visual function.

Methods: This prospective cohort study included patients with newly diagnosed neovascular AMD found eligible for treatment with Ranibizumab. Foveal morphology of both eyes was assessed using spectral-domain optical coherence tomography and all patients were interviewed using the 39-item National Eye Institute Visual Function Questionnaire (VFQ). Patients were re-interviewed 3 and 12 months after initiation of treatment with Ranibizumab. We evaluated foveal morphology at baseline in relation to VFQ scores at baseline and clinically meaningful changes in VFQ after 3 and 12 months.

Results: VFQ scores correlated with central foveal thickness, central foveal thickness of neuroretina (CFN), foveal RPE elevation, foveal integrity of the photoreceptor inner segment/outer segment junction (IS/OS), and external limiting membrane. In a multiple linear regression model, only best-corrected visual acuity of the better eye ($p<0.001$) and the IS/OS status in the better eye ($p = 0.012$) remained significant (Adjusted $R^2 = 0.418$). Lower baseline VFQ and a baseline CFN within 170–270 μm in the better eye were both associated with a clinically meaningful increase in the VFQ scores after 3 and 12 months. An absent foveal IS/OS band in the better eye was associated with a clinically meaningful decrease in the VFQ scores at 12 months.

Conclusions: Foveal morphology in the better eye influences the self-perceived visual function in patients with neovascular AMD and possesses a predictive value for change in the self-perceived visual function at 3 and 12 months after initiation of treatment. These findings may help clinicians provide patients more individualized information of their disease and treatment prognosis from a patient-perceived point-of-view.

Editor: Yingfeng Zheng, Zhongshan Ophthalmic Center, China

Funding: This work is supported by the Region Zealand Research Foundation. The funders had no role in study design, data collection and analysis, decision to publish, or preparation of the manuscript.

Competing Interests: Gitte Ø. Henningsen and Charlotte T. Larsen have received payment for lectures from Novartis. This does not alter our adherence to PLOS ONE policies on sharing data and materials.

* E-mail: torbenls@dadlnet.dk

Introduction

Age-related macular degeneration (AMD) is the leading cause of visual impairment among the elderly in the western world, and the late stages of the disease often lead to a severe negative impact on visual function. Hence, many patients experience a decreased ability to perform simple daily tasks and preserve social as well as mental function [1], [2]. Disease progression is traditionally monitored using visual acuity charts, which are unable to capture abstract dimensions of patient-perceived visual functioning [3]. Underscoring the importance of other measures of treatment effect than solely visual acuity, patient-perceived outcomes have become a common endpoint in clinical trials in medicine [4], and the National Eye Institute Visual Function Questionnaire (VFQ) is widely used and included in hallmark clinical studies in ophthalmology [5–8]. VFQ is validated in patients with AMD [9–11], and studies indicate that anti-vascular endothelial growth factor (anti-VEGF) treatment may maintain and in some cases improve the self-perceived visual function [5–8].

Emergence of high-resolution spectral-domain optical coherence tomography systems (OCT) have enabled detailed characterization of the foveal morphology in patients with neovascular AMD [12], [13]. Characteristics of foveal morphology assist in predicting treatment response of anti-VEGF in the management of wet AMD, e.g. smaller lesion size at baseline predicts of a good treatment response, and interruptions in certain hyperreflective bands such as the photoreceptor inner segment/outer segment junction (IS/OS) and external limiting membrane (ELM) predicts a bad treatment response [14–19]. Treatment response in these studies is measured as the change in visual acuity, which to the patient may be less relevant than the self-perceived visual function. Visual acuity and self-perceived visual function correlates only moderately and may not always go together [9], [20], [21]. Thus, we need studies investigating disease impact and prognosis from a patient-perceived point-of-view.

In this prospective cohort-study, we explored the relationship between baseline foveal characteristics and self-perceived visual function in patients with newly diagnosed neovascular AMD, and how baseline foveal characteristics are related to the self-perceived visual function after anti-VEGF treatment.

Methods

Study Population and Design

We included 200 consecutive patients newly diagnosed with neovascular AMD and eligible for treatment with intravitreal Ranibizumab from our outpatient clinic within the period of December 2009 and August 2011. All included patients were examined and interviewed at diagnosis and initiation of treatment, and re-examined and re-interviewed after 3 and 12 months. All patients received standard care. The Regional Committee of Ethics in Research of the Region of Zealand reviewed our study and waived further processing since the use of questionnaires within normal clinical practice does not, according to Danish law, require formal approval. Verbal and written informed consent was obtained from all participants prior to inclusion.

Retinal Diagnosis and Ranibizumab Treatment

Best-corrected visual acuity (BCVA) was measured using Early Treatment Diabetic Retinopathy Study (ETDRS) chart. Retinal imaging was made using Spectral-Domain HRA-OCT (Heidelberg Engineering, Heidelberg, Germany) and images were examined using Heidelberg Eye Explorer version 1.7.0.0 (Heidelberg Engineering, Heidelberg, Germany). Fluorescein and indocyanine-green angiography were performed on all patients to confirm the diagnosis and to exclude other causes of maculopathy. In addition, we decided to exclude polypoidal chorioretinopathy due to its difference in clinical course and treatment response [22]. Initial treatment was given as a loading dose over three months with monthly intravitral injections of 0.5 mg Ranibizumab (Lucentis). Patients were re-examined at follow-ups 4 to 6 weeks after the third injection and the patients were prescribed additional injections based on signs of activity (retinal hemorrhages, presence of intra- and/or subretinal fluid) (PRN protocol) [23].

Clinical Data

Horizontal cross-sectional Spectral-Domain HRA-OCT scans of the foveal region of both eyes were examined to: measure the central foveal thickness (CFT), measure the central foveal thickness of the neuroretina (including any serous detachment) (CFN), determine if RPE elevation is present and then measure the central foveal sub-RPE space (CFE), and categorize the foveal integrity of the IS/OS and the ELM as either complete, interrupted, or absent (**Figure 1**) [12].

Assessment of Self-Perceived Visual Function

We utilized the Danish version of the 39-item VFQ, recently translated and validated for use in patients with AMD [9]. A trained interviewer presented the 39-item VFQ after the ophthalmic examination and diagnosis of neovascular AMD.

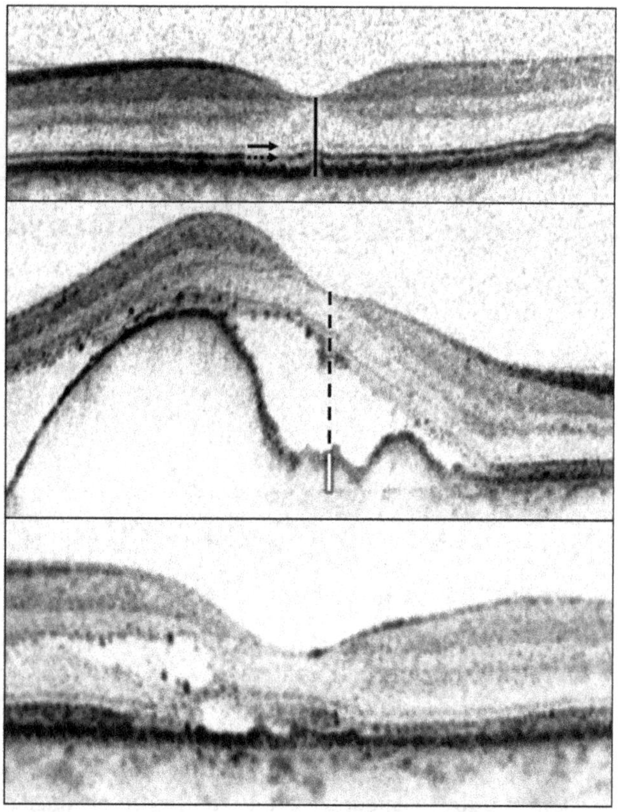

Figure 1. Optical coherence tomography images depicting measured foveal characteristics. We categorized the foveal status of external limiting membrane (ELM) (arrow) and inner segment/outer segment junction (IS/OS) (dotted arrow) as either complete, interrupted, or absent. We measured central foveal thickness (CFT) (black line), central foveal thickness of neuroretina including any serous detachment (CFN) (black dashed line), and central foveal thickness of RPE elevation in case of RPE elevation (CFE) (white line). (Top) Here, ELM and IS/OS were both complete, CFT and CFN were both 241 μm, and RPE was not elevated. (Middle) Here, ELM was complete, IS/OS was absent, CFT was 618 μm, CFN was 529 μm, RPE was elevated and CFE was 89 μm. (Bottom) Here, ELM and IS/OS were both interrupted, CFT and CFN were both 207 μm, and RPE was not elevated.

The 39-item VFQ is composed by 39 questions grouped into 12 subscales, of which one is related to general health and the rest to different aspects of visual-functioning: general vision, ocular pain, near activities, distance activities, social function, mental health, role difficulties, dependency on others, driving, color vision, peripheral vision. Each subscale is scored between 0 (the worst) and 100 (the best), and the mean of all subscales (excluding general health) is the final composite VFQ score. As the Danish 39-item VFQ could not validate the subscales pertaining to ocular pain and driving, these subscales were not included in our study and therefore not part of the composite score. All interviews were performed without the presence of a relative or friend. The interviewer neither wore a uniform nor was part of the treating team, and followed a stringent predesigned interview guideline instructing adequate responses to patients when doubts arouse about a question. Furthermore, a questionnaire log was kept to record any deviations from normal protocol.

Table 1. Patient characteristics.

Characteristics (n = 197)	
Age, median (IQR), years	79 (74–84)
Sex (male), n (%)	61 (31)
Neovascular AMD in eyes, n (%)	
In better eye only	65 (33)
In worse eye only	115 (58)
In both eyes	17 (9)

Statistical Analysis

We correlated composite VFQ scores with BCVA of the better eye and BCVA of the worse eye using Spearman's Rank Correlation. Then, composite VFQ scores were transformed into normal distribution and used as the dependent variable in a backward multiple regression analysis. We used the Kolmogorov-Smirnov Test to check the transformed values for normal distribution. We used age, sex, BCVA of the better eye, and BCVA of the worse eye as co-variates in this model.

We analyzed the foveal morphological characteristics in the better eye, and when both eyes had same visual acuity, we repeated our analyses using the data from the right eye and the left eye separately. We found this to be an issue in three patients, and as these differences did not affect our results significantly, we simply choose to report the data from the right eye in these three cases. Examination of the horizontal cross-sectional scans were repeated by the examiner after three months to calculate intra-rater reliability using Cohen's unweighted kappa for categorical data and intraclass correlation coefficient (ICC) (two-way consistency model) for continuous data.

The relationship between continuous morphological data and VFQ scores were explored using scatter plots with a lowess curve. We correlated continuous morphological data with VFQ scores using Spearman's Rank Correlation. Patients were stratified into groups by RPE elevation, IS/OS status, and ELM status; and non-parametric tests (Kruskal-Wallis Test and Mann-Whitney-U Test) were used to compare VFQ scores.

We repeated our multiple regression analysis with the transformed composite VFQ scores and included foveal morphological characteristics in the better eye to investigate 1) whether inclusion of foveal characteristics would give a better model fit suggesting an additive value, and 2) whether we can identify and distinguish one or more foveal morphological characteristics which affects self-perceived visual function. Thus, we used the following co-variates: age, sex, BCVA of the better eye, BCVA of the worse eye, CFT in the better eye, CFN in the better eye, RPE elevation status in the better eye, IS/OS status in the better eye, and ELM status in the better eye. As the relationship between CFT and CFN values and VFQ scores was found to be non-linear in lowess curves, CFT and CFN values were converted into dummy variables with two possible values when used in the regression analysis: either 1) within the peak area defined as ≥170 and <270 μm or 2) outside of the peak area defined as <170 and ≥270 μm.

Changes in VFQ scores were grouped into one of three categories: *clinically meaningful increase*, *clinically meaningful decrease*, and *no clinically meaningful change*. A 5-point or more change in the composite VFQ score is regarded as a clinically meaningful change [20], [21]. We compared these changes in relation to baseline values including foveal morphological characteristics using Kruskal-Wallis Test and Chi-square Test (Fischer's Exact Test when dealing with small numbers). We then used a multinomial logistic regression to investigate whether any baseline characteristics were associated with a *clinically meaningful increase* or a *clinically meaningful decrease* in composite VFQ score at 3 and 12 months, using the *no clinically meaningful change* category as the reference category. We included the following baseline characteristics: composite VFQ score, CFT in the better eye, CFN in the better eye, RPE elevation status in the better eye, IS/OS status in the better eye, ELM status in the better eye, BCVA of the better eye, and BCVA of the worse eye. Due to the inverse U-shaped relation of CFT and CFN in the better eye with VFQ scores, and small numbers in the <150 μm groups, CFT and CFN in the better eye were included as dummy variables with two possible values: either 1) within the peak area defined as ≥170 and < 270 μm or 2) outside of the peak area defined as <170 and ≥ 270 μm.

A p-value below 0.05 is considered significant, which was Bonferroni-adjusted to a p-value below 0.005 when testing VFQ subscores. Data were analyzed using SPSS 20 (IBM, Chicago, IL, USA) and Prism 6 (GraphPad Software, La Jolla, CA, USA).

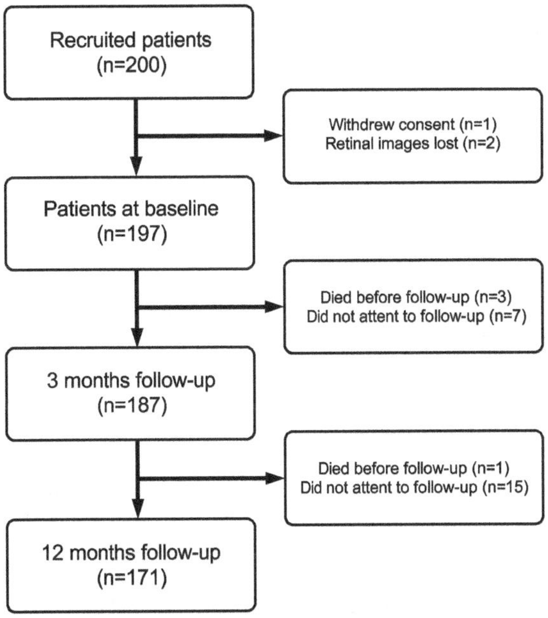

Figure 2. Study flow diagram with number of participants at each stage and reasons for non-participation.

Table 2. Foveal morphological characteristics in the better eye of study participants.

Characteristics (n = 197)	
CFT, median (IQR), µm	261 (223–375)
CFN, median (IQR), µm	237 (202–281)
RPE elevation, n (%)	
Not present	121 (61)
Present	76 (39)
CFE, median (IQR), µm	102 (56–173)
IS/OS status, n (%)	
Complete	84 (43)
Interrupted	40 (20)
Absent	73 (37)
ELM status, n (%)	
Complete	95 (48)
Interrupted	40 (20)
Absent	62 (32)

Abbreviations used: CFT = total central foveal thickness, IQR = interquartile range, CFN = central foveal thickness of the neuroretina, RPE = retinal pigment epithelium, CFE = central foveal thickness of the retinal pigment epithelium elevation, IS/OS = inner segment/outer segment junction, ELM = external limiting membrane.

Results

We enrolled 200 patients in our cohort, but one withdrew consent and in two patients the OCTs from one time-point were lost, leaving 197 patients. Patient characteristics are summarized in **Table 1**. Of the included patients, 187 completed the 3 months follow-up, and 171 completed the 12 months follow-up (**Figure 2**).

Composite VFQ scores correlated stronger with BCVA of the better eye ($\rho = 0.605$; $p < .001$) compared to BCVA of the worse eye ($\rho = .405$; $p < 0.001$). In our multiple regression analysis, we found BCVA of the better eye to be a significant co-variate ($p < 0.001$), but not BCVA of the worse eye ($p = 0.362$), age ($p = 0.526$), and sex ($p = 0.850$) (Adjusted $R^2 = 0.398$).

Self-Perceived Visual Function and Foveal Morphology in the Better Eye

Foveal morphological characteristics in the better eye are summarized in **Table 2**. Intra-rater reliability was high for all measured aspects of foveal characteristics: CFT in the better eye (ICC = 0.996), CFN in the better eye (ICC = 0.983), RPE elevation in the better eye ($\kappa = 1.000$), IS/OS status in the better eye ($\kappa = 0.964$), ELM status in the better eye ($\kappa = 0.935$).

CFT and CFN in the better eye correlated with composite VFQ scores in an inverted U-shaped fashion peaking at approximately 220 µm (**Figure 3**). RPE elevation in the better eye was associated with lower composite VFQ scores, but CFE in the better eye did not correlate with composite VFQ scores (**Figure 4**). Better IS/OS and ELM status in the better eye were both associated with higher composite VFQ scores (**Figure 5**).

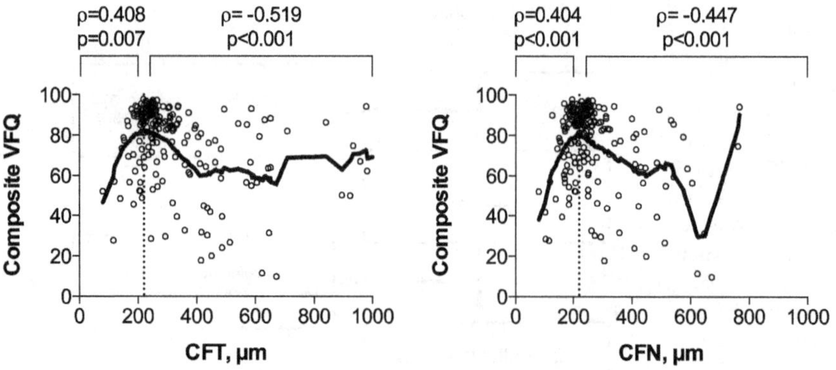

Figure 3. Composite VFQ scores in relation to foveal thickness in the better eye. Scatterplots with a lowess curve (thick line) to explore the relationship between composite VFQ scores and total central foveal thickness (CFT) in the better eye (left) and central foveal thickness of the neuroretina (CFN) in the better eye (right). Both CFT and CFN correlated with composite VFQ scores in an inverted U-shaped fashion peaking at approximately 220 µm (dotted line). ρ = Spearman's rank correlation coefficient, p = p-value.

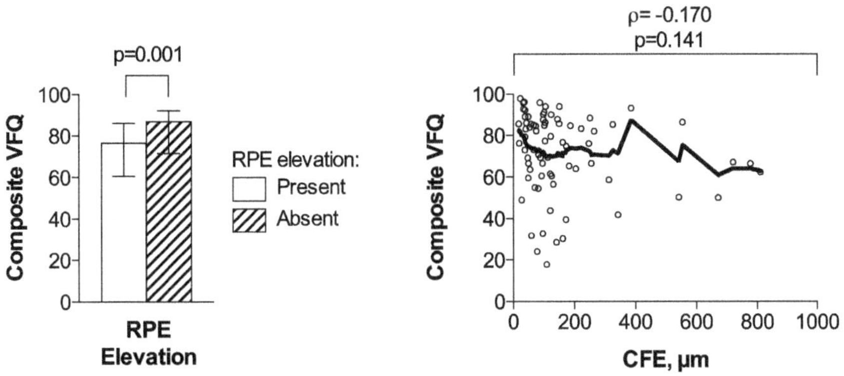

Figure 4. Composite VFQ scores in relation to retinal pigment epithelium status. Composite VFQ scores are compared between patients with or without retinal pigment epithelium (RPE) elevation in better eye (left). A scatterplot with a lowess curve (thick line) is used to explore the relationship between composite VFQ scores and central foveal thickness of the RPE elevation (CFE) (n = 76) (right). RPE elevation in the better eye was associated with lower composite VFQ scores; however, the level of RPE elevation — measured as CFE — did not correlate significantly with composite VFQ scores. The height of bars represents the median, and the whiskers represent the interquartile range. ρ = Spearman's rank correlation coefficient; p = p-value.

Low CFT values (<220 µm) in the better eye correlated positively with near activities, mental health, and dependency; and high CFT values (≥220 µm) correlated negatively with general vision, near activities, distance activities, social function, mental health, role difficulties, dependency, and color vision (**Table 3**). Low CFN values (<220 µm) in the better eye correlated positively with general vision, near activities, distance activities, social function, mental health, role difficulties, and dependency; and high CFN values (≥220 µm) correlated negatively with general vision, near activities, distance activities, social function, mental health, role difficulties, dependency, and color vision (**Table 3**). Presence of RPE elevation in the better eye was associated with lower near vision (**Figure 6**), but CFE did not correlate with any subscores (**Table 3**). Better IS/OS and ELM status in the better eye were both associated with better general vision, near activities, distance activities, social function, mental health, role difficulties, dependency, and color vision (**Figure 6**).

Including foveal characteristics in our multiple regression analysis gave a better model fit (Adjusted $R^2 = 0.418$) compared to the previous model which only included age, sex, BCVA of the better eye, and BCVA of the worse eye. In this model, BCVA of the better eye ($p<0.001$) and IS/OS status in the better eye ($p = 0.005$) were significant, while the other co-variates did not reach significance: age ($p = 0.592$), sex ($p = 0.685$), BCVA of the worse eye ($p = 0.501$), CFT in the better eye ($p = 0.702$), CFN in the better eye ($p = 0.343$), RPE elevation status in the better eye ($p = 0.887$), and ELM status in the better eye ($p = 0.633$).

Self-Perceived Visual Function and Morphology Status in the Worse Eye

We re-ran our analyses on patients only unilaterally affected by neovascular AMD in order to evaluate the impact of worse eye morphology status on self-perceived visual function. We did not find a correlation between composite VFQ scores and CFT or CFN (Figure 7). Elevated RPE in the worse eye had a significant impact on composite VFQ scores (Figure 8), but the extent of RPE elevation did not correlate with composite VFQ scores ($\rho = -0.153$, $p = 0.159$, Spearman's Rank Correlation). Status of IS/OS or ELM in the worse eye did not contribute to composite VFQ scores (Figure 8).

Clinically Meaningful Changes in Self-Perceived Visual Function at 3 and 12 Months

BCVA of the treated eyes did not change significantly during the study period; however, composite VFQ scores increased from baseline to 3 months, but fell at 12 months to a level similar to baseline (**Table 4**). Clinically meaningful changes in composite VFQ at 3 months were associated with baseline composite VFQ score, baseline BCVA of the better eye, baseline IS/OS status in the better eye, and baseline ELM status in the better eye (**Table 5**). Clinically meaningful changes in composite VFQ at 12 months were associated with baseline composite VFQ scores, baseline BCVA of the better eye, baseline BCVA of the worse eye, baseline CFT in the better eye, and baseline IS/OS status in the better eye (**Table 5**). When these values were included in multinomial logistic regression analyses, we found a clinically meaningful increase at 3 months to be associated with a lower baseline composite VFQ ($p<0.001$) and a baseline CFN <170 µm or ≥ 270 µm in the better eye ($p = 0.043$); a clinically meaningful increase at 12 months to be associated with a lower baseline composite VFQ ($p<0.001$); a clinically meaningful decrease at 3 months not to be associated with any baseline variables; and a

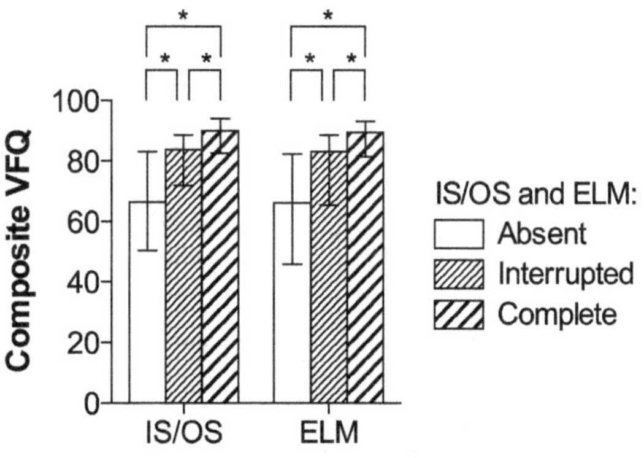

Figure 5. Comparison of composite VFQ scores between patients stratified by the foveal status of IS/OS and ELM in the better eye. A better IS/OS or ELM status in the better eye was associated with a higher composite VFQ score. * = significant ($p<0.05$).

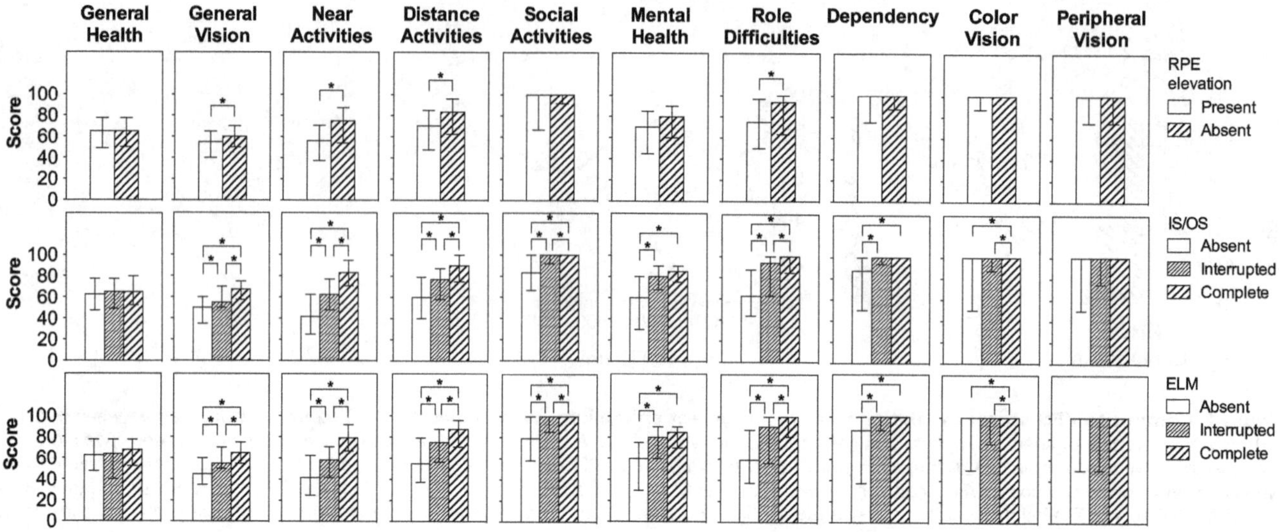

Figure 6. VFQ subscores in relation to foveal status of IS/OS, ELM, and presence of RPE elevation. Presence of retinal pigment epithelium (RPE) elevation was associated with lower general vision, lower near activities, lower distance activities, and lower role difficulties (top). Better inner segment/outer segment junction (IS/OS) (middle) and better external limiting membrane (ELM) (bottom) status were both associated with higher general vision, near activities, distance activities, social activities, mental health, role difficulties, dependency, and color vision. * = significant ($p<0.005$).

clinically meaningful decrease to be associated with an absent IS/OS line in the better eye at baseline ($p=0.018$) (**Table 6**).

Discussion

BCVA of the better eye correlated with the VFQ scores at a level similar to previous studies ($\rho=0.605$), which indicates an only moderate level of correlation between BCVA and self-perceived visual function [9], [20], [24]. Hence, the self-perceived visual function is not just another measure of BCVA, but an important addition to the overall assessment of treatment response. Previous studies have mainly focused on the predictive value of retinal morphology on visual acuity, and some have investigated self-perceived visual function in relation to treatment response. In our prospective study, we investigated the relationship between foveal morphology and self-perceived visual function, and the predictive value of foveal morphology on changes in self-perceived visual function. We found IS/OS status of the better eye to contribute to the self-perceived visual function independent of BCVA of the better eye, and we identified three baseline factors which were associated with clinically meaningful changes in self-perceived visual function.

Foveal morphology and its effect on self-perceived visual function has not previously been studied; however, some studies

Table 3. Spearman's rank correlation coefficient of the correlation between foveal thickness parameters in the better eye and Visual Function Questionnaire subscores.

	CFT <220 μm (n = 43)	CFT ≥220 μm (n = 154)	CFN <220 μm (n = 74)	CFN ≥220 μm (n = 123)	CFE (n = 76)
General health	0.110	−0.103	−0.013	−0.054	−0.064
General vision	0.350	−0.524[a]	0.268	−0.457[a]	−0.094
Near activities	0.382	−0.560[a]	0.449[a]	−0.498[a]	−0.213
Distance activities	0.357	−0.489[a]	0.325[b]	−0.374[a]	−0.221
Social function	0.282	−0.457[a]	0.265	−0.488[a]	−0.067
Mental health	0.425[b]	−0.349[a]	0.398[a]	−0.337[a]	−0.060
Role difficulties	0.365	−0.450[a]	0.397[a]	−0.381[a]	−0.185
Dependency	0.285	−0.379[a]	0.374[c]	−0.343[a]	−0.157
Color vision	0.293	−0.312[a]	0.297	−0.356[a]	−0.123
Peripheral vision	0.355	−0.150	0.261	−0.196	0.057

Abbreviations used: CFT = total central foveal thickness, CFN = central foveal thickness of the neuroretina, CFE = central foveal thickness of the retinal pigment epithelium elevation.
[a]Significant correlation, $p<0.001$.
[b]Significant correlation, $p=0.005$.
[c]Significant correlation, $p=0.001$.

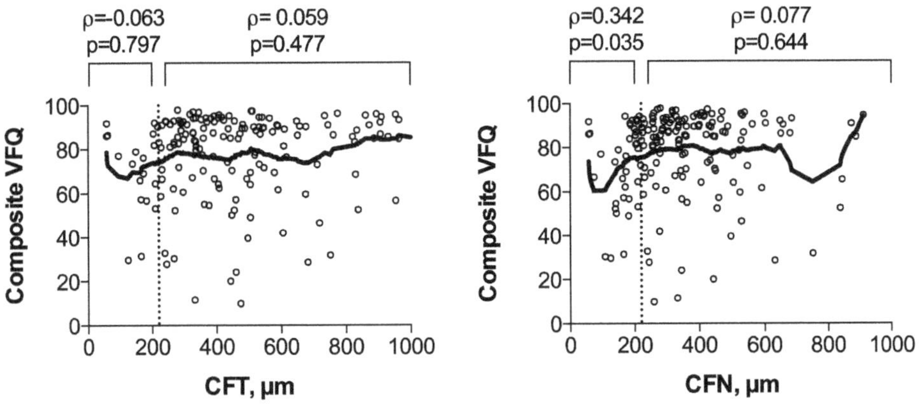

Figure 7. Composite VFQ scores in relation to foveal thickness in patients with neovascular AMD in their worse eye. Scatterplots with a lowess curve (thick line) to explore the relationship between composite VFQ scores and total central foveal thickness (CFT) in the worse eye (left) and central foveal thickness of the neuroretina (CFN) in the worse eye (right). We divided the cases into groups at 220 µm (dotted line) as previously and found no correlation between VFQ and CFT or CFN ≥220 µm, and we found a small correlation between VFQ and CFN <220 µm. ρ = Spearman's rank correlation coefficient, p = p-value.

have reported on foveal morphology and its impact on visual acuity. In eyes with neovascular AMD, foveal thickness correlated in a V-shaped fashion with visual acuity measured in logMAR, and IS/OS and ELM status had a significant impact on visual acuity in patients with neovascular AMD [12], [13]. The extent of foveal IS/OS distruption has also been linked to lower visual acuity in eyes with dry age-related macular degeneration and neovascular AMD [14], [25]. Similar findings are observed in eyes with other retinal diseases, so there is strong data supporting that photoreceptor integrity, represented by the IS/OS layer, has a significant impact on the visual acuity [26–28]. In our study, we found foveal thickness and foveal integrity of IS/OS and ELM to be related to the self-perceived visual function. However, visual acuity and self-perceived visual function correlates only moderately and does not always go together, and therefore one cannot assume that the impact of foveal morphology on the self-perceived visual function is equal to findings on visual acuity. One particularly interesting finding in our study is that the IS/OS status in the better eye contributed independently of the BCVA of the better eye to the self-perceived visual function, which indicates that visual acuity does not always capture the self-perceived visual function. This is perhaps unsurprising, as the self-perceived visual function measured by the VFQ reflects the patient-experienced visual function and vision-related quality-of-life, and contributes with a more complex and subjective dimension of visual function compared to visual acuity [29]. This is exemplified by one study which showed that anti-VEGF treatment of eyes with neovascular AMD could improve the ability to read although treatment did not improve the visual acuity [30]. In another study, reading was significantly impaired in patients with subretinal fibrosis after choroidal neovascularization, and underestimated when only considering the visual acuity [31].

Ranibizumab phase III trials MARINA and ANCHOR showed a significant increase in visual acuity after 3, 12, and 24 months [5]. These studies also investigated the self-perceived visual function using the VFQ-25 and found significant higher VFQ scores at 3, 12, and 24 months, excluding cases in the ANCHOR study, where the study eye was the worse eye [5]. Unlike these controlled clinical trials, studies based on daily clinical practice tend to show a lower effect of treatment, although still much better compared to the sham group in MARINA and ANCHOR studies [6], [23], [32], [33]. Less is known on how the self-perceived visual function changes in daily clinical practice. Using the VFQ-39, we

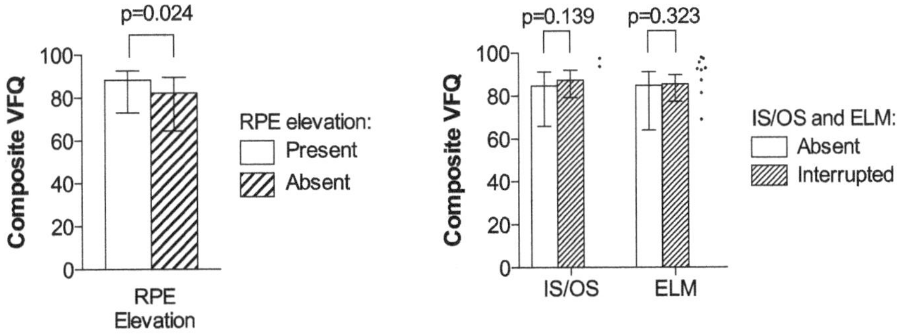

Figure 8. Comparison of composite VFQ scores in patients with neovascular AMD in their worse eye, stratified by the foveal status of RPE elevation, IS/OS and ELM. Composite VFQ scores were lower in patients with elevated retinal pigment epithelium (RPE) (left). IS/OS or ELM status did not affect composite VFQ scores significantly (right). Due to very few cases, worse eyes with complete IS/OS (n = 2) and complete ELM status (n = 9) are shown as dots and not included in statistical analyses. p = p-value.

Table 4. Best-corrected visual acuity of the treated eye and composite Visual Function Questionnaire scores throughout the study period.

	Baseline (197 patients, 214 eyes)	3 Months Follow-up (187 patients, 202 eyes)	12 Months Follow-up (n = 171 patients, 186 eyes)
BCVA of the treated eye, median (IQR), ETDRS letters	59 (48–70)	62 (48–72)	62 (47–72)
Composite VFQ Scores, median (IQR)[a]	84 (67–91)	85 (68–92)[b]	83 (65–90)[c]

Abbreviations used: BCVA = best-corrected visual acuity, IQR = interquartile range, ETDRS = Early Treatment Diabetic Retinopathy Study, VFQ = Visual Function Questionnaire.
[a]Significant change throughout the study period, $p<0.001$ in Friedman's two-way analysis of variance by ranks.
[b]Significant change between baseline and 3 months follow-up, $p = 0.004$ in Wilcoxon signed rank test.
[c]Significant change between 3 and 12 months follow-up, $p<0.001$ in Wilcoxon signed rank test.

found that the VFQ scores increased significantly at 3 months, which returned to a level similar to baseline after 12 months. This is in line with the only other study, which also found a minor increase in VFQ-25 composite score after 3 months, which returned to a level similar to baseline after one year [6]. In the majority of our patients, changes in VFQ scores were small and studies suggest that a clinically meaningful change in the VFQ score is at least 4 to 6 points [20], [21]. No previous studies have investigated predictive factors of clinical meaningful change in VFQ; however, certain baseline predictors have been associated with a clinically meaningful improvement in visual acuity (≥15 letters) 1 year after anti-VEGF treatment: lower baseline BCVA and smaller lesion size at baseline is associated with an improvement in visual acuity at 1 year [15–17]. Also, IS/OS and ELM status at baseline are shown to influence visual acuity after 1 year of treatment [14], [18], [19]. When we used a 5-point change limit to identify cases with a clinically meaningful change at 3 and 12 months, we could observe several associated baseline characteristics: baseline VFQ score, baseline BCVA, baseline CFT value, baseline IS/OS status, and baseline ELM status. In our multinomial logistic regression analysis, we found a lower baseline VFQ to be positively associated with an increase at 3 and 12 months, a baseline CFN <170 μm or ≥270 μm in the better eye to be negatively associated with an increase at 12 months, and an absent IS/OS line in the better eye to be positively associated with a decrease at 12 months. Visual acuity and self-perceived visual function does not necessarily go together; however, in the prediction of clinically meaningful changes in self-perceived visual function, we find similar factors to possess a predictive value.

This study has several strengths. We used the VFQ-39 with trained interviewers, which provide more valid and accurate data in patients with neovascular AMD [9–11]. Validity of the VFQ has been questioned as some VFQ subscales are found to be psychometrically flawed [34]. Studies on the validity of the VFQ and its subscales have determined that the VFQ-25, including the 14 question appendix (VFQ-39) and excluding subscales concerning ocular pain and driving, is valid when studying Danish patients with AMD [9–11], [35]. We included patients with neovascular AMD consecutively to minimize any selection bias. Finally, our clinic receives all patients in Region Zealand (~820.000 citizens) for neovascular AMD diagnosis and treatment without any self-payment; therefore, our results are based on a general non-selected population, which strengthens its relevance for daily clinical practice. One should also note the limitations of our study. BCVA of the worse eye did not contribute significantly to the self-perceived visual function. This is not surprising, especially in light of a previous study by Rubin et al., which investigated the visual acuity in the elderly and found that only the better eye is of importance to vision-related tasks, such as reading and face-discrimination, suggesting that the contribution from the worse eye may be small at most [36]. Our similar findings confirm that the better eye is the primary contributor to the self-perceived visual function. However, we found that elevated RPE in the worse eye contributed to the composite VFQ scores, which suggest that foveal morphology in the worse eye may influence the self-perceived visual function albeit subtler and less significant compared to the better eye. The details on how and when the foveal morphology of the worse eye influences the self-perceived visual function remain to be investigated. The VFQ scores range from 0 to 100, which limit any prediction of clinically meaningful changes near the range borders due to flooring or ceiling effect. Another important aspect is our sample size, which may large and sufficient to reveal factors with a high contribution to the self-perceived visual function, but may be too small for detecting factors with a more subtle contribution to the self-perceived visual function. For example, clinically meaningful decrease at 12 months is almost significantly associated with an interrupted IS/OS line (OR 5.1, $p = 0.07$); therefore, future studies should consider larger sample sizes when investigating clinically meaningful changes, as anti-VEGF treatment may be able to preserve the self-perceived visual function in the majority of patients with neovascular AMD.

In conclusion, foveal morphology is related to the self-perceived visual function, and the foveal IS/OS status in the better eye may influence on the self-perceived visual function independently of visual acuity. Lower VFQ score and baseline CFN in the better eye within 170 μm to 270 μm are both associated with a clinically meaningful increase in the self-perceived visual function. Absent foveal IS/OS line in the better eye is associated with a clinically meaningful decrease in the self-perceived visual function 12 months after treatment start. These associations should not discourage the use of anti-VEGF in patients with an absent IS/OS line, as some patients may experience a clinically meaningful increase. Instead, these novel findings can help clinicians provide patients more individualized information on the prognosis and what to expect on a vision-related quality-of-life perspective. Prediction of patients at risk of impaired vision-related quality-of-life may help us better target support and rehabilitation, especially considering the increasing number of elderly and the economical impact of the future prevalence of neovascular AMD [37–39]. Future studies need to investigate which aspects of the self-perceived visual function are affected, how treatment response on foveal morphology affects the self-perceived visual function, and whether identification of

Table 5. Baseline characteristics in relation to clinical meaningful changes in composite Visual Function Questionnaire scores at 3 and 12 months.

	3 months follow-up				12 months follow-up			
	Increase (n = 62)	**No change (n = 86)**	**Decrease (n = 39)**	**P-value**	**Increase (n = 41)**	**No change (n = 81)**	**Decrease (n = 49)**	**P-value**
Age, median (IQR), years	77 (73–82)	79 (75–85)	80 (76–84)	0.22[a]	78 (74–82)	78 (74–83)	79 (75–84)	0.43[a]
Sex (male), n (%)	20 (32)	24 (28)	14 (36)	0.65[b]	13 (32)	22 (27)	15 (31)	0.85[b]
Composite VFQ score	72 (57–82)	89 (81–93)	83 (60–91)	<0.001[a]	69 (53–80)	89 (79–93)	86 (69–90)	<0.001[a]
BCVA of the better eye, ETDRS letters	74 (56–81)	78 (70–85)	71 (63–78)	0.03[a]	76 (54–80)	78 (71–85)	71 (64–78)	0.005[a]
BCVA of the worse eye, ETDRS letters	48 (22–66)	50 (31–67)	48 (29–57)	0.48[a]	50 (22–67)	55 (41–68)	46 (26–60)	0.05[a]
Foveal morphology in the better eye								
CFT, n (%)								
<170 μm	7 (11)	2 (2)	1 (3)		6 (15)	1 (1)	2 (4)	
≥170 μm and <270 μm	27 (44)	47 (55)	16 (41)	0.10[c]	20 (49)	48 (59)	18 (37)	0.004[c]
≥270 μm	28 (45)	37 (43)	22 (56)		15 (37)	32 (40)	29 (59)	
CFN, n (%)								
<170 μm	8 (13)	4 (5)	4 (10)		7 (17)	3 (4)	4 (8)	
≥170 μm and <270 μm	38 (61)	59 (69)	21 (54)	0.26[c]	24 (59)	59 (73)	29 (59)	0.09[c]
≥270 μm	16 (26)	23 (27)	14 (36)		10 (24)	19 (23)	16 (33)	
RPE elevation, n (%)								
Not present	39 (63)	54 (63)	21 (54)	0.59[b]	26 (63)	50 (62)	27 (55)	0.68[b]
Present	23 (37)	32 (37)	18 (46)		15 (37)	31 (38)	22 (45)	
IS/OS status, n (%)								
Complete	20 (32)	48 (56)	9 (23)		16 (39)	43 (53)	13 (27)	
Interrupted	16 (26)	15 (17)	8 (21)	0.002[b]	8 (20)	17 (21)	12 (24)	0.03[b]
Absent	26 (42)	23 (27)	22 (56)		17 (41)	21 (26)	24 (49)	
ELM status, n (%)								
Complete	25 (40)	51 (59)	12 (31)		18 (44)	46 (57)	19 (39)	
Interrupted	15 (24)	20 (23)	9 (23)	0.03[b]	9 (22)	16 (20)	11 (22)	0.29[b]
Absent	22 (35)	38 (44)	18 (46)		14 (34)	19 (23)	19 (39)	

Abbreviations used: IQR = interquartile range, VFQ = Visual Function Questionnaire, BCVA = best-corrected visual acuity, ETDRS = Early Treatment Diabetic Retinopathy Study, CFT = total central foveal thickness, CFN = central foveal thickness of the neuroretina, RPE = retinal pigment epithelium, IS/OS = inner segment/outer segment junction, ELM = external limiting membrane.

[a]Kruskal-Wallis test.

[b]Chi-square test.

[c]Fischer's Exact Test.

Table 6. Multinomial logistic regression on clinical meaningful changes in composite Visual Function Questionnaire scores at 3 and 12 months using baseline characteristics.

	3 months follow-up				12 months follow-up			
	Increase (n = 62)		Decrease (n = 39)		Increase (n = 41)		Decrease (n = 49)	
	OR (95% CI)	P-value	OR (95% CI)	P-value	OR (95% CI)	P-value	OR (95% CI)	P-value
Age	.94 (.80–1.0)	0.06	.97 (.91–1.0)	0.37	.96 (.89–1.0)	0.21	.98 (.92–1.0)	0.62
Sex (male)	.12 (.50–3.0)	0.67	1.8 (.69–4.6)	0.24	1.4 (.50–3.7)	0.55	.83 (.33–2.1)	0.69
Composite VFQ score	.92 (.89–.95)	<0.001	.99 (.95–1.0)	0.42	.93 (.90–.96)	<0.001	1.0 (.98–1.1)	0.31
BCVA of the better eye	1.0 (.99–1.1)	0.09	1.0 (.97–1.1)	0.49	.99 (.94–1.0)	0.66	.99 (.94–1.0)	0.77
BCVA of the worse eye	1.0 (.99–1.0)	0.29	1.0 (.98–1.0)	0.77	1.0 (.99–1.0)	0.26	.98 (.96–1.0)	0.09
Foveal morphology in the better eye								
CFT								
≥170 μm and <270 μm	1.0	-	1.0	-	1.0	-	1.0	-
<170 μm or ≥270 μm	2.5 (.66–9.3)	0.18	.57 (.15–2.2)	0.41	.93 (.21–4.2)	0.92	2.4 (.67–8.5)	0.18
CFN								
≥170 μm and <270 μm	1.0	-	1.0	-	1.0	-	1.0	-
<170 μm or ≥270 μm	.27 (.08–.96)	0.04	1.5 (4.7–5.0)	0.48	.89 (.21–3.8)	0.88	.81 (.27–2.5)	0.71
RPE elevation								
Not present	1.0	-	1.0	-	1.0	-	1.0	-
Present	.36 (.13–1.0)	0.06	.86 (.31–2.4)	0.77	.56 (.19–1.7)	0.31	.55 (.20–1.5)	0.23
IS/OS status								
Complete	1.0	-	1.0	-	1.0	-	1.0	-
Interrupted	4.8 (.76–31)	0.09	2.1 (.27–16)	0.48	.69 (.08–5.9)	0.74	5.1 (.90–29)	0.07
Absent	2.6 (.29–23)	0.40	6.2 (.76–50)	0.09	1.0 (.08–14)	0.994	14 (1.6–118)	0.02
ELM status								
Complete	1.0	-	1.0	-	1.0	-	1.0	-
Interrupted	.94 (.15–5.9)	0.95	1.9 (.27–14)	0.51	1.6 (.19–13)	0.67	.39 (.07–2.1)	0.28
Absent	1.2 (.13–11)	0.88	1.6 (.20–13)	0.66	.67 (.05–9.8)	0.77	.17 (.02–1.5)	0.11

Values are in odds ratio and 95% confidence interval. Age (in years), composite VFQ score, BCVA of the better eye (in ETDRS letters), and BCVA of the worse eye (in ETDRS letters) are included as continuous co-variates. The no clinical meaningful change group was used as the reference category. Intercepts are not shown.
Abbreviations used: OR = odds ratio, CI = confidence interval, VFQ = Visual Function Questionnaire, BCVA = best-corrected visual acuity, CFT = total central foveal thickness, CFN = central foveal thickness of the neuroretina, RPE = retinal pigment epithelium, IS/OS = inner segment/outer segment junction, ELM = external limiting membrane.

patients at risk may help us more rationally target eye-related care and rehabilitation.

Author Contributions

Conceived and designed the experiments: MSS TLS. Performed the experiments: YS GOH CTL. Analyzed the data: YS TLS. Contributed reagents/materials/analysis tools: GOH CTL TLS. Wrote the paper: YS GOH CTL MSS TLS.

References

1. Lim LS, Mitchell P, Seddon JM, Holz FG, Wong TY (2012) Age-related macular degeneration. Lancet 379: 1728–1738.
2. Williams RA, Brody BL, Thomas RG, Kaplan RM, Brown SI (1998) The psychosocial impact of macular degeneration. Arch Ophthalmol 116: 514–520.
3. Margolis MK, Coyne K, Kennedy-Martin T, Baker T, Schein O, et al. (2002) Vision-specific instruments for the assessment of health-related quality of life and visual functioning: a literature review. Pharmacoeconomics 20: 791–812.
4. Brundage M, Bass B, Davidson J, Queenan J, Bezjak A, et al. (2011) Patterns of reporting health-related quality of life outcomes in randomized clinical trials: implications for clinicians and quality of life researchers. Qual Life Res 20: 653–664.
5. Bressler NM, Chang TS, Suñer IJ, Fine JT, Dolan CM, et al. (2010) Vision-related function after ranibizumab treatment by better- or worse-seeing eye: clinical trial results from MARINA and ANCHOR. Ophthalmology 117: 747–756.e4.
6. Finger RP, Wiedemann P, Blumhagen F, Pohl K, Holz FG (2013) Treatment patterns, visual acuity and quality-of-life outcomes of the WAVE study - A noninterventional study of ranibizumab treatment for neovascular age-related macular degeneration in Germany. Acta Ophthalmol 91: 540–546.
7. Leys A, Zlateva G, Shah SN, Patel M (2008) Quality of life in patients with age-related macular degeneration: results from the VISION study. Eye (Lond) 22: 792–798.
8. Chang TS, Bressler NM, Fine JT, Dolan CM, Ward J, et al. (2007) Improved vision-related function after ranibizumab treatment of neovascular age-related macular degeneration: results of a randomized clinical trial. Arch Ophthalmol 125: 1460–1469.
9. Sørensen MS, Andersen S, Henningsen GO, Larsen CT, Sørensen TL (2011) Danish version of Visual Function Questionnaire-25 and its use in age-related macular degeneration. Dan Med Bull 58: A4290.
10. Orr P, Rentz AM, Margolis MK, Revicki DA, Dolan CM, et al. (2011) Validation of the National Eye Institute Visual Function Questionnaire-25 (NEI VFQ-25) in age-related macular degeneration. Invest Ophthalmol Vis Sci 52: 3354–3359.
11. Clemons TE, Chew EY, Bressler SB, McBee W, Age-Related Eye Disease Study Research Group (2003) National Eye Institute Visual Function Questionnaire in the Age-Related Eye Disease Study (AREDS): AREDS Report No. 10. Arch Ophthalmol 121: 211–217.
12. Oishi A, Hata M, Shimozono M, Mandai M, Nishida A, et al. (2010) The significance of external limiting membrane status for visual acuity in age-related macular degeneration. Am J Ophthalmol 150: 27–32.e1.
13. Akagi-Kurashige Y, Tsujikawa A, Oishi A, Ooto S, Yamashiro K, et al. (2012) Relationship between retinal morphological findings and visual function in age-related macular degeneration. Graefes Arch Clin Exp Ophthalmol 250: 1129–1136.
14. Shin HJ, Chung H, Kim HC (2011) Association between foveal microstructure and visual outcome in age-related macular degeneration. Retina 31: 1627–1636.
15. Ying GS, Huang J, Maguire MG, Jaffe GJ, Grunwald JE, et al. (2013) Baseline predictors for one-year visual outcomes with ranibizumab or bevacizumab for neovascular age-related macular degeneration. Ophthalmology 120: 122–129.
16. Kaiser PK, Brown DM, Zhang K, Hudson HL, Holz FG, et al. (2007) Ranibizumab for predominantly classic neovascular age-related macular degeneration: subgroup analysis of first-year ANCHOR results. Am J Ophthalmol 144: 850–857.
17. Boyer DS, Antoszyk AN, Awh CC, Bhisitkul RB, Shapiro H, et al. (2007) Subgroup analysis of the MARINA study of ranibizumab in neovascular age-related macular degeneration. Ophthalmology 114: 246–252.
18. Chhablani J, Kim JS, Freeman WR, Kozak I, Wang HY, et al. (2013) Predictors of visual outcome in eyes with choroidal neovascularization secondary to age related macular degeneration treated with intravitreal bevacizumab monotherapy. Int J Ophthalmol 6: 62–66.
19. Hayashi H, Yamashiro K, Tsujikawa A, Ota M, Otani A, et al. (2009) Association between foveal photoreceptor integrity and visual outcome in neovascular age-related macular degeneration. Am J Ophthalmol 148: 83–89.e1.
20. Submacular Surgery Trials Research Group (2007) Evaluation of minimum clinically meaningful changes in scores on the National Eye Institute Visual Function Questionnaire (NEI-VFQ) SST Report Number 19. Ophthalmic Epidemiol 14: 205–215.
21. Suñer IJ, Kokame GT, Yu E, Ward J, Dolan C, et al. (2009) Responsiveness of NEI VFQ-25 to changes in visual acuity in neovascular AMD: validation studies from two phase 3 clinical trials. Invest Ophthalmol Vis Sci 50: 3629–3635.
22. Gomi F, Tano Y (2008) Polypoidal choroidal vasculopathy and treatments. Curr Opin Ophthalmol 19: 208–212.
23. Krüger Falk M, Kemp H, Sørensen TL (2013) Four-year treatment results of neovascular age-related macular degeneration with ranibizumab and causes for discontinuation of treatment. Am J Ophthalmol 155: 89–95.e3.
24. Revicki DA, Rentz AM, Harnam N, Thomas VS, Lanzetta P (2010) Reliability and validity of the National Eye Institute Visual Function Questionnaire-25 in patients with age-related macular degeneration. Invest Ophthalmol Vis Sci 51: 712–717.
25. Pappuru RR, Ouyang Y, Nittala MG, Hemmati HD, Keane PA, et al. (2011) Relationship between outer retinal thickness substructures and visual acuity in eyes with dry age-related macular degeneration. Invest Ophthalmol Vis Sci 52: 6743–6748.
26. Watanabe K, Tsunoda K, Mizuno Y, Akiyama K, Noda T (2013) Outer retinal morphology and visual function in patients with idiopathic epiretinal membrane. JAMA Ophthalmol 131: 172–177.
27. Shin HJ, Lee SH, Chung H, Kim HC (2012) Association between photoreceptor integrity and visual outcome in diabetic macular edema. Graefes Arch Clin Exp Ophthalmol 250: 61–70.
28. Kurashige Y, Tsujikawa A, Murakami T, Miyamoto K, Ogino K, et al. (2012) Changes in visual acuity and foveal photoreceptor integrity in eyes with chronic cystoid macular edema associated with retinal vein occlusion. Retina 32: 792–798.
29. Mangione CM, Lee PP, Pitts J, Gutierrez P, Berry S, et al. (1998) Psychometric properties of the National Eye Institute Visual Function Questionnaire (NEI-VFQ). NEI-VFQ Field Test Investigators. Arch Ophthalmol 116: 1496–1504.
30. Sabour-Pickett S, Loughman J, Nolan JM, Stack J, Pesudovs K, et al. (2013) Visual performance in patients with neovascular age-related macular degeneration undergoing treatment with intravitreal ranibizumab. J Ophthalmol 2013: 268438.
31. Richter-Mueksch S, Stur M, Stifter E, Radner W (2006) Differences in reading performance of patients with Drusen maculopathy and subretinal fibrosis after CNV. Graefes Arch Clin Exp Ophthalmol 244: 154–162.
32. Sørensen TL, Kemp H (2011) Ranibizumab treatment in patients with neovascular age-related macular degeneration and very low vision. Acta Ophthalmol 89: e97.
33. Marques IP, Fonseca P, Luz Cachulo M, Pires I, Figueira J, et al. (2013) Treatment of exudative age-related macular degeneration with intravitreal ranibizumab in clinical practice: a 3-year follow-up. Ophthalmologica 229: 158–167.
34. Pesudovs K, Gothwal VK, Wright T, Lamoureux EL (2010) Remediating serious flaws in the National Eye Institute Visual Function Questionnaire. J Cataract Refract Surg 36: 718–732.
35. Marella M, Pesudovs K, Keeffe JE, O'Connor PM, Rees G, et al. (2010) The psychometric validity of the NEI VFQ-25 for use in a low-vision population. Invest Ophthalmol Vis Sci 51: 2878–2884.
36. Rubin GS, Muñoz B, Bandeen-Roche K, West SK (2000) Monocular versus binocular visual acuity as measures of vision impairment and predictors of visual disability. Invest Ophthalmol Vis Sci 41: 3327–3334.
37. Rein DB, Wittenborn JS, Zhang X, Honeycutt AA, Lesesne SB, et al. (2009) Forecasting age-related macular degeneration through the year 2050: the potential impact of new treatments. Arch Ophthalmol 127: 533–540.
38. Tuulonen A, Salminen H, Linna M, Perkola M (2009) The need and total cost of Finnish eyecare services: a simulation model for 2005–2040. Acta Ophthalmol 87: 820–829.
39. Bauer P, Barthelmes D, Kurz M, Fleischhauer JC, Sutter FK (2008) The potential effect of population development, smoking and antioxidant supplementation on the future epidemiology of age-related macular degeneration in Switzerland. Klin Monbl Augenheilkd 225: 376–379.

Permissions

All chapters in this book were first published in PLOS ONE, by The Public Library of Science; hereby published with permission under the Creative Commons Attribution License or equivalent. Every chapter published in this book has been scrutinized by our experts. Their significance has been extensively debated. The topics covered herein carry significant findings which will fuel the growth of the discipline. They may even be implemented as practical applications or may be referred to as a beginning point for another development.

The contributors of this book come from diverse backgrounds, making this book a truly international effort. This book will bring forth new frontiers with its revolutionizing research information and detailed analysis of the nascent developments around the world.

We would like to thank all the contributing authors for lending their expertise to make the book truly unique. They have played a crucial role in the development of this book. Without their invaluable contributions this book wouldn't have been possible. They have made vital efforts to compile up to date information on the varied aspects of this subject to make this book a valuable addition to the collection of many professionals and students.

This book was conceptualized with the vision of imparting up-to-date information and advanced data in this field. To ensure the same, a matchless editorial board was set up. Every individual on the board went through rigorous rounds of assessment to prove their worth. After which they invested a large part of their time researching and compiling the most relevant data for our readers.

The editorial board has been involved in producing this book since its inception. They have spent rigorous hours researching and exploring the diverse topics which have resulted in the successful publishing of this book. They have passed on their knowledge of decades through this book. To expedite this challenging task, the publisher supported the team at every step. A small team of assistant editors was also appointed to further simplify the editing procedure and attain best results for the readers.

Apart from the editorial board, the designing team has also invested a significant amount of their time in understanding the subject and creating the most relevant covers. They scrutinized every image to scout for the most suitable representation of the subject and create an appropriate cover for the book.

The publishing team has been an ardent support to the editorial, designing and production team. Their endless efforts to recruit the best for this project, has resulted in the accomplishment of this book. They are a veteran in the field of academics and their pool of knowledge is as vast as their experience in printing. Their expertise and guidance has proved useful at every step. Their uncompromising quality standards have made this book an exceptional effort. Their encouragement from time to time has been an inspiration for everyone.

The publisher and the editorial board hope that this book will prove to be a valuable piece of knowledge for researchers, students, practitioners and scholars across the globe.

List of Contributors

Peng Zhou, Ram Kannan, Parameswaran G. Sreekumar and Guorui Dou
Doheny Eye Institute, Los Angeles, California, United States of America

Christine Spee
Ophthalmology, Keck School of Medicine of the University of Southern California, Los Angeles, California, United States of America

David R. Hinton
Departments of Pathology, Keck School of Medicine of the University of Southern California, Los Angeles, California, United States of America
Ophthalmology, Keck School of Medicine of the University of Southern California, Los Angeles, California, United States of America

Christine Schmucker and Gerd Antes
German Cochrane Institute, Institute of Medical Biometry and Medical Informatics, Department of Medical Biometry and Statistics, University Medical Centre Freiburg, Freiburg, Germany

Christoph Ehlken and Hansjuergen T. Agostini
University Eye Hospital, University Medical Centre Freiburg, Freiburg, Germany

Gerta Ruecker
Institute of Medical Biometry and Medical Informatics, Department of Medical Biometry and Statistics, University Medical Centre Freiburg, Freiburg, Germany

Monika Lelgemann
Medical Advisory Service of the German Health Insurance Funds, Essen, Germany

Yoon K. Loke
School of Medicine, University of East Anglia, Norwich, United Kingdom

Chui Ming Gemmy Cheung and Tien Yin Wong
Vitreoretinal Service, Singapore National Eye Centre, Singapore, Singapore
Singapore Eye Research Institute, Singapore, Singapore
Department of Ophthalmology, Yong Loo Lin School of Medicine, National University of Singapore, Singapore, Singapore
Ophthalmology Academic Clinical Program, Duke-NUS Graduate Medical School, Singapore, Singapore

Xiang Li
Singapore Eye Research Institute, Singapore, Singapore
Department of Statistics and Applied Probability, National University of Singapore, Singapore, Singapore

Ranjana Mathur, Shu Yen Lee, Choi Mun Chan, Ian Yeo, Boon Kwang Loh, Edmund Yick-Mun Wong and Doric Wong
Vitreoretinal Service, Singapore National Eye Centre, Singapore, Singapore

Rachel Williams
Worldwide Epidemiology, R and D Projects, Clinical Platforms and Sciences, GlaxoSmithKline, Pennsylvania, United States of America

Prajitha Thampi, Haripriya Vittal Rao, Sayak K. Mitter, Jun Cai, Xiaoping Qi and Michael E. Boulton
Department of Anatomy and Cell Biology, University of Florida, Gainesville, Florida, United States of America

Haoyu Mao, Alfred S. Lewin, Hong Li and Soojung Seo
Department of Molecular Genetics and Microbiology, University of Florida, Gainesville, Florida, United States of America

Carl Romano
Retina Research, Alcon Laboratories, Inc, Fort Worth, Texas, United States of America

Jennifer H. Acton
Department of Ophthalmology, New York University, New York, New York, United States of America
Ophthalmic Research Group, Optometry and Vision Sciences, School of Life and Health Sciences, Aston University, Birmingham, United Kingdom

Jonathan M. Gibson
Ophthalmic Research Group, Optometry and Vision Sciences, School of Life and Health Sciences, Aston University, Birmingham, United Kingdom
Birmingham and Midland Eye Centre, Birmingham, United Kingdom

Robert P. Cubbidge
Ophthalmic Research Group, Optometry and Vision Sciences, School of Life and Health Sciences, Aston University, Birmingham, United Kingdom

Marieh Esmaeelpour
Ludwig Boltzmann Institute of Retinology and Biomicroscopic Laser Surgery, Department of Ophthalmology, Rudolf Foundation Clinic, Vienna, Austria

Center for Medical Physics and Biomedical Engineering, Medical University of Vienna, Vienna, Austria

Vedran Kajic, Behrooz Zabihian, Richu Othara and Wolfgang Drexler
Center for Medical Physics and Biomedical Engineering, Medical University of Vienna, Vienna, Austria

Siamak Ansari-Shahrezaei, Lukas Kellner, Ilse Krebs and Susanne Binder
Ludwig Boltzmann Institute of Retinology and Biomicroscopic Laser Surgery, Department of Ophthalmology, Rudolf Foundation Clinic, Vienna, Austria

Susanne Nemetz
OptikNemetz, Vienna, Austria

Martin F. Kraus and Joachim Hornegger
Pattern Recognition Lab and School of Advanced Optical Technologies (SAOT), Friedrich-Alexander University Erlangen-Nuremberg, Erlangen, Bavaria, Germany

James G. Fujimoto
Department of Electrical Engineering and Computer Science, Massachusetts Institute of Technology, Cambridge, Massachusetts, United States of America

Ahjoku Amadi-Obi, Cheng-Rong Yu, Ivy Dambuza, Sung-Hye Kim, Bernadette Marrero and Charles E. Egwuagu
Molecular Immunology Section, National Eye Institute, National Institutes of Health, Bethesda, Maryland, United States of America

Yaoyao Sun, Wenzhen Yu, Lvzhen Huang, Jing Hou, Mingwei Zhao and Xiaoxin Li
Department of Ophthalmology, Peking University People's Hospital, Beijing, China
Key Laboratory of Vision Loss and Restoration, Ministry of Education, Beijing, China

Peihua Gong
Department of Respiration, Peking University People's Hospital, Beijing, China

Yi Zheng
Department of Immunology, School of Basic Medical Sciences, Peking University, Beijing, China

Peng Zhou
Department of Ophthalmology, Peking University People's Hospital, Beijing, China
Key Laboratory of Vision Loss and Restoration, Ministry of Education, Beijing, China
Department of Ophthalmology, Eye and ENT, Hospital Affiliated to Fudan University, Shanghai, China

Gergely Losonczy, Attila Vajas, Lili Takács, Éva Márhoffer and András Berta
Department of Ophthalmology, University of Debrecen, Debrecen, Hungary

Erika Dzsudzsák and István Balogh
Department of Laboratory Medicine, University of Debrecen, Debrecen, Hungary

Ágnes Fekete
Department of Anesthesiology and Intensive Care, University of Debrecen, Debrecen, Hungary

László Kardos
Hygiene and Infection Control Services, Kenézy Gyula County Hospital, Debrecen, Hungary

Éva Ajzner
Central Laboratory, Jósa András Teaching Hospital, Nyíregyháza, Hungary

Begoña Hurtado and Pablo Garcia de Frutos
Department of Cell Death and Proliferation, Institute of Biomedical Research of Barcelona (IIBB-CSIC, IDIBAPS), Barcelona, Spain

Bin Wu, Xiaoyan Liu and Houwen Lin
Department of Pharmacy, Ren Ji Hospital, affiliated with the School of Medicine, Shanghai Jiao tong University, Shanghai, China

Haixiang Wu
Department of Ophthalmology, and Visual Science, Eye, and ENT Hospital, Shanghai Medical College, Fudan University, Shanghai, China

Jin Li
Department of Ophthalmology, Ren Ji Hospital, affiliated with the School of Medicine, Shanghai Jiao tong University, Shanghai, China

Deepika Malik, Tiffany Hsu, Payam Falatoonzadeh, Javier Cáceres-del-Carpio, Marilyn Chwa, Shari R. Atilano, Claudio Ramirez, Baruch D. Kuppermann and Nitin Udar
Gavin Herbert Eye Institute, University California Irvine, Irvine, California, United States of America

Mohamed Tarek
Gavin Herbert Eye Institute, University California Irvine, Irvine, California, United States of America
Department of Ophthalmology, El-Minya University, El-Minya, Egypt

Anthony B. Nesburn
Gavin Herbert Eye Institute, University California Irvine, Irvine, California, United States of America

Cedars-Sinai Medical Center, Los Angeles, California, United States of America

David S. Boyer
Retina-Vitreous Associates Medical Group; Beverly Hills, California, United States of America

S. Michal Jazwinski and Michael V. Miceli
Tulane Center for Aging, Tulane University, New Orleans, Louisiana, United States of America

Douglas C. Wallace
Center for Mitochondrial and Epigenomic Medicine, Children's Hospital of Philadelphia and Department of Pathology and Laboratory Medicine, University of Pennsylvania, Philadelphia, Pennsylvania, United States of America

M. Cristina Kenney
Gavin Herbert Eye Institute, University California Irvine, Irvine, California, United States of America
Department of Pathology and Laboratory Medicine, University California Irvine, Irvine, California, United States of America

Toshio Hisatomi and Ryo Asato
Department of Ophthalmology, Graduate School of Medical Sciences, Kyushu University, Fukuoka, Japan
Clinical Research Institute, National Hospital Organization Kyushu Medical Center, Fukuoka, Japan

Shoji Notomi, Yusuke Murakami, Atsunobu Takeda, Yasuhiro Ikeda, Hiroshi Enaida and Tatsuro Ishibashi
Department of Ophthalmology, Graduate School of Medical Sciences, Kyushu University, Fukuoka, Japan

Hiroto Terasaki, Shozo Sonoda and Taiji Sakamoto
Department of Ophthalmology, Graduate School of Medical Sciences, Kagoshima University, Kagoshima, Japan

William Raoul, Sophie Lavalette, Bertrand Calippe and Xavier Guillonneau
INSERM, U968, Paris, France
University Pierre and Marie Curie, Institut de la Vision, Paris, France
Centre National de la Recherche Scientifique, Paris, France

Lucie Poupel
INSERM, UMR S945, Laboratory of Immunity and Infection, Paris, France
University Pierre and Marie Curie, Laboratory of Immunity and Infection, Paris, France

David-Alexandre Tregouet
University Pierre and Marie Curie, Paris, France
INSERM, UMR S 937, Faculté de Médecine La Pitié-Salpêtrière, Paris, France

Serge Camelo and Nicole Keller
INSERM, UMR S 872, Centre de Recherche des Cordeliers, Paris, France
University Pierre and Marie Curie, Paris, France
Université Paris Descartes, Paris, France

Sophie Krumeich and Clotilde Théry
INSERM, U932, Paris, France
Institut Curie, Centre de Recherche, Paris, France

Francine Behar-Cohen
Assistance Publique-Hôpitaux de Paris, Hôtel Dieu, Service d'Ophtalmologie, Paris, France
INSERM, UMR S 872, Centre de Recherche des Cordeliers, Paris, France
University Pierre and Marie Curie, Paris, France
Université Paris Descartes, Paris, France

Salomon-Yves Cohen
Centre d'Angiographie et de Laser, Paris, France

Holger Baatz
Augenärztliche Gemeinschaftspraxis, Augenzentrum Recklinghausen und Zentrum der Augenheilkunde, J-W Goethe Universität Frankfurt am Main, Frankfurt, Germany

Christophe Combadière
INSERM, UMR S945, Laboratory of Immunity and Infection, Paris, France
University Pierre and Marie Curie, Laboratory of Immunity and Infection, Paris, France
Assistance Publique-Hôpitaux de Paris, Groupe Hospitalier Pitié-Salpétriè re, Service d'Immunologie, Paris, France

Florian Sennlaub
INSERM, U968, Paris, France
University Pierre and Marie Curie, Institut de la Vision, Paris, France
Centre National de la Recherche Scientifique, Paris, France
Assistance Publique-Hôpitaux de Paris, Hôtel Dieu, Service d'Ophtalmologie, Paris, France

Richard A. I. Bethlehem
Experimental Psychology, Helmholtz Institute, Utrecht University, Utrecht, The Netherlands
Autism Research Centre, Department of Psychiatry, University of Cambridge, Cambridge, United Kingdom

Serge O. Dumoulin, Edwin S. Dalmaijer and Stefan Van der Stigchel
Experimental Psychology, Helmholtz Institute, Utrecht University, Utrecht, The Netherlands

Miranda Smit and Tanja C. W. Nijboer
Experimental Psychology, Helmholtz Institute, Utrecht University, Utrecht, The Netherlands
Rudolf Magnus Institute of Neuroscience and Centre of Excellence for Rehabilitation Medicine, University Medical Centre Utrecht and Rehabilitation Centre De Hoogstraat, Utrecht, The Netherlands

Tos T. J. M. Berendschot
University Eye Clinic Maastricht, Maastricht, The Netherlands

Jin-Wei Cheng and Rui-Li Wei
Department of Ophthalmology, Shanghai Changzheng Hospital, Second Military Medical University, Shanghai, China

Shi-Wei Cheng
School of Life Sciences, Ludong University, Yantai, China

Guo-Cai Lu
Center for New Drug Evaluation, Institute of Basic Medical Science, Second Military Medical University, Shanghai, China

Todd E. Scheetz and Terry A. Braun
Department of Ophthalmology and Visual Sciences, The University of Iowa, Iowa City, Iowa, United States of America
Department of Biomedical Engineering, The University of Iowa, Iowa City, Iowa, United States of America
Center for Bioinformatics and Computational Biology, The University of Iowa, Iowa City, Iowa, United States of America

John H. Fingert, Markus H. Kuehn, Wallace L. M. Alward, H. Culver Boldt, Stephen R. Russell and James C. Folk
Department of Ophthalmology and Visual Sciences, The University of Iowa, Iowa City, Iowa, United States of America

Kai Wang
Department of Biostatistics, The University of Iowa, Iowa City, Iowa, United States of America

Kevin L. Knudtson
DNA Core Facility, The University of Iowa, Iowa City, Iowa, United States of America

Thomas L. Casavant
Department of Ophthalmology and Visual Sciences, The University of Iowa, Iowa City, Iowa, United States of America
Department of Biomedical Engineering, The University of Iowa, Iowa City, Iowa, United States of America
Center for Bioinformatics and Computational Biology, The University of Iowa, Iowa City, Iowa, United States of America
Department of Electrical and Computer Engineering, The University of Iowa, Iowa City, Iowa, United States of America

Abbot F. Clark
Department of Cell Biology and Anatomy, The University of Iowa, Iowa City, Iowa, United States of America
North Texas Eye Research Institute, University of North Texas Health Sciences Center, Fort Worth, Texas, United States of America

Edwin M. Stone
Department of Ophthalmology and Visual Sciences, The University of Iowa, Iowa City, Iowa, United States of America
Department of Pediatrics, Howard Hughes Medical Institute, Iowa City, Iowa, United States of America
Howard Hughes Medical Institute, Iowa City, Iowa, United States of America

Val C. Sheffield
Department of Ophthalmology and Visual Sciences, The University of Iowa, Iowa City, Iowa, United States of America
Department of Pediatrics, Howard Hughes Medical Institute, Iowa City, Iowa, United States of America
Howard Hughes Medical Institute, Iowa City, Iowa, United States of America

Tina Ristau, Lebriz Ersoy, Bernd Kirchhof and Sascha Fauser
Department of Ophthalmology, University Hospital of Cologne, Cologne, Germany

Constantin Paun, Yara Lechanteur, Carel Hoyng, Eiko K. de Jong and Anneke I. den Hollander
Department of Ophthalmology, Radboud University Nijmegen Medical Centre, Nijmegen, the Netherlands

Moritz Hahn
Institute of Medical Statistics, Informatics and Epidemiology, University of Cologne, Cologne, Germany

Mohamed R. Daha
Department of Nephrology, Leiden University Nijmegen Medical Center, Leiden, the Netherlands

Zhao-Yang Wang
Department of Ophthalmology, Xinhua Hospital, Shanghai Jiaotong University School of Medicine, Shanghai, China
Departments of Molecular Genetics, University of Florida, Gainesville, Florida, United States of America

Keke Zhao, Brian Rossmiller, Cristhian Ildefonso and Manas Biswal
Departments of Molecular Genetics, University of Florida, Gainesville, Florida, United States of America

Jingwei Zheng
Eye Hospital, Wenzhou Medical University, Wenzhou, Zhejiang, China

Pei-quan Zhao
Department of Ophthalmology, Xinhua Hospital, Shanghai Jiaotong University School of Medicine, Shanghai, China

Audrey Cougnard-Grégoire, Mélanie Le Goff, Jean-François Dartigues, Pascale Barberger-Gateau and Cécile Delcourt
Université de Bordeaux, Bordeaux, France
INSERM (Institut National de la Santé Et de la Recherche Médicale), ISPED (Institut de Santé Publique d'Épidémiologie et de Développement), Centre INSERM U897-Epidemiologie-Biostatistique, Bordeaux, France

Marie-Noëlle Delyfer and Jean-François Korobelnik
Université de Bordeaux, Bordeaux, France
INSERM (Institut National de la Santé Et de la Recherche Médicale), ISPED (Institut de Santé Publique d'Épidémiologie et de Développement), Centre INSERM U897-Epidemiologie-Biostatistique, Bordeaux, France
Centre Hospitalier Universitaire (CHU) de Bordeaux, Service d'Ophtalmologie, Bordeaux, France

Marie-Bénédicte Rougier
Centre Hospitalier Universitaire (CHU) de Bordeaux, Service d'Ophtalmologie, Bordeaux, France

Matt Rutar
The John Curtin School of Medical Research, The Australian National University (ANU), Canberra, Australian Capital Territory, Australia

Krisztina Valter, Riccardo Natoli and Jan M. Provis
The John Curtin School of Medical Research, The Australian National University (ANU), Canberra, Australian Capital Territory, Australia
ANU Medical School, The Australian National University (ANU), Canberra, Australian Capital Territory, Australia

Huayi Lu
Departments of Ophthalmology and Visual Sciences, University of Louisville School of Medicine, Louisville, Kentucky, United States of America
Second Hospital of Jilin University, Changchun, Jilin Province, P.R. China

Qingxian Lu, Subhash Gaddipati and Qiutang Li
Departments of Ophthalmology and Visual Sciences, University of Louisville School of Medicine, Louisville, Kentucky, United States of America
James Graham Brown Cancer Center, University of Louisville School of Medicine, Louisville, Kentucky, United States of America

Ramesh Babu Kasetti, Wei Wang and Henry J. Kaplan
Departments of Ophthalmology and Visual Sciences, University of Louisville School of Medicine, Louisville, Kentucky, United States of America

Manolis Pasparakis
Institute for Genetics, University of Cologne, Cologne, Germany

Daniel Ardeljan
Immunopathology Section, Laboratory of Immunology, National Eye Institute, National Institutes of Health, Bethesda, Maryland, United States of America
School of Medicine, Johns Hopkins University, Baltimore, Maryland, United States of America

Yujuan Wang
Immunopathology Section, Laboratory of Immunology, National Eye Institute, National Institutes of Health, Bethesda, Maryland, United States of America
Zhongshan Ophthalmic Center, Sun Yat-sen University, Guangzhou, China

Stanley Park
Immunopathology Section, Laboratory of Immunology, National Eye Institute, National Institutes of Health, Bethesda, Maryland, United States of America
Howard Hughes Medical Institute, Chevy Chase, Maryland, United States of America

Defen Shen, Xi Kathy Chu, Jingsheng Tuo and Chi-Chao Chan
Immunopathology Section, Laboratory of Immunology, National Eye Institute, National Institutes of Health, Bethesda, Maryland, United States of America

Cheng-Rong Yu
Molecular Immunology Section, Laboratory of Immunology, National Eye Institute, National Institutes of Health, Bethesda, Maryland, United States of America

Mones Abu-Asab
Histology Core, Laboratory of Immunology, National Eye Institute, National Institutes of Health, Bethesda, Maryland, United States of America

Charles G. Eberhart
Department of Pathology, Johns Hopkins University, Baltimore, Maryland, United States of America

Timothy W. Olsen
Department of Ophthalmology, Emory University, Atlanta, Georgia, United States of America

Robert F. Mullins
Department of Ophthalmology and Visual Sciences, University of Iowa Carver College of Medicine, Iowa City, Iowa, United States of America

Gary White, Sam Wadsworth and Abraham Scaria
Genzyme Corporation, Framingham, Massachusetts, United States of America

Avraham Dishy
Department of Ophthalmology, Cantonal Hospital Aarau, Aarau, Switzerland

Anja Frei
Institute of General Practice and Health Service Research, University of Zurich, University Hospital of Zurich, Zurich, Switzerland
Institute of Social and Preventive Medicine, University of Zurich, Zurich, Switzerland

Ashley Wood and Thomas Margrain
School of Optometry and Vision Sciences, Cardiff University, Cardiff, United Kingdom

Alison Mary Binns
Division of Optometry and Visual Science, School of Health Sciences, City University London, London, United Kingdom

Juan Wu
Department of Nutrition, Harvard School of Public Health, Boston, Massachusetts, United States of America

Miki Uchino
Department of Ophthalmology, Keio University School of Medicine, Tokyo, Japan

Srinivas M. Sastry
Suburban Hospital, Bethesda, Maryland, United States of America

Debra A. Schaumberg
Division of Preventive Medicine, Brigham and Women's Hospital, Harvard Medical School, Boston, Massachusetts, United States of America
Moran Center for Translational Medicine, John A. Moran Eye Center, Department of Ophthalmology and Visual Sciences, University of Utah School of Medicine, Salt Lake City, Utah, United States of America Department of Epidemiology, Harvard School of Public Health, Boston, Massachusetts, United States of America
Schepens Eye Research Institute, Boston, Massachusetts, United States of America

Mei Chen, Jose R. Hombrebueno, Chang Luo, Rosana Penalva, Jiawu Zhao, Liza Colhoun, Sudha Pirya Soundara Pandi and Heping Xu
Centre for Vision and Vascular Science, School of Medicine, Dentistry and Biomedical Sciences, Queen's University Belfast, Belfast, Northern Ireland, United Kingdom

John V Forrester
Ocular Immunology Group, Section of Immunology and Infection, School of Medicine and Dentistry, University of Aberdeen, Aberdeen, Scotland, United Kingdom

Stefan Markun, Elisabeth Brändle and Thomas Rosemann
Institute of General Practice and Health Service Research, University of Zurich, University Hospital of Zurich, Zurich, Switzerland

Yousif Subhi and Torben L. Sørensen
Clinical Eye Research Unit, Department of Ophthalmology, Copenhagen University Hospital Roskilde, Roskilde, Denmark
University of Copenhagen, Copenhagen, Denmark

Gitte Ø. Henningsen, Charlotte T. Larsen and Mette S. Sørensen
Clinical Eye Research Unit, Department of Ophthalmology, Copenhagen University Hospital Roskilde, Roskilde, Denmark

Index

Index

R

S

T

U

V

CPSIA information can be obtained
at www.ICGtesting.com
Printed in the USA
BVHW011356160220
572492BV00003B/7

9 781632 427557